Practical Guide to Surgical Pathology with Cytologic Correlation

Kitai Kim   Bernard Naylor

Practical Guide to Surgical Pathology with Cytologic Correlation

A Text and Color Atlas

With 397 Figures in 806 Parts, 777 in Full Color

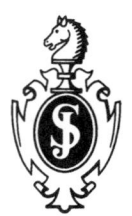

Springer-Verlag

New York Berlin Heidelberg London Paris
Tokyo Hong Kong Barcelona Budapest

Kitai Kim, MD
Professor of Pathology, Medical College of Ohio
and
Director of Cytology and Surgical Pathology, Medical College Hospitals
Toledo, OH 43699-0008, USA

Bernard Naylor, MD
Professor of Pathology, The University of Michigan
Director of Cytology, The University of Michigan Hospitals
Ann Arbor, MI 48109, USA

Library of Congress Cataloging-in-Publication Data
Kim, Kitai.
    Practical guide to surgical pathology with cytologic correlation
a text and color atlas / Kitai Kim, Bernard Naylor.
       p.   cm.
    Includes bibliographical references and index.

    ISBN-13: 978-1-4612-7658-6   e-ISBN-13: 978-1-4612-2764-9
    DOI: 10.1007/978-1-4612-2764-9

paper)
    1. Pathology, Surgical—Atlases.   2. Cytodiagnosis—Atlases.
3. Histology, Pathological—Atlases.   I. Naylor, Bernard, 1926–
II. Title.
    [DNLM: 1. Cytology—atlases.   2. Pathology, Surgical—atlases.
WO 517 K49p]
RD57.K56   1991
616.07'582—dc20
DNLM/DLC
for Library of Congress   91-5000

Printed on acid-free paper.

©1992 Springer-Verlag New York, Inc.
Softcover reprint of the hardcover 1st edition 1992

Typeset by Publishers Service of Montana, Bozeman, MT.

9 8 7 6 5 4 3 2 1

*We dedicate this book
to our patients, students,
teachers and families*

Preface

Although new concepts and new techniques are constantly being developed in the medical sciences, certain approaches to the elucidation of medical disorders vary little from decade to decade. This is well exemplified by the application of the complementary disciplines of surgical pathology and cytopathology to the problems of pathogenesis and diagnosis of human diseases.

In this book we have sought to demonstrate the interdependence of surgical pathology and cytopathology by emphasizing their role in the diagnosis of neoplasms, although nonneoplastic diseases have not been neglected. The text is supplemented with numerous illustrations of radiographs, gross specimens, histopathologic sections and cytologic specimens. We intend this book to provide information not only about the morphologic appearance of various lesions under the microscope, either as histopathologic sections or as cytologic preparations, but also to remind the reader that the techniques of surgical pathology and cytopathology, used either separately or together, achieve a high degree of specificity and sensitivity in the diagnosis of human disease.

We believe it is now especially important to stress the role of cytopathology in the diagnosis of human disease. Not only may it supplement the findings of surgical pathology but, in these days of cost containment, it provides one of the least expensive and least invasive methods of morphologic diagnosis, especially of neoplasms.

We have designed this book so that the text and its corresponding illustrations face each other. With this convenient layout we hope that this text will prove useful for practicing pathologists as a quick desk reference, for clinicians as a guide to the approach to diagnosis, to medical students desirous of learning about the morphologic basis of the diseases they are encountering, and to residents in all medical specialties as a guide to clinicopathologic concepts and as an aid to preparing for specialty board examinations.

Kitai Kim
Bernard Naylor

Acknowledgments

We wish to express our indebtedness and appreciation to the pathologists and clinicians who provided us with sample materials and clinical information. We sincerely appreciate the technical help of Carrie Greenway (cytology), Emily Duran (histology), and Judy Meredith (histology) and the secretarial help of Marilyn Hartkopf, Terrie Latta and Lisa Nikkila, members of the staffs of The Medical College of Ohio and The University of Michigan. The technical and professional help of Drs. Jonathan Myles and Manuel E. Velasco of The Medical College of Ohio and Dr. Sharon W. Weiss of The University of Michigan are gratefully appreciated. We acknowledge the valuable assistance given to us by our publisher, Springer-Verlag New York. And lastly, we have a special word of gratitude to Marilyn Cline, who typed the entire manuscript with patience and a smile. Without her unflagging efforts, this book would not exist.

Kitai Kim
Bernard Naylor

Contents

Contributors

Amira F. Gohara, MD

Professor of Pathology, Medical College of Ohio; Director of Clinical Laboratory, Medical College Hospitals, Toledo, Ohio 43699, USA

Contributed to Chapter 13, Kidney

Peter J. Goldblatt, MD

Professor and Chairman, Department of Pathology, Medical College of Ohio, Toledo, Ohio 43699, USA

Contributed to Chapter 13, Kidney

Yong-Il Kim, MD, PhD

Professor and Chairman, Department of Pathology, Seoul National University, College of Medicine, Seoul 110-460, Korea

Contributed to Chapter 8, Liver

Edwin R. Phillips, MD, PhD

Associate Professor of Pathology, Medical College of Ohio, Toledo, Ohio 43699, USA

Contributed to Chapter 2, Skin

Edward R. Savolaine, MD

Professor of Radiology, Medical College of Ohio, Toledo, Ohio 43699, USA

Contributed radiographs throughout the book

1

Introduction to Cytopathology and Histopathology

Cytopathology and histopathology supplement and complement each other. Cytologic evaluation should identify altered cells and from these cells one may be able to recognize a disease process. In fact, from this evaluation one may be able to synthesize the histopathologic picture.

However, in order to do this, the following are desired:

1. pertinent clinical information
2. an appropriate sample containing satisfactory cellular material
3. a microscopist skilled enough to identify and synthesize the cellular changes into a histopathologic picture.

Diagnostic Approach to Cytology

Smears of cellular material should be examined thoroughly in a systematic manner under a ×10 objective lens. Such screening should identify the general cell population and the presence of any altered cells. Such cells should then be scrutinized under the high dry (×40) objective lens. The final interpretation, based on an evaluation of the cellular findings in relation to clinical data, may provide a specific diagnosis.[1]

General Features of Cell Smears

Normal smears usually show single cells or sheets of uniform cells in a "clean" background. Smears from malignant neoplasms typically show abundant cells in a granular proteinaceous background comprising disintegrated necrotic cells, a feature of the so-called tumor diathesis. Their abundance is a result of their loss of mutual cohesiveness, a feature typical of cancer cells.

Cell Arrangement

Most benign cells shed spontaneously as isolated cells. If the cells are obtained by mechanical force, for example by aspiration or scraping, normal or non-neoplastic abnormal cells may occur in sheets. A sheet of cells is a grouping in which the component cells are regularly arranged in relation to one another and possess distinct cell boundaries (Fig. 1.1). In contrast, cells from malignant neoplasms occur usually in a syncytium, which is a group of cells arranged irregularly with respect to one another and with indistinct cell boundaries. This arrangement is rarely observed without an abnormality in the parent tissue, in which the corresponding cells or their nuclei are characterized by altered polarity (Fig. 1.2). A cell cluster is a more or less three-dimensional grouping of cells with altered polarity and usually poorly defined cell boundaries. Such an arrangement is generally associated with cells having a glandular origin and is most often characteristic of adenocarcinoma (Fig. 1.3). Cells arising from nonlymphomatous sarcomas occur in loose and irregular aggregates and as isolated cells. They tend to be pleomorphic (Fig. 1.4). Cells of lymphomas characteristically are isolated from each other (Fig. 1.5).

Identification and evaluation of abnormal cells in terms of malignant neoplasm should, for the most part, be based on individual cells. Isolated cells are best for such evaluation.

Cell Characteristics

Non-neoplastic cells tend to be isodiametric (polygonal, cuboidal, or round) with distinct cell borders. The size of the cells of a particular type varies only slightly. It is practical to estimate the size of abnormal cells or their nuclei against known standards, for example, against the size of lymphocytes, red blood cells, or the nuclei of the intermediate squamous cells. The nuclei of non-neoplastic cells tend to be small, round, or kidney-shaped and have finely granular chromatin, of "bland" or "transparent" texture.

In contrast, atypical cells or malignant neoplastic cells tend to vary in size and shape. Such pleomorphism includes non-isodiametric forms (elongated, spindle-shaped, caudate, or tadpole shaped). Their nuclei tend to be large and pleomorphic, and have coarsely granular and irregularly dispersed chromatin. The relative nuclear area (nucleocytoplasmic ratio) is usually high; for example, the nucleocytoplasmic ratio of cells of squamous cell carcinoma is high compared with that of superficial squamous cells.

Nucleoli are composed mainly of ribonucleic acid (RNA) protein, and their size is closely related to the metabolic activity of the cells. They are referred to as micronucleoli or macronucleoli. Macronucleoli are usually round with an acidophilic (eosinophilic) staining reaction. The presence of a macronucleolus is frequently suggestive of active cellular regeneration or invasive carcinoma. It is a useful criterion in distinguishing between carcinoma in situ and invasive squamous cell carcinoma of the uterine cervix. However, since proliferating non-neoplastic cells may have prominent macronucleoli, the presence of macronucleoli alone cannot be a reliable diagnostic criterion of malignancy. Similarly, the presence of mitotic figures alone should not be interpreted as denoting malignancy.

In summary, the arrangement of cells and their cytoplasm provides useful information about the origin and differentiation of a cell, whereas the nucleus provides the most useful information in terms of its biologic or malignant potential.

Cytologic Sampling and Preparation

An adequate population of cells, evenly spread smears, and good cell preservation and staining are prerequisites for cytologic evaluation. Sampling techniques for cytopathology will be discussed for each organ site.

Procedures and Techniques of Fine Needle Aspiration

Fine needle aspiration (FNA) biopsy obtains material for cytologic evaluation by the use of thin needles (21–25 gauge). This is a much less traumatic procedure than a large core needle biopsy, which obtains a core of tissue. FNA can be applied to palpable superficial lesions (breast, lymph nodes, thyroid, cutaneous and subcutaneous soft tissue lesions, and salivary glands) and to deeply situated lesions visible by imaging techniques.

Instruments

1. Needle. Short thin needles (22–25 gauge) may be used for the superficial, palpable lesions. For deeply situated lesions, the following are usually used: 20- to 23-gauge Chiba needles (Cook, Bloomington, IN), 20-gauge Westcott needles (Becton Dickinson, Rutherford, NJ), 20- to 22-gauge Turner cutting needles (Cook, Bloomington, IN)
2. Syringe (20–50 ml size)
3. Single hand-grip syringe holder
4. Frosted end slides
5. Fixative: 95% ethanol or spray fixative
6. 20 to 30 ml of physiologic saline solution for rinsing the syringe
7. Culture medium for microbiology

Technique

The sampling techniques of FNA are essentially the same for superficial and deeply situated lesions.

Technique for Superficial Sites.
1. The needle should be inserted into the lesion and moved forward and backward in different directions to obtain a sample from the different areas of the lesion. During the aspiration, maintain a strong negative pressure in the syringe. Before withdrawing the needle from the lesion, it is important to release the negative pressure; otherwise, the cell material will be sucked into the syringe.

2. Detach the needle from the syringe, fill the syringe with air, reconnect the needle to the syringe, and expel the cell material on to the center of the slide.
3. Place another glass slide on top of the slide with the expelled aspirate, quickly pulling the two slides apart. Fix the slides in 95% ethanol or with a spray fixative.

Technique for Deeply Situated Lesions.
Fine needle aspiration is performed under the guidance of computed tomography, ultrasonography, or fluoroscopy, with image intensification. The patient is placed on the table in the supine or prone position, depending on the location of the lesion. Local anesthesia is applied to the body wall and a small nick is made in the skin with a scalpel to facilitate insertion of the needle. The needle (20–23 gauge) is inserted perpendicularly over the lesion until the needle tip is in the lesion. The stylet is partly withdrawn and the needle is moved back and forth in the lesion. The stylet is then removed and suction is applied by using a 20-ml syringe attached to the needle. Before withdrawing the needle from the lesion, the negative pressure in the syringe is released. The needle is then detached from the syringe, the syringe is filled with air, the needle is reattached, and the cellular material is expelled onto the frosted slides. If there is suspicion of infection, a portion of the aspirate should be expelled into a culture tube. The smears are fixed in 95% ethanol or a spray fixative. For rapid on-site evaluation a portion of the aspirate may be stained with Diff-Quik stain (Harleco, Gibbstown, NJ) or by a wet-film technique. For the former stain, the smears should be air dried.

Staining Procedures. Several different methods are used for fixing and staining cytologic specimens. Whereas some methods are standard universally, others are a matter of individual preference.

1. Fixation in 95% ethanol or with a spray fixative and staining with a rapid hematoxylin and eosin stain for stat reports, or with the Papanicolaou stain for regular reports. These procedures are widely used in the United States.
2. May-Gruenwald-Giemsa (MGG) and Diff-Quick stain for air-dried smears. These stains are widely used in Europe. Since the cytologic features of specimens processed by these methods are different from those of alcohol-fixed Papanicolaou stained smears, it is important to be familiar with the differences. These methods are quite useful for lymph-proliferative disorders.

Reporting of Results. Reports should be succinct and provide effective communication between the cytopathologist and clinician. Avoid ambiguous reports. Reports of "atypical" cells are almost as useless as no report at all. If appropriate, a report in which there is some diagnostic uncertainty may include a recommendation regarding further evaluation of the lesion.

Biopsy and Imprint Cytology

Biopsy is a procedure to obtain tissue samples of abnormal lesions detected by the clinical examination or radiologic imaging method. Biopsy is the last resort of diagnosis. On the

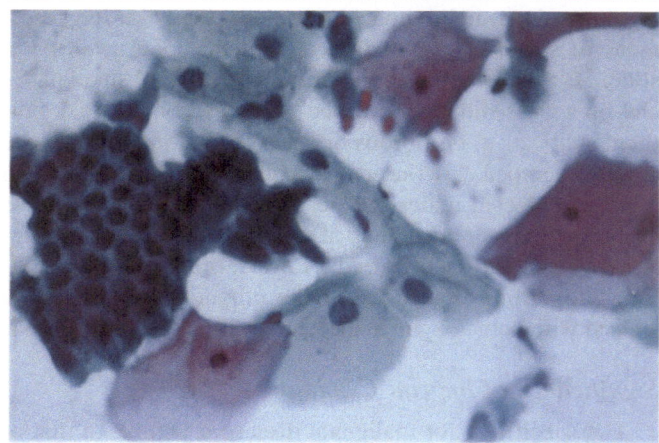

FIGURE 1.1 Normal squamous epithelial and endocervical gland cells. The endocervical cells arranged in sheets are uniform in shape and size. The superficial and intermediate squamous cells occur singly (Papanicolaou stain).

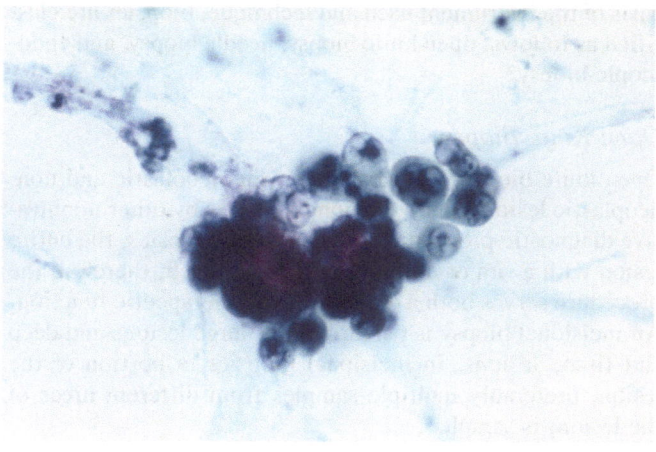

FIGURE 1.3 Adenocarcinoma. Neoplastic cells arranged in three-dimensional clusters (Papanicolaou stain).

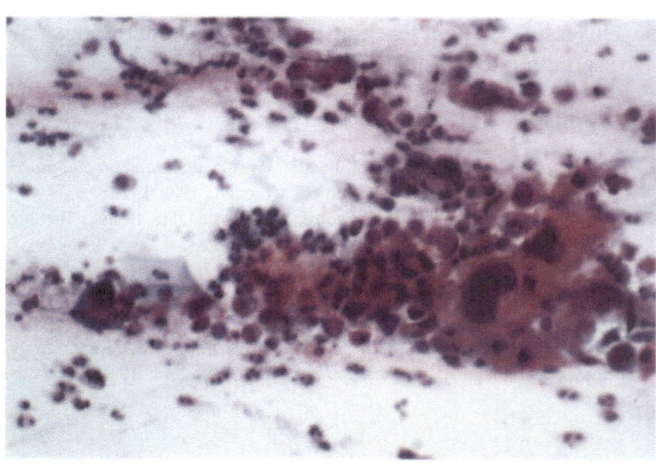

FIGURE 1.2 Squamous cell carcinoma. Neoplastic squamous cells arranged in a syncytium with loss of cell polarity (Papanicolaou stain).

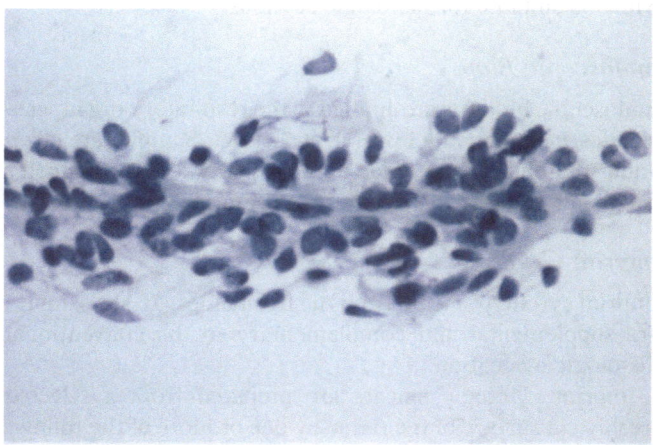

FIGURE 1.4 Sarcoma. Pleomorphic neoplastic cells occurring in loose and irregular aggregates (Papanicolaou stain).

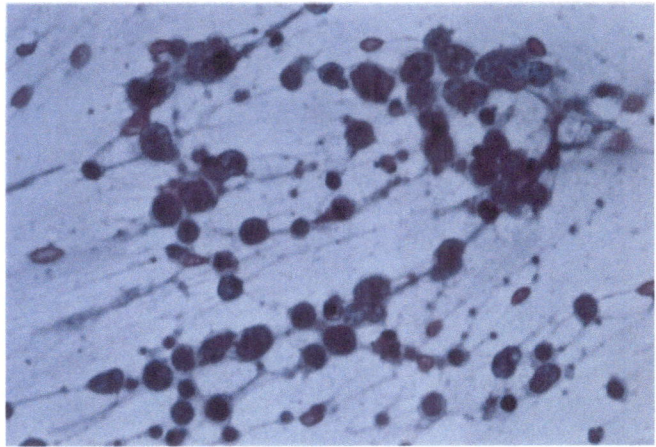

FIGURE 1.5 Lymphoma. Large neoplastic lymphocytes occurring as isolated cells (H&E stain).

basis of the instrument used and technique, biopsies are classified as follows: open knife biopsy, needle biopsy, and endoscopic biopsy.[2]

Open Knife Biopsy

Open knife biopsy is performed on the neoplastic and non-neoplastic lesions that were nondiagnostic by other noninvasive diagnostic procedures. In excisional biopsies, the entire lesion with a rim of normal tissue is removed; therefore the procedure serves both a diagnostic and therapeutic function. An incisional biopsy is performed for large lesions and deep soft tissue lesions. In incisional biopsies, a portion of the lesion, preferably multiple samples from different areas of the lesion, is sampled.

Core-Needle Biopsy

Core-needle biopsy is applied to the lesions of the superficial sites, solid visceral organs, and blind sampling in neoplastic work-up. The procedure provides 15 to 20 mm of tissue core, which is suitable for histologic sections.

Endoscopic Biopsy

Endoscopic biopsies are applied to the respiratory organ, gastrointestinal tract, and lower urinary tract. Samples are taken under the endoscopic guide and consist of a few millimeter fragments suitable for histologic sections.

Imprint Cytology

Imprint cytology smears from the fresh biopsy tissue samples are supplemental and complementary to the conventional histologic evaluation.[3,4]

Imprint cytologic smears are prepared from a selected freshly cut surface of the tissue by one or more of the following methods: a) lightly touching a glass slide with the specimen, b) smearing the surface of the specimen against the slide, c) "rolling" small specimens on the slide, d) small particles on a glass slide are "crushed" with a second slide to pull them apart, or e) on fibrous or sclerotic lesions, the surface could be scraped with the edge of a glass slide or scalpel blade and the collected material smeared on a slide. All of these smears are fixed immediately in 95% ethanol. One or two air-dried smears may be prepared for evaluation of lymphoma or intracytoplasmic lipid. One of the ethanol-fixed smears is stained with hematoxylin and eosin for immediate evaluation.

Significance of Imprint Cytology

1. The specificity for malignant disease is similar to that of frozen section.
2. A simple preparation provides diagnosis more quickly than a frozen section.
3. Imprint smears can provide a diagnosis in some cases in which a small sample size or composition (e.g. bone) precludes adequate frozen section.
4. Ancillary information is provided that contributes to the final diagnosis on permanent sections.
5. This is an excellent teaching exercise in cytopathology corresponding to histopathology.

References

1. Wied GL, Keebler CM, Koss LG, Reagan JW. *Compendium on Diagnostic Cytology. Tutorials of Cytology.* 6th ed. Chicago: 1988:1–23.
2. Rosai J. *Ackerman's Surgical Pathology.* 7th ed. St. Louis, Toronto, Washington, DC: The CV Mosby Co; 1989:1–12.
3. Nochomovitz L, Sidawy M, Jannotta F, Silverberg S, Schwartz A. *Intra-operative Consultation: A Guide to Smears, Imprints and Frozen Sections.* ASCP Press; 1990.
4. Kim K, Phillips E, Paolino M. Intra-operative imprint cytology: its significance as a diagnostic adjunct. *Diagnostic Cytopathol.* 1990;6:304–307

2
Neoplasms of the Skin

The integument may give rise to a wide variety of neoplasms, partly because of the plethora of specialized structures that compose the organ. A complete exposition of these is far beyond the scope of this chapter, which will be devoted to the most common tumors, or to neoplasms that serve as examples of categories of these lesions.

Pathologic diagnosis of skin neoplasms rests principally on histologic preparations from incisional or excisional biopsies. Aspiration cytopathology plays a comparatively small role in this area, but may be of use in diagnosis of recurrent tumors or neoplasms metastatic to the skin.

A precise standard of classification of skin tumors has not been widely adopted. However, the following fractionation (Table 2.1) complies with the conventional listings encountered in most of the more extensive treatises on the subject.[1,2] Categories in this classification are assigned according to the structure of the histogenetic parent of the tumor.

Table 2.1. Tumors of the integument.

Tumors of the epidermis
Melanocytic tumors
Adnexal (appendage) tumors
Hair follicular
Sebaceous
Apocrine
Eccrine
Tumors of the Dermis

Tumors of the Epidermis

Non-Neoplastic Processes Mimicking Neoplasms

Epidermal Inclusion Cysts

Epidermal inclusion cysts are probably the most common examples of this type of lesion. They arise by aberrant growth of epidermis within the dermis. They are of two types, depending on whether they arise from epidermal or pilar (hair follicular) structures. These cysts create benign, slowly growing masses arising anywhere, but often on the trunk or head and neck. The wall is lined by cutaneous squamous epithelium, filling the lumen with the anucleate keratin product (Fig. 2.1). The pilar variety is of appendageal (hair follicular) origin rather than epidermal.

Benign Epidermal Tumors

Verruca Vulgaris

Some viral infections may produce tumors of the epidermis. The most common of these is verruca vulgaris, induced by the human papilloma virus. The virus creates a proliferative effect on the infected keratinocytes, resulting in a papillary thickening (acanthosis) of the epidermis (Fig. 2.2). The lesions are infectious and may be transmitted between individuals or spread by autoinoculation.

These may occur anywhere on the skin, but are especially common on the face and hands. The tips of the papillae typically display cytoplasmic vacuolization, loss of keratohyalin granules, and parakeratosis, whereas the intervening epidermis exhibits an increased granular cell layer and hyperkeratosis.

Molluscum Contagiosum

Molluscum contagiasum usually manifests by firm, waxy papules, a few millimeters in diameter, which, when mature, have umbilicated centers from which whitish keratin material may be expressed. These are the results of virus infection by a large poxlike virus. It is usually self-limited, except in the immunosuppressed individual, in whom the lesions may be more numerous and may persist indefinitely.

Histologically, a downward lobular proliferation of the epidermis is seen, such that the underlying dermis is pushed downward and outward. The epidermal cells, as they differentiate upward, show the development of large eosinophilic viral inclusions, sometimes nearly the size of the cell itself. As they reach the granular cell layer they become basophilic and eventually are extruded into the keratin layer (Fig. 2.3).

Seborrheic Keratosis

Other benign proliferations of the epidermis are also common. Seborrheic keratoses are greasy, elevated, often pigmented, well circumscribed lesions. They arise on virtually any portion of the skin except the palms or soles and occur principally in middle age and beyond. They can assume a variety of histologic patterns but characteristically comprise a thickened epidermis that rises above the plane of the surrounding dermal–epidermal interface. The cells have predominantly basaloid features. Frequent intratumoral inclusions composed of round whorls of keratin (pseudohorn cysts) are usually present (Fig. 2.4).

Keratoacanthoma

Keratoacanthoma generally occurs on hair-bearing skin, most often in exposed areas. It probably arises from one or several hair follicular infundibula and might be appropriately classified among appendageal tumors. It is 3 to 4 times more common in men than women. In its natural history, it progresses rapidly in size and may grow quite large. However, it tends to regress spontaneously over a long period. Grossly, it presents as an elevated, symmetrical nodule with a central keratin-filled crater. Histologically, this is reflected in an upward displacement of neighboring epidermis accompanied by epidermal proliferation surrounding the keratin-filled crater. The keratinocytes frequently assume a glassy keratinized cytoplasm and may have atypical cytologic features. Mitoses may be startlingly frequent. Often a pseudoinfiltrative pattern is apparent at the base (Fig. 2.5). Differentiation from well differentiated squamous cell carcinoma presents the chief diagnostic problem,[3,4] although keratoacanthoma tends to occur in a younger population.

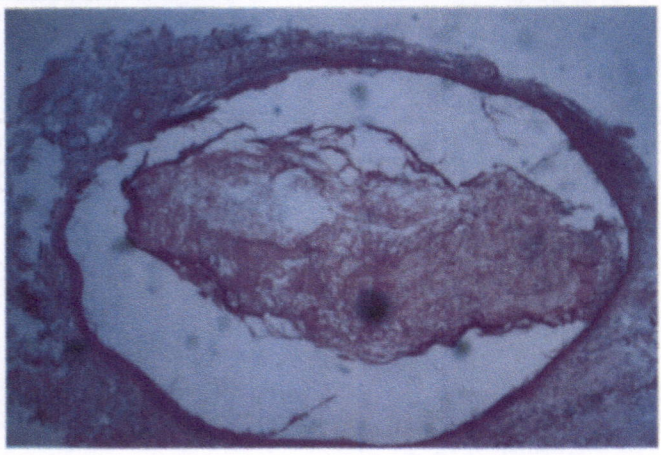

FIGURE 2.1 **Epidermal inclusion cysts.** A cystic structure in the dermis is lined by stratified squamous epithelium and filled with laminated keratin.

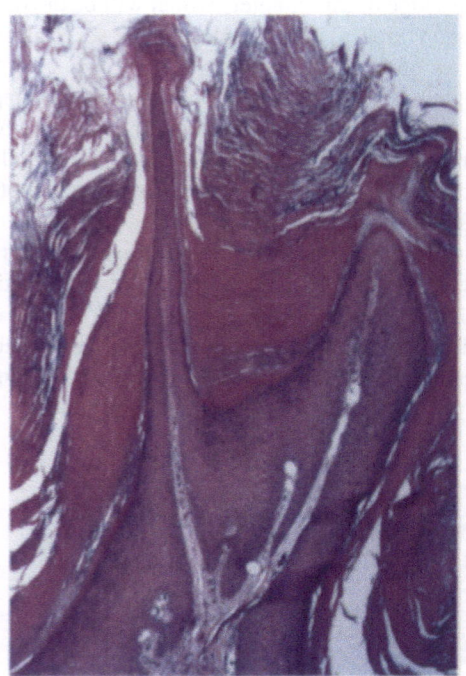

FIGURE 2.2 **Viral verruca (verruca vulgaris).** Acanthosis, with papillomatous spires that often terminate in a stack (tier) of parakeratosis. The intervening cornified layer is densely hyperkeratotic.

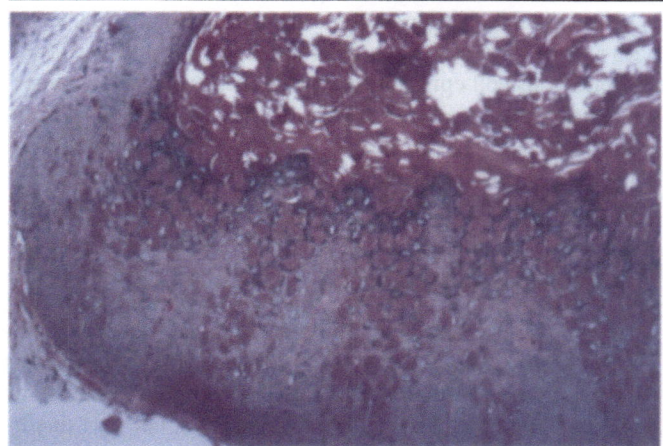

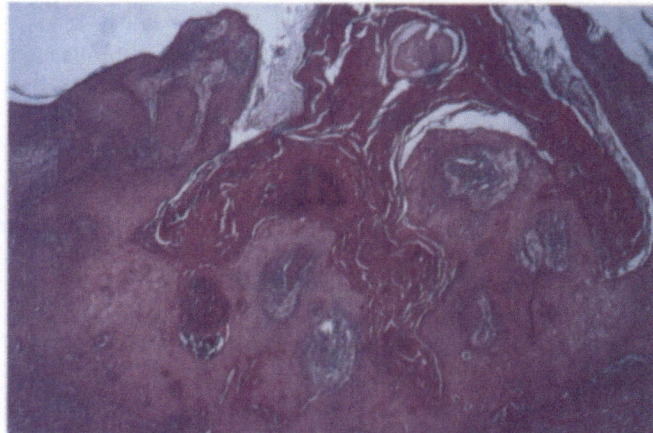

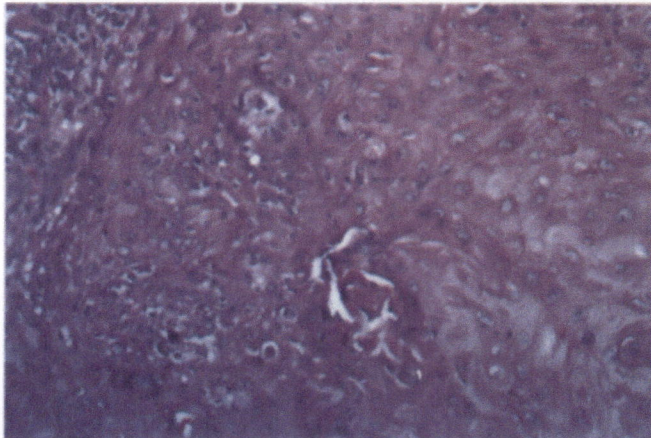

FIGURE 2.3 Molluscum contagiosum. The cup-shaped, thickened epidermis pushes into the dermis. The inclusion bodies can be seen in the deep layers of the epidermis extending upward toward the cornified lumen of the cup.

FIGURE 2.5 Keratoacanthoma. The lesion is symmetrical with a keratin-filled crater. The cells contain glassy pink cytoplasm and appear to infiltrate the dermis.

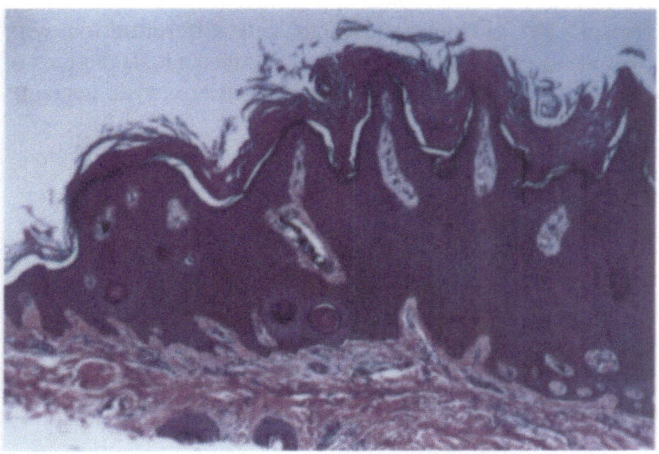

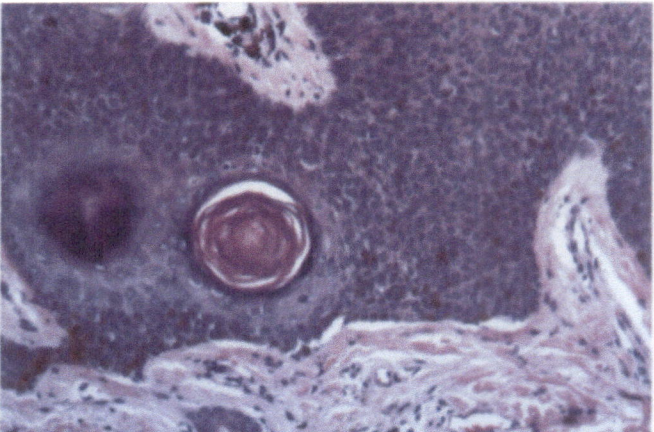

FIGURE 2.4 Seborrheic keratosis. There is acanthosis, papillomatosis, hyperkeratosis, and variable parakeratosis accompanying the proliferation of basaloid cells above the dermal–epidermal junction. Seemingly entrapped spheres of keratin form "pseudohorn cysts."

Squamous Intraepithelial Neoplasia

Squamous intraepithelial neoplasia (SIN) is an umbrella term that includes premalignant and malignant lesions confined to the epidermis. Dysplasia, including actinic keratosis, belongs in this category. At its worst, it is "squamous cell carcinoma in situ."

Actinic Keratosis (Solar Keratosis)

In skin exposed to solar radiation, the effects of exposure are manifested by degenerative changes in the dermis followed by atrophic changes and by dysplastic and hyperplastic effects in the epidermis. These premalignant features are found principally in exposed areas on persons of middle or late life, and are present as multifocal areas of erythema, which may become scaly or even crusted. If sufficient hyperkeratosis follows, a so-called cutaneous horn may develop. Histologically, the solar effect is reflected by basophilic ("elastotic") degeneration of the dermal collagen. With increasing exposure, the epidermis, beginning in the basal zone, will show increasing atypia and proliferative capacity (Fig. 2.6). Progressive dysplasia may eventuate in full blown squamous carcinoma, but invasion is slow to occur and metastases are rare.[5]

Carcinoma In Situ

Carcinoma in situ also arises on skin not exposed to the sun, where it is referred to as Bowen's disease. This latter entity appears as a well demarcated erythematous plaque, often with a finely scaled surface. Histologically, these show atypical squamous cell epithelium over the full span of the epidermal compartment. Scattered cells with vacuolated cytoplasm (Bowen's cells) may be present (Fig. 2.7). Histologically similar lesions in sun-exposed areas are designated as actinic keratosis or as SIN "Bowenoid" type.

Squamous Cell Carcinoma

As the neoplastic process exceeds the limits of SIN, by violating the basement membrane, it becomes invasive squamous cell carcinoma. Predictably, these lesions occur in the same epidemiologic population as actinic keratosis. The vast majority appear in sun-exposed skin; fair-skinned persons with a history of excessive exposure are at high risk. Most frequently, these lesions present as a limited ulcer, circumscribed by a diffuse elevated border. The ulcer bed often has a granular, "dirty" appearance. Some may instead exhibit a nonulcerated wartlike surface. Histologically, a variety of growth patterns may be seen, including acantholytic (pseudoglandular), spindle cell, or verrucous types. However, by far the most typical appearance is that which reflects deviant, but obvious, squamous cell differentiation with infiltration of the dermis (Fig. 2.8). Although all degrees of differentiation occur, the well differentiated type accounts for the great majority.

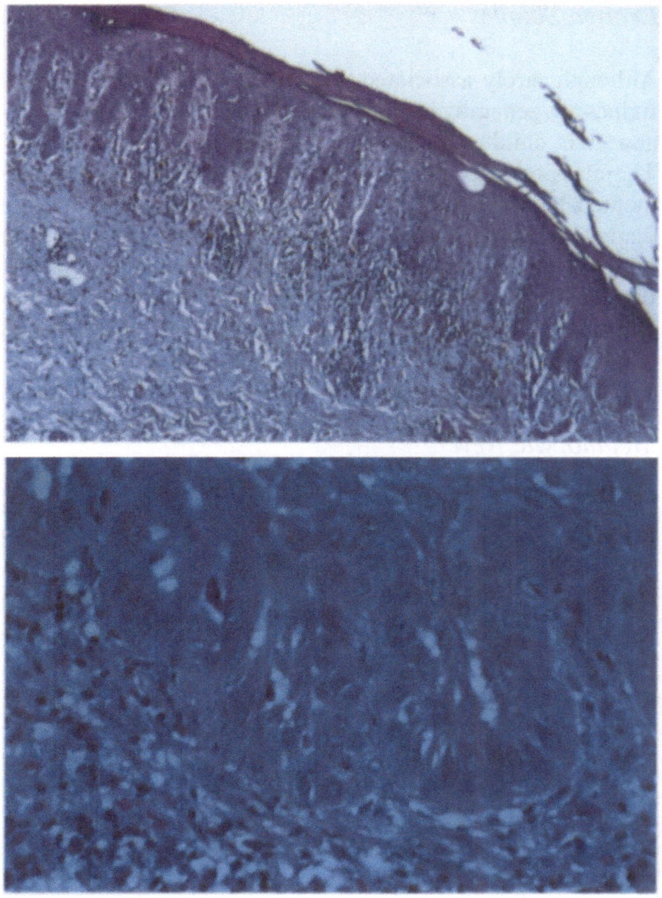

FIGURE 2.6 Actinic keratosis. The dermis displays the homogenized bluish tinge of actinically damaged collagen. The hyperplastic epidermis displays prolonged rete ridges and compact hyperkeratosis with segmental parakeratosis. Atypia in the parakeratinocytes is substantial, especially in the basal layer.

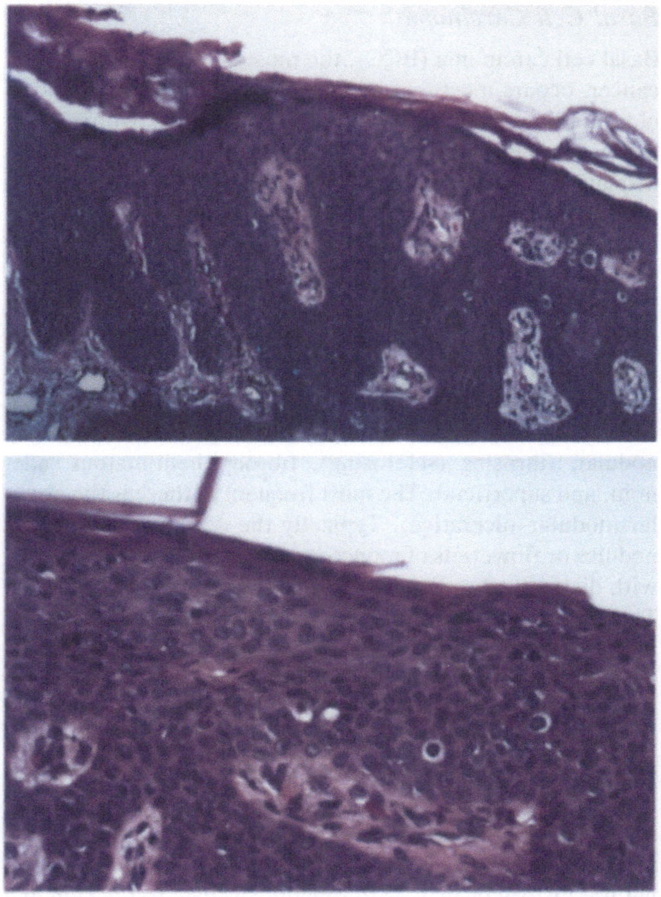

FIGURE 2.7 Squamous cell carcinoma in situ (Bowen's disease). Dysplastic cytologic features are seen throughout the span of the epidermis, along with increased mitotic activity and improper maturation. The dermis lacks evidence of actinic damage (nonexposed skin).

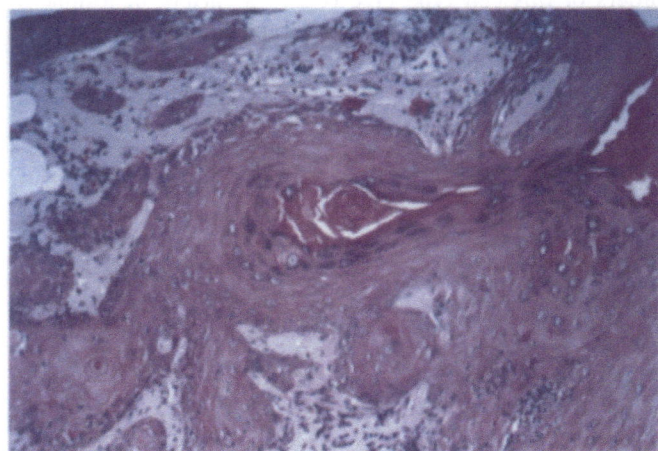

FIGURE 2.8 Squamous cell carcinoma (invasive). Proliferating atypical keratinocytes invade the underlying actinically damaged and inflamed dermis. The neoplastic cells are well differentiated, closely mimicking those of the epidermis.

Basal Cell Carcinoma

Basal cell carcinoma (BCC), the most common form of skin cancer, occurs most frequently on sun-exposed areas and in older individuals or fair-skinned persons in whom solar injury has been long-standing or more intense. The neoplasm displays differentiation features similar to the basal cells in normal epidermis and in the pilosebaceous apparatus. It could be considered histogenetically derived from epidermis or from skin appendages. Clinically, the appearance of the lesion is variable, typically producing ulcerating lesions with raised pearly margins. The "superficial" variety of BCC may present clinically as a crusted or scaly erythematous patch much like squamous cell carcinoma in situ.

Histologically, a number of patterns may be seen, including nodular, fibrosing (sclerosing), fibroepitheliomatous, adenoid, and superficial. The most frequent of these is the nodular (nodular–ulcerative). Typically the dermis is invaded by nodules or flowerlets of monotonous basophilic basaloid cells with distinct palisading by those at the periphery (Fig. 2.9). There is variable reactive fibrosis and chronic inflammation in the environs. Other types of special significance are superficial basal cell carcinoma, in which numerous independent foci of neoplasm appear to "bud" from the basal zone of the epidermis and the sclerosing or "morphealike" variant in which small strands and cords of basal cells are suspended in a voluminous background of fibrous tissue. These two types are particularly important because the boundaries of the tumor are difficult to define clinically or histologically. The natural history of BCC is to remain confined to the skin and adjacent structures. If left untreated it may infiltrate extensively but it has little or no ability to metastasize.

Tumors of Melanocytic Origin

Pigment production in the skin is the province of the melanocyte, a neural crest-derived migrant cell that populates principally the lower levels of the epidermis. Proliferative disorders of this cell type give rise to a variety of lesions of highly variable import and clinical appearance.

Lentigo Simplex

Although rarely associated with a systemic syndrome, lentigines are generally isolated and few in number. They usually appear in childhood, but may also appear at any other age. The classical appearance is that of a small, uniformly pigmented brown or black macule, only a few millimeters in diameter, unrelated to sun exposure. Histologically, the "pure lentigo" comprises an increased number of melanocytes in the basal layer, with increased pigmentation of basal keratinocytes in the company of modestly elongated rete ridges (Fig. 2.10).

Melanocytic Nevi

Melanocytic or nevocellular nevi are exceedingly common lesions—so common that they might be considered, in small numbers, normal variations in the skin. Most arise in childhood or early adulthood and rarely later. The appearance of the lesions is largely related to the location and to the structural type, of which there are basically three: junctional, compound, and intradermal.

The junctional (intraepidermal) melanocytic nevus comprises nests of melanocytes at the junctional zone of the epidermis (Fig. 2.11), confined above the basement membrane. Grossly (clinically), it is usually a brown flat lesion, often difficult to distinguish from lentigo. Occasionally it is slightly elevated.

Intradermal nevi, as the name implies, confine the nevus cells to the dermis where they occur in a variety of arrangements: in nests, cords, or individually. Cellular features also vary. Some comprise cells with typical melanocytic features; others may show evidence of Schwannian or "neuroid" differentiation. Multinucleated cells, especially superficially, are common (Fig. 2.12). Although there are occasionally flat lesions they are more often elevated and may even be pedunculated. Pigment may vary from none to deep brown or black. (*Discussion continued on p. 12*)

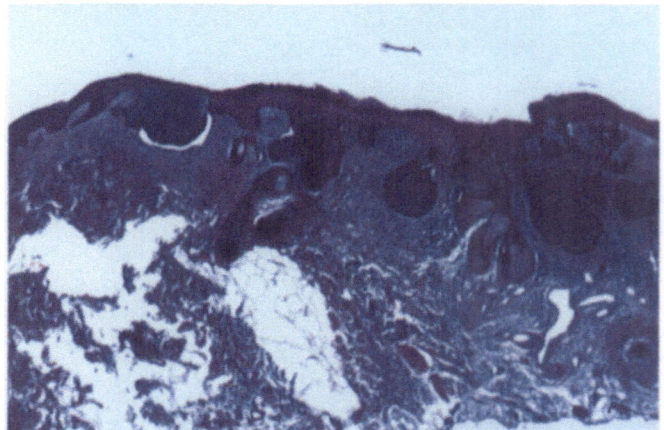

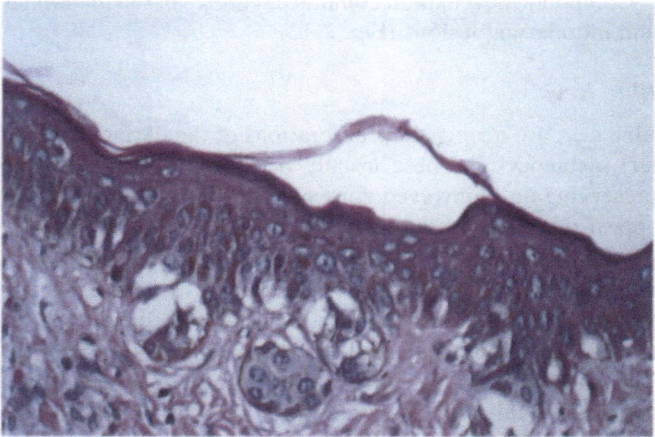

FIGURE 2.11 Junctional nevus. Well circumscribed rounded nests of nevus cells are seen at the junctional zone of the epidermis.

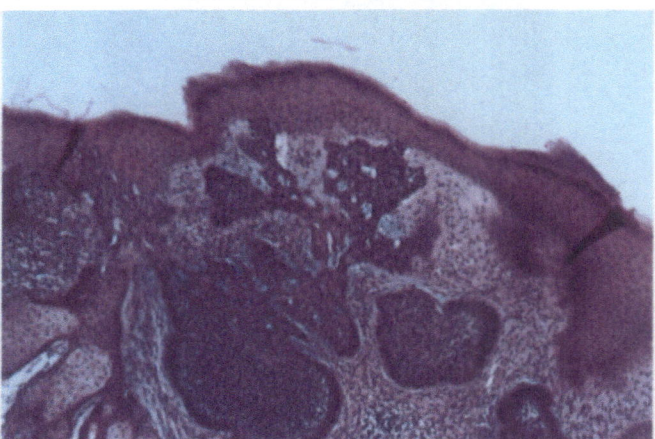

FIGURE 2.9 Basal cell carcinoma. The dermis is penetrated by many islands of darkly staining basaloid cells that show palisading at their periphery.

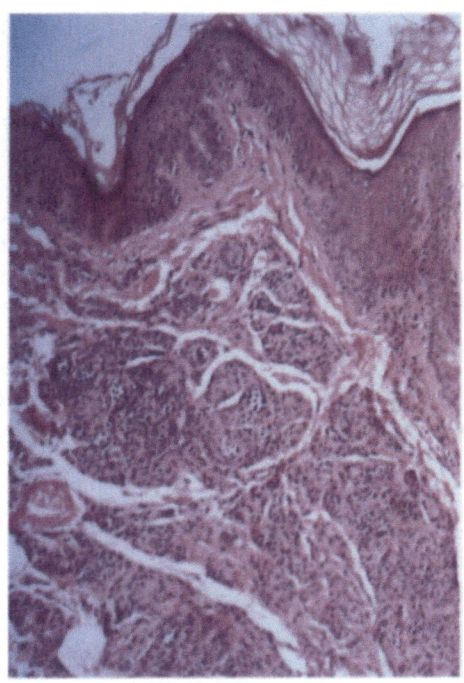

FIGURE 2.12 Intradermal nevus. Nevus cells in sheets and nests are confined to the dermis.

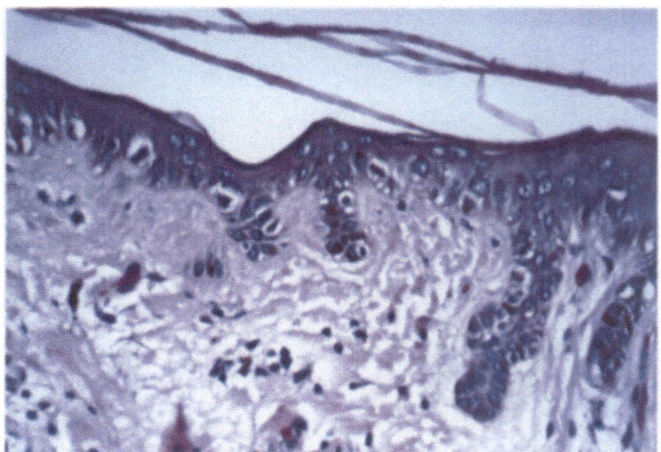

FIGURE 2.10 Lentigo. There is elongation and slight broadening of tips of the rete ridges accompanied by increased melanocytes and pigment in the basal cells.

Compound nevi exhibit combined features of the junctional and intradermal lesions (Fig. 2.13).

Blue Nevi

Blue nevi are neoplastic proliferations of the dermal (reticular) melanocytes. These usually occur only in the dermis, preserving an uninvolved zone of superficial dermis. These appear microscopically as spindle cells or cells with multiple processes, that contain variable, but frequently abundant pigment (Fig. 2.14). They are named *blue nevi* because the localization in the dermis gives a blue color on clinical inspection. Conventional blue nevi are relatively low in cellularity. The so-called cellular blue nevus displays a much higher degree of cellularity. They are often heavily pigmented and blue nevus may occur in combination with a nevocellular component, therefore so-called combined nevus. Most are benign but malignant forms do occur.

Spitz Nevus

Most Spitz nevi (spindle and epithelioid cell nevi) arise in juveniles although they may occur at any age. Typically they are elevated nodular lesions not heavily pigmented but quite vascular, providing a reddish, raspberrylike appearance, clinically. Histologically, they comprise epithelioid or spindle cells or both, which have an "active" appearance with large nuclei and frequent prominent nucleoli. Mitoses also may be fairly frequent. These features may be readily misinterpreted as malignant; differentiation between this lesion and malignant melanoma often is a diagnostic challenge. Spitz nevi are generally highly symmetrical and display a vertical orientation of spindle cells, tending to "cleavage artifact" with respect to neighboring structures. Although pseudoinfiltration of the dermis may occur, true invasion and infiltration of the epidermis are lacking (Fig. 2.15).

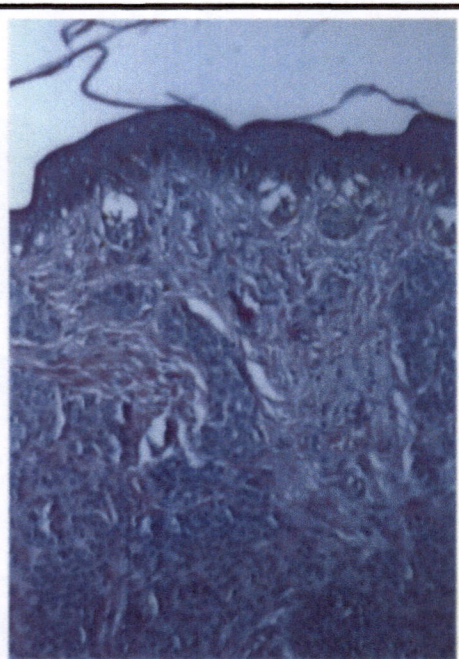

FIGURE 2.13 **Compound nevus.** Nevus cells occur in both epidermis at the junction with the dermis and in the midsuperficial dermis.

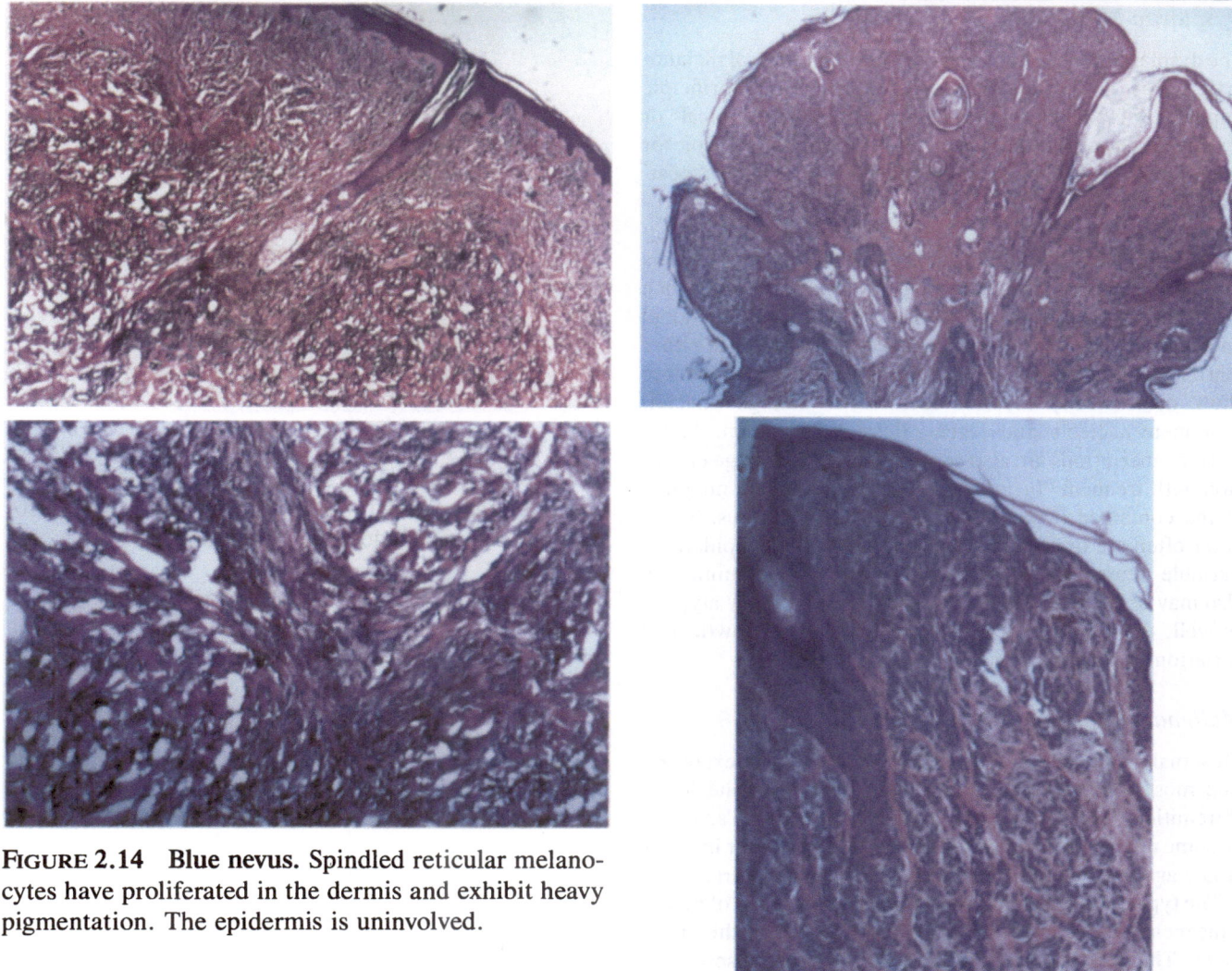

FIGURE 2.14 **Blue nevus.** Spindled reticular melanocytes have proliferated in the dermis and exhibit heavy pigmentation. The epidermis is uninvolved.

FIGURE 2.15 **Spitz nevus.** There is symmetrical expansion by spindled and epithelioid nevus cells. Spindled cells tend to orient perpendicularly to skin; pigment is focal and superficial. Secondary papillary changes of the epidermis are seen.

Dysplastic Nevus

The dysplastic nevus is a rather controversial form of melanocytic nevus, both clinically and pathologically. Of principle importance is the occurrence of such nevi with "atypical" or dysplastic features in persons with a genetic disposition for development of malignant melanoma. These persons repeatedly develop nevi with a dysplastic character or which progress with time, almost inevitably eventuating in a malignant lesion. However, such lesions can also occur in sporadic or isolated fashion. In this setting, the significance is much less clear.[6] Most dysplastic nevi are compound or junctional nevi with hyperplasia of the interface melanocytes in either lentiginous or nevocellular pattern. These nevus cells often show cytologically atypical features of enlarged nuclei, prominent nucleoli, and vaguely defined cytoplasm. Architectural aberrations are also seen, including rete ridge expansion with frequent "fusion" of adjoining ridges and mingling of the contained hyperplastic spindled melanocytes. These latter often are oriented in the same plane as the epidermis. Variable degrees of subepithelial fibrosis or inflammation also may be present (Fig. 2.16). These are clinically atypical as well, exhibiting an irregular outline, radial growth, and variation in pigmentation.

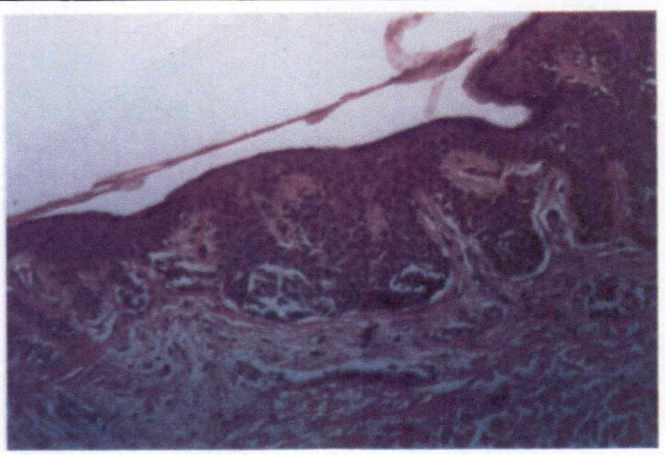

FIGURE 2.16 **Dysplastic nevus.** There is complex downward hyperplasia of rete ridges with a tendency to fusion accompanied by a lentiginous proliferation of melanocytes with mildly atypical features.

Malignant Melanoma

Most malignant melanomas arise on the areas of sun exposure. The most common sites are the head and neck and lower extremities, but they may arise anywhere on the skin and even on some mucous membranes. The vast majority occur in adults at any age, but rarely melanomas can occur in children.

The types and patterns of morphologic expression of malignant melanoma are far too numerous to cover in this treatment. The most common form is the superficial spreading type. This type begins as a junctional atypical melanocytic proliferation with a strong tendency to radial growth and an upward infiltration into the epidermis to provide the so-called pagetoid appearance, after the pattern seen in Paget's disease of the skin. At this point, it is malignant melanoma in situ. With continued growth, the tumor enters a "vertical phase" in which underlying dermis is invaded by the malignant melanocytes (Fig. 2.17). Penetration depth (assessed as Clark level or as Breslow measurement) is an important index in assessing the progress of the disease and the prognosis.[7] Other types of melanomas include nodular, acrolentiginous, and desmoplastic melanomas.

Lentigo maligna refers to a type of melanoma in situ. It presents as a slowly enlarging flat brown to black lesion almost always on sun-exposed regions, especially the face. Microscopically, a lentiginous proliferation of atypical, often spindled melanocytes is seen (Fig. 2.18). Focally, as the lesion progresses there may be nesting, particularly at sites ultimately becoming invasive. Development occurs over a number of years, and most often in older individuals, eventuating in invasion if untreated. At this point, the designation changes to "lentigo maligna melanoma." However, even with this occurrence, growth usually continues to be indolent and slow.

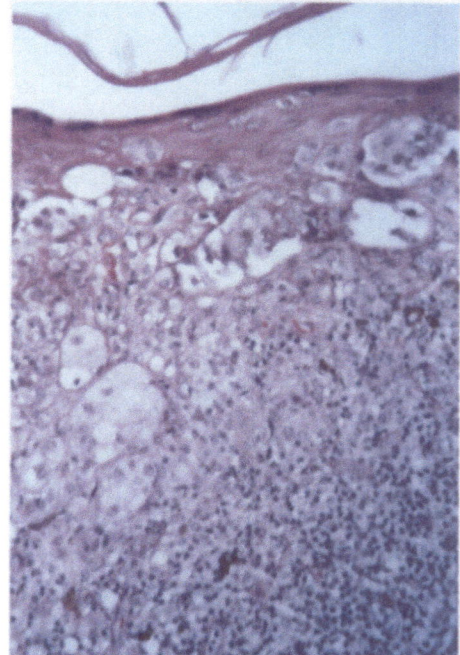

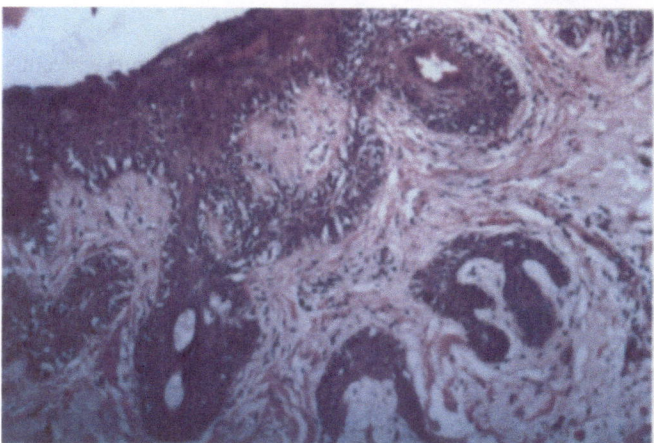

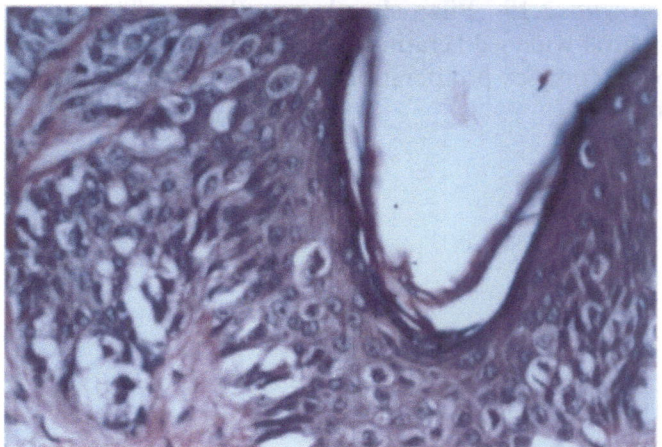

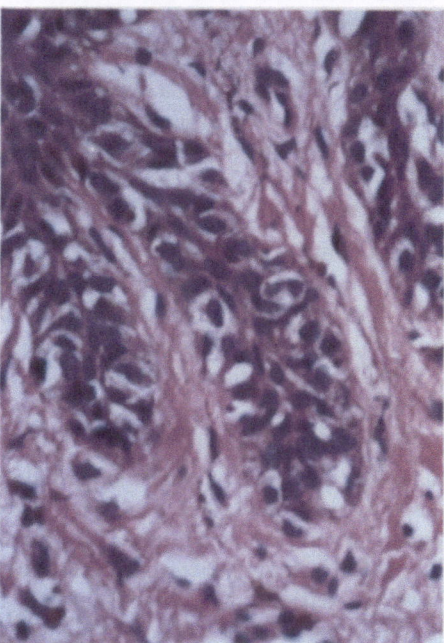

FIGURE 2.17   **Superficial spreading malignant melanoma.** The epidermis contains atypical or neoplastic melanocytes that infiltrate the epidermis in "pagetoid" fashion. Infiltration of the dermis is seen along with a brisk inflammatory response.

FIGURE 2.18   **Lentigo maligna.** The lesion is at a relatively early stage and shows a lentiginous proliferation of atypical melanocytes at the junctional zone with a tendency to track along the appendages. There is mild host inflammatory response.

Adnexal Tumors

The cutaneous appendages include hair follicle and sebaceous glands (pilosebaceous apparatus), sweat glands and their ducts (eccrine apparatus), and apocrine glands and ducts. Each of these forms a fairly complex functional and anatomic system within the integument, so that they may give rise to a great variety of neoplastic expressions. Only a few of these will be demonstrated as exemplary of this histogenetic process. Each structure can produce benign or malignant neoplasms; the emphasis here will be on the benign because of the greater frequency and the more obvious resemblance to the parent structure.

Hair Follicular Neoplasms

Hair follicular neoplasms include an extensive list of tumors, most of which are benign, including trichoepithelioma, pilar sheath acanthoma, trichofolliculoma, pilar cysts, warty dyskeratoma, pilar tumor (of the scalp), and pilomatricoma. Pilar sheath acanthoma and pilomatricoma are discussed below.

Pilar Sheath Acanthoma

Pilar sheath acanthoma occurs most often on the lip, presenting as a flesh-colored papule with a central umbilication. Histologically, it displays a proliferation of keratinocytes of pilar sheath differentiation, around a widened follicular infundibulum containing laminated keratin (Fig. 2.19).

Pilomatricoma (Calcifying Epithelioma of Malherbe)

Pilomatricoma may present as a rather large nodule (up to 5 cm) covered by normal epidermis, occurring mostly on the face and upper extremities of children and young adults. Histologically, it is found in the deep dermis and subcutis and comprises two populations of epithelial cells in a cellular stroma. The epithelial cells are sheets of indistinctly separated compact basaloid cells (basophilic cells) with dark nuclei and scant cytoplasm, and "shadow cells"–large cells with pale ghosts where nuclei have been. Calcification is frequent, as the alternate eponym implies (Fig. 2.20).

Proliferating Trichilemmal Tumor (Cyst)

Proliferating trichilemmal tumor usually is a cystic lesion, occurring principally in the scalp of elderly women. Beginning in a subcutaneous location, they may attain considerable size and even ulcerate. Histologically, it is well demarcated from the surrounding soft tissue. It comprises lobules of proliferating squamous cells that undergo amorphous (pilar-type) keratinization (Fig. 2.21). Some nuclear atypia may be present. The lesion is generally considered benign, although malignant forms have been described.

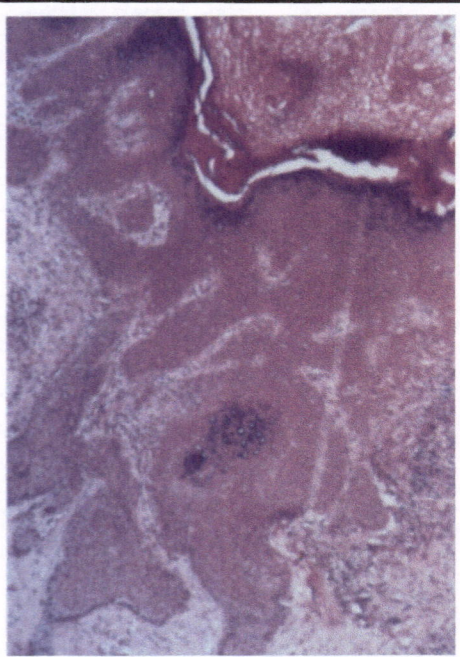

FIGURE 2.19 **Pilar sheath acanthoma.** There is a central widened keratin-filled follicular opening (pore) with complex proliferation of pilar sheath components beneath.

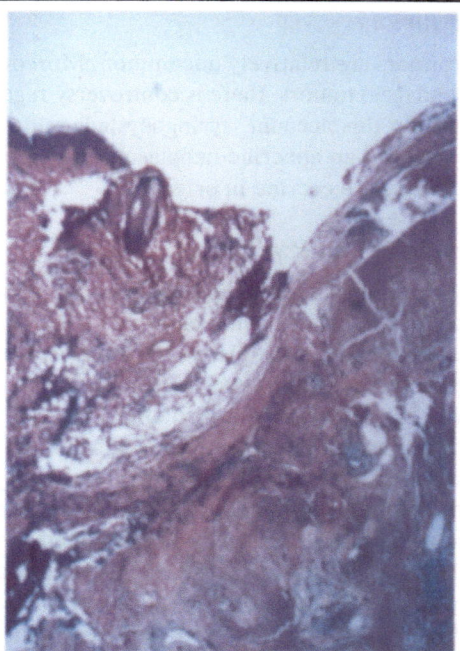

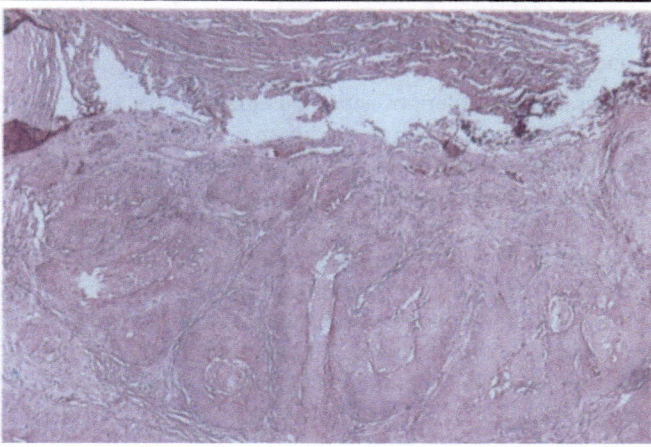

FIGURE 2.21 **Proliferating trichilemmal tumor (cyst).** The well demarcated tumor comprises proliferating squamous eddies with central pilar keratinization.

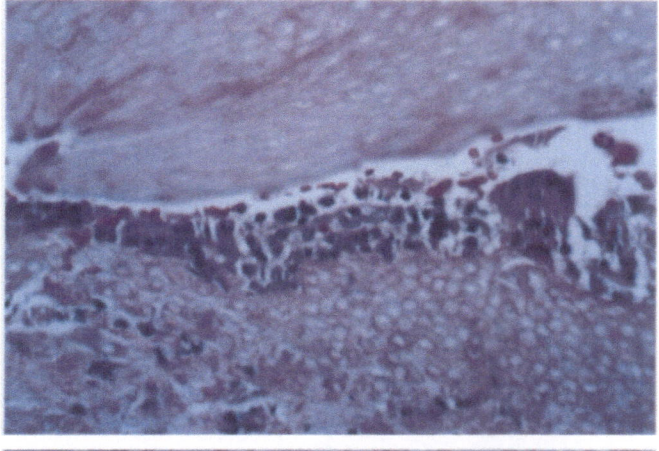

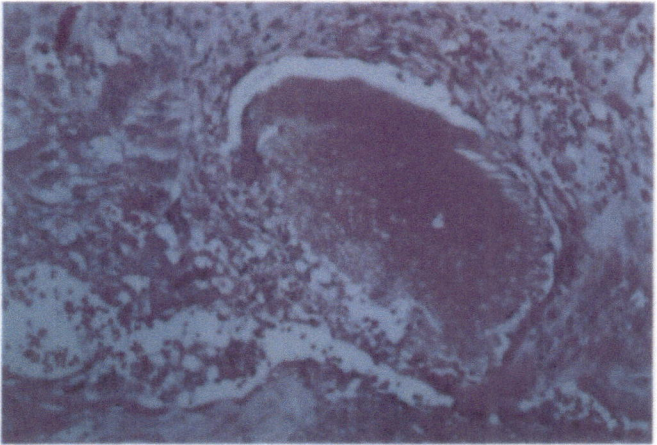

FIGURE 2.20 **Pilomatricoma.** Two cellular elements are seen: "dark" cells in the lower field and "shadow" cells in a central focus. Surrounding there is a granulomatous reaction to keratin.

Sebaceous Neoplasms

Sebaceous Adenoma

Proliferative disorders of sebaceous glands vary, from sebaceous hyperplasia to frank carcinoma. Sebaceous adenoma serves as an example of sebaceous neoplasia. It appears clinically as a nodule of variable location. Although usually isolated, multiple adenomas may occur and have been reported as accompaniments of multiple visceral carcinomas (Torre's syndrome). Histologically, the lesion is well circumscribed and is formed by lobules of sebaceous tissue of variable size and shape, lacking complete differentiation. Both differentiated fat (sebum)-containing cells and germinative cells are present (Fig. 2.22).

Apocrine Tumors

Apocrine tumors are relatively uncommon. Moreover, as for many appendageal tumors, there is controversy regarding the histogenesis. In this account, syringocystadenoma papilliferum is considered an apocrine neoplasm, although it is also argued that they are eccrine in origin.[8]

Syringocystadenoma Papilliferum

Syringocystadenoma papilliferum is most common on the face or scalp of infants or small children. It may present as one or more papules or as a plaque. Growth occurs with the onset of puberty, at which time it may assume a verrucous appearance. Histologically the epidermis is papillomatous. Invaginating sinuses are present, in which the necks of the sinuses are squamous-lined, but the depths show cystic features and a papillary lining of double layered glandular epithelium (Fig. 2.23). There may be associated surrounding tubular glands in the stroma and these, as well as the lining cells, may show evidence of apocrine secretion. A plasmocytic infiltrate in the stroma is a virtually constant feature.

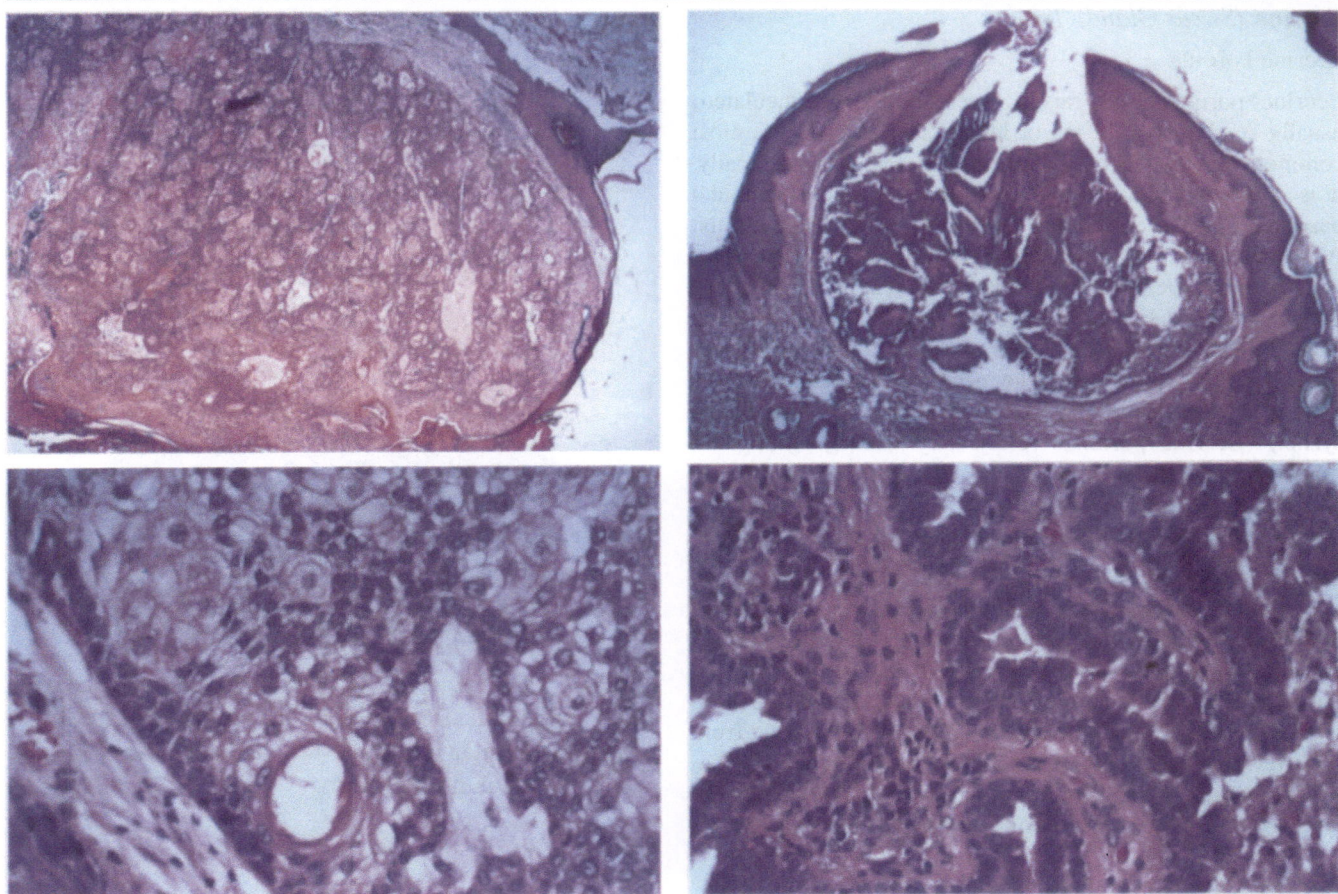

FIGURE 2.22 Sebaceous adenoma. Well demarcated lobules of incompletely differentiated sebaceous structures are present. Dark cells are the germinative component and the pale cells are differentiated sebaceous elements.

FIGURE 2.23 Syringocystadenoma papilliferum. The lesion opens to the surface with a small sinus lined by squamous epithelium. The deeper contents are papillary with two rows of lining cells; the dermis contains a plasma cell infiltrate.

Eccrine (Sweat Gland) Tumors

Eccrine Poroma

Eccrine poroma is a raised, occasionally pedunculated, usually single lesion, 2 cm or less in size, that occurs most commonly on the feet of middle-aged persons. Histologically, it is composed of a proliferation of monotonous cuboidal basophilic cells emanating from the lower epidermis. Although there is little tendency to keratinize, intercellular bridges are evident. The appearance of cells is basaloid but the peripheral palisading of basal cell carcinoma is lacking (Fig. 2.24). Occasionally, small or cystic ductal lumen are formed within the tumor. The neoplasm probably derives from the intraepidermal portion of the eccrine duct (acrosyrinx). Eccrine poromas rarely may undergo malignant transformation after a long period.

Clear Cell Hidradenoma (Eccrine Acrospiroma)

The site of origin of clear cell hidradenoma in the eccrine apparatus is unclear. It occurs as a nodule covered by normal skin. Histologically, the tumor is usually well circumscribed and comprises lobules of closely packed cells. Tubular lumina are present; there are quite commonly cystic changes in these tubular elements. The proliferation is usually separated from the overlying epidermis. Two cellular elements are characteristic; a small basophilic cell and a larger cell with abundant clear cytoplasm. Focal keratinization may occur (Fig. 2.25).

Adenoid Cystic Carcinoma

Adenoid cystic carcinoma is an uncommon example of a sweat gland carcinoma that parallels that seen in salivary glands. Metastases are unusual. The histoanatomy is that of cellular accumulations with glandular differentiation alternating with more solid areas. The glandular spaces appear to distend with secretory products, forming small or large cystic spaces (Fig. 2.26).

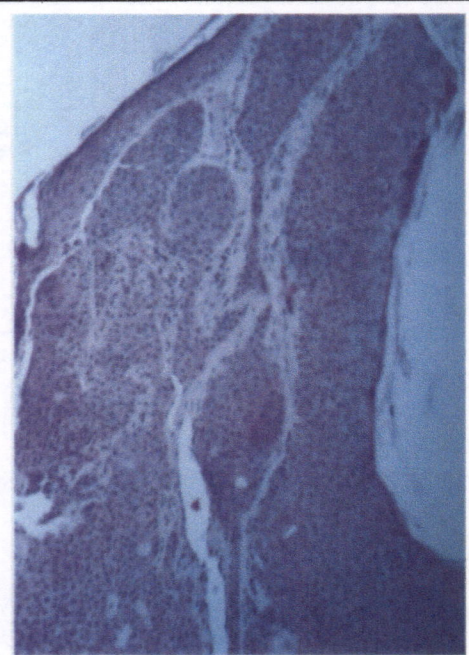

FIGURE 2.24 **Eccrine poroma.** Sheets of relatively small polygonal or cuboidal cells are punctuated by a few small tubular lumina, a few of which have become cystic. There is no palisading.

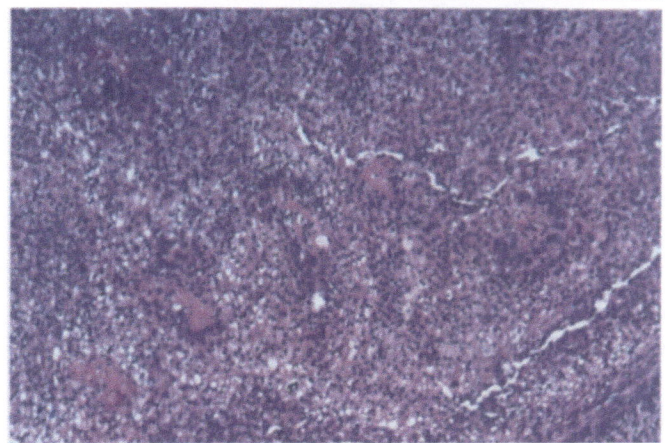

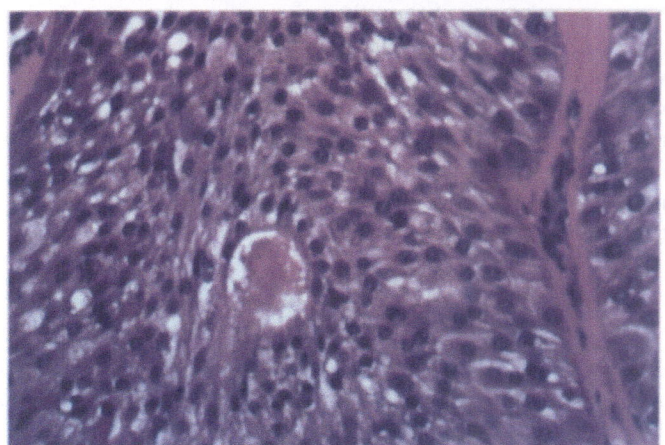

FIGURE 2.25   **Clear cell hidradenoma.** Sheets of clear cells are punctuated by a few tubular lumina lined by cuboidal cells and contain eosinophilic material.

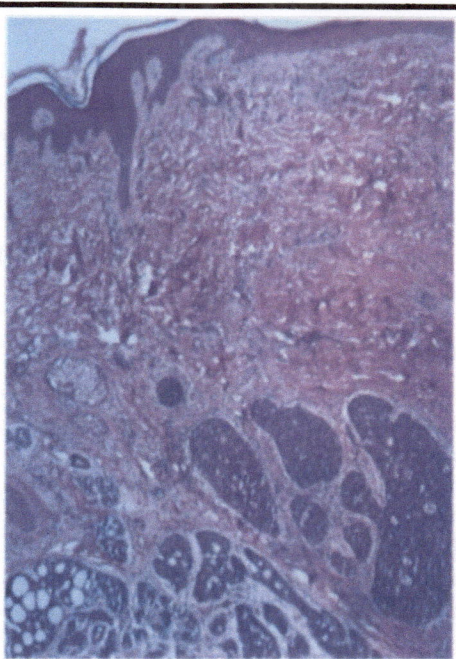

FIGURE 2.26   **Adenoid cystic carcinoma.** Sheets of darkly staining cells show a "Swiss cheese" appearance resulting from a gland formation with occasional distension.

Tumors of the Dermis

The cellular elements that occupy the dermis (i.e., fibrocytes, lymphoid cells, endothelial cells, nerve sheath cells, etc.) are, to a large extent, the same as those that form tissue stroma elsewhere. Thus, most of the neoplasms, derived from these elements, are similar to those in other organs. There are some of these, however, in which cutaneous expression is common or presentation is peculiar to the skin. A few of these will be illustrated.

Fibroepithelial Polyp

Fibroepithial polyp is an extremely common lesion. Frequently called "skin tag" or "acrochordon," the most common variety occurs as multiple small polypoid structures, most frequently in the neck or axillae. They are generally but a few millimeters in size although they may possess a rather elongated stalk. The histologic appearance is more that of a fibrous growth abnormality than of a true neoplasm. The epidermis is often mildly hyperplastic and the fibrous dermis beneath is loose with prominent capillary vascularity (Fig. 2.27).

Tumors of Fibrocytic/Histiocytic Origin

Dermatofibroma

Dermatofibromas are common tumors that are also known as benign fibrous histiocytomas and sclerosing hemangiomas. This plurality of designations results from the varying composition by fibrocytes, histiocytes, collagen, and capillaries. Often the overlying epidermis exhibits a hyperplastic reaction, and hyperpigmentation of the basal layer is not unusual. Hemosiderin accumulation in the lesion also occurs, especially in those with a more vascular content. The principle cell type is a spindle cell, and these characteristically deposit immature collagen fibers providing a hazy, bluish background. The growth is often poorly demarcated and may frequently show extension into the subcutis (Fig. 2.28). Clinically, the lesion may occur at any age or site but is most common on the extremities, especially the legs. When fully developed, they are raised nodules, usually 1 to 2 cm in size with a brown or reddish brown surface.

Xanthomas

Xanthomas are common lesions that may occur in persons with lipid metabolism abnormalities, but also in apparently normal persons. The xanthelasmata are among the most common expressions of this, occurring largely as multiple yellowish small plaques, especially on the eyelids. Histologically, xanthelasmata comprise collections of foamy histiocytes with small, usually single nuclei in abundant clear, "wrinkled" cytoplasm (Fig. 2.29).

Dermatofibrosarcoma Protuberans

Dermatofibrosarcoma protuberans is best considered a tumor of low grade, mostly local, malignant potential. It generally resembles dermatofibroma but with greater size, cellularity, frequent nuclear atypical changes, and invasive behavior. The hallmark of this lesion is often considered the "storiform pattern"—a woven arrangement of the neoplastic cells and their collagenous support (Fig. 2.30).

Clinically the lesion is a firm, often multinodular tumor, with a reddish or bluish color. The trunk is the most common site; proximal extremities are also favored.

Vascular Neoplasms

Many types of vascular proliferation or neoplasms occur in the skin, with varying clinical significance. These include vessel disorders of various size and various components of vessels. Some angiomatous lesions are associated with systemic disease or disease of other organ systems such as the chondromatosis of Maffucci's syndrome or leptomeningeal involvement with Sturge-Weber syndrome.
(Discussion continued on p. 24)

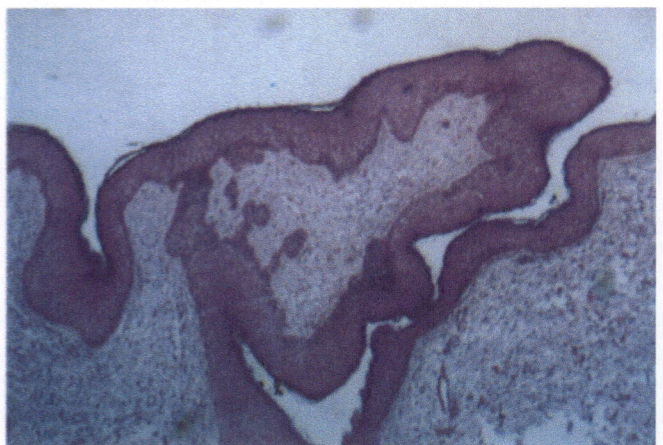

FIGURE 2.27 **Fibroepithelial polyp.** A segment of a polypoid acrochordon shows a hyperplastic epidermis over a moderately vascular fibrous stroma.

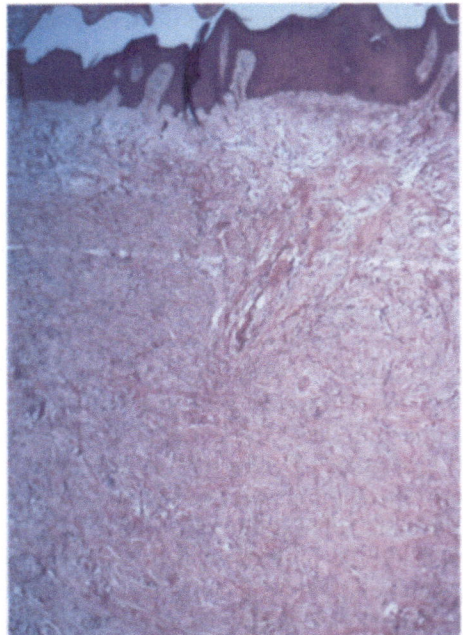

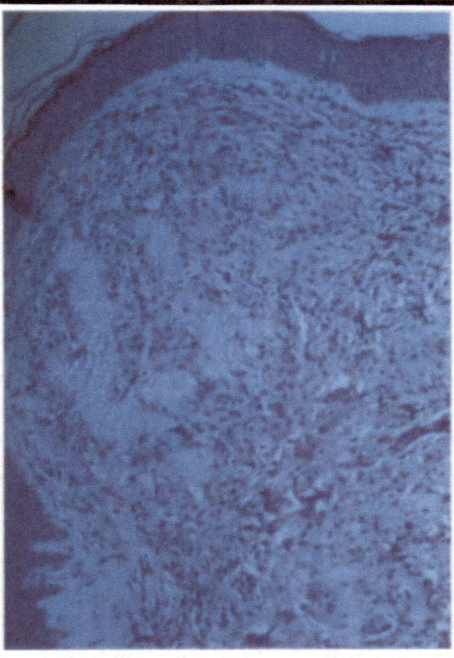

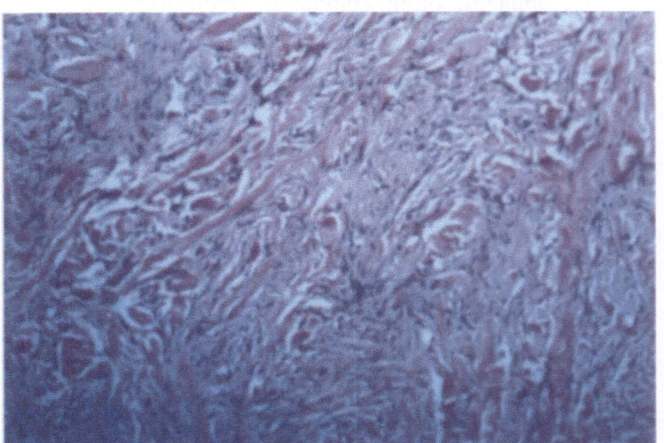

FIGURE 2.29 **Xanthoma.** Closely placed histiocytes show expansive pink foamy cytoplasm.

FIGURE 2.28 **Dermatofibroma.** The spindle cell proliferation with collagen deposition lies in the dermis beneath the hyperplastic epidermis.

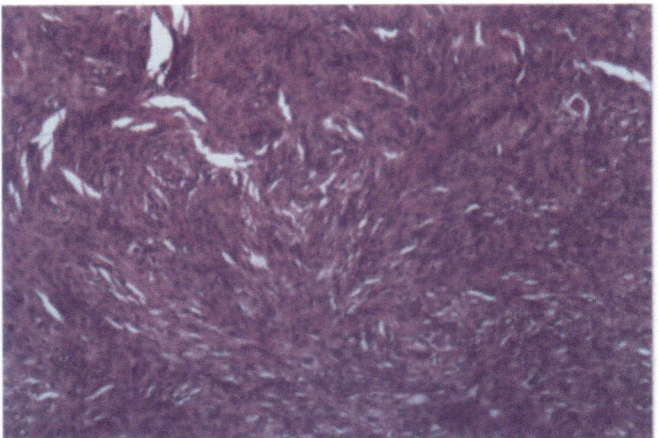

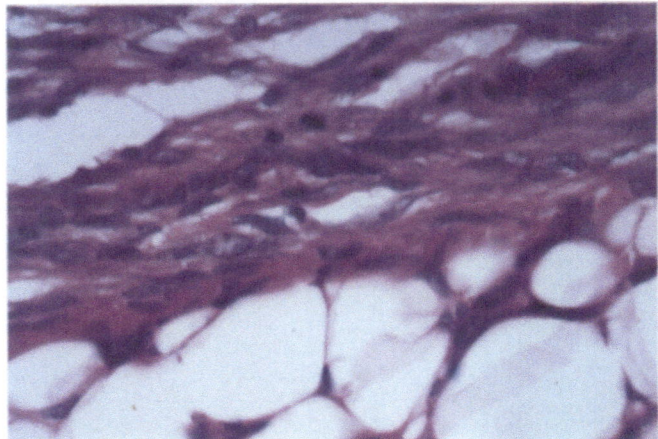

FIGURE 2.30 **Dermatofibrosarcoma protuberans.** There is a dense population of spindle cells exhibiting a woven storiform pattern. Scattered mitotic figures are present.

The most commonly encountered vascular neoplasm is formed principally of proliferating capillaries and small venules. It is so common that it is virtually within the spectrum of normal variation. They occur as congenital lesions, which usually regress spontaneously (strawberry mark), and as small cherry-red papules that crop up in middle life (cherry hemangiomas). Histologically, they comprise closely placed vessels of capillary or venular dimension with variable intervening stroma (Fig. 2.31)

Angiosarcoma

Cutaneous angiosarcomas are, except for rare circumstances, limited to the head and neck of the elderly population. They may begin as an erythematous or purplish patch, eventually becoming nodular and ulcerating. Histologically, the neoplasm is seen to extend deceptively into the soft tissues beyond the limits of the grossly defined lesion. They may vary considerably in differentiation; the well differentiated tumors resembling granulation tissue and the more anaplastic lesions may have lost the resemblance to their vascular origins. In many cases, the discrimination from benign vascular lesions may prove difficult (Fig. 2.32). Although the growth rate is generally slow, the disease is relentless, ultimately resulting in metastases to cervical lymph nodes and distant sites. These neoplasms respond poorly to surgical therapy or radiotherapy.

Kaposi's Sarcoma

Formerly a rare neoplastic condition in the United States, this has become much more commonplace as a result of its association with immunosuppression, particularly with acquired immune deficiency syndrome (AIDS). In this setting, the lesions may appear at any site, may involve viscera, and have an aggressive course. Grossly, they present as multiple purplish, hemorrhagic nodules. It is debated whether it represents true clonal neoplasia or is a multifocal proliferative disorder. The histogenesis is not entirely certain, but it probably stems from a vasoformative mesenchymal element, quite possibly the endothelial cell.

Histologically, the fully developed lesions are characterized by spindle cells that form slits containing red blood cells. There is a variable accompanying presence of lymphocytes and macrophages, often containing hemosiderin pigment (Fig. 2.33).

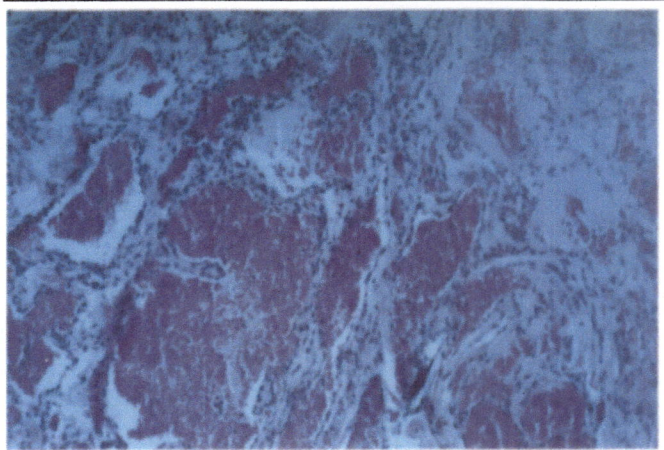

FIGURE 2.31 **Hemangioma.** Closely placed dilated capillaries and venules occupy the mid-dermis and superficial dermis. The endothelial layer is somewhat pronounced and the overlying epidermis is focally thinned.

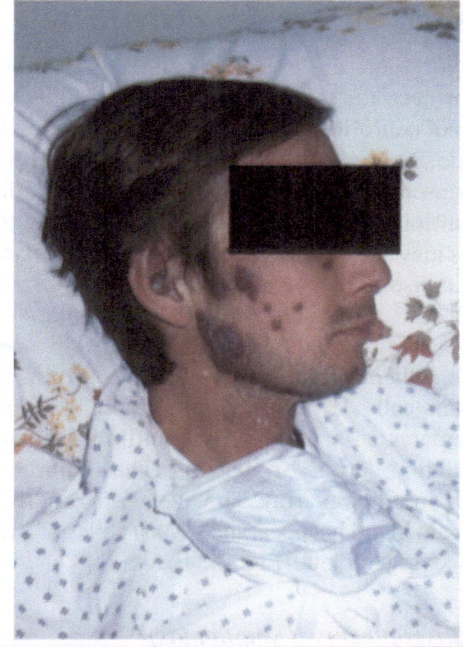

A

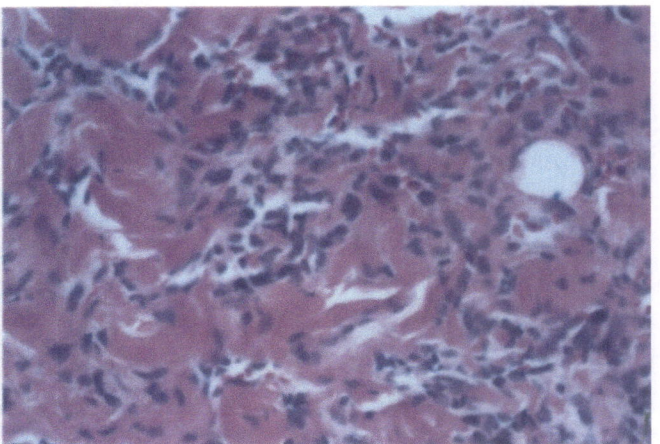

FIGURE 2.32 **Angiosarcoma.** The dermis contains many slits lined by atypical endothelial cells with scattered red blood cells within.

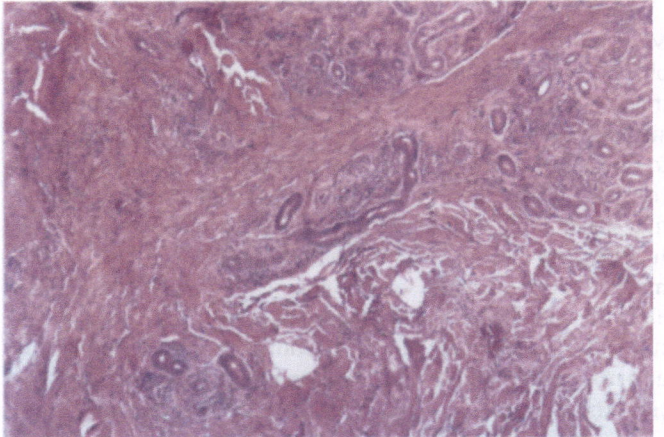

B

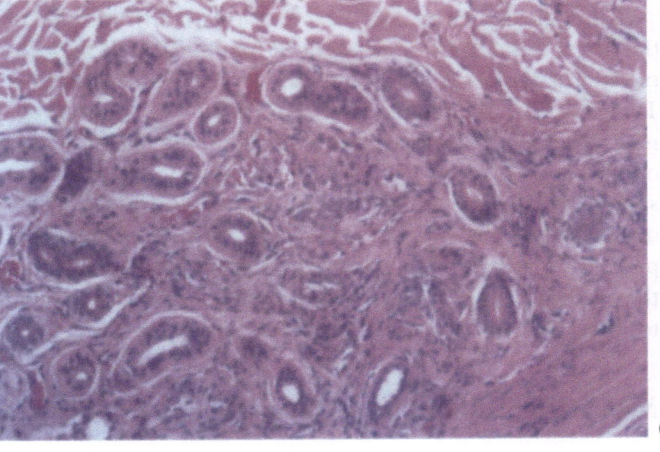

C

FIGURE 2.33 **Kaposi's sarcoma. A:** Multiple purplish hemorrhagic nodules on the face (clinical). **B, C:** An early tumor showing bland-appearing spindle cells in the dermis dissecting into appendages, splaying apart the elements of the eccrine coil. Extravasated red cells are in the dermis.

Neural Tumors

Neural skin tumors are essentially the same as those else-where. However, the skin is a particularly prominent site for expression of neurofibromas, especially as a manifestation of the autosomal dominant disorder neurofibromatosis (Von Recklinghausen's disease). In this disorder most patients also exhibit multiple brown macules (café-au-lait spots). Neurofibromas may also occur on an isolated basis, separate from this genetic disorder.

In either case, the lesions present most commonly as protuberant flesh-colored nodules, often attached to a peripheral nerve. The cells of origin probably include both fibroblasts and Schwann cells. Histologically, this common tumor may be well demarcated or may have an infiltrative pattern into the surrounding dermis or subcutis. The tumors comprise wavy fibers in random array. The nuclei are oval to elongate and wavy, and bland in appearance. Mast cells are a relatively frequent accompaniment (Fig. 2.34).

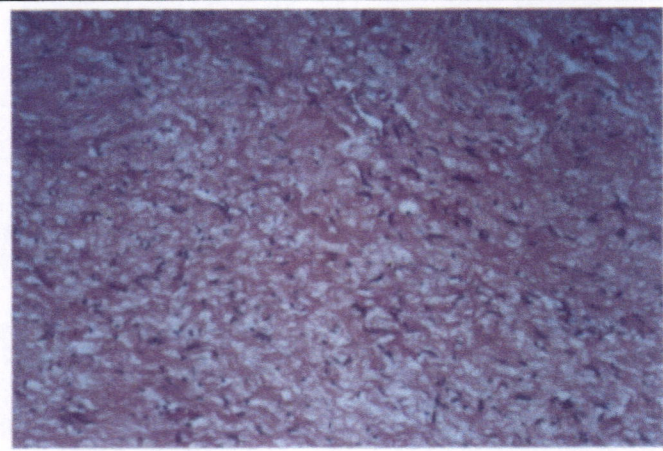

FIGURE 2.34 Neurofibroma. Wavy nuclei are scattered in the collagenous matrix. Round mast cells are also present.

Lymphoid Neoplasms (Lymphomas)

Most malignant lymphomas arise in lymph nodes or in lymphoid tissue of nonlymphoid structures (i.e, gastrointestinal tract). Chiefly, they involve the skin by extension or metastasis. However, certain lymphomas of T-cell origin are peculiar to the skin as a primary site. The cutaneous T-cell lymphoma (mycosis fungoides) is an indolent progressive neoplasm that may affect large skin areas and ultimately becomes systemic. It undergoes development through three stages. In the erythematous stage, a patchy eruption appears, later evolving into elevated lesions during the plaque stage. In the third stage, the tumor stage, irregular elevated reddish brown tumors occur and may undergo necrosis and ulceration. During this evolution there is generally progressive involvement of lymph nodes and viscera.

Histologically, in the early stage, distinction from some of the dermatidites may be difficult. Often the dermis is occupied by a lymphoid infiltrate and mixed with histiocytes. Typically, the lymphoid cells demonstrate "epidermotropism"—a proclivity for infiltration of the intercellular spaces of the epidermis. As the disease progresses, the infiltrate shows increasing cytologic atypicality of lymphocytes, frequently displaying enlarged nuclei with complex twisted morphologic features, and increased epidermotropism. Within the epidermis, aggregates of tumor lymphocytes may develop to form "Pautrier abscesses" (Fig. 2.35).

Metastatic Tumors

Although not a chief site for metastases, the frequency of metastasis to the skin generally reflects the occurrence of the primary neoplasm. Thus, breast (in females), lung, colon, melanoma, kidney, and ovary are among the leading sources of primary neoplasms that find their way to the skin. Metastatic skin tumors usually occupy the subcutis or dermis, and often leave the epidermis uninvolved or appear to involve it secondarily from beneath. Grossly, they frequently present

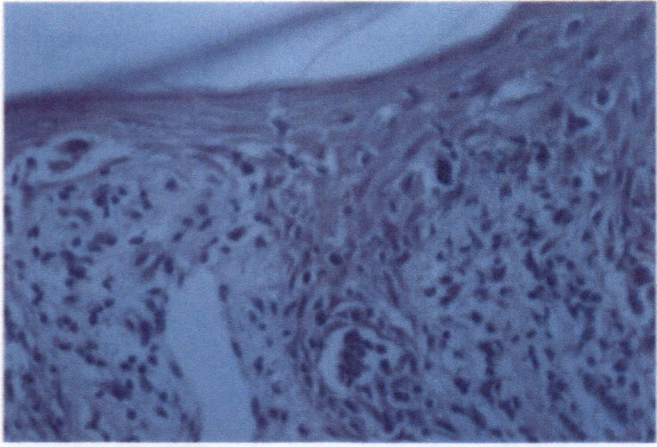
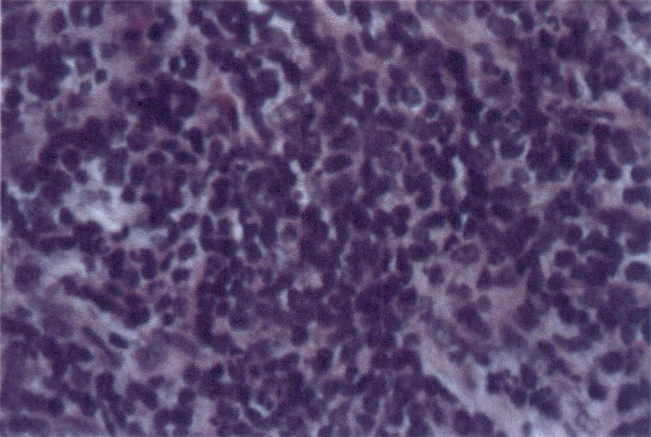

FIGURE 2.35 Cutaneous T-cell lymphoma. Atypical lymphoid cells lie in the dermis and permeate the epidermis, forming small collections (Pautrier's abscesses).

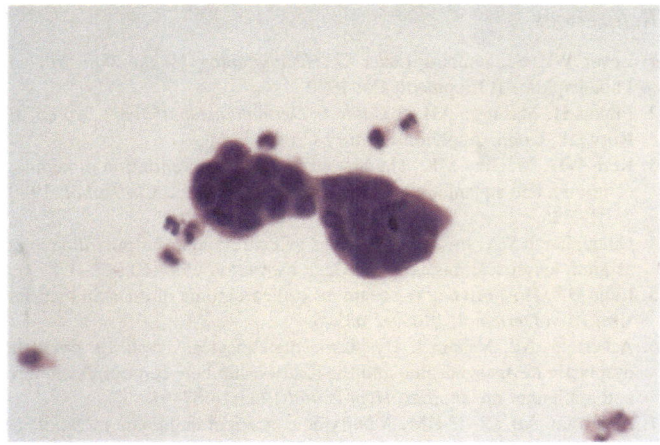

A

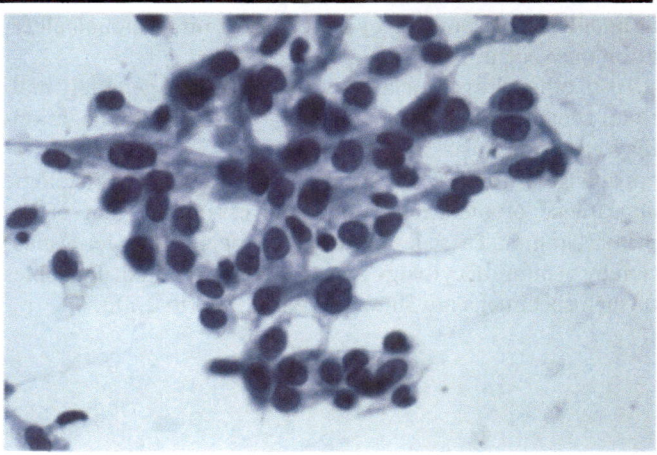

FIGURE 2.38 Metastatic renal cell carcinoma to the skin. Mildly pleomorphic cells with epithelial character and pale cytoplasm are present (FNA smear).

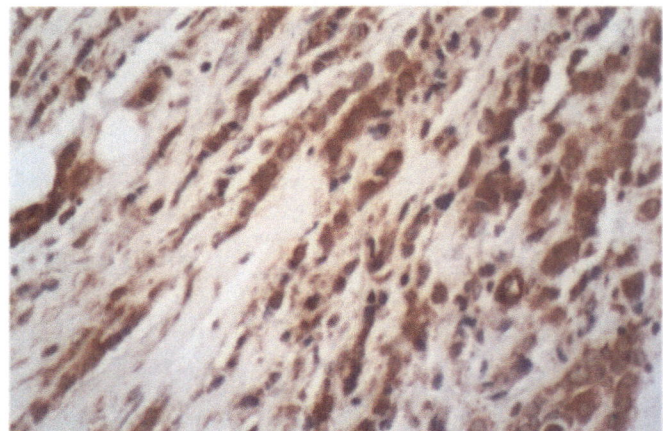

B

FIGURE 2.36 Metastatic breast carcinoma metastatic to skin. A: Tight clusters of atypical epithelial cells are seen along with a few isolated individual cells (FNA smear). **B:** Immunostain of the biopsy section showing the neoplastic cells reactive to alpha lactoalbumin.

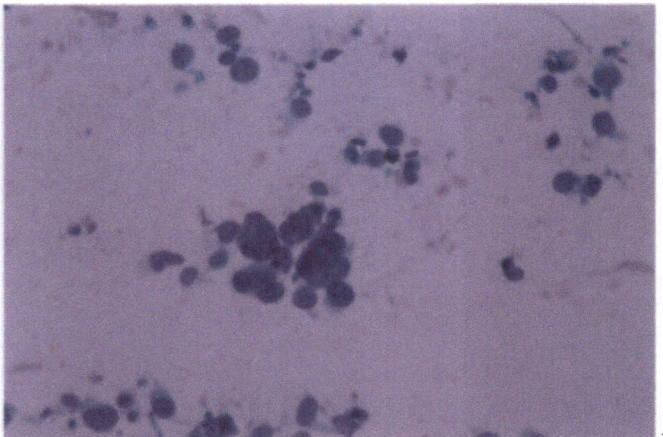

A

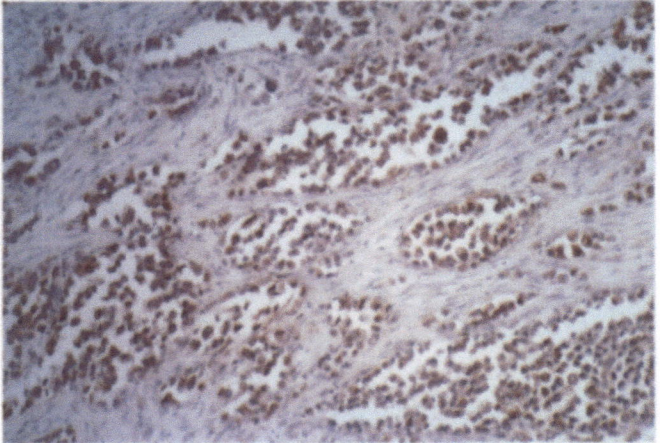

B

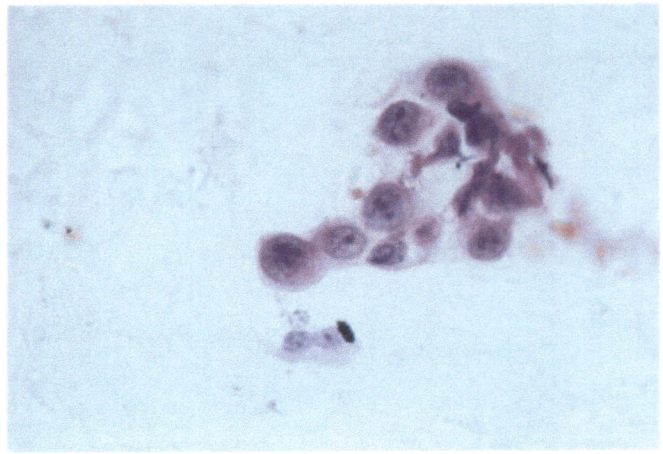

FIGURE 2.37 Metastatic adenocarcinoma involving skin from an unspecified primary site. Fairly loosely associated epithelial cells contain enlarged nuclei with prominent macronucleoli (FNA smear).

FIGURE 2.39 Metastatic melanoma to the skin. A: Neoplastic cells in cluster and isolated (FNA smear). **B:** Immunostain of the biopsy section showing the neoplastic cells positive for S-100 protein.

as nodules, often covered by intact epidermis, although ulceration may occur.

As in other sites of metastasis, the lesions are generally multiple, a feature assisting in diagnosis. When single, the lesions may easily be mistaken for primary tumors, particularly for appendageal tumors because of location. The histologic appearance of metastatic tumors is essentially that of the primary tumor. These lesions afford an opportunity for evaluation by aspiration cytology as a diagnostic method. Examples of such specimens are shown (Figures 2.36 to 2.38).

References

1. Lever WF, Schaumburg-Lever G. *Histopathology of the skin*. 7th ed. Philadelphia: JB Lippincott Co; 1990.
2. Pinkus H, Mehrgun AH. *A Guide to Dermatohistopathology*. 3rd ed. E. Norwalk, Conn: Appleton-Century-Crofts; 1981.
3. Kern WH, McGray MK. The histopathologic differentiation of keratoacanthoma and squamous cell carcinoma of the skin. *J Cut Pathol*. 1980; 7:318–325.
4. Goldenhersh WA. Invasive squamous cell carcinoma, initially diagnosed as giant keratoacanthoma. *J Am Acad Dermatol*. 1984;10:372–378.
5. Lund HZ. How often does squamous cell carcinoma of the skin metastasize? *Arch Dermatol*. 1965;92:635–637.
6. Ackerman AB, Mihara I. Dysplastic melanocytes, dysplastic nevi, the dysplastic nevus syndrome and the relationship between dysplastic nevi and malignant melanomas. *Hum Pathol* 1985;16:87–91.
7. Ackerman AB, David KM. A unifying concept of malignant melanomas: biologic aspects. *Hum Pathol*. 1986;17:432–440.
8. Helwig EB, Hackney VC. Syringoadenoma papilliferum. *Arch Dermatol*. 1955;71:361–372.

3
Salivary Glands and Oral Cavity

There are three distinct pairs of major salivary glands: parotid, submandibular, and sublingual. Minor salivary glands are scattered in the lips, buccal mucosa, palate, and tongue. The major salivary glands are lobulated structures comprising lobules separated by fibrous connective tissue (Fig. 3.1A).

The lobules, comprising serous and mucus-secreting cells, are the primary secretory units (Fig. 3.1B). The secretion drains into intralobular ducts from where it is conveyed via interlobular ducts to the main secretory duct.

Because salivary gland tumors are relatively uncommon and their cytologic presentation is complex, fine needle aspiration (FNA) cytology of salivary glands is not widely used in North America. Most non-neoplastic lesions of salivary glands can be diagnosed with reasonable certainty on clinical and radiologic findings. Most neoplastic lesions can be delineated by physical findings and computed tomography (CT), but for identification of their benign or malignant nature, FNA cytology may be useful. If the cytologic features are equivocal, open biopsy is required.

Non-Neoplastic Lesions

Sialolithiasis

Stones in salivary ducts are common, especially in the submandibular gland. Typically, the patient complains of pain, particularly at meal times when the gland swells in response to the stimulus of food. Chronic sialadenitis is a potential complication.

Sialadenitis

Mumps (epidemic parotitis) is a contagious viral infectious disease seen most often in children. Bacterial or suppurative sialadenitis occurs among elderly patients and is clinically characterized by unilateral painful swelling of the gland.

The aspirate from suppurative parotitis contains inflammatory exudate with a few aggregates of acinar cells (Fig. 3.2).

Granulomatous Sailadenitis

Granulomatous sialadenitis may be observed in tuberculosis or sarcoidosis. It is rare in the United States (Fig. 3.3A).

Lymphoproliferative Lesions

Lymphoproliferative lesions are usually solitary palpable masses showing partial replacement of the parenchyma by a polymorphous infiltrate of lymphoid cells, with or without germinal centers (Fig. 3.4). These lesions may be bilateral (Mikulicz syndrome). When they are accompanied by dryness of the mouth, keratoconjunctivitis sicca, or rheumatoid arthritis, the condition is termed Sjögren's syndrome. If the lymphoid cell populations is monomorphic, it suggests lymphoma.

Neoplasms

More than 90% of salivary gland tumors occur in the parotid gland and more than 80% are benign. Fewer than 10% of all salivary gland tumors occur in the submandibular gland and more than 30% to 40% are malignant. Minor salivary gland tumors are rare, but show an equal distribution of benign or malignant lesions.

Benign Neoplasms

Three types of benign neoplasms commonly arise in major and minor salivary glands, with the parotid gland being affected more commonly than the other glands.

Pleomorphic Adenoma (Benign Mixed Tumor)

Pleomorphic adenomas occur most often in the parotid gland and represent 70% of all neoplasms of the parotid gland. Clinically, they present as movable preauricular swellings involving the gland superficially. They are encapsulated and solid and exhibit a wide variety of histologic patterns; they probably comprise cells of ductal myoepithelial origin. These neoplasms consist of solid sheets and nests of uniform epithelial cells interspersed with myxomatous, adipose, and chondroid elements (Fig. 3.5A). Fine needle aspiration cytology shows sheets and occasional clusters of uniform, bland epithelial cells, isolated elongated cells, and basophilic amorphous material (the chondroid element) (Fig. 3.5B).

Warthin's Tumor (Papillary Cystadenoma Lymphomatosum)

Warthin's tumors are encapsulated and partly cystic and are easily dissected from the surrounding glands. Histologically,

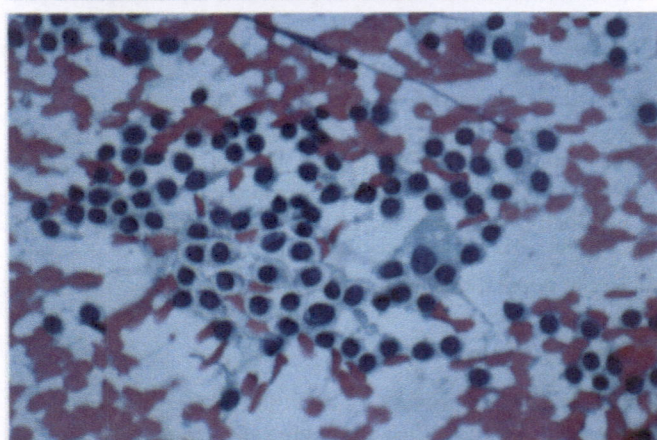

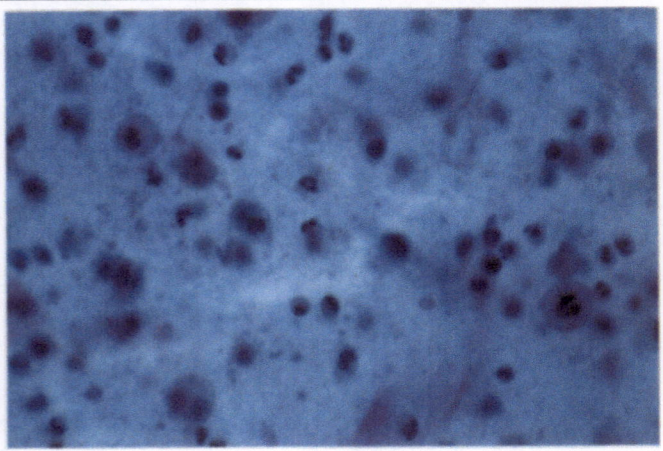

FIGURE 3.2 **Suppurative parotitis.** FNA smear showing scattered acinar cells in a background of suppurative inflammation.

FIGURE 3.1   **Normal salivary gland. A**: Lobules separated by delicate fibroconnective stroma. They consist of serous and mucous acini and intralobular ducts. **B**: FNA smear showing normal serous and mucus-secreting cells arranged in sheets.

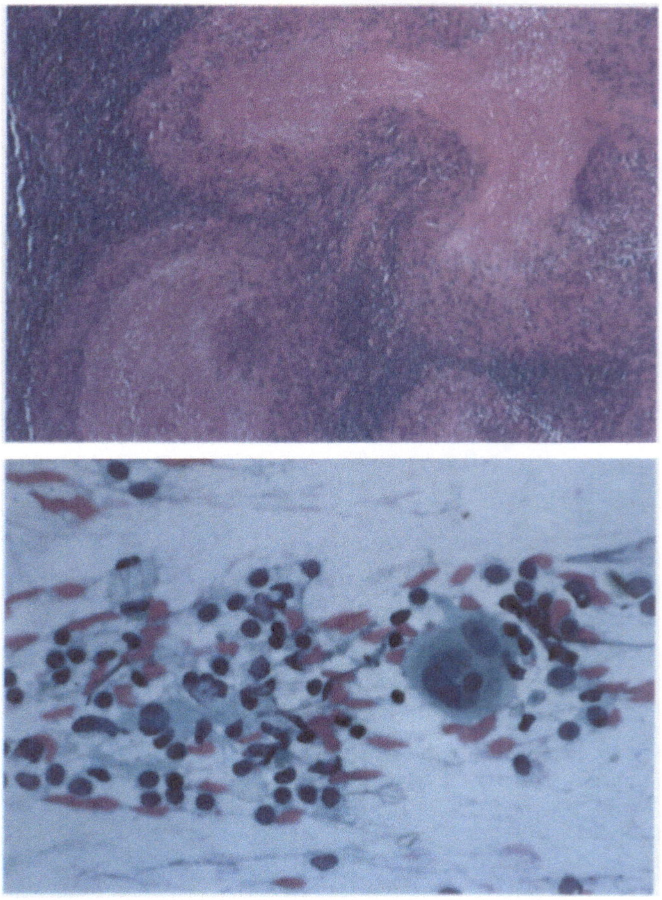

A

B

FIGURE 3.3 Tuberculosis of parotid gland. A: Granuloma with central caseous necrosis and a peripheral layer of epithelioid cells. B: FNA aspirate showing Langerhans' giant cells, comma-shaped epithelioid cells, and lymphocytes.

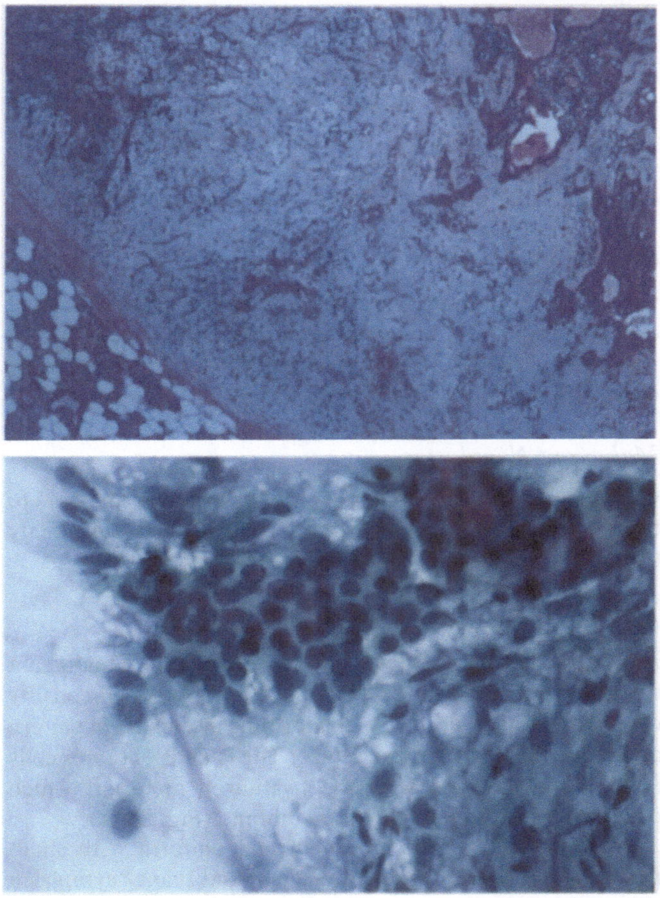

A

B

FIGURE 3.5 Pleomorphic adenoma. A: Solid nests and sheets of acinar cells mixed with myxoid and chondroid stroma. B: FNA smear showing sheets of acinar cells in a chondroid and myxoid background.

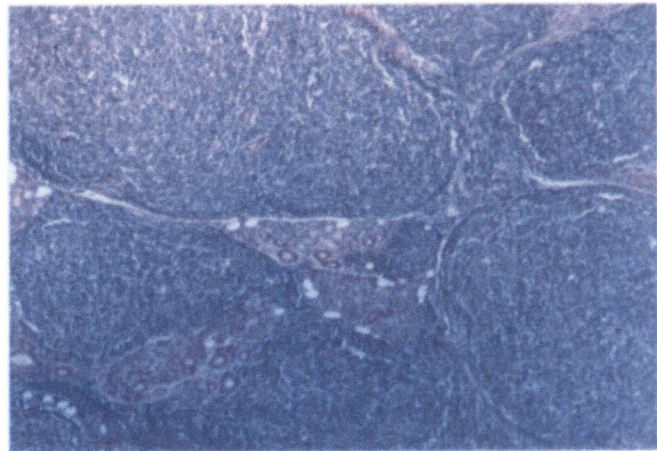

FIGURE 3.4 Mikulicz disease of parotid gland. An extensive lymphocytic proliferation compressing acini.

they consist of multiple cystlike spaces lined by crowded papillary structures covered by a single layer of columnar oncocytes, beneath which are compact sheets of mature lymphocytes (Fig. 3.6A). Fine needle aspiration cytology shows sheets of bland oncocytes with scattered small lymphocytes. Oncocytes are columnar to polygonal and have abundant eosinophilic cytoplasm and small round nuclei (Fig. 3.6B).

Oncocytoma

Oncytoma is an encapsulated solid tumor comprising sheets and cords of polygonal eosinophilic epithelial cells (oncocytes), surrounded by fibrous stroma. Fine needle aspiration cytology shows sheets of polygonal eosinophilic epithelial cells.

Malignant Neoplasms

Clinically, the malignant tumors are firm masses that tend to become fixed to adjacent tissues. They metastasize mainly through lymphatics.

Adenoid Cystic Carcinoma (Cylindroma)

Adenoid cystic carcinoma is a relatively common malignant neoplasm of the salivary glands. Microscopically, it consists of islands of small uniform cells forming a cribriform pattern and separated by hyalinized septae. The islands of tumor cells enclose spaces filled with the hyalinized material, which originates from the basement membrane (Fig. 3.7A).

In aspirates the cells are small and uniform with small round nuclei, with prominent nucleoli and scanty cytoplasm (Fig. 3.7B). Cells surrounding balls of hyalinized material may be found.

Acinic Cell Carcinoma

Acinic cell carcinoma is a relatively rare malignant neoplasm of the salivary gland. It is slowly growing and consists of cells in sheets or forming acini. The cells are uniform and polygonal and have basophilic granular cytoplasm, resembling normal serous cells and round hyperchromatic nuclei. Mitotic figures are rare (Fig. 3.8).

Mucoepidermoid Tumor

Mucoepidermoid tumor is classified into low, intermediate, and high grades. Low-grade tumors show large cystic spaces lined by epidermoid and mucous-secreting cells as well as transitional forms. High–grade tumors are generally solid and consist predominantly of squamoid and intermediate cells (Fig. 3.9A). Aspirates show sheets of neoplastic squamous cells and clusters of acinar cells (Fig. 3.9B).

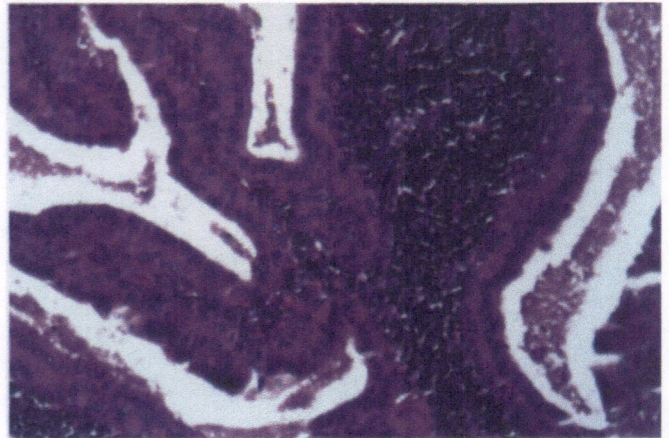

A

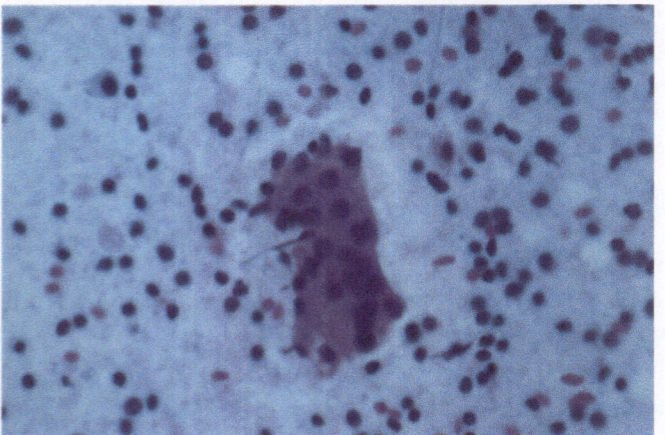

B

FIGURE 3.6 Warthin's tumor. A: Irregular cystlike spaces lined by papillary structures covered with a single layer of columnar oncocytes. B: FNA smear showing sheets or strips of oncocytes and scattered lymphocytes.

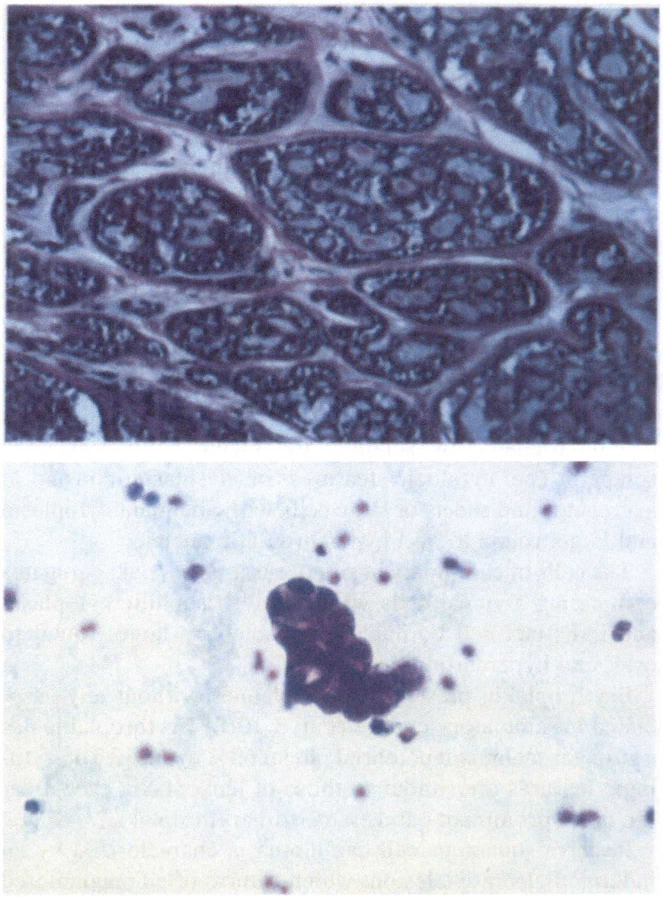

FIGURE 3.7 **Adenoid cystic carcinoma. A**: Islands of neoplastic cells arranged in a cribriform pattern. **B**: FNA smear showing cluster of neoplastic cells.

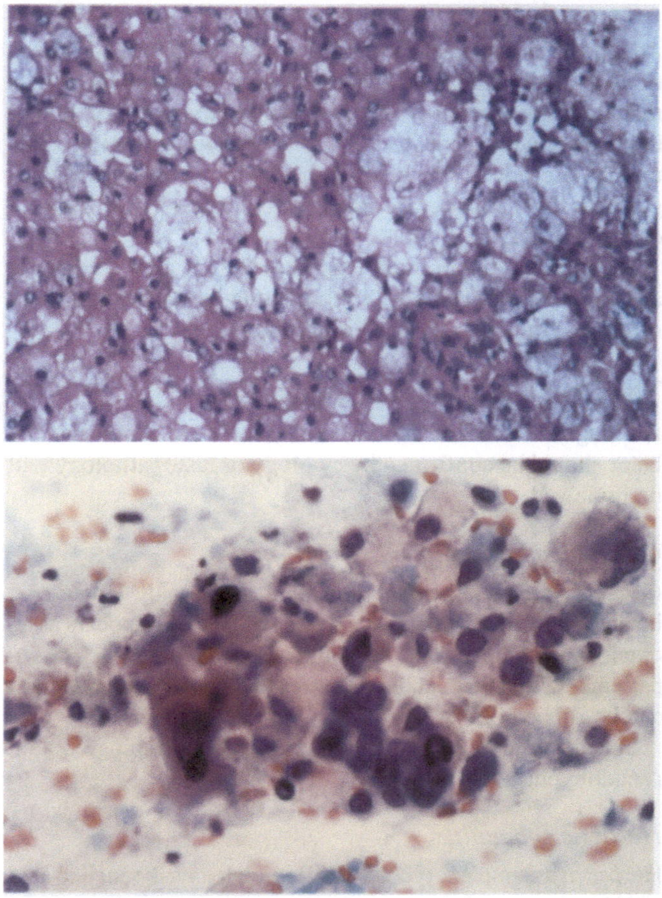

FIGURE 3.9 **Mucoepidermoid carcinoma. A**: Sheets of epidermoid and mucous-secreting cells as well as transitional forms. **B**: FNA smear showing atypical squamous cells and acinar cell clusters.

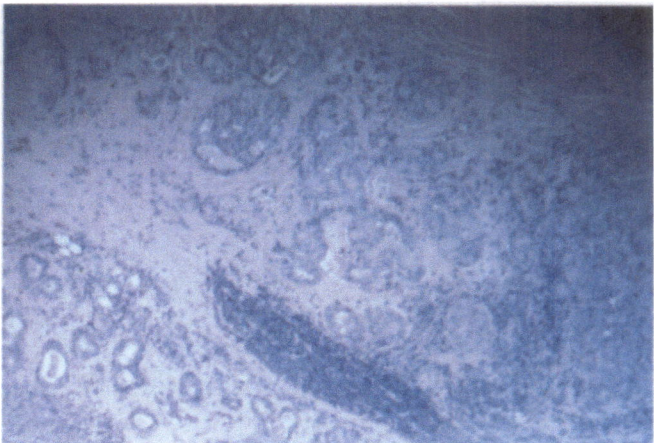

FIGURE 3.8 **Acinic cell carcinoma.** Nests and acini of polygonal cells.

Adenocarcinoma

Adenocarcinoma consists of tubules or papillary gland formations of malignant cells. The cells are pleomorphic, with a moderate amount of cytoplasm, and have pleomorphic and hyperchromatic eccentric nuclei. Mucous-secreting cells may be present in adenocarcinoma, which should be distinguished from mucoepidermoid carcinoma on the basis of overall architecture.

Squamous cell carcinoma and undifferentiated carcinoma are rare in salivary glands. Their histologic and cytologic features are similar to those of other organs.

The Oral Cavity and Nasopharynx

Although there are many oral cavity diseases, those that can be or should be confirmed by cytology or histopathology will be reviewed.

Candidiasis (Maniliasis, Thrush)

Candida species, a normal inhabitant, is the only fungus that involves the mouth with any frequency. It usually appears as an opportunistic infection in debilitated or immunosuppressed patients. Clinically, candidiasis presents as a white patch that can be rubbed off.

Smears prepared from a white patch by scraping contain pseudohyphae or yeast forms, or both.

Herpetic Stomatitis

Herpesvirus simplex, types I and II, and deoxyribonucleic acid (DNA) viruses infect the oral mucosa, with type I being far more prevalent. Primary infection is uncommon. The vesicles typically develop on the gingiva, lips, palate, and tongue. Recurrent or secondary herpes simplex is quite common.

Cytologic preparations are made by scraping a deroofed vesicle, the Tzanck test. The smears show multinucleated giant cells with intranuclear inclusions, similar to those occurring in other organs.

Premalignant and Malignant Lesions

Oral cancer accounts for about 5% of all malignancies and usually occurs in men over 50 years of age who smoke or use smokeless tobacco. Almost all oral cancers are squamous cell carcinomas. Next in frequency are adenocarcinomas of the minor salivary glands. The evolution of oral squamous cell carcinoma is similar to that of squamous cell carcinomas in other organs.

The precancerous changes of oral squamous cell carcinoma present in two distinct forms: leukoplakia and erythroplakia. Leukoplakia presents as flat, white plaques that fail to rub away and that are not associated with an identifiable cause (Fig. 3.10A). Twenty percent of examples of oral leukoplakia exhibit cytologic atypia, ranging from dysplasia to carcinoma in situ and superficial squamous cell carcinoma.[1-3]

The cytologic and histologic features of oral precancerous changes are similar to those of the uterine cervix, and smears can be prepared by scraping the plaque with a wooden scraper. The cytologic features of dysplasia consist of aggregates and sheets of large cells with abundant cytoplasm and large, round to oval hyperchromatic nuclei.

The cells of carcinoma in situ occur as syncytial aggregates comprising atypical cells with faintly basophilic cytoplasm and indistinct cell borders. The nuclei are large, round to oval, and hyperchromatic.

Erythroplakia presents as red plaques without any associated inflammatory change (Fig. 3.10B). Erythroplakia has a stronger malignant potential, about 60% to 90%.[3] The cytologic features are similar to those of leukoplakia except for the more prominent parakeratosis in erythroplakia.

Invasive squamous cell carcinoma is characterized by an indurated ulcerative lesion, which is most often encountered on the lateral border of the tongue and floor of the mouth (Fig. 3.11A). Since it metastasizes primarily through lymphatics, palpable cervical lymph nodes may present when the oral lesion is first discovered.

Smears prepared by scraping the ulcerated area show large, pleomorphic atypical squamous cells arranged either in aggregates or singly. The cells have lightly cyanophilic or eosinophilic cytoplasm and pleomorphic, large, hyperchromatic nuclei with coarse chromatin (Fig. 3.11B).

Histologically, invasive squamous cell carcinoma consists of atypical squamous cell sheets or nests that infiltrate the submucosa (Fig. 3.11C).

(*Discussion continued on p. 36*)

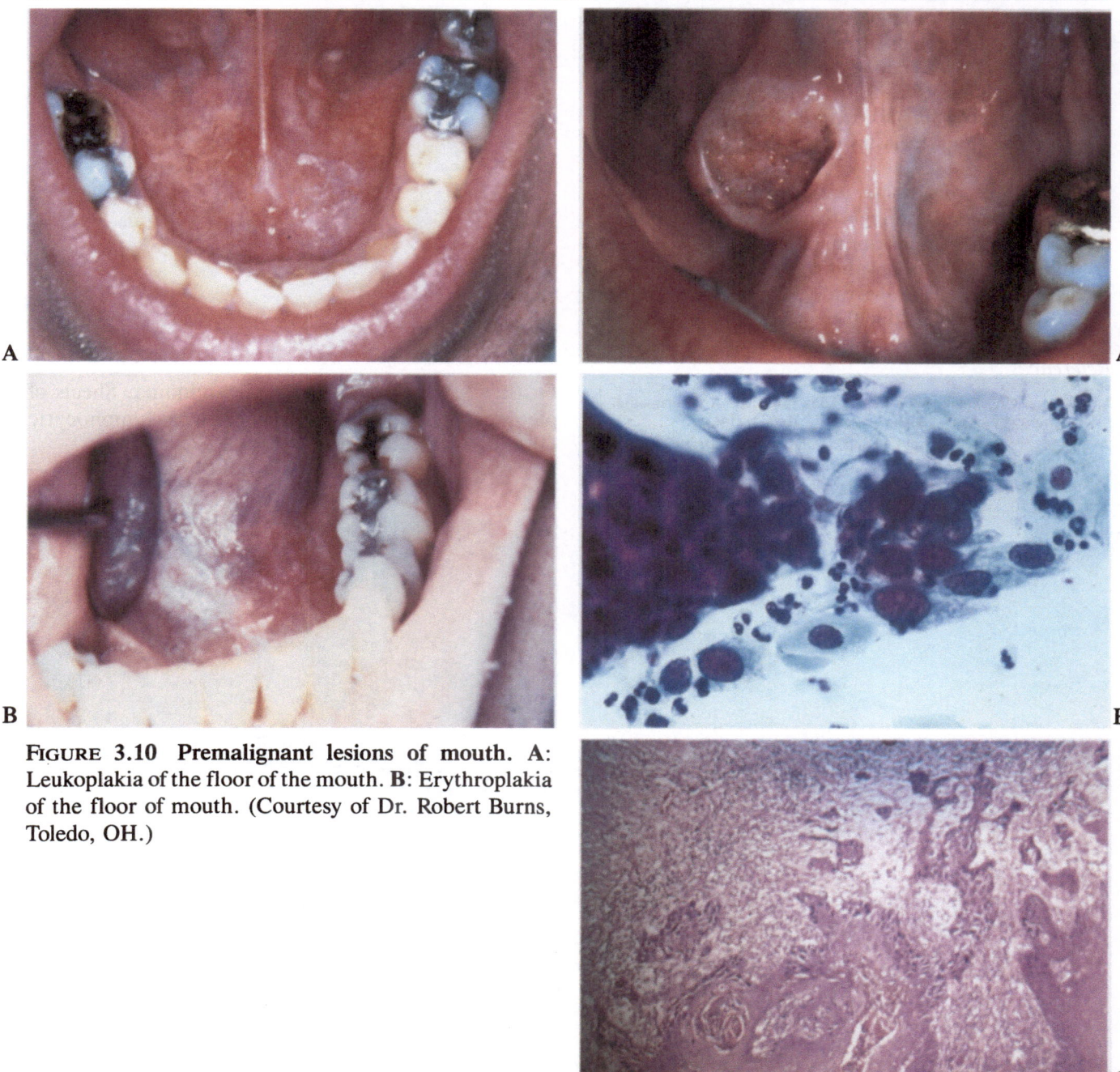

FIGURE 3.10 Premalignant lesions of mouth. A: Leukoplakia of the floor of the mouth. B: Erythroplakia of the floor of mouth. (Courtesy of Dr. Robert Burns, Toledo, OH.)

FIGURE 3.11 Squamous cell carcinoma of the floor of the mouth. A: Ulcerated mass in the right side of the floor of the mouth. (Courtesy of Dr. Robert Burns, Toledo, OH.) B: Smear prepared by scraping the lesion, thus showing pleomorphic carcinoma cells arranged in syncytial aggregates. C: Squamous cell carcinoma. The neoplasm infiltrates the submucosa in cords and sheets.

Nasopharyngeal carcinomas are squamous cell carcinomas. Those that comprise squamous cell carcinoma mixed with an abundant infiltrate of lymphoid cells are designated lymphoepithelioma (Fig. 3.12). These neoplasms may be closely associated with infection with the Epstein-Barr virus. They are common neoplasms in southern China. Many are radiosensitive.

Olfactory neuroblastoma (esthesioneuroblastoma) is a neoplasm of neural crest origin that arises from the olfactory mucosa covering the superior third of the nasal septum and cribriform plate. The neoplasms consist of small round cells arranged haphazardly in sheets (Fig. 3.13). The neoplasm is highly sensitive to radiation therapy.

References

1. Walderon CA, Shafer WG. Leukoplakia revisited. A clinicopathologic study of 3256 oral leukoplakias. *Cancer.* 1975;36:1386.
2. Silverman S Jr, et al. Oral leukoplakia and malignant transformation. A followup study of 257 patients. *Cancer.* 1984;53:565.
3. Shafer WG, Walderon CA. Erythroplakia of the oral cavity. *Cancer.* 1975;36:1021.

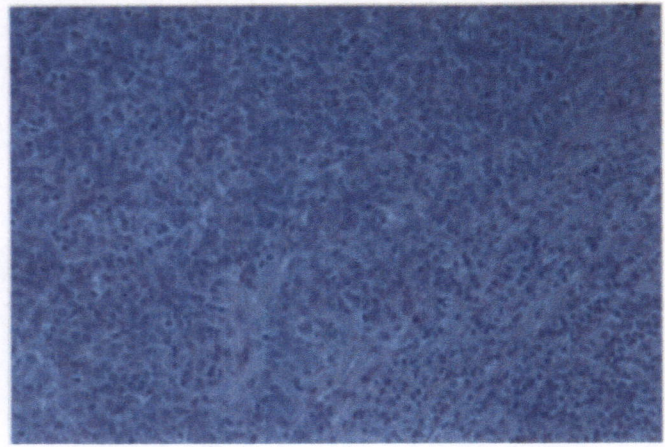

FIGURE 3.12 **Nasopharyngeal carcinoma.** Sheets of pleomorphic squamous cells with a lymphocytic infiltrate.

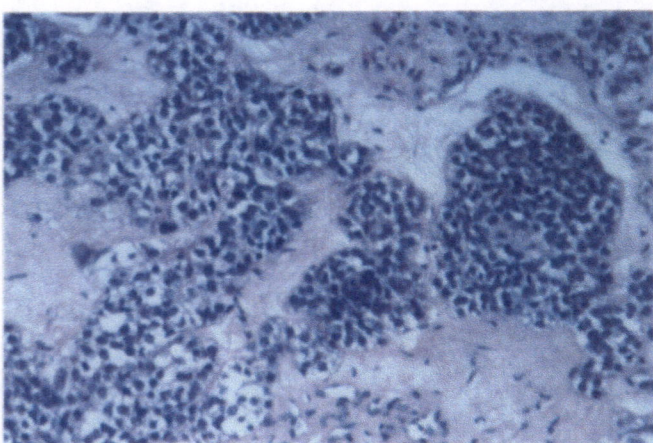

FIGURE 3.13 **Olfactory neuroblastoma.** Small round cells arranged in sheets.

4

Thyroid and Parathyroid Glands

Thyroid Gland

Enlargement of the thyroid gland (goiter) is a common clinical problem, with most goiters being of nodular pattern type. Radionuclide or ultrasound imaging of the thyroid are sufficiently accurate to eliminate the need for surgical exploration in most cases. Since the mid-1970s, fine needle aspiration (FNA) has become a highly cost-effective diagnostic test for thyroid nodules.[1] Solitary nonfunctioning "cold" nodules raise a high suspicion of cancer.

The following non-neoplastic lesions of the thyroid gland will be considered with reference to their frequency and their clinical presentation, which may simulate neoplasm.

Hashimoto's Thyroiditis

Hashimoto's thyroiditis is the most common type of inflammatory thyroid disease. It is characterized by symmetrical lobular enlargement of the gland. It is predominantly a disease of women, with a female:male ratio of 10:1. Most cases occur between the ages of 30 and 50 years. Hashimoto's thyroiditis has an autoimmune origin. A variety of auto-antibodies (thyrotropinreceptor antibodies and thyroid microsomal antibodies) against thyroid-cell antigens can be identified in almost all patients with this condition.

Clinically, this condition presents as a symmetrically enlarged firm thyroid with slight to marked hypothyroidism. As hypothyroidism becomes more established, the radioactive iodine uptake (RAIU), and thyroxine T_4 and triiodo thyronine T_3 levels decline.

Cytology

Fine needle aspiration biopsy is recommended to establish diagnosis. Aspiration samples should be taken from both lobes to exclude coexisting lymphoma.

Fine needle aspiration smears contain small and large activated lymphocytes, plasma cells, and clusters of follicular cells sharing oxyphilic change (oncocytes). Oncocytes are round to polygonal and have abundant, finely granular, eosinophilic cytoplasm and large round nuclei (Fig. 4.1A).

Histology

The gland is replaced by dense infiltrates of small and large lymphocytes containing germinal centers. Many thyroid follicles are distorted, with their epithelium showing oxyphilic change (Fig. 4.1B,C).

Hyperthyroidism (Graves' or Basedow's Diseases)

Hyperthyroidism is usually diagnosed by clinical and laboratory findings. Even though the diagnosis of this disease is not made on cytologic specimens, we include for comparison a brief description of its histologic appearance. The untreated hyperactive thyroid gland shows diffuse hyperplasia of thyroid follicles. They are lined by tall columnar cells and papillary projections. Colloid is usually scanty (Fig. 4.2).

Diffuse and Nodular Goiter

Diffuse and multinodular goiter have a common origin. The multinodular variant is a later development from the diffuse lesion because of repeated cycles of hyperplasia and involution creating nodules of varying size. The intermittent or persistent hyperplasia or diffuse multinodular goiters is a response to thyroid-stimulating hormone or thyroid growth immunoglobulin, whose production is stimulated by hypothyroxinemia related to iodine deficiency, environmental goitrogens, or unknown factors. Solitary nodular goiter is the most common benign condition mistaken for a thyroid tumor. Goiters come to clinical attention because of progressive enlargement of the thyroid. Occasionally, the thyromegaly may extend downward substernally and compress the trachea, esophagus, or superior vena cava (Fig. 4.3).

Most of the patients are euthyroid. It is of major importance to distinguish a solitary nodular goiter from a neoplasm. Ultrasonography and computed tomography (CT) scans can be of great help in this. Fine needle aspiration smears contain small follicular cells, isolated and in loose aggregates, in a background of colloid (Fig. 4.4A,B). Histologically, the thyroid follicles are dilated, filled with colloid, and lined by flat follicular cells (Fig. 4.4C). There may be focal or diffuse hyperplastic follicles (Fig. 4.4D).

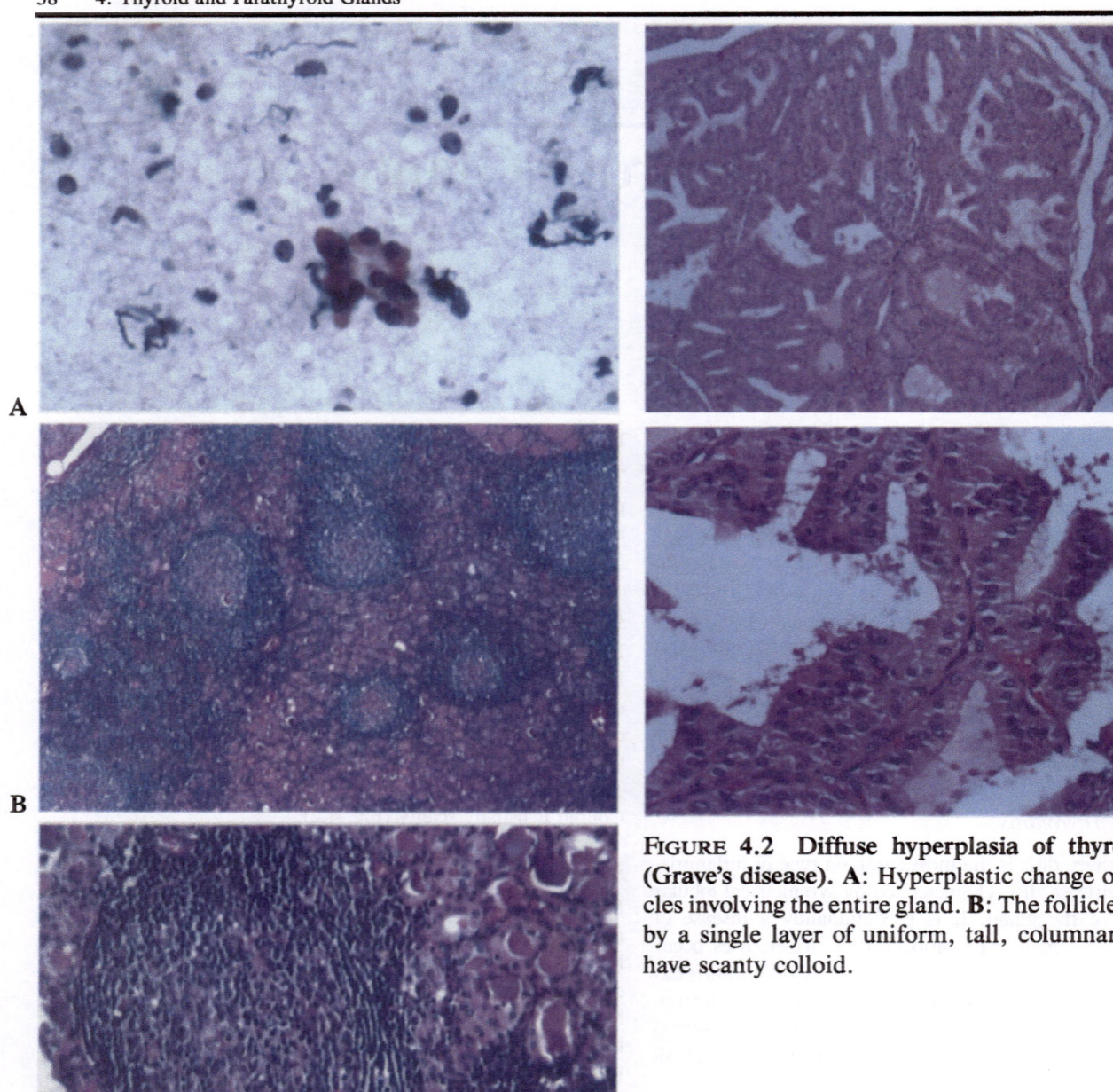

A

B

C

A

B

FIGURE 4.2 Diffuse hyperplasia of thyroid gland (Grave's disease). A: Hyperplastic change of the follicles involving the entire gland. **B**: The follicles are lined by a single layer of uniform, tall, columnar cells and have scanty colloid.

FIGURE 4.1 Hashimoto's thyroiditis. A: FNA smear showing aggregates of follicular cells with oxyphilic change, and scattered lymphocytes. **B**: Histologic section of the same case showing dense lymphocytic infiltration with lymphoid follicles. **B,C**: Distorted small follicles with oxyphilic change.

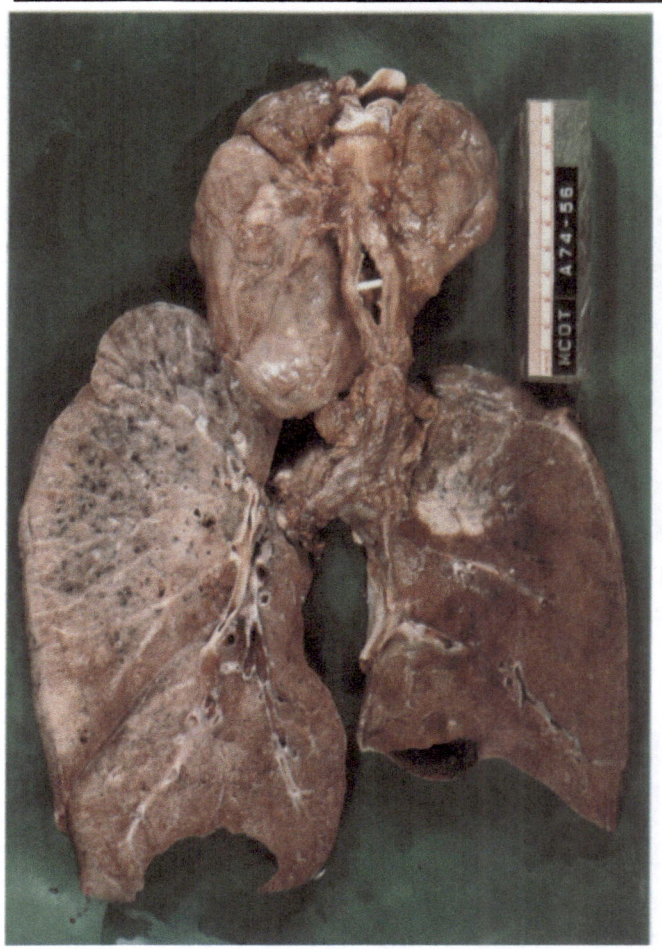

FIGURE 4.3 Substernal goiter. Goiter grows behind the sternum (necropsy).

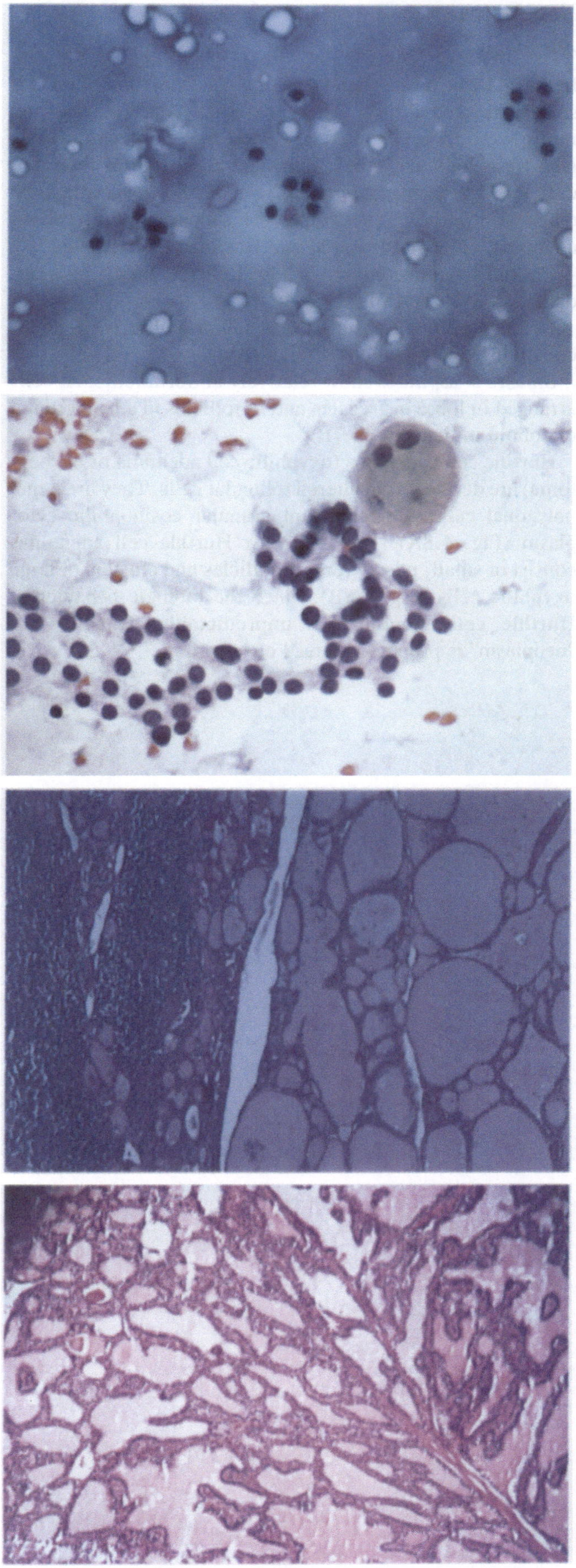

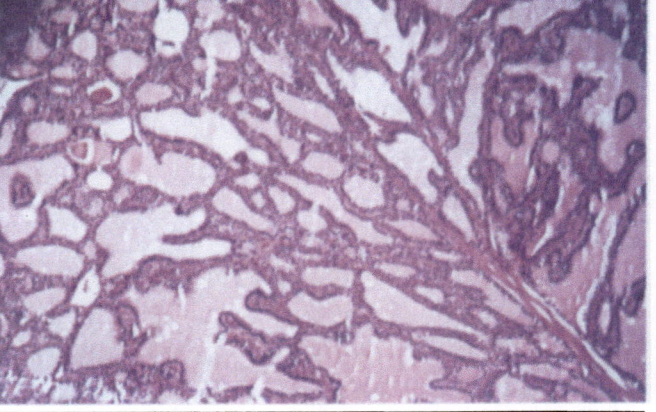

FIGURE 4.4 Nontoxic goiter. A: Colloid goiter. Aggregates of small follicle cells in colloid background (FNA). **B**: Hyperplastic nodular goiter. Sheets of follicular cells and histiocytes (FNA). **C**: Colloid goiter. Dilated follicles containing abundant colloid and compressed follicular cells (histology). **D**: Hyperplastic nodular goiter. Small and large follicles in active proliferation and scanty colloid (histology).

Neoplasms

Adenomas

In nonendemic areas, adenoma is the most common cause of a solitary thyroid nodule. They are usually encapsulated and rarely exceed 4 cm in diameter (Fig. 4.5). Adenomas are derived from follicular epithelium, and almost all of them are designated follicular adenomas. For simple cytopathologic diagnostic purposes, adenomas are subclassified as colloid adenoma, cellular adenoma, and Hurthle cell adenoma.

Colloid adenomas consist of large follicles containing abundant colloid (Fig. 4.6).

Cellular adenomas consist of small and abortive follicles containing scanty colloid (Fig. 4.7A).

Smears of aspirates show relatively uniform follicular cells arranged in loose aggregates and in follicles in a background of colloid milieu (Fig. 4.7B).

Hurthle cell adenomas (oxyphilic cell adenoma or oncocytoma) are derived from altered follicular cells. They are large, polygonal cells with abundant granular eosinophilic cytoplasm (Fig. 4.8A). Histologically, Hurthle cell adenomas consist of small, poorly formed follicles and clusters of large oxyphilic cells (Fig. 4.8B). Since the biologic behavior of Hurthle cell adenomas is unpredictable, Hurthle cell "neoplasm" is proposed instead of "adenoma."

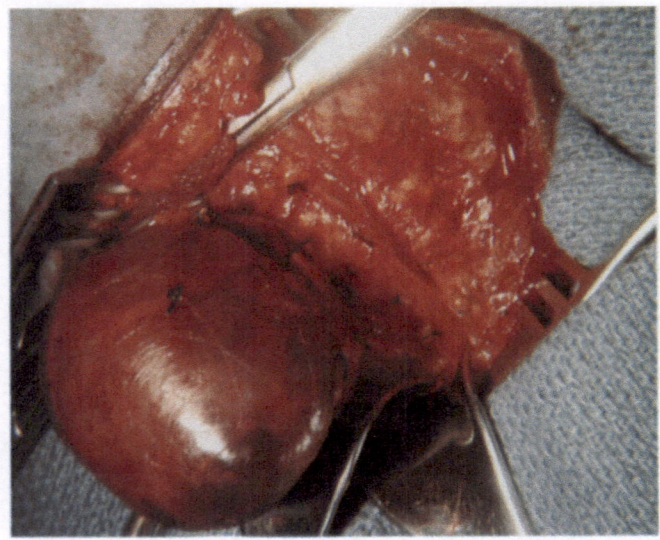

FIGURE 4.5   Follicular adenoma of thyroid. Nodular encapsulated mass (gross).

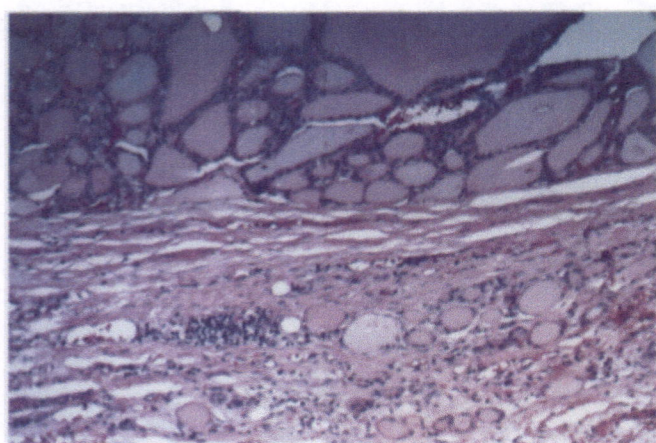

FIGURE 4.6   Colloid adenoma. Small and large follicles with active follicle cells and abundant colloid, and normal follicles outside the capsule in the lower portion.

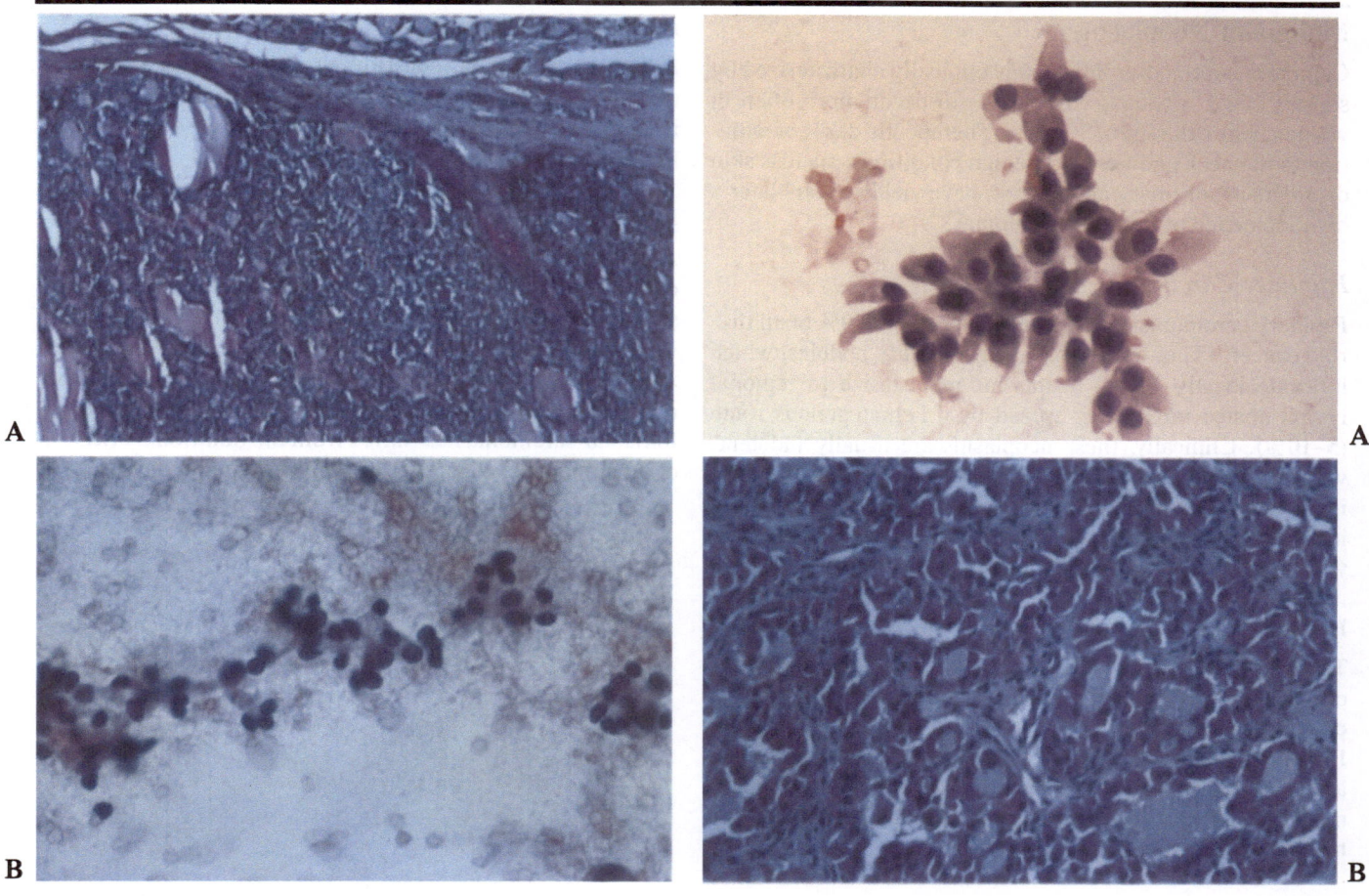

FIGURE 4.7 **Cellular adenoma. A**: Encapsulated nodule with compact hyperplastic follicles (histology). **B**: FNA smear from the same tumor showing aggreates of follicle cells with follicular arrangement in some.

FIGURE 4.8 **Hurthle cell "neoplasm." A**: Aggregates of large polygonal cells with abundant eosinophilic cytoplasm (FNA). **B**: Histologic section from the same tumor showing poorly formed follicles and clusters of oxyphilic cells.

Malignant Neoplasms

Carcinoma of the thyroid gland is clinically characterized by solitary "cold" nodule, which tends to occur more often in women before the age of 30 years. Therapeutic doses of radiation to the neck and head for benign conditions, such as skin disorders or tonsillar enlargement, have yielded years later a high incidence of thyroid carcinomas.[2]

Papillary Carcinoma

Papillary carcinomas constitute about 60% to 70% of all thyroid cancers. They are almost always solitary nodules, which infiltrate locally. These neoplasms metastasize to regional lymph nodes; rarely they spread by a hematogenous route (5–10%). Clinically, these neoplasms are usually indolent, with a 70% to 85% overall 10-year survival rate. Surprisingly, cervical lymph node metastasis does not significantly influence the prognosis. Favorable prognostic features are young age, small tumor size, and encapsulation.

Histology

The neoplasms consist of papillary structures, irregular follicles, or both. The papillae are covered by a single layer of cuboidal cells and have central delicate fibrovascular stalk. Psammoma bodies are seen in half of the cases. These nuclei are vesicular because of peripheral distribution of chromatin or intranuclear cytoplasmic invagination, a characteristic microscopic feature (Fig. 4.9A).

Cytology

In smears, the cells occur singly, in papillary clusters, or sheets. The cells are cuboidal or polygonal, with variable amounts of pale cytoplasm. The nuclei are round to oval with finely granular, powdery chromatin. Micronucleoli are frequently observed. Intranuclear cytoplasmic inclusions resulting from invagination of cytoplasm are often observed (Fig. 4.9B,C).

Follicular Carcinoma

Follicular carcinoma, constituting about 20% of all thyroid cancers, presents as solitary nodules up to a few centimeters in diameter, usually extending to the capsule or into extrathyroid tissue.

Histology

Although to the naked eye these neoplasms appear well circumscribed, microscopically they usually infiltrate the capsule (Fig. 4.10A). These neoplasms exhibit great histologic variation. The cells can be arranged in small follicles containing colloid, in trabecular cords, or solid sheets. The emphasis in the histologic distinction between papillary carcinoma and follicular carcinoma has shifted from the traditional criterion of predominance of papillae in papillary carcinoma to a set of

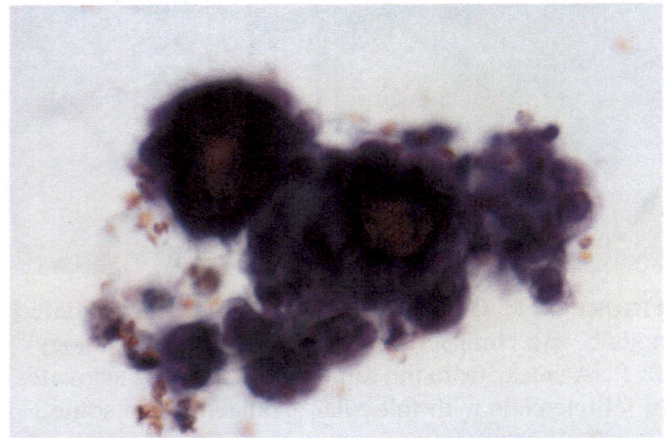

B

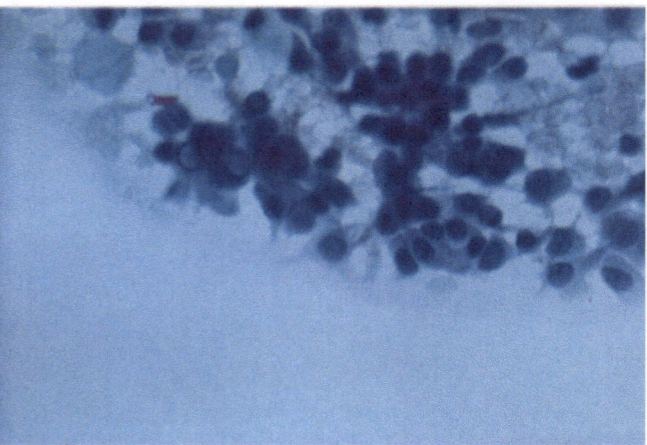

C

FIGURE 4.9 **Papillary carcinoma of thyroid. A**: Poorly formed follicles and papillary structures supported by delicate fibrovascular core. Papillae are surrounded by single layer of cuboidal cells with vesicular nuclei. Note psammoma body in the right portion (histology). **B**: Papillary clusters with psammoma bodies (FNA). **C**: Sheets of round to cuboidal cells with intranuclear inclusions "Orphan Annie eye" (FNA).

A

cytologic parameters, notably the presence of overlapping nuclei with a "ground-glass" quality to their chromatin. When ground-glass nuclei or even sparsely distributed papillae are present, the lesion is papillary carcinoma.[3]

Cytology

Aspirates of follicular carcinomas exhibit a spectrum of cytologic changes depending on the degree of differentiation. In differentiated follicular carcinomas, the cells occur as loose aggregates with a rosettelike pattern. They are relatively uniform and moderately enlarged, with hyperchromatic round nuclei (Fig. 4.10B). In poorly differentiated follicular carcinomas, the cells occur in a syncytium with overlapping of nuclei and they are pleomorphic, with a scanty to slight amount of pale, granular cytoplasm. Most nuclei are irregular in shape, with irregular contours and prominent nucleoli (Fig. 4.11).

Immunocytochemical study may be of help in differential diagnosis of poorly differentiated carcinomas. Most thyroid follicular carcinomas are strongly positive for thyroglobulin.

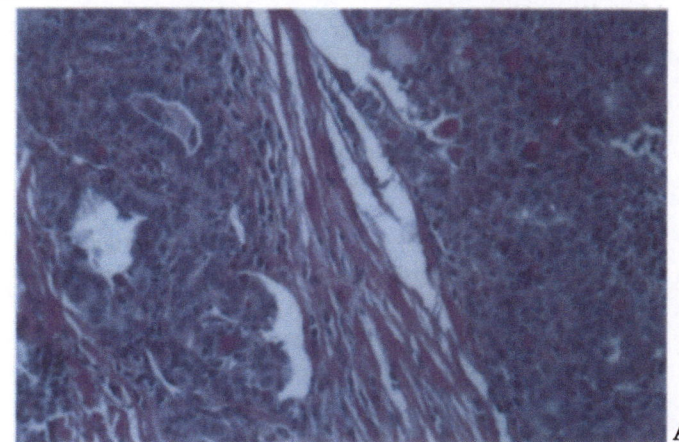

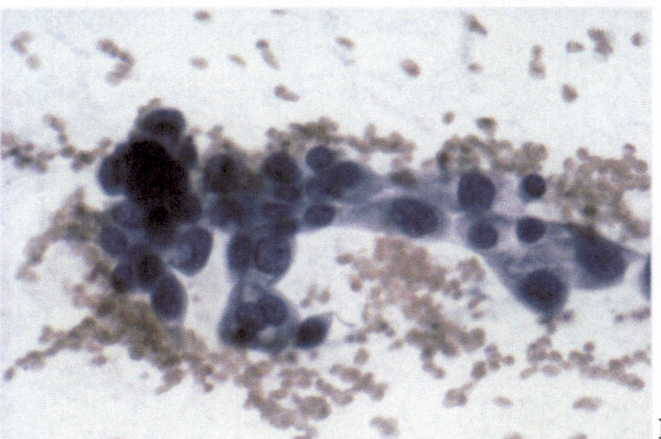

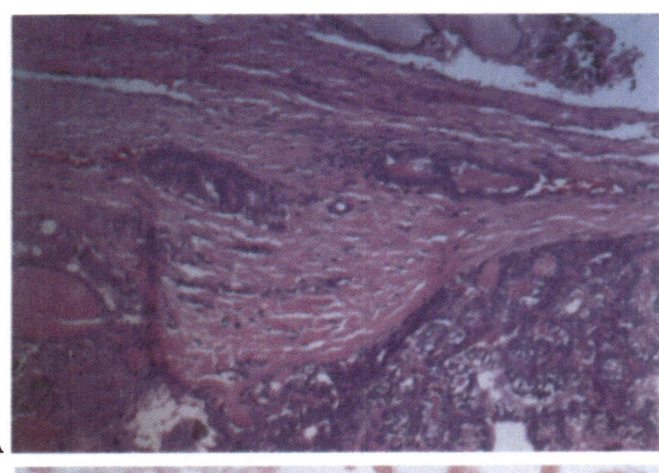

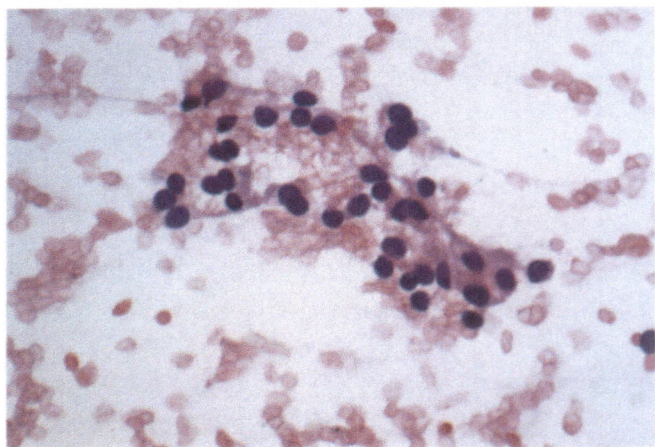

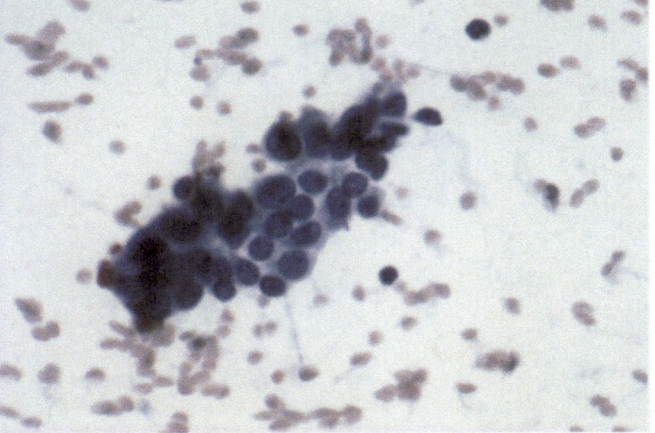

FIGURE **4.11 Poorly differentiated follicular carcinoma. A**: Sheets and poorly formed follicles with scanty colloid (histology). **B, C**: FNA smear showing syncytial aggregates and clusters of enlarged follicle cells.

FIGURE **4.10 Follicular carcinoma of thyroid. A**: Compactly arranged follicles with capsular invasion (histology). **B**: FNA smear showing enlarged follicular cells arranged in follicles.

Medullary Carcinoma

Medullary carcinoma is less common than other types of carcinoma of the thyroid. These tumors belong to the group of endocrine neoplasms producing polypeptide hormones and amines characterized by the presence of cytoplasmic neurosecretory granules.[4] The neoplasm arises from the parafollicular cells (C cells) producing calcitonin. About 10% of these neoplasms occur in familial syndromes having autosomal dominant transmission; the remainder arise sporadically. The overall 10-year survival of patients with sporadic disease is 40%, compared with 70% in patients with familial syndromes.

The sporadic tumors tend to be large, solitary, and well circumscribed (Fig. 4.12A). The neoplasms occurring in familial syndromes tend to involve both lobes multifocally.

Histologically, medullary carcinoma comprises nests and sheets of polygonal to spindle-shaped cells embedded in fibrovascular stroma, which has deposits of amyloid (Fig. 4.12B).

Using anticalcitonin antibodies, immunocytochemistry may demonstrate calcitonin in the tumor cells (Fig. 4.12C). Electron microscopy reveals membrane-delineated dense core of neurosecretory granules (Fig. 4.12D).

Aspirates show the tumor cells in loose aggregates and singly. The cells are round, oval, or spindle-shaped, and frequently multinucleated. Their nuclei are hyperchromatic and have evenly distributed, finely granular chromatin. Nucleoli are not conspicuous (Fig. 4-12E,F).

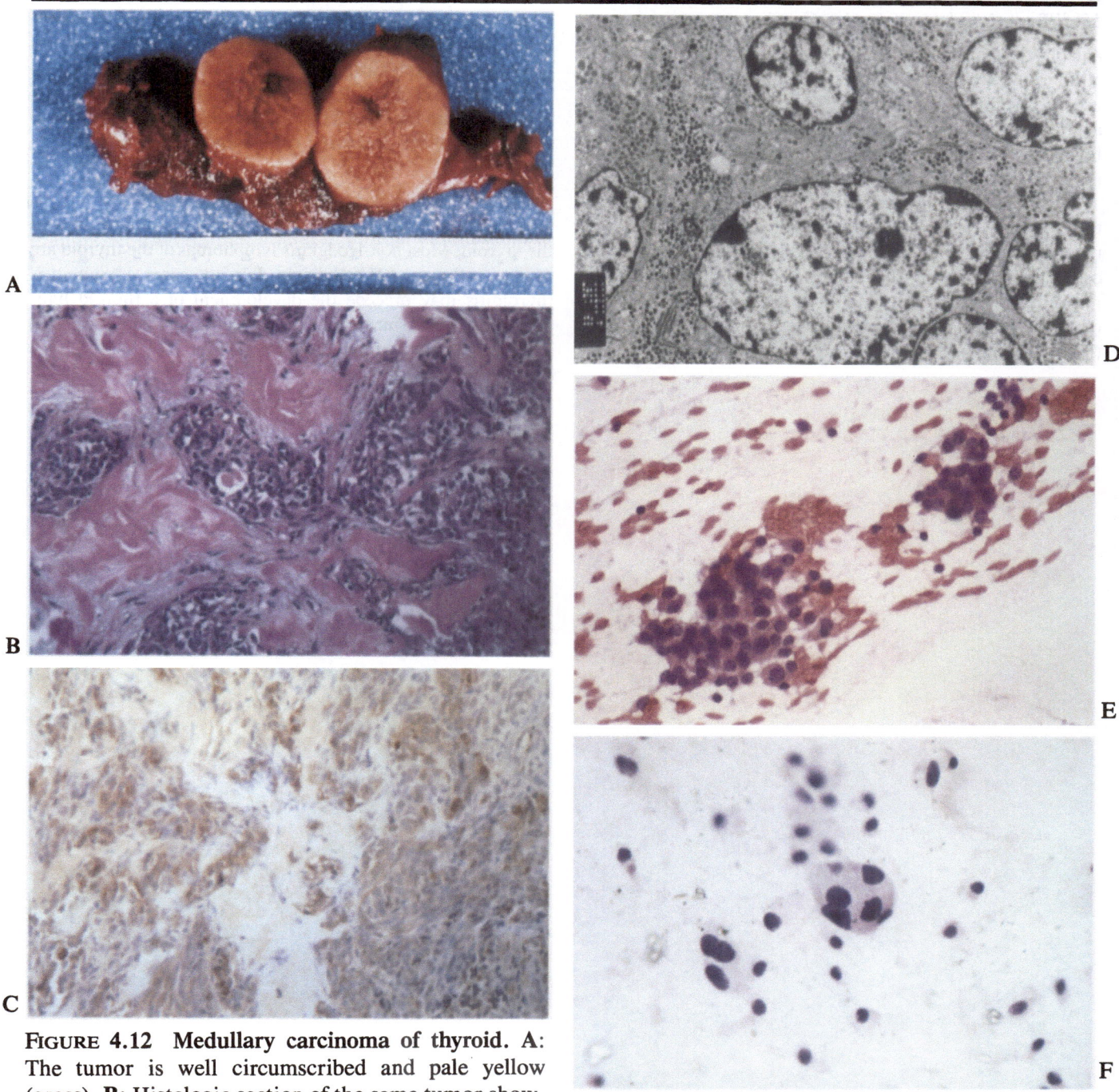

FIGURE 4.12 Medullary carcinoma of thyroid. A: The tumor is well circumscribed and pale yellow (gross). **B:** Histologic section of the same tumor showing nests of cells separated by amyloid stroma. **C:** Positive calcitonin granules in the tumor cells by immunoperoxidase stain. **D:** Dense-core neurosecretory granules in the tumor cells (EM). **E, F:** Medullary carcinoma of thyroid (FNA). The cells are variable in their arrangement and their shape. They occur in loose aggregates and clusters.

Undifferentiated (Anaplastic) Carcinomas

Anaplastic carcinomas of the thyroid compose 5% to 15% of all thyroid carcinomas. They are found in older individuals, usually over 60 years of age. The neoplasm is extremely aggressive, with almost 100% metastasis within months or a few years. This neoplasm usually presents as a rapidly growing, painful thyroid nodule and pressure symptoms.[5,6]

At the time of diagnosis, both lobes of the thyroid and the adjacent tissues are usually involved. Histologically, the neoplasms are most poorly differentiated and indiscriminately infiltrate the adjacent tissues. The cells are markedly pleomorphic, with their size ranging from that of giant cells to small anaplastic carcinomas of other organs (Fig. 4.13A).

In aspirate smears, the cells occur singly or in loose aggregates. The cells of the giant cell type are large, variable in shape, and multinucleated (Fig. 4.13B).

The small cell undifferentiated carcinomas are pleomorphic with hyperchromatic nuclei and are similar in many respects to those of small cell anaplastic carcinoma of other organs.

Lymphoma

Both Hodgkin's and non-Hodgkin's lymphomas may involve the thyroid. Most non-Hodgkin's lymphomas of the thyroid are of large cell type of B-cell origin. In some cases, Hashimoto's thyroiditis may precede the development of a thyroid lymphoma.[7] In FNA smears, the cells occur singly and have large nuclei with prominent macronucleoli (Fig. 4.14).

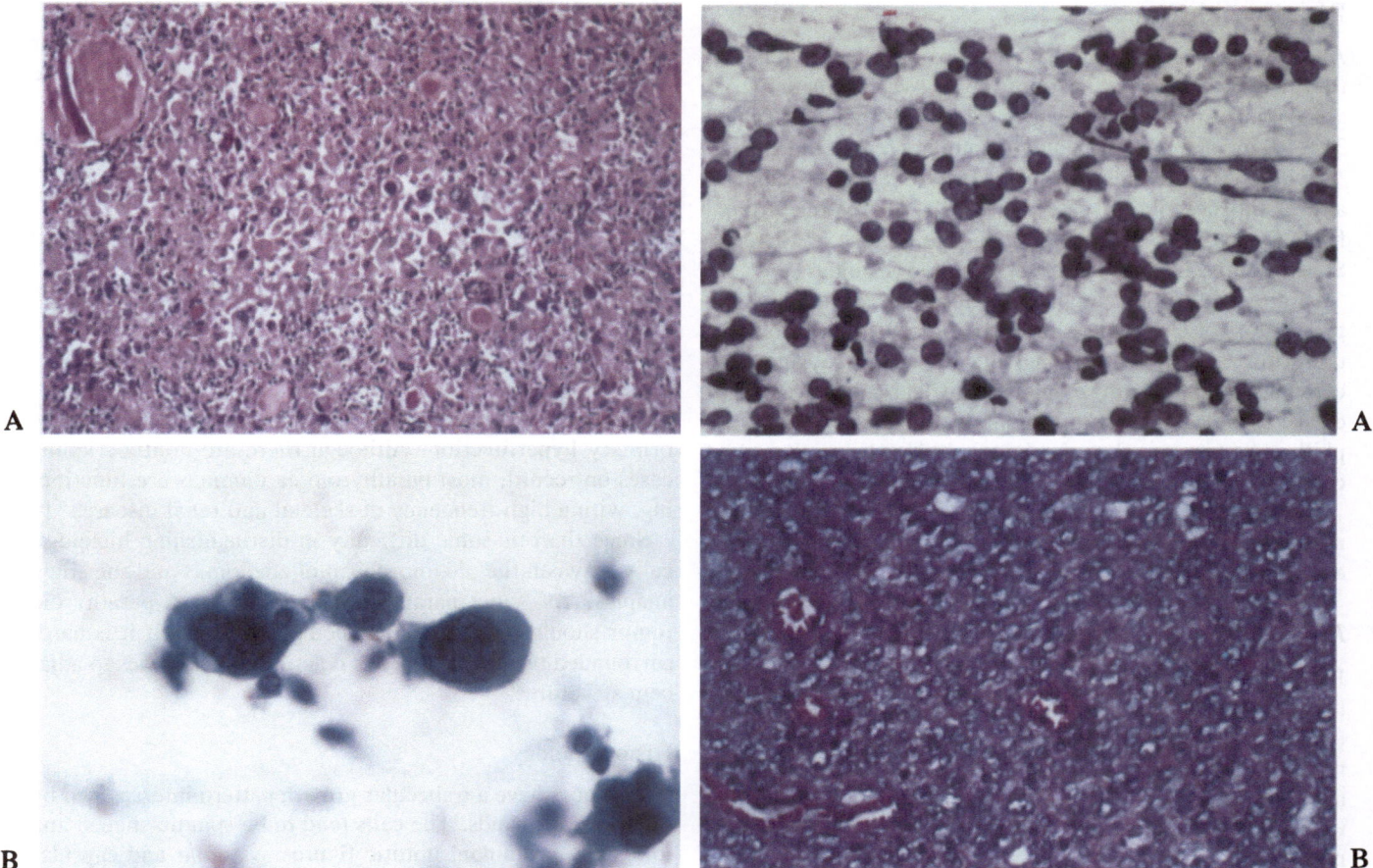

FIGURE 4.13   Undifferentiated carcinoma of thyroid. A: Sheets of large giant cells replace the thyroid entirely (histology). **B**: FNA smear from the tumor showing large pleomorphic cells in loose aggregates.

FIGURE 4.14   Large cell lymphoma of thyroid. A: The cells occur singly and have large nuclei with nucleoli (FNA smear). **B**: Histologic section from the tumor.

Parathyroid Glands

About 90% of individuals have four parathyroid glands, but they may be as many as six or as few as two. The parathyroid gland is an oval, yellow-brown, encapsulated nodule, weighing 35 to 40 mg and measuring up to 4 mm in greatest dimension.

In infancy and childhood, the parathyroid glands comprise almost entirely solid sheets of chief cells. Thereafter, stromal fat increases up to 30% of the glands at the age of 25 years. Subsequently, the amount of fat is quite variable.

Parathyroid glands comprise mainly chief cells, which are progenitors of clear cells and oxyphilic cells. Chief cells are uniformly round to polygonal and have pale eosinophilic cytoplasm and uniform round nuclei. Clear cells have "water clear" cytoplasm because of large glycogen content. Oxyphilic cells occur singly or in clusters and are larger than chief cells. They have a bright eosinophilic granular cytoplasm.

The parathyroid glands produce a peptide hormone that regulates and maintains normal levels of ionized calcium in extracellular fluid.

Primary Hyperparathyroidism

Primary hyperparathyroidism results from disorders intrinsic to the glands, causing hypersecretion of parathyroid hormone (PTH) with hypercalcemia and hypophosphatemia. The major biochemical features of primary hyperparathyroidism are elevated PTH serum level, hypercalcemia, hypophosphatemia, and excessive urinary secretion of calcium. Neuromuscular weakness and fatigue are early symptoms.

In advanced and severe cases, increased mobilization of skeletal calcium followed by bone resorption and remodeling may give rise to osteitis fibrosa cystica, which is diagnostic of hyperparathyroidism. Other causes of hypercalcemia are nonparathyroid malignancy, vitamin D excess, hyperthyroidism, milk-alkali syndrome, immobilization, idiopathic origin, and sarcoidosis.

The most common cause of primary hyperparathyroidism is parathyroid adenoma (80%), followed by primary parathyroid hyperplasia (15%) and parathyroid carcinomas (3%).[8]

Adenoma

Parathyroid adenomas can occur at any age, but most occur in the fourth decade of life. They average 0.5 to 5 g in weight and rarely are as large as 20 g. They are well encapsulated, yellow to tan, soft lesions.

Histologically, the tumors consist of a single cell type or mixed cell population in sheets with focal glandular areas. Clear cells or oxyphilic cells may be present in scattered patterns or in aggregates (Fig. 4.15A). Sometimes there may be a part of a normal, non-neoplastic, parathyroid gland outside the capsule. In parathyroid exploration, other parathyroid glands in individuals with single adenomas are normal or atrophic.

Smears of aspirates or imprints show slightly enlarged chief, clear, or oxyphilic cells in loose aggregates or follicles. The cells are uniformly round and have pale, eosinophilic, clear or dense eosinophilic cytoplasm and round, uniform, bland nuclei (Fig. 4.15B). Imprint cytology is valuable in distinguishing parathyroid glands from lymph nodes during parathyroid exploration.

Carcinoma

Carcinoma of the parathyroid glands is rare. It may cause primary hyperfunction. Although there are nonfunctioning cases on record, most parathyroid carcinomas are functioning, with a high frequency of skeletal and renal diseases.[9,10]

Since there is some difficulty in distinguishing histologically between the pleomorphism of adenomas and the slight anaplasia of some parathyroid carcinomas, a parathyroid tumor should be suspected of being carcinoma if it is hard, surrounded by a dense fibrous reaction, and adheres to adjacent structures.

Histopathology

The tumors have a trabecular growth pattern interspersed by thick fibrous bands. The cells tend to be spindle-shaped and to display prominent mitotic figures. Vascular and capsular invasion may be observed. These carcinomas may metastasize to regional lymph nodes but rarely to distant organs. Long-term survival is the rule, and death results more often from the complications of hyperparathyroidism than from spread of the carcinoma.

Primary Hyperplasia

Primary hyperplasia of the parathyroid glands is diffuse enlargement of all four parathyroid glands (Fig. 4.16A). The cause of the primary hyperplasia is unknown.

Histopathology

There are two types of hyperplasia, with the more common chief cell type and less common clear cell type. The chief cells are arranged in cords and sheets and rarely glandular patterns. Chief cell hyperplasia may comprise a mixture of groups of chief cells, oxyphilic cells, and transitional cells. The parenchyme adjacent to hyperplasia shows hyperplasia (Fig. 4.16B).

Clear cell hyperplasia tends to be larger than the chief cell type.

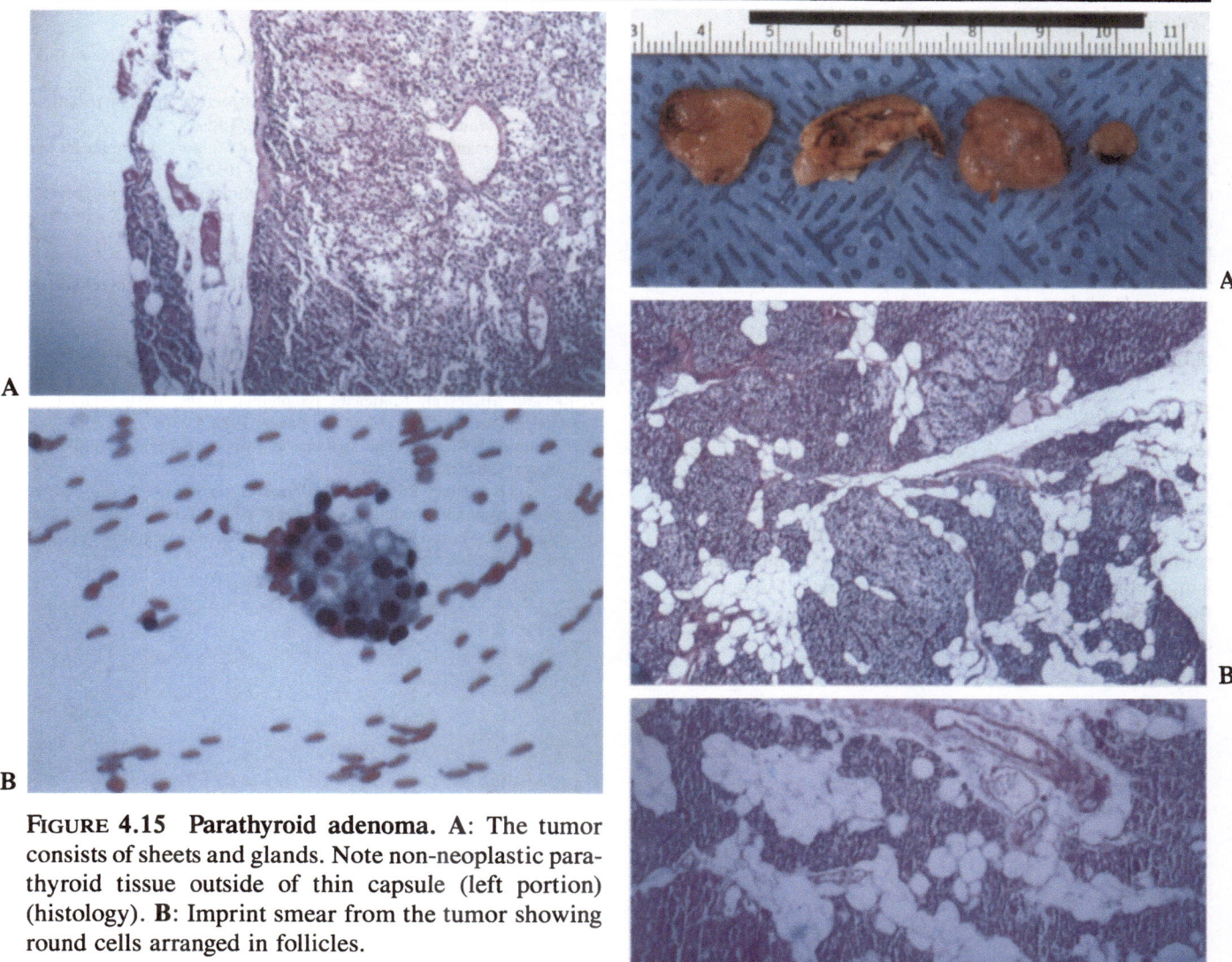

FIGURE 4.15 **Parathyroid adenoma. A**: The tumor consists of sheets and glands. Note non-neoplastic parathyroid tissue outside of thin capsule (left portion) (histology). **B**: Imprint smear from the tumor showing round cells arranged in follicles.

FIGURE 4.16 **Hyperplasia of parathyroid gland. A**: All four parathyroid glands are enlarged. **B**: Hyperplastic change is diffuse and replaces fat cells. **C**: Normal parathyroid gland for comparison.

Secondary Hyperparathyroidism

Secondary hyperparathyroidism is characterized by compensatory hypersecretion of PTH in response to end-organ resistance to PTH, resulting in depressed blood calcium levels. Chronic renal failure, vitamin D deficiency, and intestinal malabsorption syndromes are important known causes of secondary hyperparathyroidism. The parathyroid glands affect all glands with chief cell hyperplasia. Usually, the glands revert to normal if the basic clinical causes are corrected. However, with long-standing secondary hyperplasia and persistent glandular enlargement, it may convert into autonomous primary hyperplasia, referred to as tertiary hyperparathyroidism.

Hypoparathyroidism

Hypoparathyroidism occurs under the circumstances in which there is an inadequate secretion of PTH, biologically ineffective PTH, or reduced end-organ sensitivity to PTH. The common clinical causes are postsurgical hypoparathyroidism after thyroidectomy, surgery for hyperparathyroidism, and radical neck dissections for cancer. Also, a familial form of hypoparathyroidism is thought to represent a form of autoimmune disease.

References

1. Kini SR. *Guides to Clinical Aspiration Biopsy. Thyroid.* New York, Tokyo: Igaku-Shoin; 1987;1–5.
2. DeGroot LJ, et al. Retrospective and prospective study of radiation-induced thyroid disease. *Am J Med.* 1983;74:852.
3. Rosai J, Carcangiu ML. Pathology of thyroid tumors: Some recent and old questions. *Hum Pathol.* 1984;15:1008–1012.
4. Pearse AGE. The cytochemistry and ultrastructure of polypeptide hormone-secreting cells of the APUD series and the embryologic, physiologic, and pathologic implications of the concept. *J Histochem Cytochem.* 1969;17:303.
5. Carcangiu ML, Steeper T, Zampi G, Rosai J. Anaplastic thyroid carcinoma. *Am J Clin Pathol.* 1985;83:135–158.
6. Nel CJC, vanHeerden JA, Goeliner JR, et al. Anaplastic carcinoma of the thyroid: A clinicopathologic study of 82 cases. *Mayo Clin Proc.* 1985;60:51–58.
7. Kapadia SB, et al. Malignant lymphoma of the thyroid gland: A clinicopathologic study. *Head Neck Surg.* 1982;4:270.
8. Thompson NW, et al. The anatomy of primary hyperparathyroidism. *Surgery.* 1982;92:814.
9. Aldinger KA, Hicky RC, et al. Parathyroid carcinoma. A clinical study of seven cases of nonfunctioning parathyroid cancer. *Cancer.* 1982;49: 388.
10. Holmes EC, Marton DL, Ketcham AS. Parathyroid carcinoma. A collective review. *Ann Surg.* 1969;169:631.

5

Lymph Nodes

Fine needle aspiration (FNA) of lymph nodes is applied primarily to palpable lymph nodes in patients with persistently enlarged lymph nodes that cannot be readily explained on clinical grounds. Such enlargement of lymph nodes could be a manifestation of hyperplasia, Hodgkin's or non-Hodgkin's lymphoma, or metastatic neoplasm. Aspiration of a palpable lymph node containing metastatic carcinoma is usually a straightforward interpretative exercise in establishing diagnosis and from a practical standpoint is a most rewarding procedure. Metastatic carcinoma cells usually stand out as cohesive clusters or loose aggregates of alien cells in a background of lymphoid cells.

In fine needle aspirates, the distinction between lymphoid hyperplasia and lymphoma is often not as clear-cut as in the diagnosis of metastatic neoplasm.

If the enlarged lymph nodes are in the thoracic or abdominal cavities, FNA is performed under the guidance of computer tomography (CT) or ultrasonography; its diagnostic accuracy depends heavily on the accuracy of cell sampling.

The following two entities are the common non-neoplastic disease of lymph node.

1. *Lymph node hyperplasia*. The cell population is polymorphous, consisting of small normal lymphocytes, large activated lymphocytes, histiocytes that may contain phagocytosed particles, and, possibly, plasma cells (Fig. 5.1).
2. *Granulomatous lymphadenitis*. The cell population may be similar to that above but also includes epithelioid cells and/or benign giant multinucleated histiocytes (Fig. 5.2). Tuberculosis and sarcoidosis are the common causes of granulomatous lymphadenitis. The distinction between sarcoidosis and tuberculosis is based on the cultured isolation of mycobacteria.

Non-Hodgkin's Lymphoma

Non-Hodgkin's lymphoma (NHL) is a malignant neoplasm characterized by a proliferation of atypical lymphoid cells. Most lymphomas arise in lymph nodes, and less often in the lymphoid tissue of the parenchyma of other organs.

Most patients with lymphoma present with painless enlargement of either a single node or a group of nodes. Hepatosplenomegaly and the systemic manifestations of fever, weight loss, weakness, and anemia subsequently may occur.

For decades the classification of NHL has been controversial. The Rappaport classification is based on the growth pattern of the lymphoma and morphologic features of the cells.[1] The Lukes-Collins classification is based on immunologic and cytochemical markers in addition to the usual morphologic features of the cells.[2] The Working Formulation for Clinical Usage for the Classification of NHL was proposed by an international panel of experts in 1982 (Table 5.1).

Non-Hodgkin's lymphomas exhibit two distinct growth patterns: nodular and diffuse. Even though the cytologic features of nodular and diffuse lymphomas are similar, the nodular lymphomas have a better prognosis.

Histologically, nodular lymphomas are characterized by uniform lymphomatous nodules dispersed throughout the cortex and medulla, a distinct contrast to follicular hyperplasia with its haphazardly dispersed, irregularly shaped, and variably sized follicles (Fig. 5.3). Diffuse lymphomas are characterized by a diffuse proliferation of neoplastic cells without any notable nodular pattern (Fig. 5.4).

Table 5.1. A working formulation of non-Hodgkin's lymphomas for clinical usage.

Working formulation	Rappaport classification
Low grade	
Small lymphocytic	Lymphocytic, well differentiated
Follicular, small cleaved cell	Nodular, poorly differentiated, lymphocytic
Follicular, mixed small cleaved and large cleaved cell	Nodular, mixed lymphocytic-histiocytic
Intermediate Grade	
Follicular, large cell	Nodular, histiocytic
Diffuse, small cleaved cell	Diffuse, poorly differentiated, lymphocytic
Diffuse, mixed large and small cell	Diffuse, mixed lymphocytic-histiocytic
Diffuse, large cell	Diffuse histiocytic
High Grade	
Large cell, immunoblastic	Diffuse histiocytic
Lymphoblastic	Lymphoblastic lymphoma
Small noncleaved cell	Undifferentiated, Burkitt's and non-Burkitt's

From the National Cancer Institute: Sponsored study of classifications of non-Hodgkin's lymphomas. Summary and description of Working Formulation for Clinical Usage. *Cancer* 49:2112, 1982.[3]

Imprint or FNA smears prepared from the cut surface of fresh specimens demonstrate cytomorphologic features to the best advantage. The cardinal cytologic feature of lymphomas is a monomorphic population of single cells that are isolated from each other. In contrast, the cells from hyperplastic lymph nodes are polymorphous, including large and small lymphocytes and histiocytes.

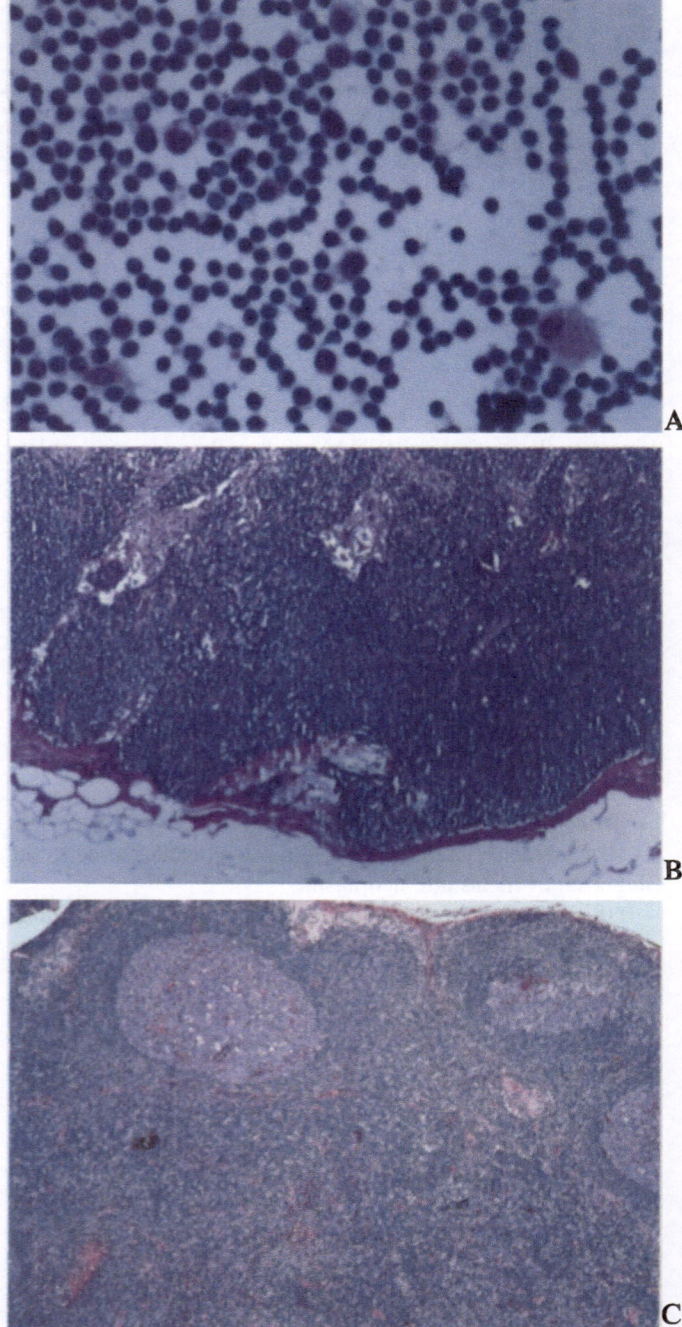

FIGURE 5.1 **Hyperplasia of lymph node. A**: FNA smear showing small and large activated lymphocytes and histiocytes occurring singly. **B**: Sinus histiocytosis. Dilated sinuses engorged with histiocytes. **C**: Follicular hyperplasia. Prominent germinal follicles with phagocytic cells.

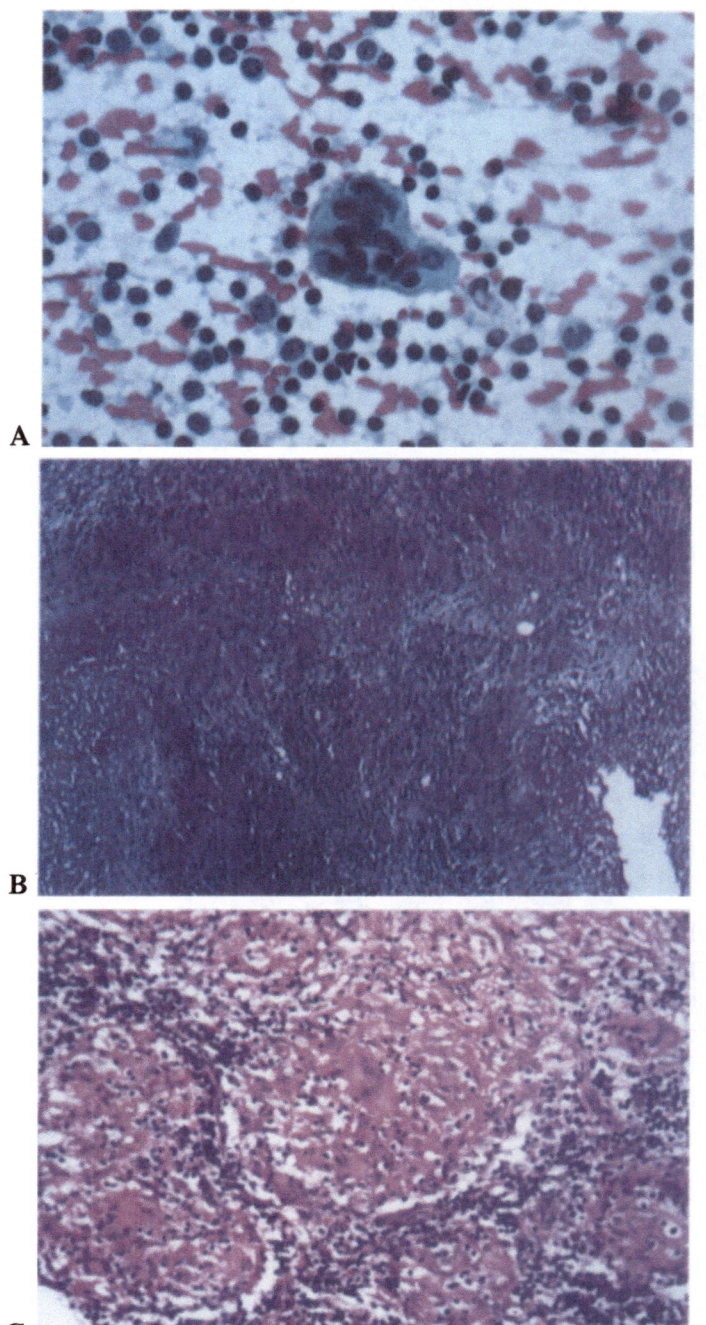

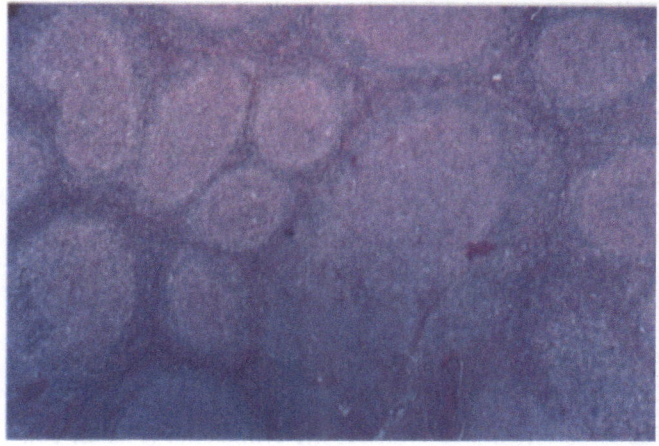

FIGURE 5.3 **Nodular lymphoma.** Relatively uniform size and shape of lymphoid nodules (follicles) involving the cortex and medulla. Compare this to Fig. 5.1C.

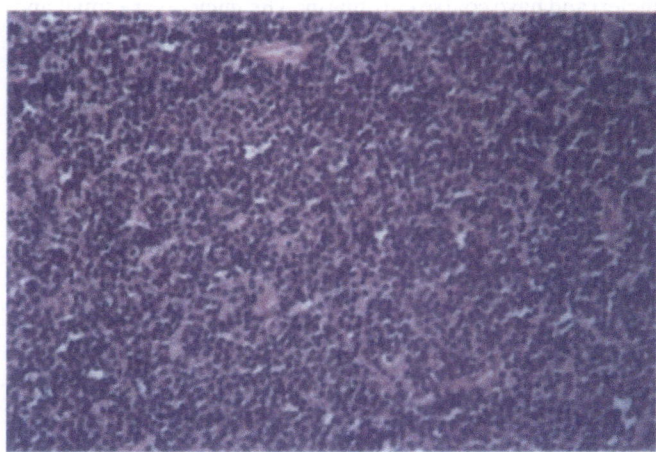

FIGURE 5.4 **Diffuse lymphoma.** Diffuse infiltration of lymph node with effacement of nodal architecture. No discernible nodular pattern is present.

FIGURE 5.2 **Granulomatous lymphadenitis (tuberculosis).** **A**: Langerhans' giant cell, singly isolated epithelioid cells, and lymphocytes. **B**: Caseating granuloma of lymph node (tuberculosis). Caseating granuloma with central caseation and a peripheral layer of epithelioid and Langerhans' giant cells. **C**: Noncaseating granuloma of lymph node (sarcoidosis). Granuloma composed of epithelioid cells and giant cells.

Well Differentiated Lymphocytic Lymphoma (Small Lymphocytic Lymphoma)

Well differentiated lymphocytic lymphoma (WDLL) occurs primarily in the old-age group and is characterized clinically by generalized or localized lymph node enlargement. The cells are a uniform population of small lymphocytes. The cells have scanty cytoplasm and small, round, hyperchromatic nuclei (Fig. 5.5A). Histologically, WDLL occurs in only a diffuse pattern, with the proliferation of small lymphocytes diffusely effacing the nodal architecture (Fig. 5.5B).

Poorly Differentiated Lymphocytic Lymphoma (Small Cleaved Cell Lymphoma)

Poorly differentiated lymphocytic lymphoma (PDLL) consists of small atypical B lymphocytes that may form nodules or diffuse infiltrate and that may involve bone marrow, although less frequently than in WDLL. The cells are similar to or slightly larger than those of WDLL. The nuclei are pleomorphic with irregular indentations and infoldings (cleaved nuclei) and have coarse chromatin. The nucleoli are small and often inconspicuous. Mitotic figures are scanty (Fig. 5.6).

"Histiocytic" Lymphoma (Large Cleaved and Large Noncleaved Cell Lymphoma)

Histiocytic lymphoma (HL) occurs in nodular and diffuse forms, with the latter being the more frequent as well as the most common form of NHL. "Histiocytic" lymphomas are aggressive neoplasms with a high frequency of extranodal involvement, particularly of the gastrointestinal tract, skin, bone, and brain. "Histiocytic" lymphomas are not of true histiocytic origin. Immunologic phenotyping has revealed that 60% originate from B cells and 10% to 15% from T cells. The remaining 20% to 30% do not display any cell markers.[4] Recently, analysis of DNA extracted from the histiocytic lymphomas without B or T markers revealed immunoglobulin gene rearrangements that firmly assign them to B-cell lineage.[5] Histiocytic lymphomas of true histiocytic origin are extremely rare.

In FNA smears or imprints, the cells have scanty and poorly defined cytoplasm and large nuclei. The nuclei are large and round with indentations or cleavages (large, cleaved cells), large and round with smooth nuclear contour (large, noncleaved cells), or large and pleomorphic. The nuclei are hyperchromatic with coarsely granular, irregularly dispersed chromatin resulting in a vesicular pattern. Most nuclei have single or multiple prominent nucleoli. Mitotic figures are frequently observed (Fig. 5.7).

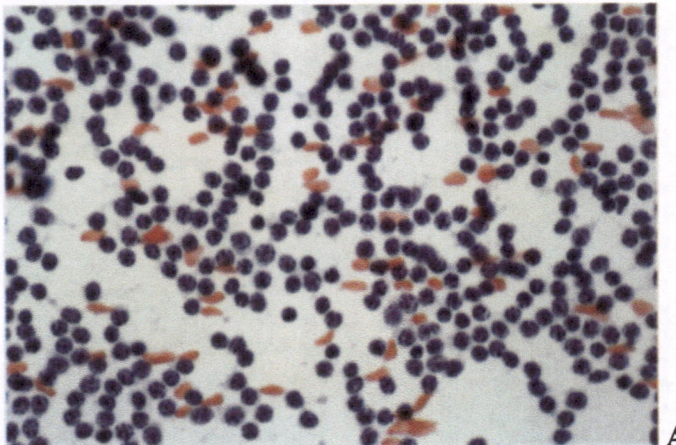

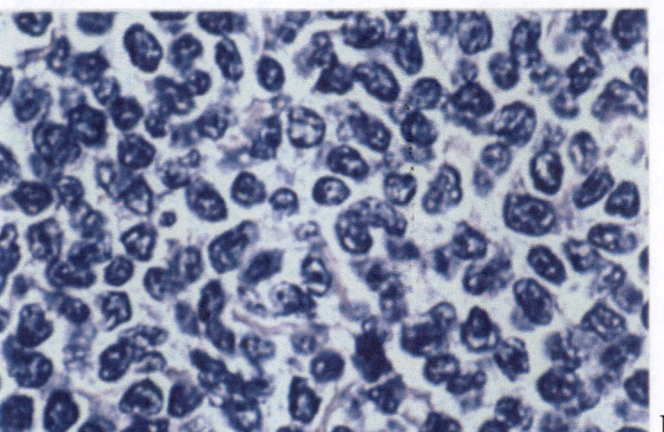

FIGURE 5.5 **Well differentiated lymphocytic lymphoma. A**: The cells in this FNA smear are uniform, small lymphocytes (Papanicolaou stain, ×500). **B**: Well differentiated lymphocytic lymphoma. Diffuse infiltrate of small lymphocytes (H&E stain, ×900). (Courtesy of Dr. Hun Kim, Los Angeles, Calif.)

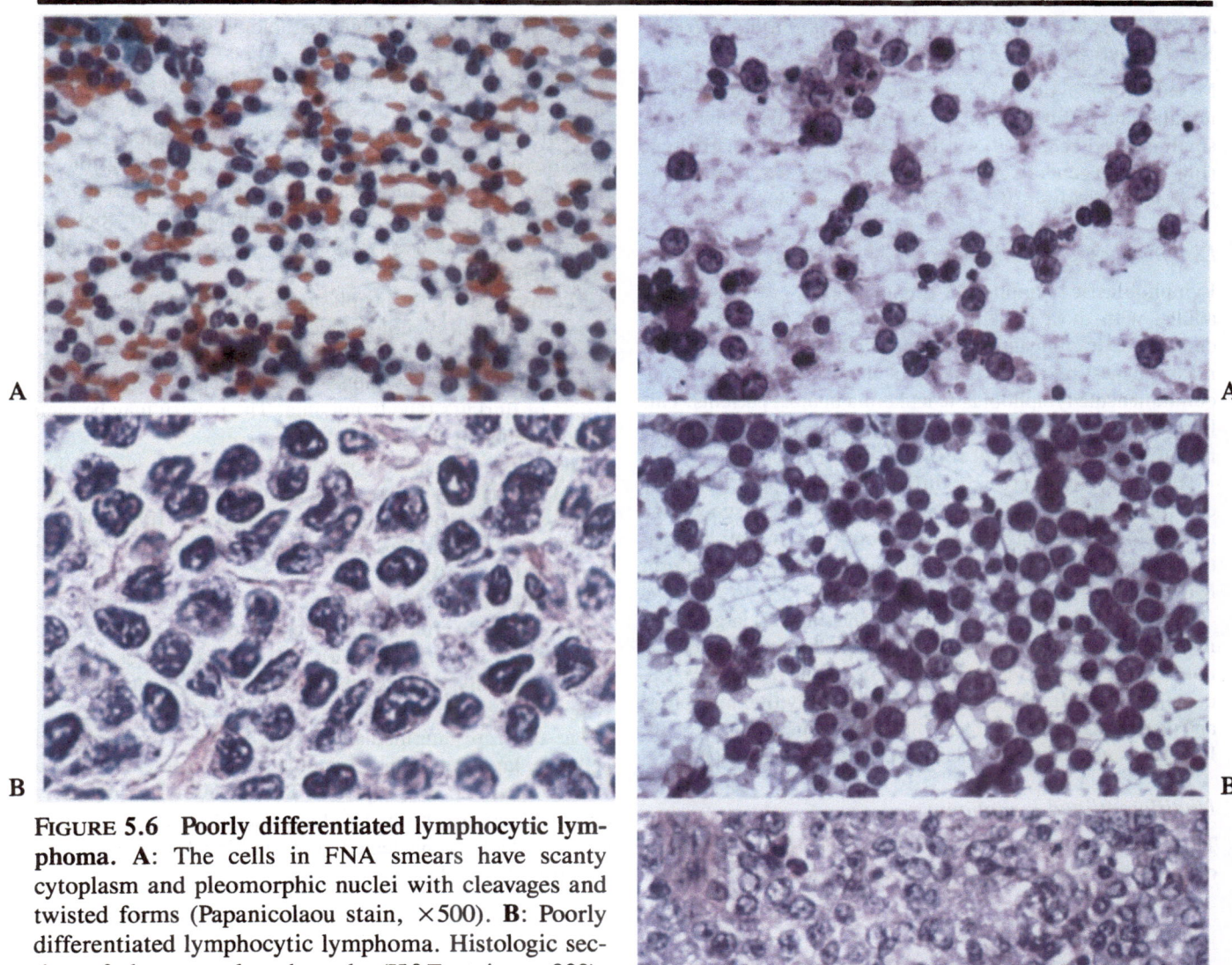

FIGURE 5.6 **Poorly differentiated lymphocytic lymphoma. A**: The cells in FNA smears have scanty cytoplasm and pleomorphic nuclei with cleavages and twisted forms (Papanicolaou stain, ×500). **B**: Poorly differentiated lymphocytic lymphoma. Histologic section of the same lymph node (H&E stain, ×900). (Courtesy of Dr. Hun Kim, Los Angeles, Calif.)

FIGURE 5.7 **"Histiocytic" lymphoma. A**: The cells in this FNA smear have large, round nuclei with prominent macronucleoli (Papanicolaou stain, ×500). **B**: Histiocytic lymphoma (large cleaved cells). The cells in this FNA smear have large nuclei with indentations and cleavages and prominent macronucleoli (Papanicolaou stain, ×500). **C**: Histiocytic lymphoma. Histologic section of large, noncleaved cell type (H&E stain, ×500).

Mixed Lymphocytic and Histiocytic Lymphoma (Mixed Small Cleaved Cell and Large Cell Type)

Mixed lymphocytic and histiocytic lymphoma occurs in both nodular and diffuse forms. It comprises two dissimilar cells, small cleaved cells of PDLL type and large cells of HL type (Fig. 5.8). In general, a lymphoma is classified as mixed if the large cells constitute 30% to 50% of the total number of cells.

Lymphoblastic Lymphoma

Lymphoblastic lymphoma predominantly affects young adults, with most patients being under 20 years of age. A characteristic clinical feature in most patients is a mediastinal mass, suggesting thymic origin of the lymphoma, and concomitant acute lymphoblastic leukemia in most patients. This lymphoma is quite aggressive with high mortality, although a recent treatment protocol seems to be encouraging.

Histologically, there is a diffuse monomorphic lymphoid cell proliferation. Macrophages containing phagocytosed nuclear material (tingible body macrophages) may be scattered through the lymphoma to impart a "starry sky" pattern. Mitotic figures are frequent.

The lymphoma cells have scanty cytoplasm and a large, round nucleus with smooth contours. On close examination under oil immersion, delicate deep convolution of the nuclei are frequently identified. The nuclei have a relatively thin membrane and dispersed chromatin. Nucleoli are inconspicuous (Fig. 5.9). In most examples, the neoplastic cells have T-cell markers.

Undifferentiated Lymphoma

This type of lymphoma of B-cell origin is defined on the basis of its lack of "maturation." The neoplasm occurs predominantly in children. On clinicopathologic grounds, there are two distinct subgroups.

Undifferentiated Burkitt's lymphoma was described initially in Africa, but it also occurs sporadically in non-endemic areas. In African cases, the lymphomas involve the maxilla and mandible; leukemic transformation of the tumors is rare. There is strong evidence linking Epstein-Barr virus to African Burkitt's lymphoma.[6] In contrast, non-African Burkitt's lymphomas involve predominantly the abdominal organs.

Microscopically, the neoplasms of both subgroups are similar, consisting of monomorphic, small, round cells infiltrating diffusely, and scattered tingible body macrophages imparting a "starry sky" appearance, which is not pathognomonic of Burkitt's type lymphoma. The pattern may be seen in lymphoblastic lymphomas.

The cells are small and round with distinctly identifiable cytoplasm. The nuclei are small and round with smooth contours without cleavages and have relatively thick nuclear membranes, coarse chromatin clumps, and multiple distinct nucleoli (Fig. 5.10).

Undifferentiated pleomorphic (non-Burkitt's) lymphoma more commonly affects adults (mean age 34 years) and has no evidence of association with Epstein-Barr virus (EBV). Microscopically, there is a diffuse infiltration of pleomorphic lymphoma cells.

The cells are intermediate in size, between small cleaved cells and large cells. They are quite pleomorphic and have a well-defined rim of cytoplasm. The nuclei have irregularly dispersed, coarse chromatin clumps and distinct eosinophilic macronucleoli. Binucleated and multinucleated cells are common (Fig. 5.11).

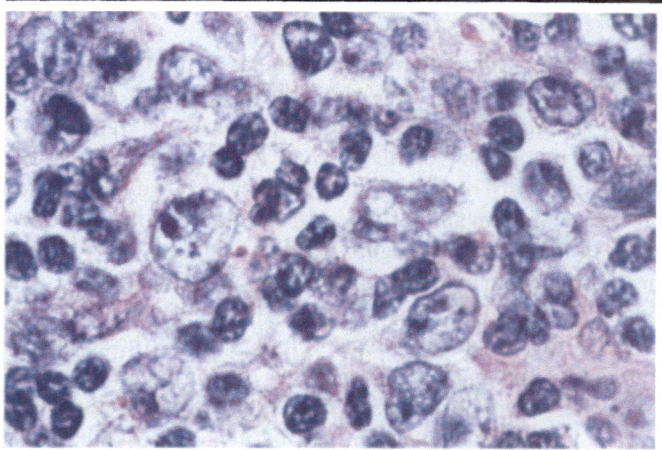

FIGURE 5.8   **Mixed lymphocytic and histiocytic lymphoma.** Histologic section showing mixture of small cleaved cells and large cells (H&E stain, ×900).

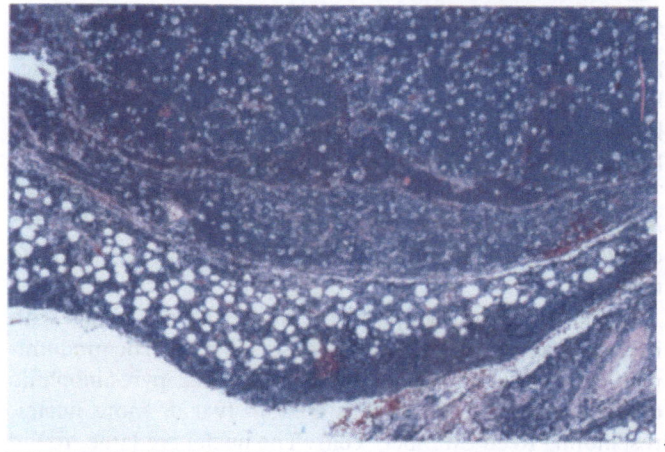

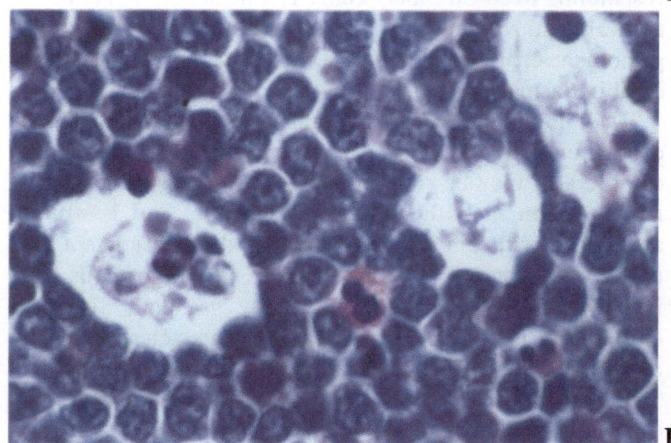

FIGURE 5.10   **Undifferentiated lymphoma, Burkitt's type. A**: Scattered tingible body macrophages impart a "starry sky" appearance (H&E stain, ×80). **B**: Small noncleaved cells with distinct nucleoli and tingible body macrophages (H&E stain, ×900). (Courtesy of Dr. Hun Kim, Los Angeles, Calif.)

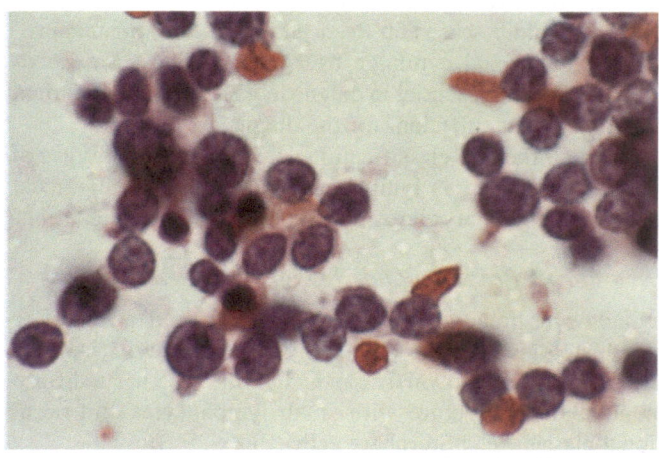

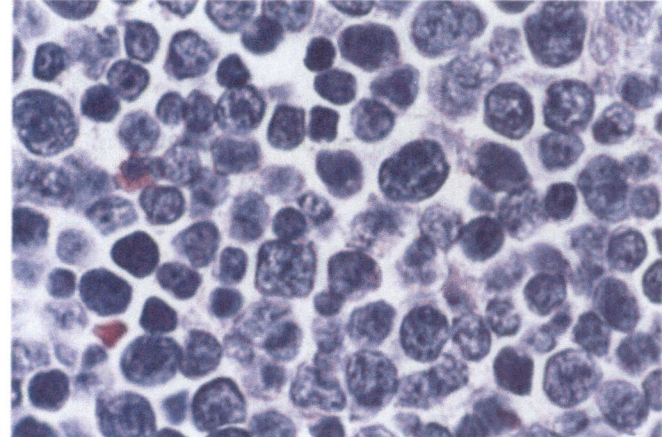

FIGURE 5.9   **Lymphoblastic lymphoma. A**: The cells in this FNA smear show large nuclei with convolutions (Papanicolaou stain, ×500). **B**: Histologic section (H&E stain, ×900).

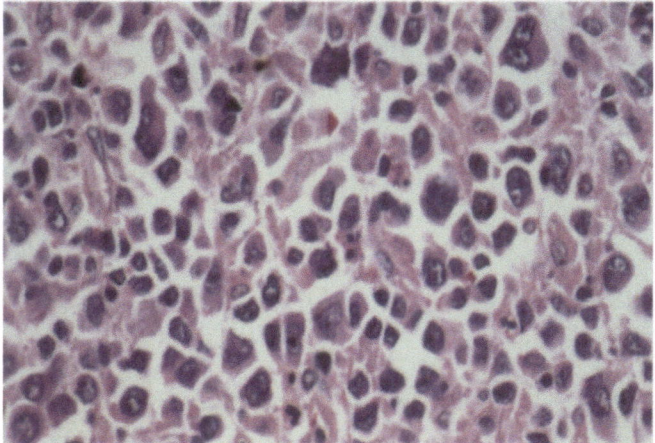

FIGURE 5.11   **Undifferentiated lymphoma, pleomorphic type.** The cells are pleomorphic and intermediate in size between small cleaved cells and large cells (H&E stain, ×500).

Immunoblastic Lymphoma

Immunoblastic lymphomas used to be called "histiocytic" lymphoma in the Rappaport classification. However, these lymphomas are dissimilar to other large cell ("histiocytic") lymphomas in terms of their clinicopathologic features. They comprise cells having morphologic features of immunoblasts (transformed lymphocytes). There are two categories, corresponding to the two major lymphocyte types.[7-11]

B-immunoblastic lymphoma is frequently associated with immunologic disorders. The prognosis is poor. The predominant cells are large immunoblasts with dense pyroninophilic cytoplasm. Some of the cells contain two or more nuclei, resembling Reed-Sternberg cells. The nuclei are large, round to oval, and vesicular with thick nuclear membranes and prominent central nucleoli (Fig. 5.12). Some of these cells exhibit plasmacytoid features.

T-cell immunoblastic lymphoma is less common than its B-cell counterpart and is usually not preceded by immunologic disorders. It may be superimposed on mycosis fungoides. It may be seen in both children and adults, and is usually associated with generalized lymph node enlargement and polyclonal hypergammaglobulinemia. The tumor cells have irregular nuclear contours and finely granular, dispersed chromatin. The cytoplasm is usually water-clear and well defined (Fig. 5.13).

Most studies show that there is a considerable morphologic overlap between B and T immunoblastic lymphomas. However, further stratification based on immunologic markers that identify T-cell and B-cell subsets may reveal clinicopathological differences.[12,13]

Hodgkin's Disease

Hodgkin's disease is a malignant lymphoma consisting of Reed-Sternberg cells in a background of reactive inflammatory cells of various types. The morphologic background in Hodgkin's disease is polymorphous, a contrast to monomorphic cell population in non-Hodgkin's lymphoma.

Clinical Features

About 40% of all malignant lymphomas in the United States are Hodgkin's disease. There is a wide range in age incidence. The major clinical presentation is painless enlargement of high cervical nodes or mediastinal lymph nodes. Constitutional symptoms of fever, night sweats, loss of weight, or pruritus are common and influence the clinical staging. The patterns of spread are contiguity (direct extension) to adjacent nodes and by the hematogenous route to the spleen, liver, and bone marrow. The classical Reed-Sternberg cell is a large binucleate or multinucleate giant cell with abundant cytoplasm and nuclei appearing as mirror images of each other. The nuclei have prominent acidophilic macronucleoli with a perinucleolar halo, imparting an "owl-eyed" appearance (Fig. 5.14A). The Reed-Sternberg cell is a distinctive neoplastic cell and is considered to be the essential neoplastic element in all forms of Hodgkin's disease. Since Reed-Sternberg–like cells have been identified in other diseases such as infectious mononucleosis and non-Hodgkin's lymphomas, the cytologic or histologic diagnosis of Hodgkin's disease should be based on Reed-Sternberg cells in an appropriate clinical and cytologic background. Thus, the Reed-Sternberg cell is essential in diagnosing Hodgkin's lymphoma but alone is not sufficient for the diagnosis.

Based on the Rye classification, there are four subtypes of Hodgkin's disease: 1) lymphocyte predominance, 2) mixed cell type, 3) nodular sclerosing, and 4) lymphocyte depletion.

Lymphocyte Predominance Hodgkin's Disease

Lymphocyte predominance Hodgkin's disease is a relatively rare histologic variant, practically never involving spleen, liver, or bone marrow. Histologically, this type has a diffuse or nodular architecture with small lymphocytes and occasional classic Reed-Sternberg cells (Fig. 5.14B).

Mixed Cell Type Hodgkin's Disease

Mixed cell type Hodgkin's disease is a relatively common type consisting of a mixture of small lymphocytes, eosinophils, plasma cells, and numerous classic Reed-Sternberg cells (Fig. 5.15).

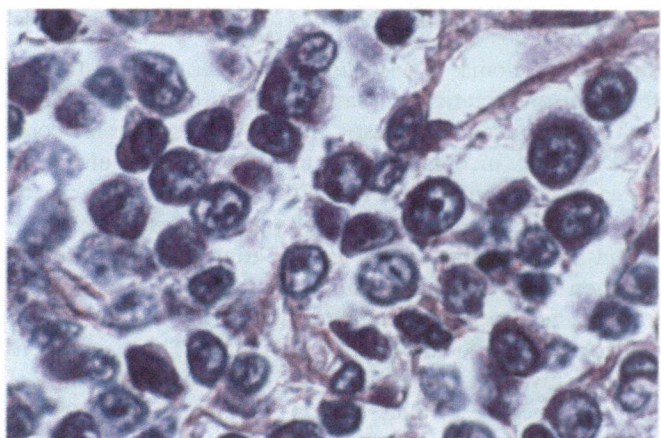

FIGURE 5.12 **B-immunoblastic lymphoma.** Large immunoblasts with pyroninophilic cytoplasm and large vesicular nuclei and nucleoli (H&E stain, ×900) (Courtesy of Dr. Hun Kim, Los Angeles, Calif).

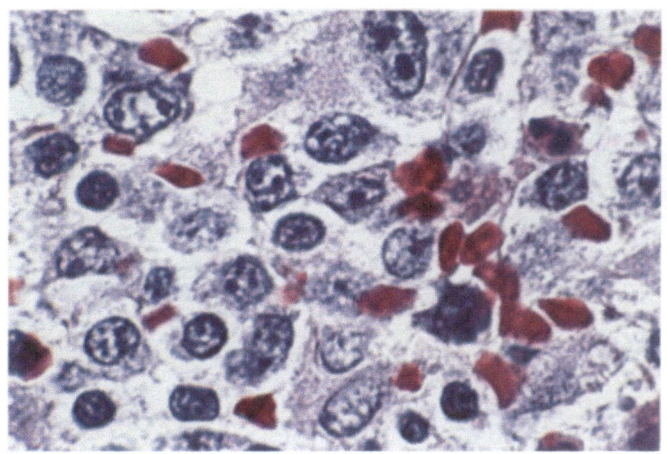

FIGURE 5.13 **T-immunoblastic lymphoma.** Large cells with large nuclei (H&E stain, ×900). (Courtesy of Dr. Hun Kim, Los Angeles, Calif.)

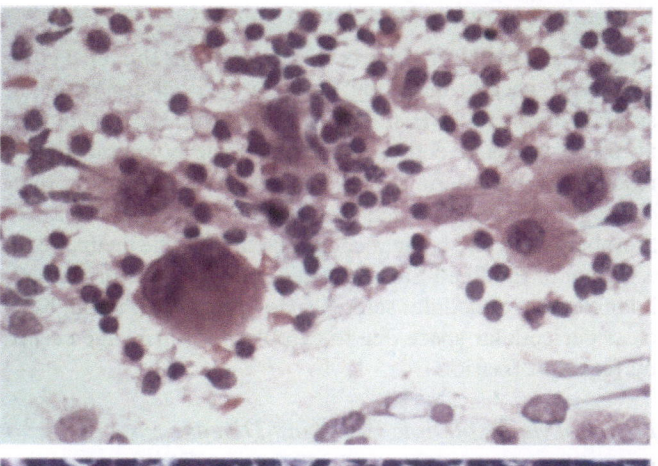

A

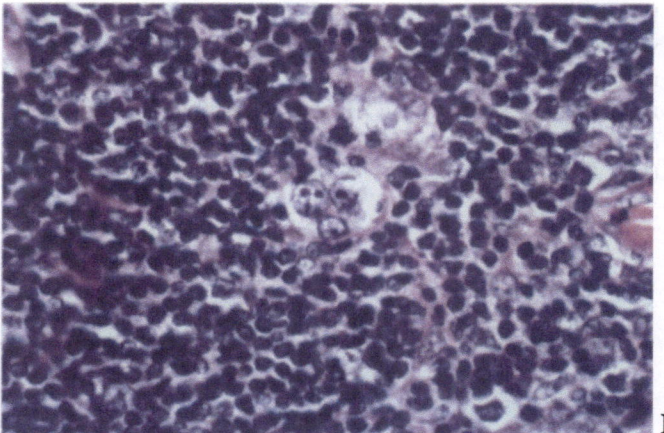

B

FIGURE 5.14 **Hodgkin's lymphoma, lymphocyte predominance. A:** Reed-Sternberg cells showing binucleated cells with the nuclei arranged as a mirror image of each other (FNA). **B:** Histologic section showing Reed-Sternberg cells (*center*) in a background comprising predominantly lymphocytes (H&E stain, ×500).

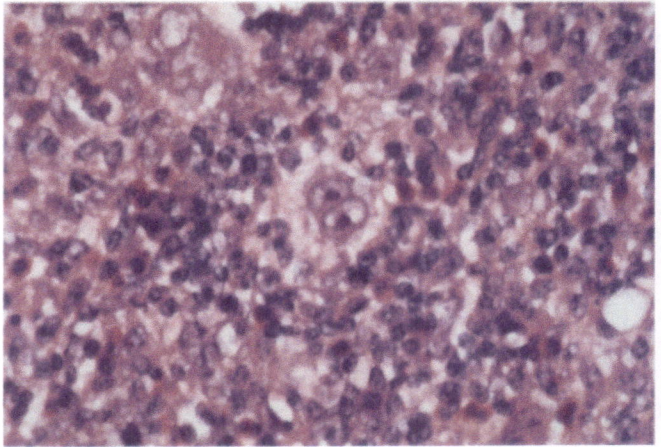

FIGURE 5.15 **Hodgkin's lymphoma, mixed cellularity.** Reed-Sternberg cells in a mixed cell background comprising lymphocytes, eosinophils, and plasma cells (H&E stain, ×500).

Nodular Sclerosing Hodgkin's Disease

Nodular sclerosing Hodgkin's disease is by far the most common type, usually involving the high cervical and/or mediastinal lymph nodes. Histologically, this type is characterized by broad bands of collagen separating the lymphoid tissue, resulting in well defined nodules. The nodules vary in their cytologic composition and contain occasional classic Reed-Sternberg cells and lacunar cells (Fig. 5.16). The lacunar cell, a variant of the Reed-Sternberg cell, and a characteristic cellular element of nodular sclerosis Hodgkin's lymphoma, has a clear pericellular space due to cytoplasmic shrinkage caused by formalin fixation.

Lymphocyte Depletion Hodgkin's Disease

Lymphocyte depletion Hodgkin's disease is a relatively rare variant, that presents in adults or elderly patients as a febrile illness with pancytopenia or hepatomegaly. Histologically, it is characterized by diffuse fibrosis, sparse lymphocytic cells, and large numbers of classic and bizarre Reed-Sternberg cells (Fig. 5.17). Clinically, this is the most aggressive type.

Multiple Myeloma (Plasma Cell Myeloma)

Multiple myeloma is a malignant neoplasm consisting of abnormal proliferation of plasma cells involving bones in a multifocal fashion. Neoplastic plasma cells synthesize complete and/or incomplete immunoglobulins, resulting in increased concentrations of one of the immunoglobulin classes in blood (M component) and urine (Bence Jones protein).

Multiple myeloma occurs usually after age 50 years. The common clinical manifestations are bone pain, pathologic fracture, recurrent infections resulting from suppression of normal immunoglobulins, and renal failure. The diagnosis of multiple myeloma is based on the radiographic features of sharply punched-out bone defects, the identification of the monoclonal nature of the serum M component by immunoelectrophoresis, and ultimately by biopsy of a lesion. Although any bone may be affected, the vertebral column, ribs, and skull are most commonly affected.

In FNA smears, the cells are oval to round with eccentric nuclei and a perinuclear halo. They range from well differentiated plasma cells to markedly atypical plasma cells (Fig. 5.18).

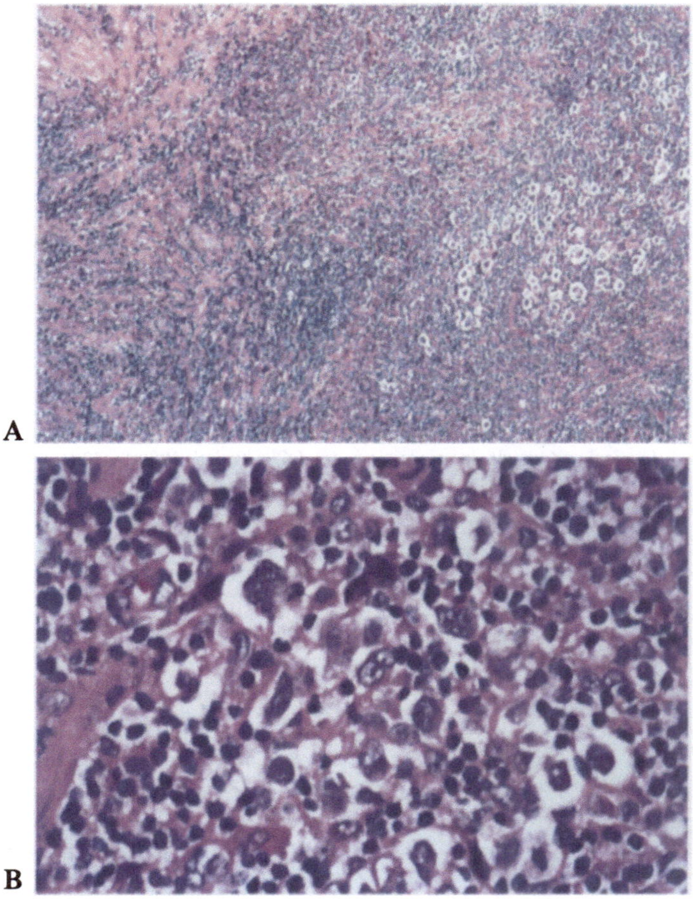

FIGURE 5.16 Hodgkin's lymphoma, nodular sclerosis. A: Irregular collagen bands dividing the lymph node and lacunar cells (H&E stain, ×80). **B**: Lacunar cells showing their clear pericellular space (H&E stain, ×300).

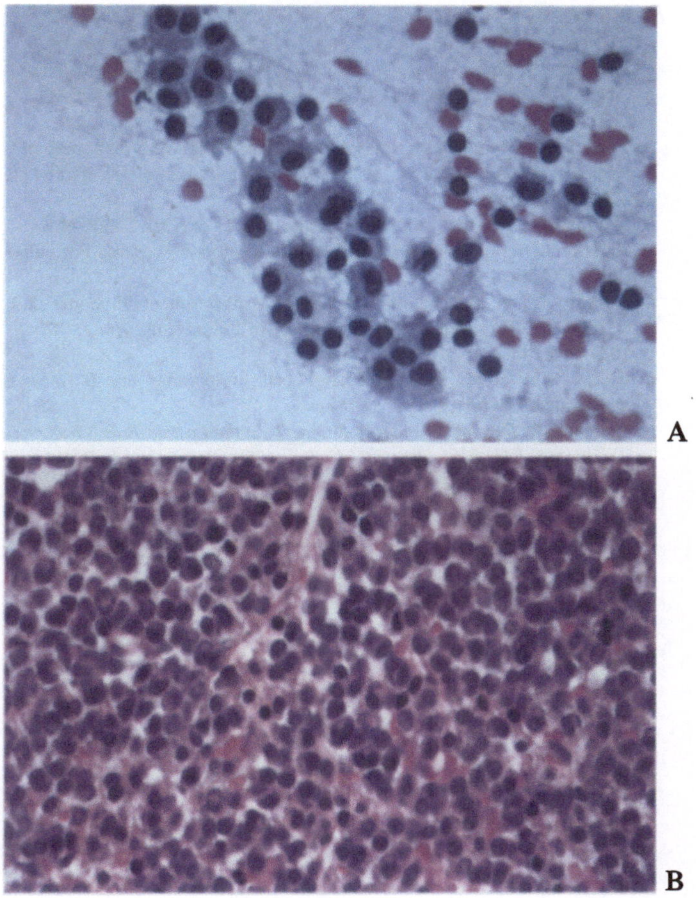

FIGURE 5.18 Multiple myeloma. A: FNA smear showing atypical plasma cells occurring singly. **B**: Histologic section showing a solid sheet of atypical plasma cells (H&E stain, ×500).

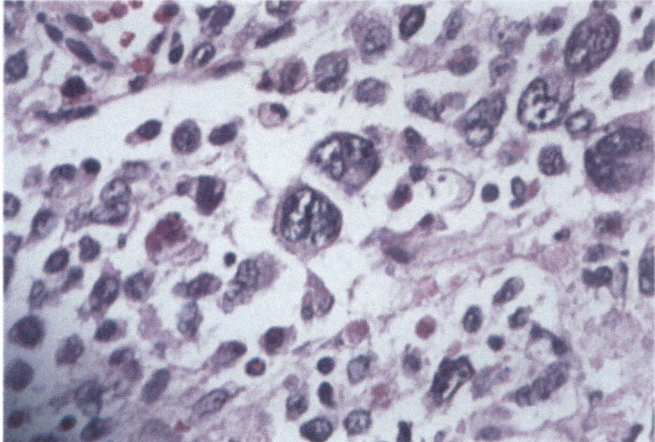

FIGURE 5.17 Hodgkin's lymphoma, lymphocyte depletion. Multiple Reed-Sternberg cells in a background of sparse lymphocytic cells (H&E stain, ×500).

References

1. Jaffe ES. *An Overview of Classification of Non-Hodgkin's Lymphomas. Surgical Pathology of Lymph Nodes and Related Organs.* Philadelphia: WB Saunders Co; 1985:135.

2. Lukes RJ, et al. Immunologic approach to non-Hodgkins lymphomas and related leukemias. Analysis of the results of multiparameter studies of 425 cases. *Semin Hematol.* 1978;15:322.

3. National Cancer Institute. Sponsored study of classifications of non-Hodgkin's lymphomas. Summary and description of Working Formulation for Clinical Usage. *Cancer.* 1982;49:2112.

4. Doggett RS, et al. The immunologic classification of 95 nodal and extranodal diffuse large cell lymphomas in 89 patients. *Am J Pathol.* 1984;115:245.

5. Cleary ML, et al. Most null large cell lymphomas are B lineage neoplasms. *Lab Invest.* 1985;53:521.

6. Pearson GR. *Recent Advances in Research on the Epstein-Barr Virus and Associated Diseases, 4th ed, Current Hematology and Oncology.* Chicago: Year Book Medical Publishers; 1986:123.

7. Neiman RS. Immunoblastic sarcoma. *Am J Surg Pathol.* 1982;6:755–760.

8. Waldron JA, Leech JH, Glick AD, Flexner JM, Collins RD. Malignant lymphoma of peripheral T-lymphocytic origin. Immunologic, pathologic and clinical features in six patients. *Cancer.* 1977;40:1604–1617.

9. Lichtenstein A, Levine AM, Lukes RJ, et al. Immunoblastic sarcoma. A clinical description. *Cancer.* 1979;43:343–352.

10. Lukes RJ, Parker JW, Taylor CR, Tindle RH, Cramer AD, Lincoln TL. Immunologic approach to non-Hodgkin's lymphomas and related leukemias. Analysis of the results of multiparameter studies of 425 cases. *Semin Hematol.* 1978;15:322–351.

11. Michel RP, Case BW, Moinuddin M. Immunoblastic lymphosarcoma. A light, immunofluorescence, and electron microscopy study. *Cancer.* 1979;43:224–236.

12. Harris NL. Lymphoma 1987. An interim approach to diagnosis and classification. *Path Annu.* 1987;22(P.T.2):1.

13. Winter JN, et al. Phenotypic analysis in diffuse large cell lymphoma. Clinical and histologic association. *Am J Clin Pathol.* 1986;86:429.

6
Lung and Mediastinum

Anatomy and Histology of the Lungs

The combined weight of the normal adult lungs is about 700 to 800 g. The lungs are divided into lobes by fissures lined by visceral pleura. The right lung has three lobes: upper, middle, and lower; the left lung has only two. The lungs are covered by the visceral pleura. The parietal pleura covers the internal surface of the chest wall and the upper surface of the diaphragm, and constitutes the lateral border of the mediastinum.

The trachea divides into the right and left main stem bronchi at the carina. On entering the lung from the hilus, each main stem bronchus divides into lobar bronchi, two on the left and three on the right. Progressive branching of the bronchi forms the terminal bronchioles. The part of the lung distal to a terminal bronchiole is called an acinus, or terminal respiratory unit. Each terminal bronchiole subdivides into respiratory bronchioles which give off the alveolar sacs.

The main stem and lobar bronchi are lined by pseudostratified ciliated columnar epithelium mixed with mucus-secreting goblet cells, nonciliated cells, and small basal or reserve cells (Fig. 6.1). Numerous submucosal mucus-secreting glands are dispersed throughout the wall of the trachea and bronchi. The walls of the bronchi consist of the inner mucosal layer, submucosal connective tissue, smooth muscle, and cartilage. The bronchial mucosa also contains neuroendocrine cells, the bronchial counterpart of the argentaffin or Kulchitsky cells of the gastrointestinal tract.

The respiratory bronchioles are lined by nonciliated epithelium containing occasional secretory clear cells known as Clara cells. The respiratory bronchioles open into the alveoli. The alveoli are lined by flat, pavement type I pneumocytes (membranous pneumocytes) and a few type II pneumocytes (granular pneumocytes) and usually contain macrophages (Fig. 6.2). The alveolar septa contain anastomosing capillaries.

Introduction

This chapter focuses on neoplasms and neoplasmlike lesions of the lungs and mediastinum.

Solitary or multiple lung nodules in an x-ray film of the chest may represent granuloma, benign neoplasm, or malignant neoplasm. Diagnostic methods encompass exfoliative cytology of sputum, fiberoptic bronchoscopy with washing or brushing cytology, punch biopsy, percutaneous transthoracic fine needle aspiration cytology, and thoracotomy for an open biopsy. On a practical basis, it is most important to distinguish a nonneoplastic lesion from a neoplastic lesion. For the past several decades, sputum cytology has been the method for screening and the first-step diagnostic and screening procedure for the lung lesions.

For central lesions involving the large caliber bronchi, identification of cancer cells by sputum cytology and localization by bronchoscopy are suitable methods of diagnosis. For the peripheral lesions, sputum cytology and washing and brushing by fiberoptic bronchoscopy often fail to give a diagnosis.[1,2]

Transthoracic fine needle aspiration (FNA) is particularly the method of choice for peripheral lung lesions and for the lesions for which an operative procedure is not suitable. The indications and contraindications of transthoracic FNA are as follows[3,4]:

Indications:
1. medical contraindications to thoracotomy, refusal of surgery by a patient, or the presence of metastatic neoplasm
2. inoperable cancer in which a pathologic diagnosis is required before radiotherapy or chemotherapy
3. for the confirmation of a suspected cancer in a patient who has a marginal surgical risk
4. for the confirmation of a clinically suspected small cell carcinoma
5. poorly resolving pneumonia
6. for the identification of the nature of an infectious process
7. for the staging work-up of malignant tumors

Contraindications:
1. hemorrhagic diathesis
2. anticoagulant therapy
3. severe pulmonary hypertension
4. uncontrolled cough
5. advanced emphysema
6. suspected arteriovenous malformation
7. uncooperative patient
8. suspicion of a pulmonary hydatid cyst

Diagnostic Procedure and Cytopreparatory Methods

Based on clinical information and with an appropriate radiological presentation, some cytodiagnostic procedure may be preferable to others.

Sputum Cytology

Sputum cytology has been a traditional cytodiagnostic method for several decades. It has been used routinely in patients with known chest lesions and also for screening a population at risk. This method is particularly useful in patients believed to have clinically advanced lung cancer, especially when it involves the large segmental bronchi. Fresh "deep cough" specimens are collected. Smears are prepared by spreading a portion of the specimen between two glass slides. These are fixed immediately in 95% ethanol or with a spray fixative.

If it is not possible to deliver the fresh sputum, the sputum may be collected in a jar containing 70% ethanol. For the Saccomanno method, collect the sputum in a container in which there is either 50% ethanol or 50% isopropanol mixed with 2% polyethylene glycol, the liquid form of carbowax.[5] This method is recommended for outpatient screening.

Bronchoscopic Samples

Flexible fiberoptic bronchoscopy is used for lesions of the primary and lobar bronchi as well as some of the segmental bronchi. It is not ideal for peripheral lesions.

This procedure is useful to localize lesions detected by sputum cytology or to diagnose clinically suspicious lesions in which the sputum cytology is negative. Bronchoscopy allows the operator to obtain brushings and biopsy specimens under direct vision. The operator or stand-by cytotechnologist rolls the brush on an alcohol-wet slide, spreading the cells evenly, and fixes it immediately in 95% ethanol or with a spray fixative. If the operator is not adept at preparing the smears, the disposable brush is cut at the end and is delivered to the laboratory in a container in which there are 5.0 to 10.0 mL of balanced salt solution. After the smears are made, the brush is shaken in 10.0 mL of balanced salt solution in a test tube and membrane filter preparations are made using Millipore or Nuclepore filters. Bronchial washing specimens should be processed by the same filter process. Turbid washing specimen can be spun down to make a cell button for direct smears.

Transthoracic Fine Needle Aspiration

Refer to Introduction.

Staining

The Papanicolaou method is the generally accepted staining method.

Diff-Quick or hematoxylin and eosin stains may be used for rapid processing. Smears can be used for special stains, for identification of infectious agents, and for immunostaining for cell markers.

Normal Cells of Lower Respiratory Tract

The principal cell components of the lower respiratory tract are ciliated columnar epithelial cells, goblet cells (mucus-producing bronchial epithelial cells), and alveolar macrophages.

The ciliated columnar cells are from the tracheobronchial mucosa and are seen in sheets, clusters, and singly. Individual cells are characterized in profile by a columnar or prismatic shape ending in a tail and by cilia attached to the terminal plate. The nuclei are small and round or oval and may occupy various positions in the cell, but usually at its base (Fig. 6.3). Multinucleated ciliated cells are common. Ciliated columnar cells are more abundant in bronchial washings and brushings.

Goblet cells are observed more often in patients with chronic bronchitis, asthma, and bronchiectasis. They are characterized by cytoplasm distended with vacuoles that distort the nucleus and push it eccentrically. They are occasionally seen in bronchial brushings.

(*Discussion continued on p. 66*)

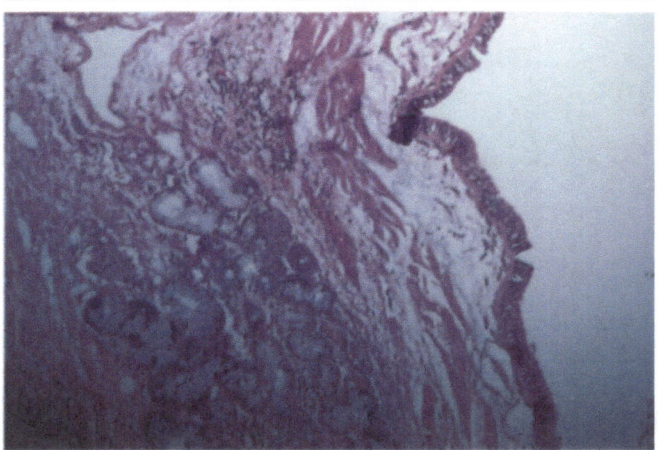

FIGURE 6.1 Normal bronchial mucosa lined by pseudostratified ciliated columnar epithelium, beneath which are the submucosal bronchial glands.

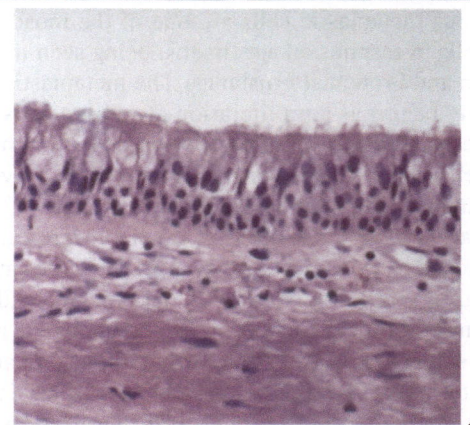

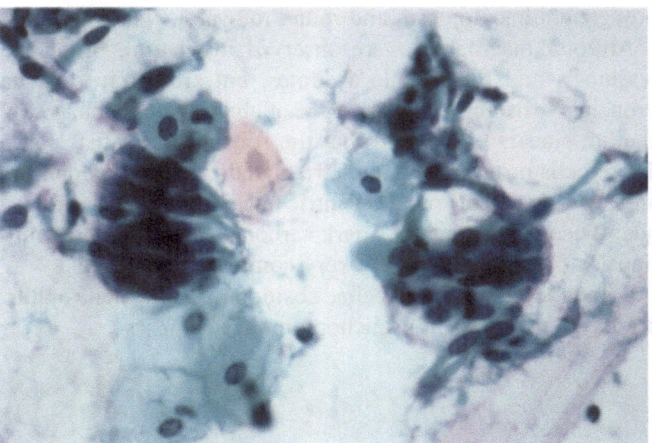

FIGURE 6.3 Normal bronchial epithelium. A: Pseudostratified ciliated epithelium with occasional goblet cells. B: Strips of ciliated bronchial epithelial cells (bronchial brushing).

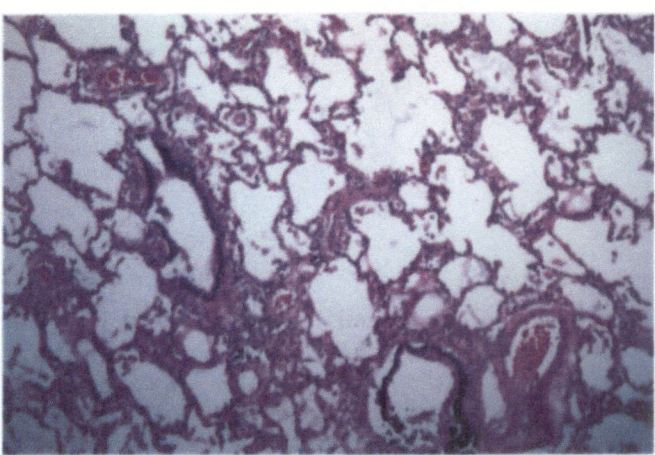

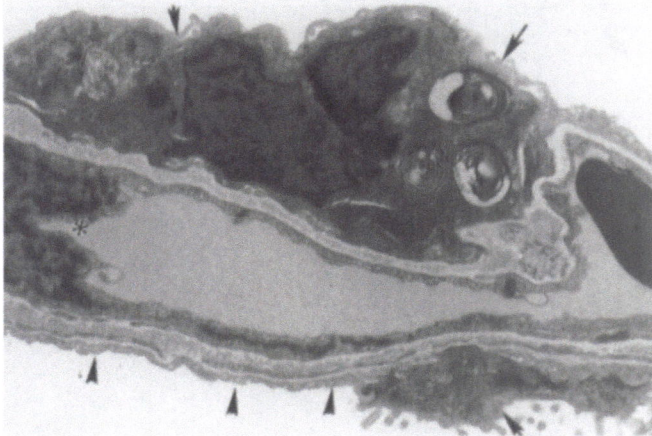

FIGURE 6.2 Normal alveoli. A: Thin alveolar septa and alveolar macrophages. B: Alveolar wall lined by type I (*arrowhead*) and type II (*arrow*) pneumocytes. The wall contains septal capillaries (*asterisk*) (EM). (Courtesy of William Gunning, Ph.D., Medical College of Ohio.)

Squamous metaplastic cells are one of the most common benign cells in respiration specimens, being seen most often in sputum and bronchial brushings. The metaplastic process most likely begins as a proliferation of reserve cells to form immature squamous epithelium beneath the columnar epithelial cells (Fig. 6.4A). As they mature, they eventually form stratified squamous epithelium.

In smears, reserve cells occur in small clusters and sheets, often attached to ciliated columnar cells. They are small, uniform, tightly coherent cells with dark nuclei and scanty cytoplasm (Fig. 6.4B). Cells from foci of squamous metaplasia occur singly or in sheets. They are smaller, compared with the cells of mature squamous epithelium, and have a higher nucleocytoplasmic ratio. The cells have dense cyanophilic or orangeophilic cytoplasm and round to oval nuclei (Fig. 6.5).

Alveolar macrophages are observed in sputum, bronchial washings, and fine needle aspirates, but are rarely seen in bronchial brushings. The presence of alveolar macrophages in sputum smears establishes that the specimen is satisfactory. These cells occur singly and have abundant foamy cytoplasm and bean-shaped or round eccentric nuclei. The cytoplasm frequently contains numerous dark carbonaceous particles. Multinucleated macrophages are very common (Fig. 6.6).

Lymphocytes, plasma cells, eosinophils, and neutrophils are frequently seen in bronchopulmonary smears.

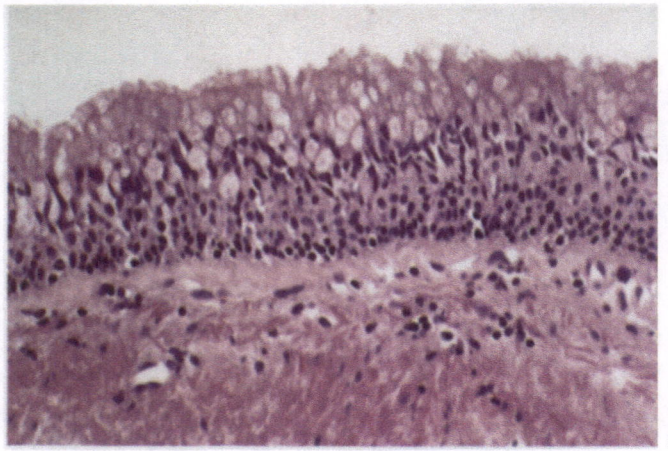

A

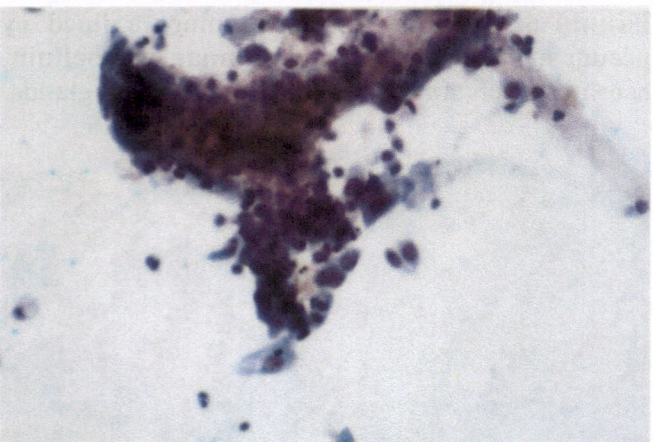

B

FIGURE 6.4 Reserve cell hyperplasia. A: Multiple layers of reserve cells between columnar cells and basement membrane. B: Cluster of reserve cells with scanty cytoplasm and small dark nuclei (bronchial brushing).

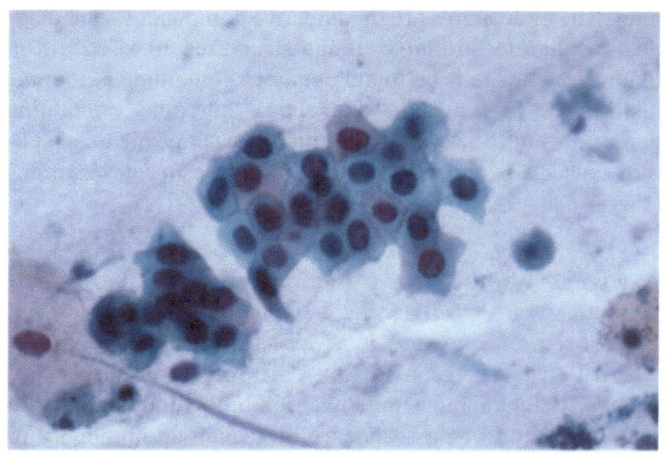

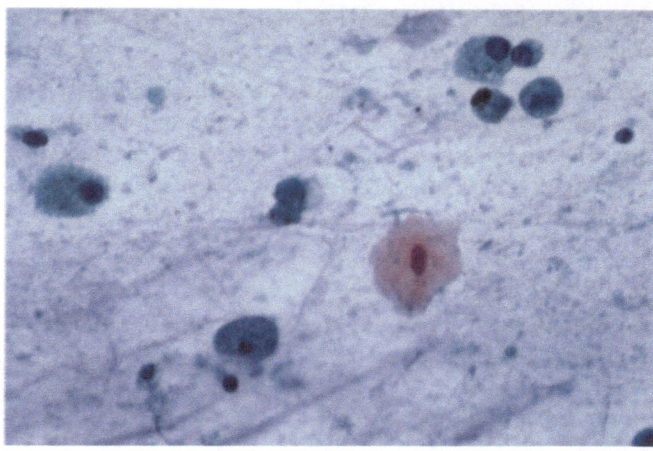

FIGURE 6.5 Squamous metaplastic cells with dense cytoplasm and round to oval nuclei (sputum).

FIGURE 6.6 Alveolar macrophages with abundant foamy cytoplasm and round eccentric nuclei (sputum).

Non-Neoplastic Lung Diseases Mimicking Cancer

Inflammatory and non-neoplastic bronchopulmonary diseases often clinically masquerade as a cancer. With highly sophisticated imaging methods and fiberoptic bronchoscopy, bronchopulmonary cytology has become essential in the diagnostic process.

Granulomatous Diseases

The following are representative disease entities causing a granulomatous change.

Tuberculosis and Sarcoidosis

Since there are no characteristic cytologic features of tuberculosis, transthoracic FNA may provide a specimen directly from the granuloma for microbial culture. Sarcoidosis has no reliable diagnostic feature. Transbronchial biopsy by fiberoptic bronchoscopy may establish the diagnosis. Multinucleated dust free giant cells are suggestive of either tuberculosis or sarcoidosis dust free in cytologic specimens.

Histoplasmosis

Histoplasma capsulatum is a dimorphic fungus occurring as a mycelial form in soil and being transformed to the yeast phase at body temperature. Histoplasmosis can occur in both healthy and in immunocompromised persons, and may present radiologically as a well circumscribed lesion mimicking cancer.

Small intracytoplasmic yeasts (2–5 μm in diameter) can be identified in histiocytes (Fig. 6.7). Definite diagnosis can be established by culture.

Coccidioidomycosis

Coccidioides immitis is a dimorphic fungus occurring as a mold in the soil, but as spherules containing endospores in man. The endospores are the infective component. The diagnostic spherules are large, round structures 30 to 60 μm in diameter. They may be found empty or containing numerous endospores (2–5 μm in diameter). Spherules containing endospores may be seen in Papanicolaou stain smears of sputum but can be better appreciated in fine needle aspirates (Fig. 6.8).

Cryptococcosis

Cryptococcus neoformans is a yeast found in soil especially where it is rich in pigeon droppings. The organism can produce primary granulomatous inflammation in the lung, although it is more likely to be a secondary invader in an immunocompromised host.

The budding organisms vary in size, ranging from 2 to 15 μm in diameter. They have a thick mucinous capsule (Fig. 6.9A). The organisms can be identified in Papanicolaou-stained smears, but are more clearly identified by silver strains, the periodic acid-Schiff stain, or in India ink preparation (Fig. 6.9B).

North American Blastomycosis

Blastomyces dermatidis is a dimorphic fungus occurring as mycelia at room temperature and as yeasts, the infectious form at body temperature. The south, south central, and Great Lakes areas of the United States are the endemic areas.

The yeast forms vary in size from 8 to 15 μm in diameter. The individual yeast cell is surrounded by a thick refractile wall and contains multiple nuclei. These yeast forms bud in a broad-based fashion, in sharp contrast to *Cryptococcus* with its thin tapering attachment (Fig. 6.10). The histologic changes of blastomycosis are variable and nonspecific.

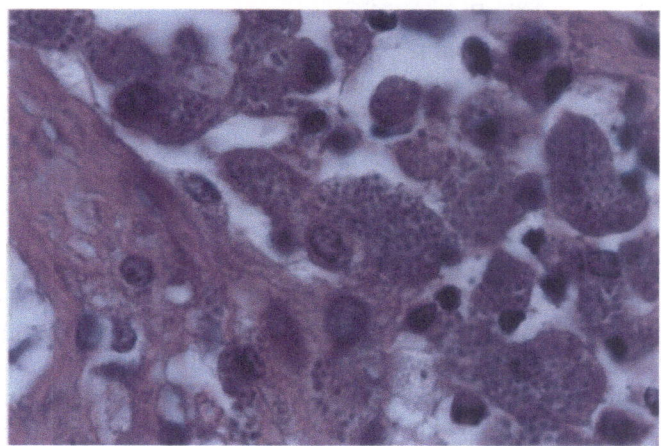

FIGURE 6.7   **Histoplasmosis.** Aspirate smear showing introcytoplasmic yeasts in histiocytes (silver stain).

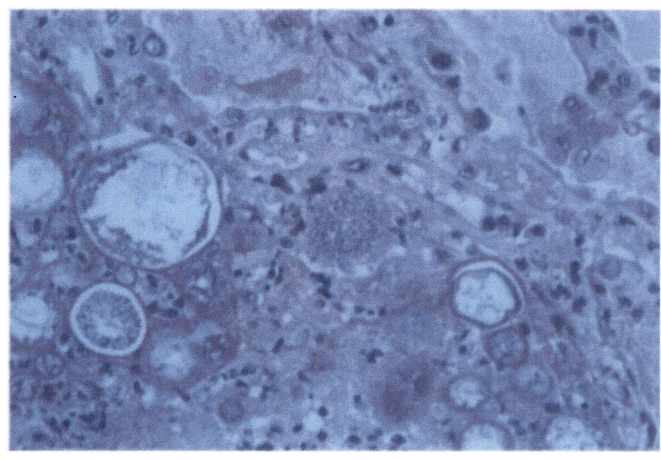

FIGURE 6.8   **Coccidioidomycosis.** Biopsy section showing spherules containing numerous endospores (silver stain).

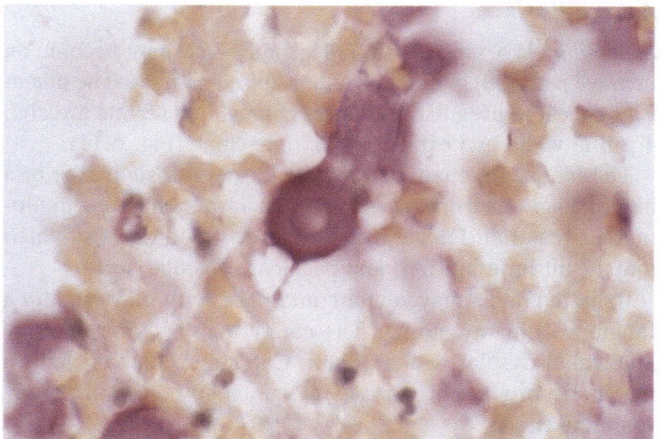

A

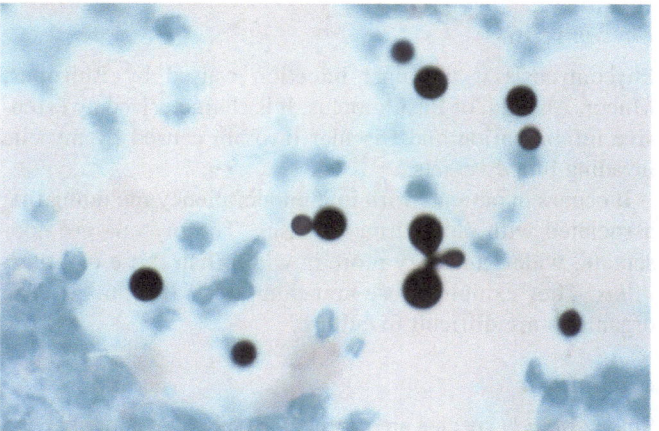

B

FIGURE 6.9   **Cryptococcosis. A**: Aspirate smear showing yeasts with thick mucoid capsule and narrow-based budding (mucicarmine stain). **B**: Aspirate smear showing yeasts with narrow-based budding (silver stain).

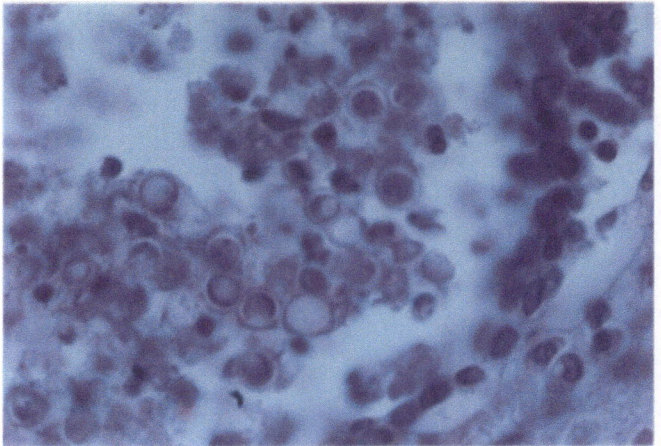

FIGURE 6.10 **North American Blastomycosis** (*Blastomyces dermatidis*). Lung biopsy showing large yeasts with double-contoured capsule and broad-based budding (Hematoxylin-eosin stain).

Aspergillosis

Aspergillus is a saprophytic organism, which may become an invasive pathogen in immunocompromised patients. The organisms appear as irregular aggregates of long, thin septate mycelia, 4 μm in width and exhibiting 45° branching (Fig. 6.11).

The histologic change in invasive aspergillosis is that of a hemorrhagic necrotizing pneumonia rather than a granulomatous reaction. Fungal hyphae invade blood vessels, which may result in infarction, and permeate alveolar septa.

Infarcted areas may cavitate and the cavity may contain a fungus ball or mycetoma. The cavity may become lined by atypical or dysplastic epithelium. Calcium oxalate crystals, a metabolic product of *Aspergillus* sp., may be found in surrounding tissue.

Phycomycosis

Phycomycosis is a fungal infection caused by Rhizopus, Mucor, Absidia, or Basidiobolus. It is characterized by extensive inflammation and vascular thrombi caused by mycelia invading blood vessels.

It occurs in patients with immunodeficiency including that associated with debilitating diseases. The mycelia are nonseptate, wider, and vary more in width than those of *Aspergillus*. They exhibit obtuse branching (90°) (Fig. 6.12). The organisms are difficult to culture.

Candidiasis

Since *Candida* species are saprophytic inhabitants of skin and oral cavity, the presence of Candida in sputum must be evaluated carefully before concluding that this fungus is the causative agent of lung disease. The clinical background and, more specifically, identification of the organism in pulmonary tissue are of importance. The presence of the organism in a fine needle aspirate is highly suggestive of invasive candidiasis.

In smears, the organisms appear as aggregates of long, slender pseudohyphae with budding yeasts (Fig. 6.13).

Pneumocystis Pneumonia

Pneumocystis carinii is a ubiquitous opportunistic organism, which is probably classifiable as a fungus.

Pneumocystis pneumonia occurs in immunosuppressed adults, especially AIDS patients, and malnourished children.

An x-ray examination shows hilar shadows expanding to the periphery often simulating the adult respiratory distress syndrome.

Histologically, the alveolar spaces are filled by foamy, amorphous, eosinophilic material comprising proliferating parasites and cell debris. The septae are widened by a mild interstitial inflammatory reaction (Fig. 6.14A).

Bronchoalveolar lavage (BAL), bronchial washings, or bronchial brushings are most suitable for detecting the organism. Sputum may be used but is not as valuable as the other specimens. Other concurrent opportunistic infectious agents should also be looked for. No reliable culture or antigenic detection method for this organism is yet available.

Papanicolaou-stained smears show foamy eosinophilic exudate, a highly diagnostic feature (Fig. 6.14B). Special stains such as Gram-Weigert, methenamine silver, or toluidine blue demonstrate small, round, or cup-shaped cystic structures about the size of a red blood cell (Fig. 6.14C).

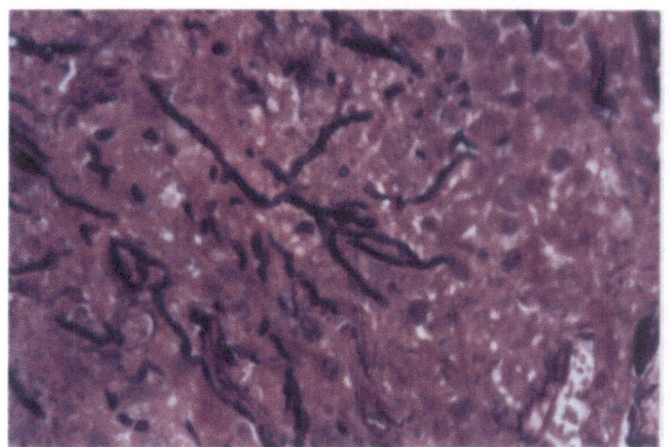

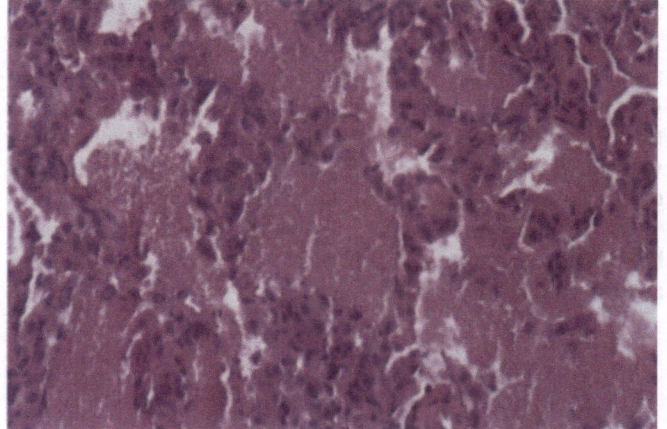

FIGURE 6.11   Aspergillosis. Biopsy sections showing thin septate mycelia with 45° branching (silver stain).

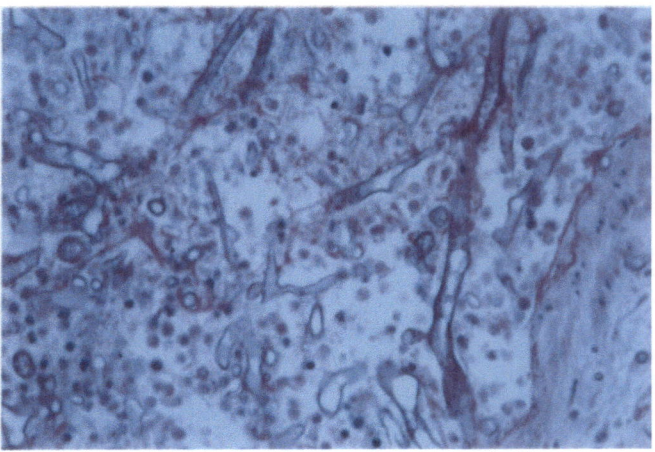

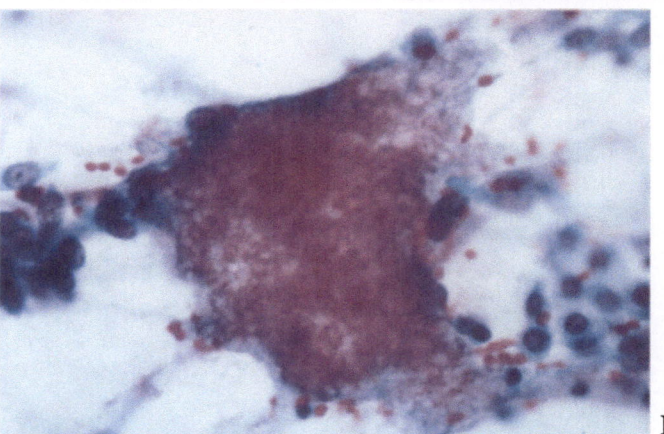

FIGURE 6.12   Phycomycosis. Biopsy section showing irregular empty-looking nonseptate hyphae with wide-angle branching. Blood vessel invasion is present (lower right corner) (silver stain).

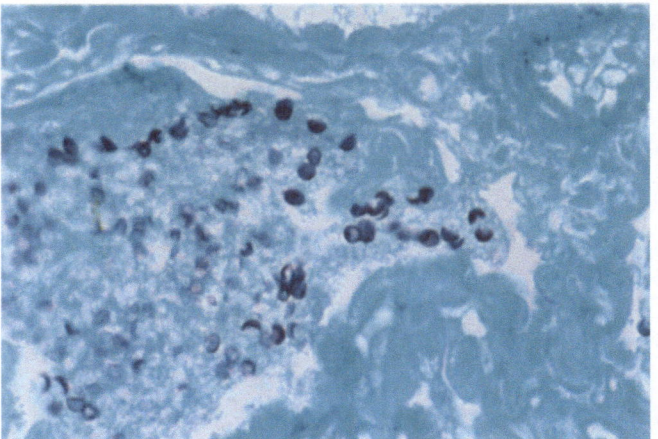

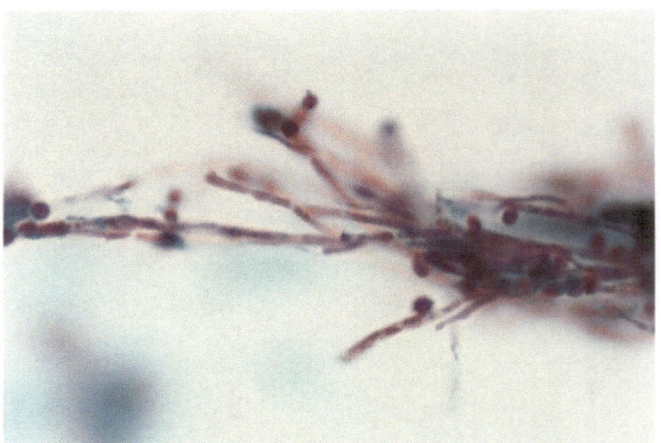

FIGURE 6.14   Pneumocystis carinii. A: Inflammatory thickening of septa and amorphous material in the alveolar spaces. **B:** Sputum smear showing foamy eosinophilic exudate (Papanicolaou stain). **C:** Bronchial lavage smear showing small round or cup-shaped cystic structures (size of red blood cells) (silver stain).

FIGURE 6.13   Candidiasis. Nonbranching pseudohyphae and yeast forms (sputum smear with Papanicolaou stain).

Actinomycosis

All infections with Actinomycetes are derived endogenously and there is no person-to-person spread. The three classic forms of actinomycosis are cervicofacial, abdominal, and thoracic. Thoracic actinomycosis causes lung abscesses, which may result in pulmonopleural fistula or empyema. The usual causative agent is *Actinomyces israelii*.

Cytology smears or tissue sections show colonies with basophilic centers surrounded by eosinophilic radially arranged filament ("sulfur granules") (Fig. 6.15).

Viral Infections

With the increasing number of immunocompromised patients, including AIDS patients, viral infections of the respiratory tract are also increasing in number.

Since certain viruses may be detected in the respiratory tract in apparently healthy persons, careful consideration of all of the related circumstances should be given before concluding that a respiratory disease is caused by viral infection.

Bronchoalveolar lavage, bronchial washings, and sputum or transthoracic FNA can provide suitable cell material for evaluation.

Figure 6.16 illustrates the cytologic features of the two most commonly detected respiratory viral diseases in cytologic preparations. These features are specific enough to initiate treatment. Cytologic diagnoses of viral diseases may be corroborated by culture, deoxyribonucleic acid (DNA) probes, or immunocytochemistry.

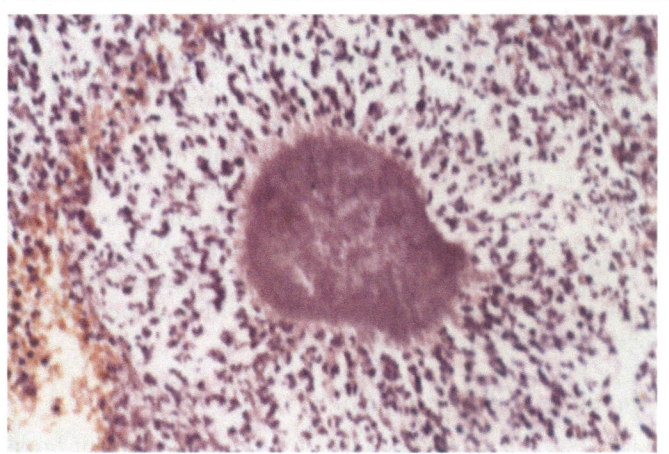

FIGURE 6.15   Actinomycosis. Aspirate smear showing colonies surrounded by eosinophilic radially arranged filaments ("sulfur granules").

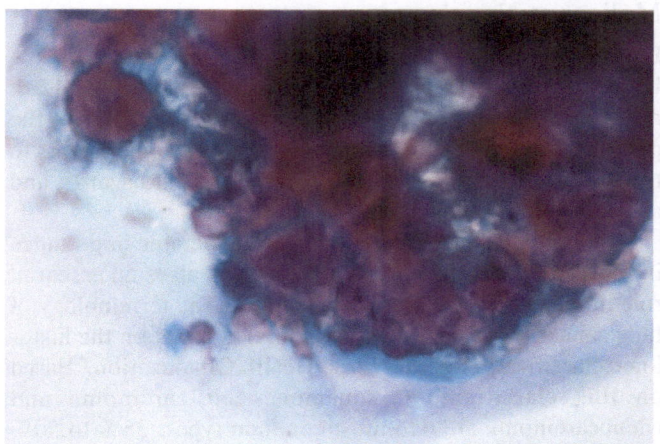

A

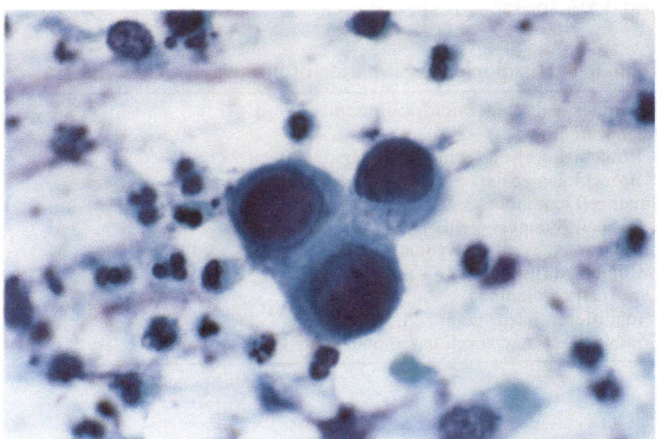

B

FIGURE 6.16   Viral infection. A: Herpes virus simplex. Bronchial lavage smear showing multinuclear herpes giant cells, "ground-glass appearance" (Papanicolaou stain). **B**: Cytomegalovirus. Bronchial lavage smear showing enlarged cells with large basophilic intranuclear inclusion surround by a clear space (Papanicolaou stain).

Malignant Neoplasms

Lung cancer is the leading cause of cancer deaths in the United States and Western countries. The age-adjusted death rate from lung cancer has been increasing steadily over the past decades, with the major contributing etiologic factors to the increase being tobacco smoking, industrial hazards, and air pollution.

Consequently, lung cancers are of considerable importance in modern medical practice, and cytology plays an essential role in their diagnosis and management. The terminology of lung cancer (bronchogenic carcinoma) is based on the histologic classification of the World Health Organization.[6] Based on this classification, squamous cell carcinoma and adenocarcinoma are two most common types, 35% to 50% and 15% to 35%, respectively.[7]

Table 6.1. Histologic classification of bronchogenic carcinoma.

Squamous cell (epidermoid) carcinoma
Adenocarcinoma
   Bronchial derived (acinar, papillary, solid)
   Bronchioloalveolar
Small cell carcinoma
   Oat cell (lymphocytelike)
   Intermediate cell (polygonal)
   Combined (usually with squamous)
Large cell carcinoma
   (undifferentiated, giant cell, clear cell)
Combined squamous cell carcinoma and adenocarcinoma

Clinical Course

Squamous cell carcinoma and adenocarcinoma have a better overall 5-year survival rate (10%) compared with small cell anaplastic carcinomas (3%). Unfortunately, most lung cancers are advanced at the time of detection, with fewer than 20% being resectable.[8,9] The common presenting complaints are cough, weight loss, chest pain, and dyspnea.

Based on the clinical presentation and radiologic examination of the chest, cytologic examination of sputum, bronchial washings or brushings, or transthoracic FNA is the principal method of diagnostic confirmation.

Squamous Cell Carcinoma

Squamous cell carcinoma tends to occur in the major bronchi, appearing on radiographs of the chest as central or hilar masses (Fig. 6.17A). Usually they exfoliate large numbers of tumor cells.

These centrally located bronchogenic carcinomas present as pale gray-yellow exophytic excrescences on the bronchial mucosa and may ultimately completely obstruct the lumen (Fig. 6.17B).

Cytology

In sputum smears, the cells tend to occur singly and in loose aggregates. Cells from well differentiated squamous carcinoma are usually pleomorphic and have abundant orangeophilic cytoplasm. The nuclei are pleomorphic and hyperchromatic, with coarse chromatin clumps. Macronucleoli are not frequent but may be conspicuous (Fig. 6.18).

(Discussion continued on p. 76)

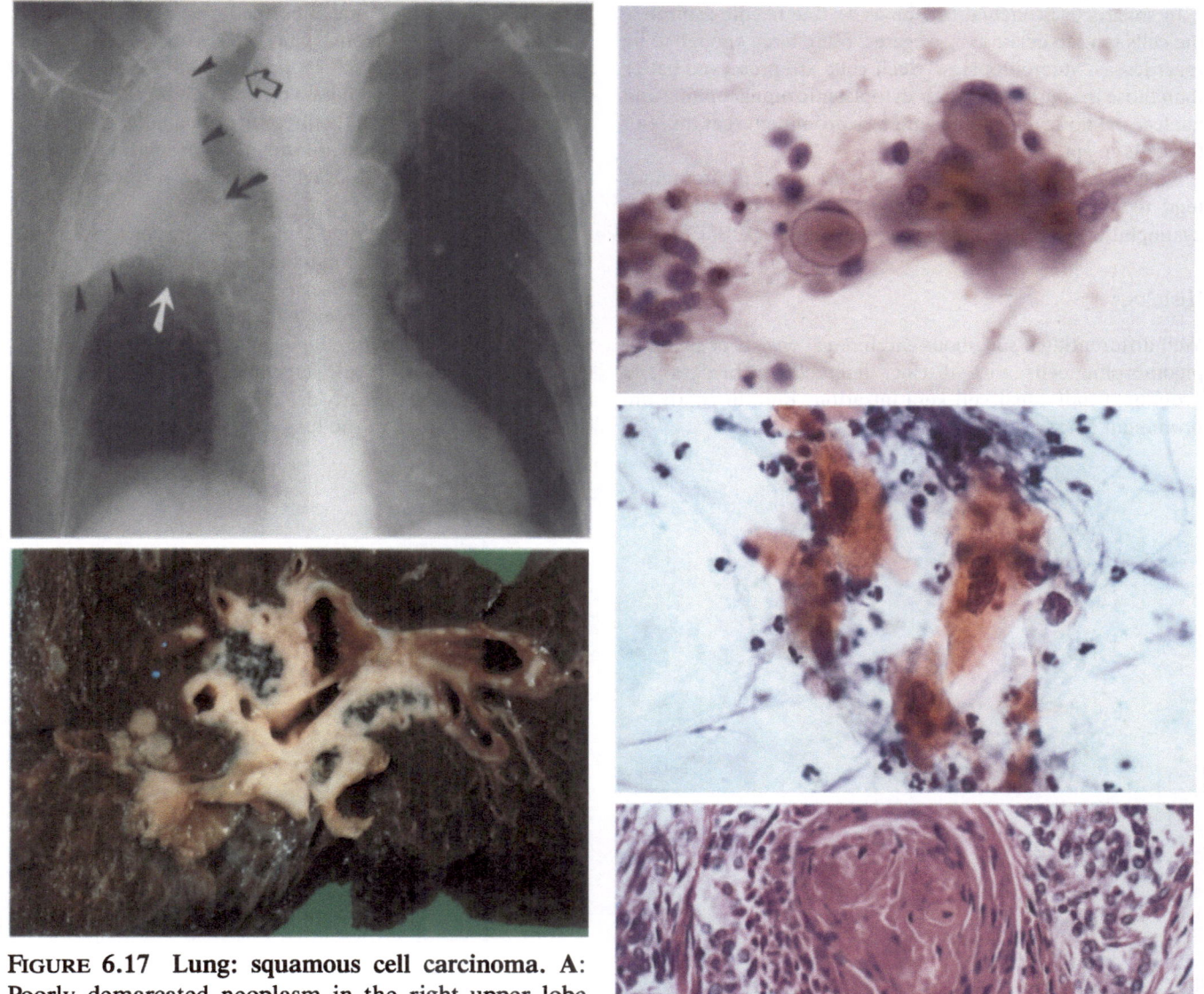

FIGURE 6.17 Lung: squamous cell carcinoma. A:
Poorly demarcated neoplasm in the right upper lobe
(*black and white arrows*) with obstruction of the bronchus causing atelectasis (*arrowheads*). Trachea (*open
arrow*) is deviated to the right because of lung volume
loss. **B**: Resected lung showing the neoplasm involving
the lower lobe bronchus, with luminal narrowing.

**FIGURE 6.18 Lung: well differentiated squamous
cell carcinoma. A:** Loose aggregates of carcinoma
cells. Squamous pearl formation is present. The cells
forming the pearl have orangeophilic cytoplasm (sputum). **B**: Pleomorphic tumor cells occurring singly.
They have abundant orangeophilic cytoplasm, suggestive of cavitating squamous cell carcinoma (sputum).
C: Histologic section showing keratin pearl formation.

In smears of bronchial brushings or fine needle aspirates, the cells tend to occur in aggregates, often large enough to be regarded as "microbiopsies." Such cells are preserved better than those in sputum and their cytoplasmic orangeophilia and nuclear pyknotic appearance are less prominent that those of the cells in sputum (Fig. 6.19A).

Cells from poorly differentiated squamous cell carcinomas tend to occur in aggregates. Their cytoplasm tends to be cyanophilic and to have sharp borders (Fig. 6.19B, C).

Histology

Well differentiated squamous carcinoma consists of sheets of pleomorphic cells with distinct intercellular bridges and prominent individual cell keratinization. Keratin pearls are prominent (Fig. 6.18C).

Poorly differentiated squamous cell carcinoma consists of sheets and cords of pleomorphic cells with less prominent intercellular bridges and individual cell keratinization. Cytoplasm of the cells tends to be cyanophilic (Fig. 6.19D).

A number of reports in the literature documented the cytologic manifestations of severe squamous dysplasia and squamous cell carcinoma in situ in the lower respiratory tract (Fig. 6.20).[10-12]

A Cooperative Early Lung Cancer Group sponsored by the National Cancer Institute demonstrated the cytologic detection of 98 in situ or early invasive squamous cell carcinomas in a group of asymptomatic men of 45 years of age or older who had an increased risk of developing lung cancer. The investigators concluded that cytologic screening of such high-risk populations is of value in the early detection of lung cancers and the consequent reduction of the lung cancer death rate.[13,14]

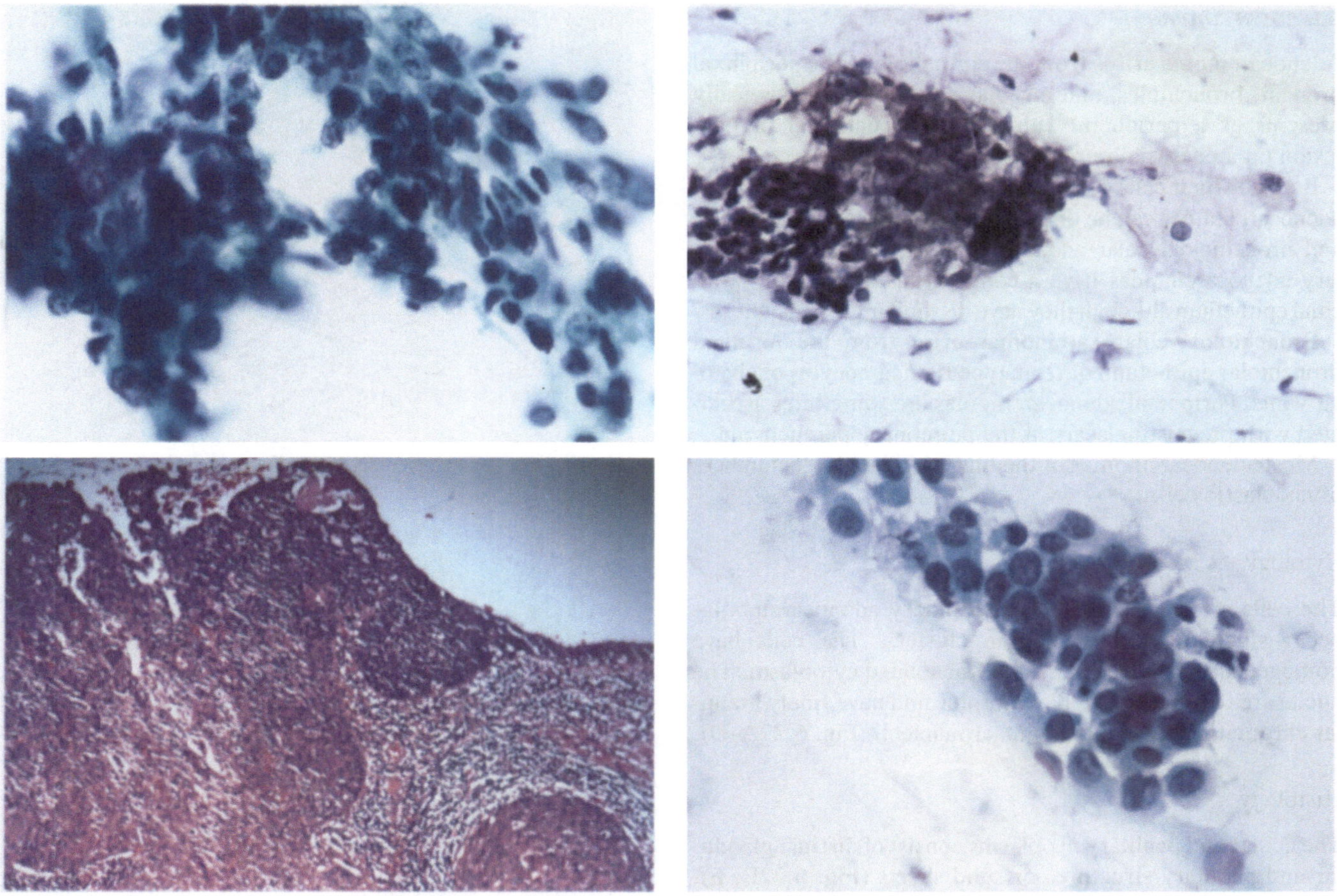

FIGURE 6.19 Lung: poorly differentiated squamous cell carcinoma. A: Syncytial aggregates of pleomorphic tumor cells with cyanophilic cytoplasm and large hyperchromatic nuclei (bronchial washing). **B**: Syncytial aggregate of pleomorphic cells. **C**: Syncytial aggregate of pleomorphic cells and normal squamous cells (sputum). **D**: Histologic section taken at the site of origin of the carcinoma.

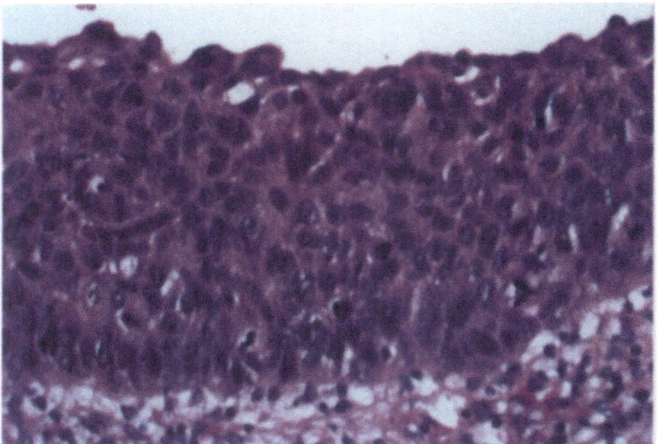

FIGURE 6.20 Carcinoma in situ of bronchus. Primitive atypical cells confined to the bronchial epithelium (bronchoscopic biopsy).

Adenocarcinoma

Adenocarcinoma arises from the epithelium of the peripheral bronchi, bronchioles, and alveolar epithelium and typically presents as a peripheral pulmonary parenchymal or coin lesion on a chest radiogram (Fig. 6.21).

Based on their cells of origin and growth pattern, pulmonary adenocarcinomas can be divided further into acinar, papillary, and bronchioloalveolar adenocarcinomas. Acinar and papillary adenocarcinomas have a common histogenesis in bronchial epithelium although they have dissimilar growth patterns.

Bronchioloalveolar carcinomas arise from the terminal bronchiolar epithelium or from type II pneumocytes of alveolar walls. Peripheral adenocarcinomas are sometimes associated with preexisting scars of the pulmonary parenchyma.

Most adenocarcinomas of the lung exfoliate large numbers of neoplastic cells.

Cytology

The cells arisen from acinar or papillary adenocarcinomas occur singly, in sheets, and in clusters. The cells have homogeneous, granular, or finely vacuolated cytoplasm. The nuclei are round, oval, or pleomorphic and have finely granular chromatin and prominent macronucleoli (Fig. 6.22A–D).

Histology

The acinar and papillary neoplasms consist of distinct glandular and papillary structures or solid sheets (Fig. 6.22E, F). Eighty percent of lung adenocarcinomas contain mucin. (*Discussion continued on p. 80*)

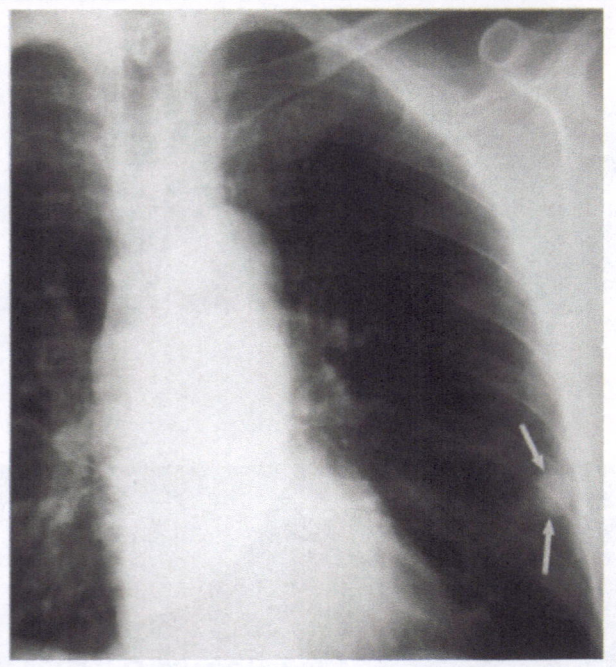

A

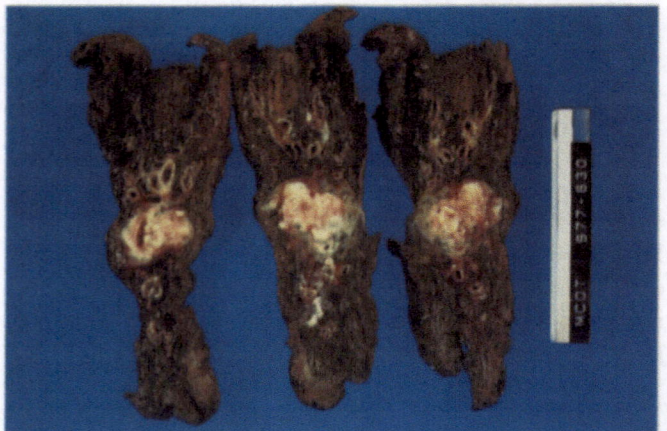

B

FIGURE 6.21 **Lung: adenocarcinoma. A**: Well circumscribed lesion in the left lower lobe (chest x ray). **B**: Resected specimen showing well circumscribed peripheral carcinoma.

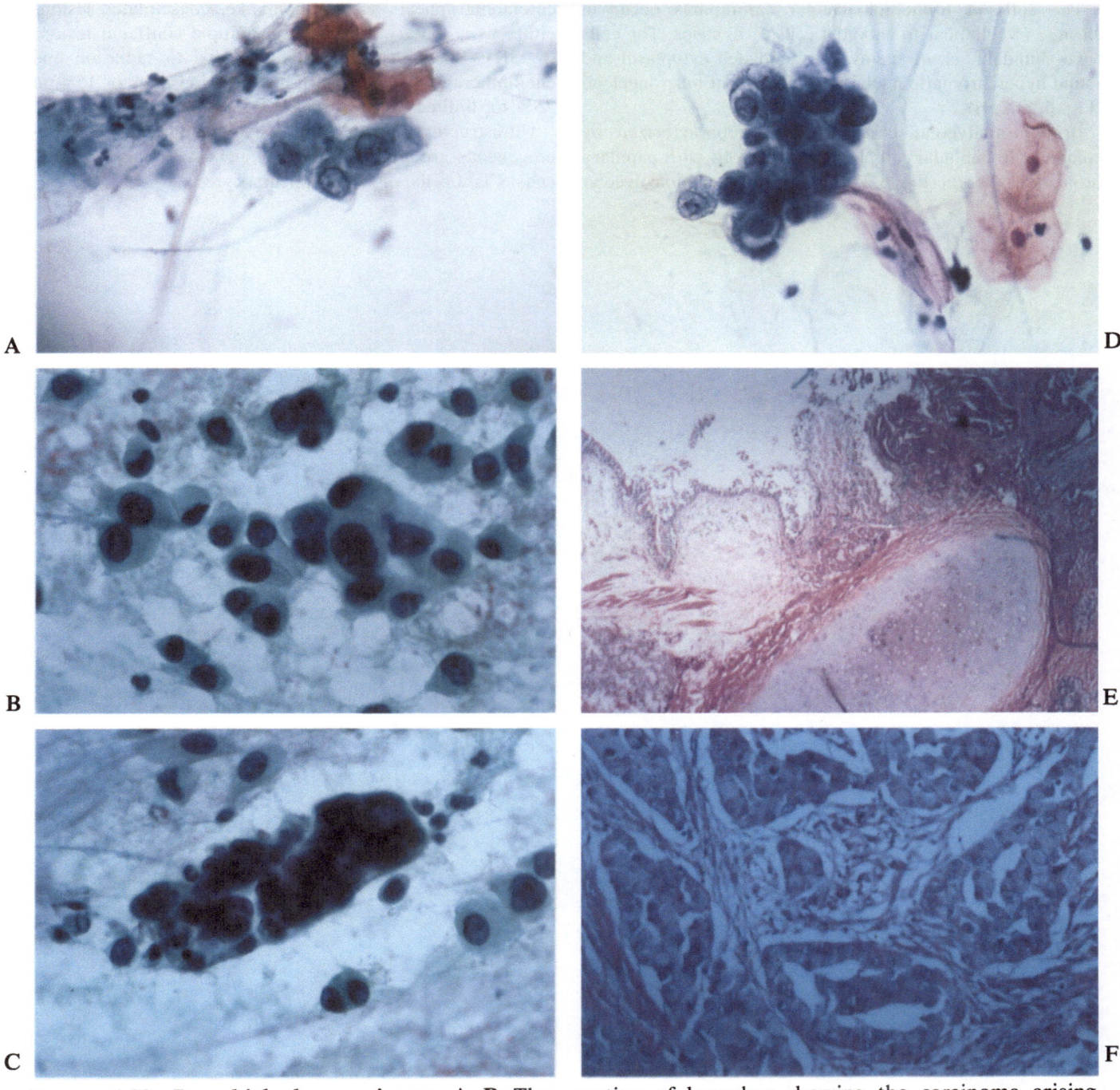

FIGURE 6.22   Bronchial adenocarcinoma. A, B: The carcinoma cells occur in loose aggregates with evidence of acinar formation. C, D: The carcinoma cells occurring in clusters and papillary formation. E: Histologic section of bronchus showing the carcinoma arising from the mucosa. F: The tumor comprising well formed acinar structures.

The cells of bronchioloalveolar carcinomas occur in clusters of columnar-to-cuboidal cells or in strips. The cells have abundant, clear, foamy, or vacuolated cytoplasm and round hyperchromatic nuclei with prominent macronucleoli (Fig. 6.23A, B).

Bronchioloalveolar carcinomas are characterized by columnar-to-cuboidal cells lining the alveoli, with papillary projections therein (Fig. 6.23C). Grossly, bronchioloalveolar carcinoma appears as pneumonialike, consolidated lesions either as a solitary lesion or as multiple confluent lesions (6.23D). Since this cancer is sensitive to radiation and chemotherapy, potential cure or remission rates of 15% to 25% for limited disease have been reported.

Ultrastructurally, bronchioloalveolar carcinomas are a heterogeneous group, derived from mucin-secreting bronchial cells, Clara cells, or type II pneumocytes.

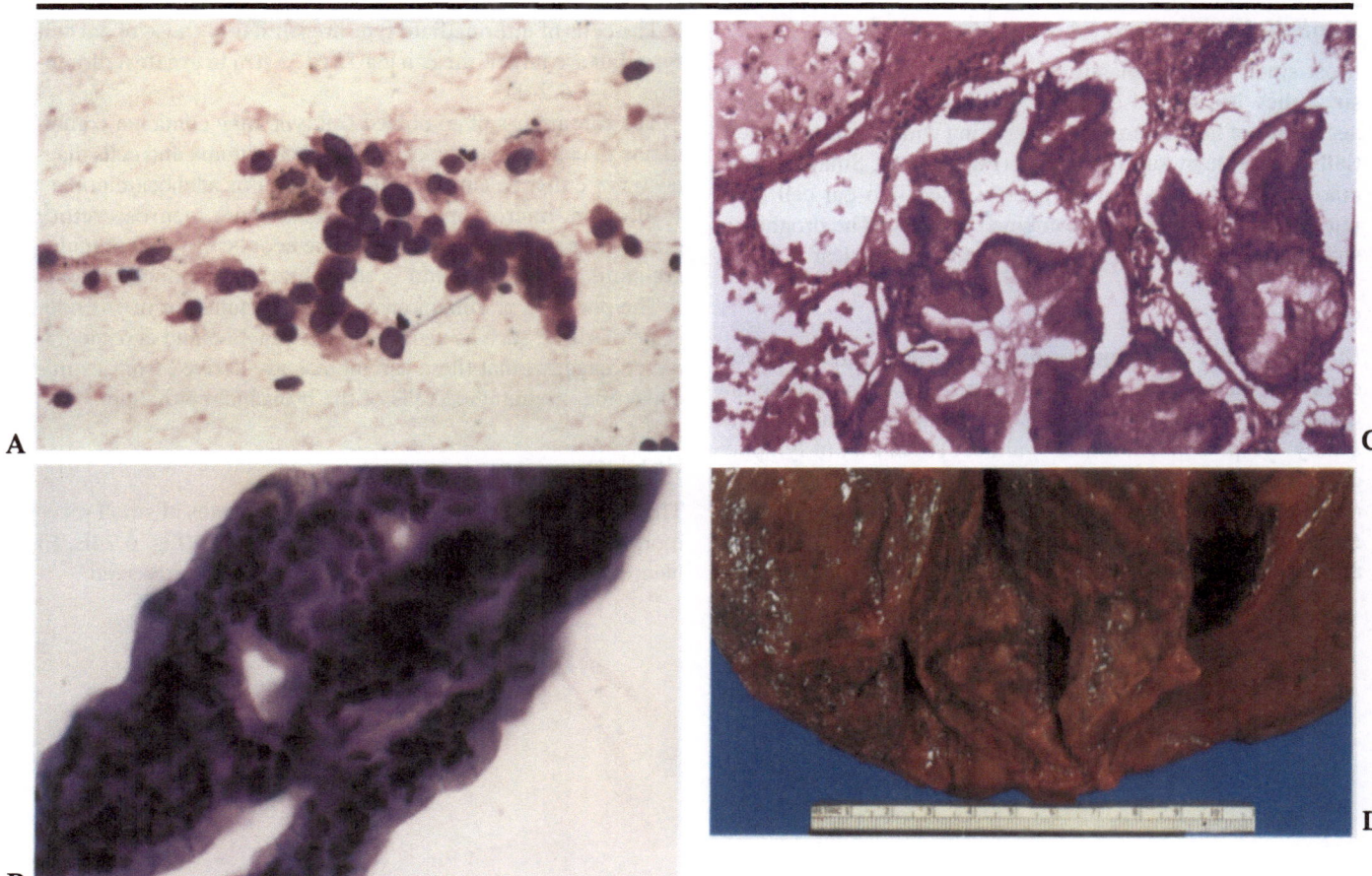

FIGURE 6.23 Bronchioloalveolar carcinoma. A: Tumor cells occurring in clusters and strips (FNA). **B:** Papillary structures covered by mucin-secreting colum-nar cells. **C:** Histologic section showing the carcinoma growing along the alveolar and bronchiolar walls. **D:** Confluent consolidated lesions in the periphery of the lung (necropsy).

Small Cell (anaplastic) Carcinoma

Most small cell (anaplastic) carcinomas are central or hilar, since they usually arise in large bronchi. They are the most aggressive of lung tumors, metastasizing widely, and are essentially incurable by surgical means (Fig. 6.24A). Small cell carcinomas of the lung may be subclassified into oat cell type, intermediate cell type, and combined cell type. The prognostic significance of the subclassification remains unclear.

Cytology

Most small cell carcinomas exfoliate a large number of tumor cells in sputum (Fig. 6.24B). The cells of oat cell type are dominated by round, oval, or spindle-shaped nuclei with scanty cytoplasm. Their size is almost twice that of lymphocytes, measuring 10 to 15 µm in greatest dimension. The cells occur in loose aggregates and in clusters, with prominent nuclear molding. The nuclei are hyperchromatic with coarse chromatin clumps; nucleoli are inconspicuous (Fig. 6.24C).

The cells of intermediate type are similar to those of oat cell type, but are larger, measuring 15 to 25 µm in greatest dimension (Fig. 6.24D).

The carcinomas of combined cell type may contain a combination of cells diagnostic of small cell carcinoma and cells diagnostic of either squamous cell carcinoma or adenocarcinoma.

Electron microscopy shows dense core neurosecretory granules in some of the cells of these neoplasms. The granules are similar to those found in the other neuroendocrine cells.

The presence of immunohistochemical stains for neuroendocrine markers, such as neuron-specific enolase and chromogranin A, suggests that these carcinomas are derived from neuroendocrine-programmed cells of the bronchial epithelium.

Histology

The neoplasms consist of sheets and aggregates of small pleomorphic cells with very little visible cytoplasm. (Fig. 6.24E, F) Necrosis and nuclear crush artefact are frequently seen.

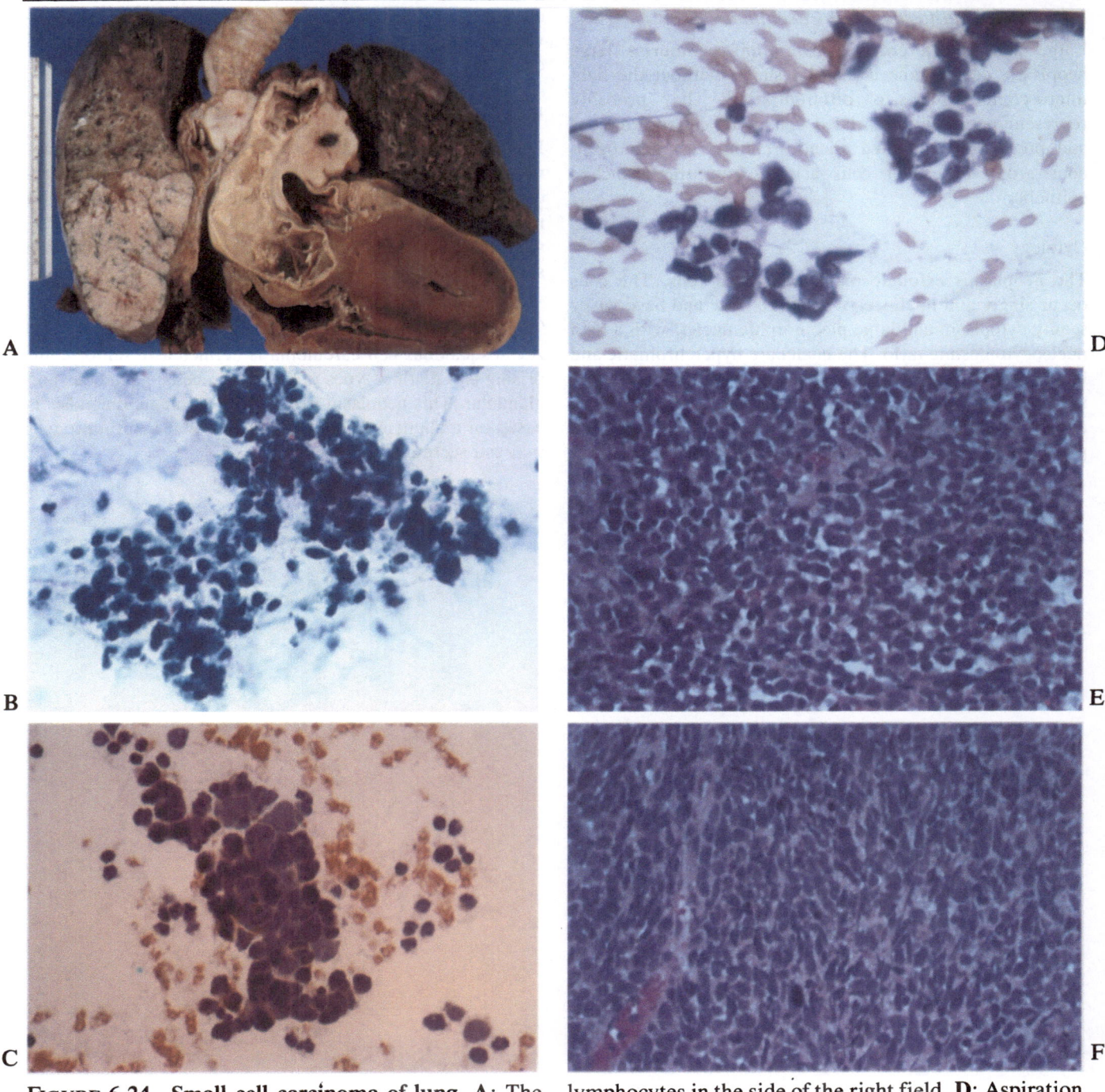

FIGURE 6.24 Small cell carcinoma of lung. A: The carcinoma involving the right lower lobe with metastasis to the mediastinal nodes (necropsy). B: The carcinoma cells in sputum showing nuclear degeneration and crushing artifact. C: Aspiration smear showing small carcinoma cells with characteristic nuclear molding (oat cell type). Tumor cells are much larger than the lymphocytes in the side of the right field. D: Aspiration smear showing polygonal to spindle-shaped carcinoma cells, larger than those of oat cell type (intermediate cell type). E: Bronchoscopic biopsy section showing sheets of carcinoma cells (oat cell type). F: Bronchoscopic biopsy sections showing sheets of spindle-shaped cells (intermediate type).

Large Cell Undifferentiated Carcinoma

Large cell undifferentiated carcinomas comprise large neoplastic cells arranged in solid sheets without the light microscopic features of differentiation. They probably represent poorly differentiated squamous cell carcinomas and poorly differentiated adenocarcinomas, a heterogeneous group of cancer cells arising from the bronchial epithelium.

Cytology

The neoplasms exfoliate many neoplastic cells. The cells occur singly and in clusters. They are large and have wispy scanty cytoplasm and large pleomorphic nuclei, with a high nucleocytoplasmic ratio. The nuclei are hyperchromatic and have irregularly dispersed chromatin and prominent macronucleoli (Fig. 6.25A). It may be difficult to classify large anaplastic cells correctly, since they may be derived from poorly differentiated squamous cell carcinoma or adeno-carcinoma, or large cell undifferentiated carcinoma. For convenience, such neoplasms may be designated as "Non-small cell carcinoma" of the lung.

Histology

Large cell undifferentiated carcinomas consist of large pleomorphic cells arranged in solid sheets. Mitotic figures are frequently observed (Fig. 6.25B). Some of these tumors exhibit many multinucleate tumor giant cells (giant cell carcinoma), some have clear cells (clear cell carcinoma), and some have spindle cell features (spindle cell carcinoma).

Adenosquamous Carcinoma

Adenosquamous cell carcinoma is defined as a tumor comprising two distinct types of neoplastic cells: squamous and glandular. This neoplasm is rare. The cytologic diagnosis is based on malignant tumor cells that exhibit keratin production and secretory activity.

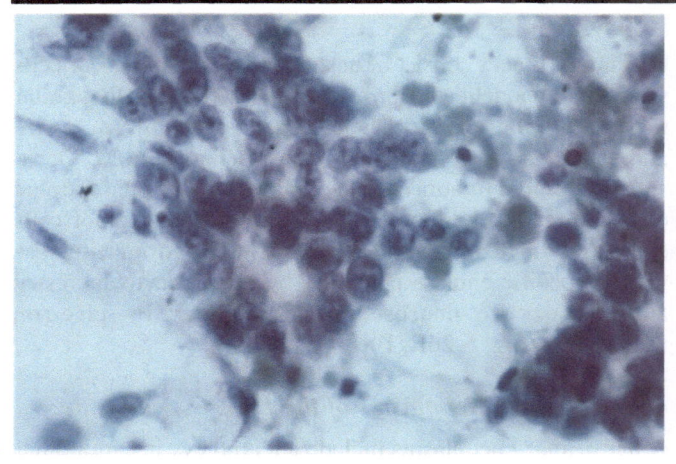

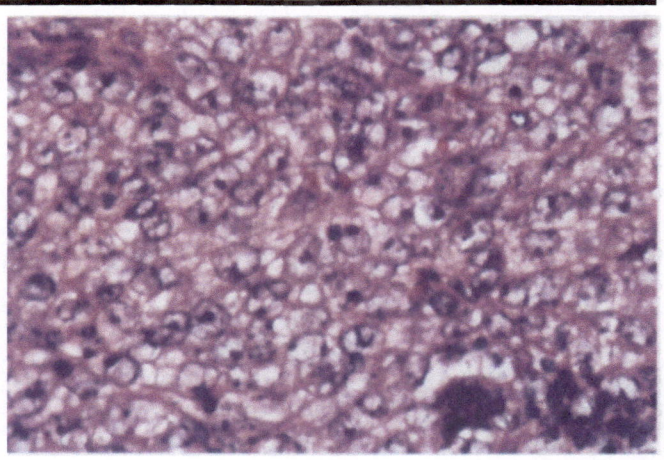

FIGURE 6.25   Large cell undifferentiated carcinoma of lung. A: Aspiration smear showing clusters and syncytial aggregates of carcinoma cells with scanty cytoplasm and pleomorphic nuclei. **B**: Histologic sections showing solid sheets of large pleomorphic cells.

Carcinoid Tumor (Bronchial Carcinoid)

Carcinoid tumors of lung represent 1% to 2% of all lung tumors.[15] Bronchial carcinoids show the neuroendocrine differentiation of the Kulchitsky cells of bronchial mucosa. Most patients with bronchial carcinoids are under 40 years of age.

The clinical manifestations of bronchial carcinoids are cough and hemoptysis; these are caused by bronchial luminal obstruction, which results in atelectasis and pneumonitis.

Bronchial carcinoids are slowly growing but may ultimately metastasize to regional lymph nodes or to the liver. Most of these tumors are resectable and curable. So-called atypical carcinoids tend to be more aggressive.[16]

Ten percent of bronchial carcinoids occur peripherally and present as peripheral coin lesions (Fig. 6.26A). The carcinoid syndrome occurs rarely with bronchial carcinoids.[17]

Cytology

Since bronchial carcinoids occur usually in the bronchial submucosal glands, their cells are rarely found in sputum specimens or bronchial washings and brushings.

Fine needle aspirates from peripheral carcinoids exhibit oval to spindle-shaped cells in aggregates or in rosette forms, in distinction to adenocarcinoma or small cell carcinomas (Fig. 6.26B, C).[18] The cells have scanty pale cytoplasm and round, oval, or spindle-shaped nuclei with bland nuclear chromatin and prominent nucleoli.

Histology

Carcinoid tumors consist of nests, cords, and masses of cells separated by a delicate fibrous stroma, histologically similar to those of other organs. The cells are fairly uniform in size and shape and have scanty cytoplasm (Fig. 6.26D). Occasional carcinoid tumors consist of more atypical pleomorphic cells and tend to be more aggressive. Carcinoid tumor cells exhibit all the features of neuroendocrine cell origin, such as neuron-specific enolase positivity by immunocytochemistry and dense core neurosecretory granules by electron microscopy (Fig. 6.26E, F).

Other Primary Neoplasms of the Lung

Other primary neoplasms include adenoid cystic carcinoma, mucoepidermoid carcinoma, pulmonary blastoma, Hodgkin's and non-Hodgkin's lymphoma, and various other sarcomas.

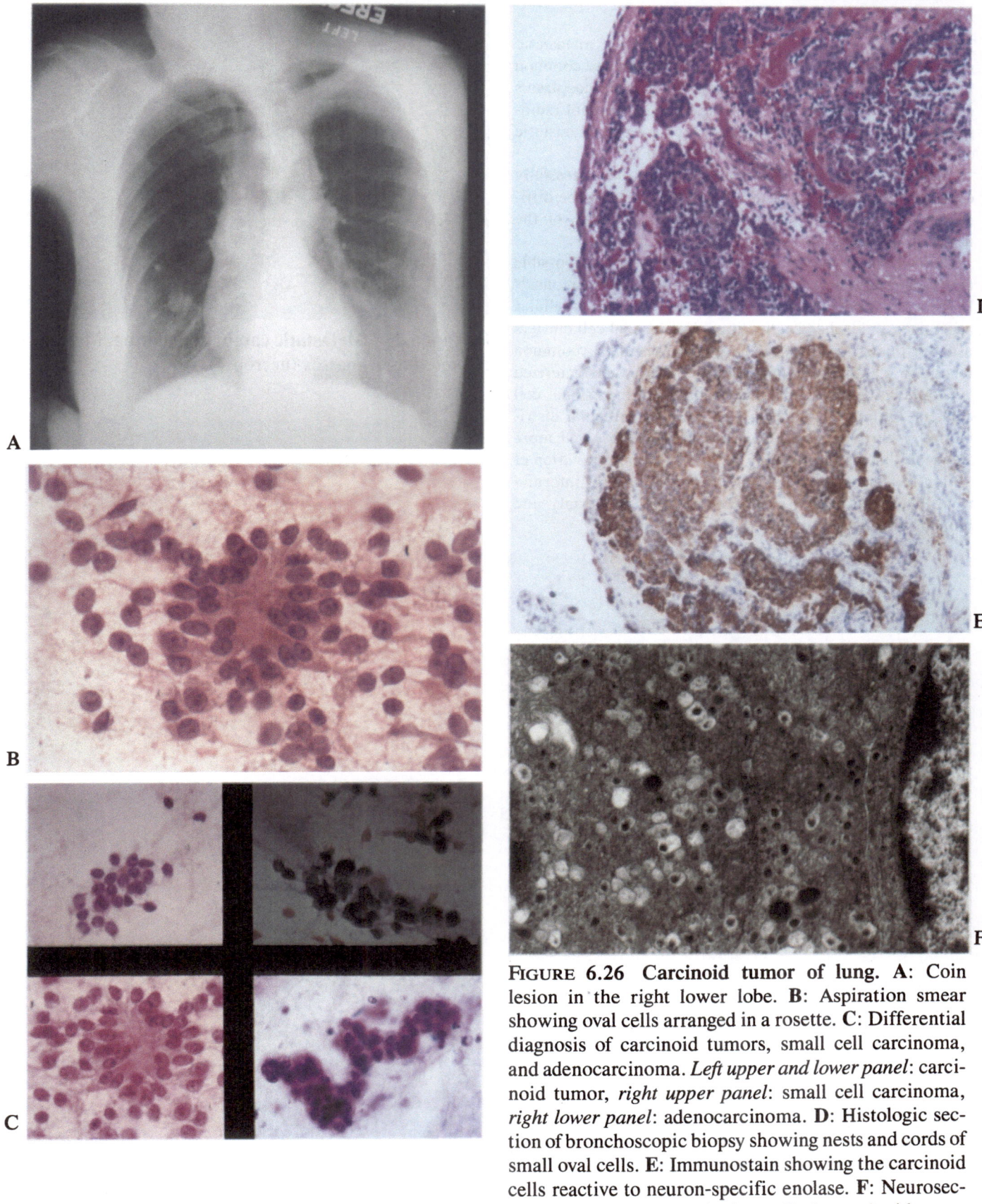

FIGURE 6.26 Carcinoid tumor of lung. A: Coin lesion in the right lower lobe. B: Aspiration smear showing oval cells arranged in a rosette. C: Differential diagnosis of carcinoid tumors, small cell carcinoma, and adenocarcinoma. *Left upper and lower panel*: carcinoid tumor, *right upper panel*: small cell carcinoma, *right lower panel*: adenocarcinoma. D: Histologic section of bronchoscopic biopsy showing nests and cords of small oval cells. E: Immunostain showing the carcinoid cells reactive to neuron-specific enolase. F: Neurosecretory dense core granules in a cell of a carcinoid tumor (EM).

Metastatic Cancers to the Lung

The lung is a common site of a wide variety of metastatic neoplasms. In fact, metastatic neoplasms are more common than primary neoplasms in the lung. Metastatic neoplasms usually involve the periphery of the lung and present radiographically as solitary or multiple discrete lesions. Metastatic deposits tend to be discrete and multiple (Fig. 6.27).

Most metastatic neoplasms in the lung may be successfully diagnosed by transthoracic FNA. However, it may be difficult or impossible to identify the primary source of the neoplasm on objective cytologic features alone.

On the basis of cytologic characteristics, it may be possible to distinguish primary lung cancer from metastatic sarcoma.[19] In general, sarcomas are characterized by loose cellular aggregates and isolated cells; three-dimensional cell clusters usually are not present. Cellular pleomorphism is a common feature (Fig. 6.28). In contrast, carcinomas are characterized by cohesive cellular aggregates and three-dimensional cell clusters. Cellular pleomorphism is variable. Irregular distribution of chromatin and macronucleoli are observed more frequently in carcinomas (Fig. 6.29).[19] The interpretation of aspiration smears is greatly facilitated by clinical information, chest radiograms, review of prior material, and immunocytochemistry.

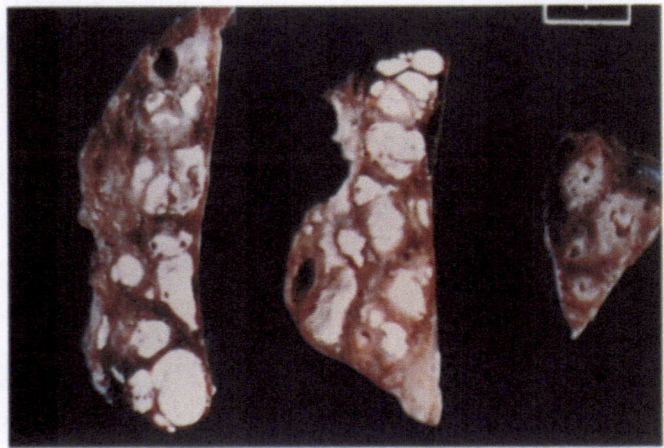

FIGURE 6.27   Metastatic carcinoma of lung. Multiple discrete tumor masses (necropsy).

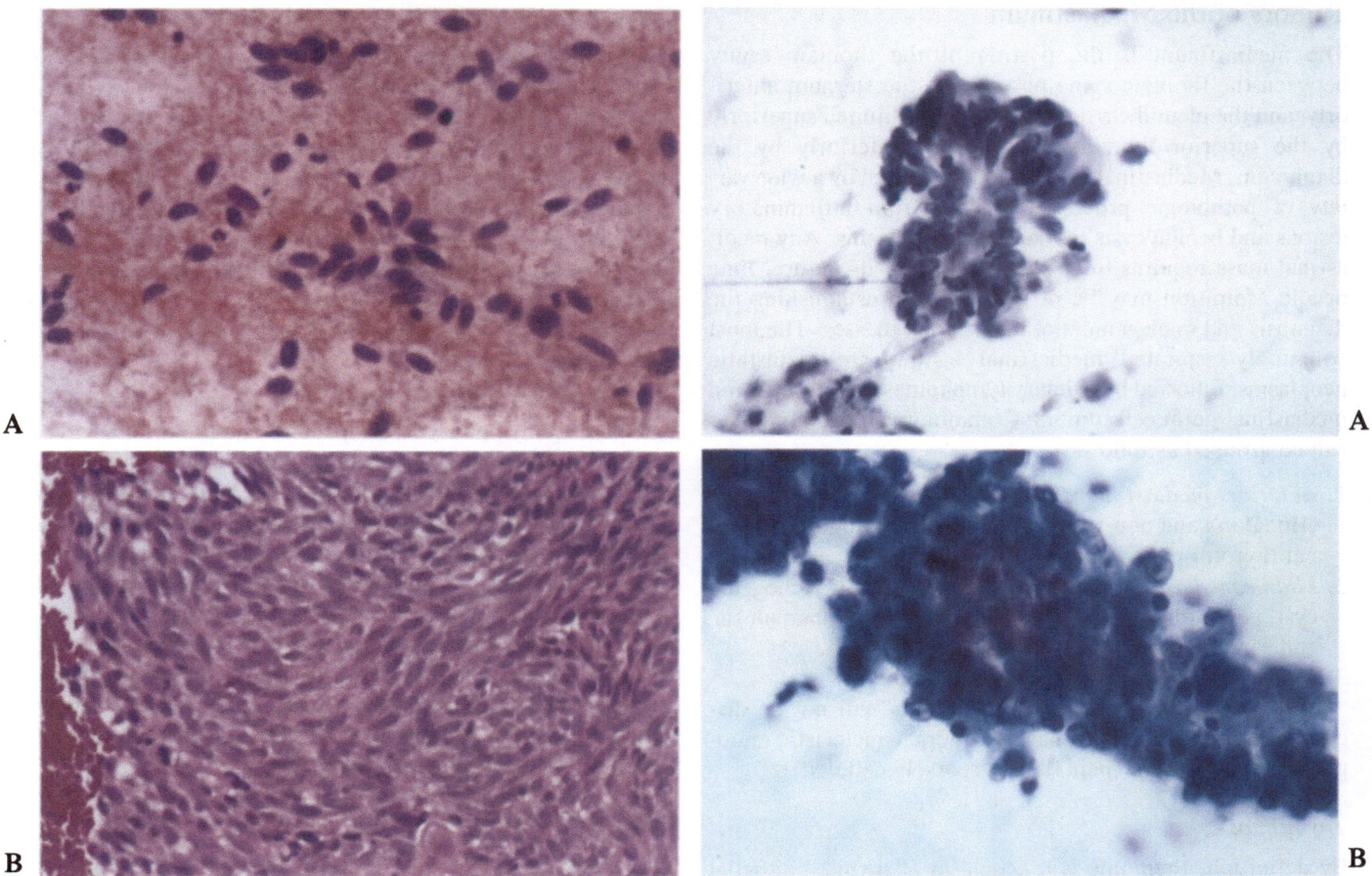

FIGURE 6.28 Metastatic sarcoma to the lung. A: Pleomorphic and spindle-shaped sarcoma cells occurring in loose aggregates and singly (aspirate). **B:** Histologic section of the sarcoma showing interlacing bundles of spindle cells.

FIGURE 6.29 Metastatic adenocarcinoma in the lung (aspirate). A, B: Carcinoma cells occurring in an acinar pattern and in clusters.

Tumors of the Mediastinum

The mediastinum is the portion of the thoracic cavity between the thoracic spine posteriorly, the sternum anteriorly, and the pleural cavities laterally. It is limited superiorly by the superior thoracic aperture and inferiorly by the diaphragm. Mediastinal masses may be caused by a wide variety of pathologic processes ranging from inflammatory lesions and benign cysts to malignant neoplasms. Any mediastinal mass requires to be identified as to its nature. Fine needle aspiration may be of great help in establishing the diagnosis and management of mediastinal masses. The most commonly aspirated mediastinal lesions are metastatic neoplasms, followed by primary lymphomas, thymomas, and mediastinal germ cell tumors. Common mediastinal masses can be grouped as follows:

1. *Anterior mediastinum*: thymoma, thymic lymphoma (Hodgkin's and non-Hodgkin's), germ cell tumor, substernal thyroid, pericardial cyst, and metastatic carcinoma.
2. *Middle mediastinum*: malignant lymphoma, bronchogenic cyst, pericardial cyst, metastatic carcinoma, tuberculosis, and sarcoidosis.
3. *Posterior mediastinum*: neurogenic tumor.

Cystic and other non-neoplastic lesions will not be discussed here. Cystic lesions have a rather characteristic radiographic appearance. Their fluid is sparsely cellular.

Thymoma

By definition, thymoma is a neoplasm of thymic epithelial cells, and may include various proportions of normal lymphocytes. These tumors may be associated with myasthenia gravis, hypogammaglobulinemia, or erythroid hypoplasia.

About 90% of thymomas are benign. Lymphocytes are almost always present in various proportions; however, they are not neoplastic.

About 10% of thymomas are malignant. Determination of their malignancy is based entirely on evidence of local invasion beyond the capsule or the presence of lymphatic or hematogenous spread by metastasis.

Grossly, all thymomas are lobulated and encapsulated, pale yellow masses, ranging from 1 to 20 cm in greatest dimension (Fig. 6.30A).

Cytology

In aspiration smears, the cells occur in loose aggregates and singly. They are highly variable in size and shape with scanty and poorly defined cytoplasm. The nuclei vary in size and shape and are round, oval, spindle-shaped, or irregularly shaped. Nuclear chromatin is usually delicate and finely granular. Coarse chromatin clumps and macronucleoli are rarely observed. Various proportions of mature benign lymphocytes are almost always mixed with the neoplastic cells (Fig. 6.30B).

Histology

The histologic features vary depending on the proportions of epithelial and lymphocytic components and the cytologic features of the epithelial component (Fig. 6.30C, D). Thymomas with a small number of small epithelial cells and abundant lymphocytes should be distinguished from lymphomas. Cells from lymphomas occur singly and are monomorphic. Thymoma with abundant large epithelial cells and a scanty amount of lymphocytes should be distinguished from metastatic carcinoma. The cells from carcinomas usually occur in cohesive clusters and the nuclear chromatin displays coarse, irregularly dispersed clumps. Neoplastic thymic epithelial cells show tonofilaments and desmosomes by electron microscopy and keratin by immunohistochemistry (Fig. 6.30E, F).

Clinical Course

The clinical presentation is variable. Some patients are asymptomatic and are discovered to have thymoma incidentally on chest radiography. Some patients have local compression signs and symptoms such as cough, dyspnea, dysphagia, or signs of vena caval compression. Thirty to 40% of patients have an associated disease, and about two thirds of such patients die of infection or another complication related to the associated disease.[20]

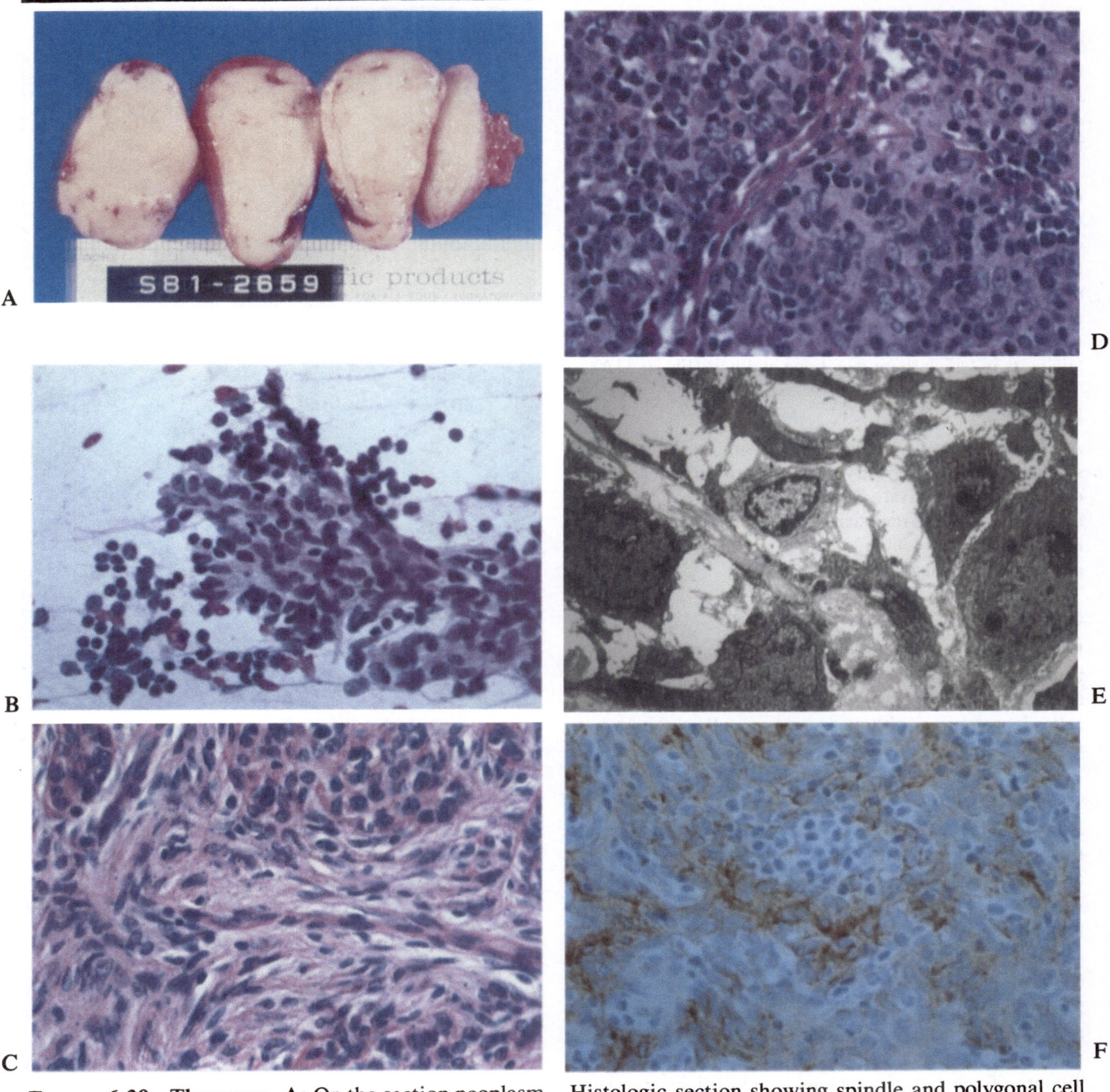

FIGURE 6.30 Thymoma. A: On the section neoplasm is encapsulated, lobulated, and pale yellow. **B:** Aspiration smear showing loose aggregates of spindle-shaped cells mixed with non-neoplastic lymphocytes. **C, D:** Histologic section showing spindle and polygonal cell types. **E:** The neoplastic cells showing tonofilaments and desmosomes (EM). **F:** Immunostain showing the neoplastic cells reactive to cytokeratin.

Teratoma

Teratoma is a germ cell tumor. The histogenesis of germ cell tumors of the mediastinum remains obscure, although it is speculated that they arise from misplaced germ cells. Some cases of mediastinal germ cell tumor occur in close association with Klinefelter's syndrome.[21]

Teratomas are the most common type of germ cell neoplasm of the mediastinum. The tumors occur in the anterior mediastinum in early adult life. Ninety percent are benign cystic teratomas, similar to those of the ovary. Whereas benign cystic teratomas occur with equal frequency in both sexes, malignant teratomas, which compose less than 5% of all mediastinal teratomas, occur almost exclusively in young men.[22] Benign cystic teratomas grow to a large size and contain cysts in which there may bone and hair (Fig. 6.31A).

Histology

All germ cell tumors of the mediastinum are histologically similar to those of the ovary. Benign cystic teratomas consist of ectodermal derivatives, such as stratified squamous epithelium, entodermal derivatives such as bronchial or intestinal type epithelium, and mesodermal derivatives such as bone and cartilage (Fig. 6.31B).

Cytology

In aspiration smears, the cells are benign squamous cells and benign glandular cells, occurring in loose aggregates (Fig. 6.31C). Aspirates of malignant teratomas contain malignant cells representing either squamous cell carcinoma or adenocarcinoma.

Seminoma

Primary seminoma of the mediastinum is a relatively rare tumor, occurring most often in young men. The histologic and cytologic features are identical to those of its testicular counterpart. Primary treatment is radiation therapy, and the prognosis is good.

Neurogenic Tumors

Neurogenic tumors of the mediastinum arise in the paravertebral region. Tumors of nerve sheath origin are neurofibroma, neurilemmoma, and malignant schwannoma. Tumors of sympathetic nervous system origin are neuroblastoma, ganglioneuroblastoma, and ganglioneuroma.

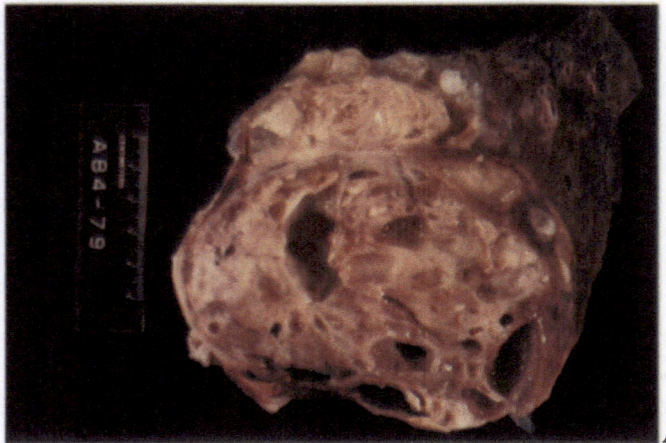

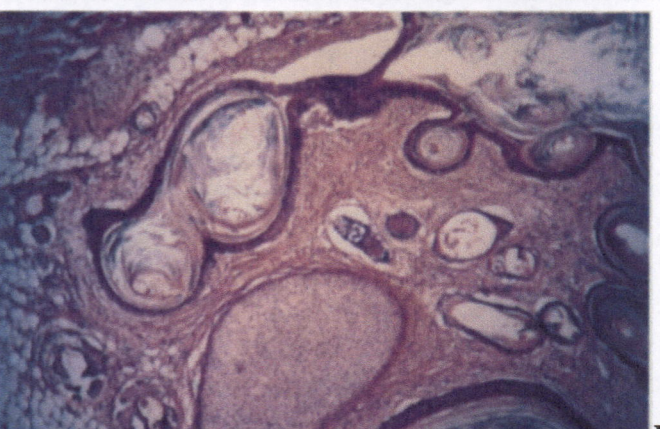

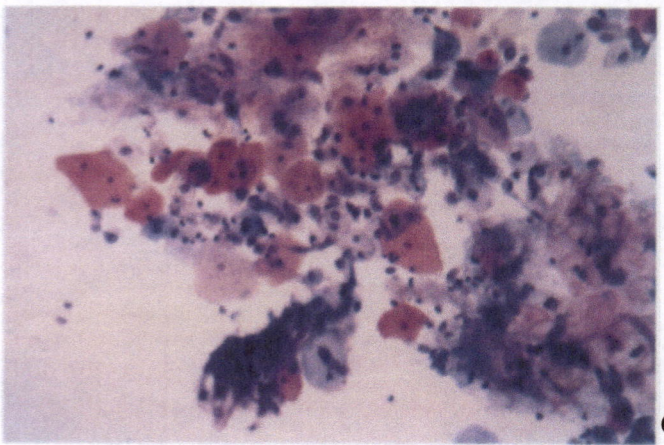

FIGURE 6.31 **Benign cystic teratoma of mediastinum. A**: Multicystic mass adherent to the lung (gross). **B**: Histologic section showing multiple cysts lined by benign squamous epithelium, cartilage, and fibroadipose tissue. **C**: Aspiration smear showing benign squamous and glandular cells.

References

1. Fontana, RS, Sanderson DR, Miller WE, et al. The Mayo lung project for early detection and localization of bronchogenic carcinoma, a status report. *Chest*. 1975;65:511–522.
2. Woolner JB, Fontana RS, et al. The Mayo lung project. Evaluation of lung cancer screening through December, 1979. *Mayo Clin Proc*. 1981;56:544–555.
3. Tao LC. *Guides to Clinical Aspiration Biopsy: Lung, Pleura, and Mediastinum*. New York, Tokyo: Igaku-Shoin; 1988:1–10.
4. Frable WJ. Thin needle aspiration biopsy. A personal experience with 469 cases. *Am J Clin Pathol*. 1972;65:168–182.
5. Saccomanno G, et al. Concentration of carcinoma or atypical cells in sputum. *Acta Cytol*. 1963;7:305–310.
6. Yesner R, et al. *International Histological Classification of Tumors. No. 1, Histologic Typing of Lung Tumors*, 2nd ed. Geneva: World Health Organization; 1982.
7. Yesner R, Carter D. Pathology of carcinoma of the lung: Changing patterns. *Clin Chest Med*. 1982;3:257.
8. Carny C, et al. *Cancer of the Lung. Pulmonary Diseases and Disorders*. 2nd ed. New York: McGraw-Hill Book Co; 1988.
9. Jett JR, et al. Lung cancer: Current concepts. *CA*. 1983;33:74.
10. Saccomanno G, Archer VE, Auerbach O, et al. Development of carcinoma of the lung as reflected in exfoliated cells. *Cancer*. 1974;33:256–270.
11. Saccomanno G, Saunders RP, Archer VE, et al. Cancer of the lung. The cytology of sputum prior to the development of carcinoma. *Acta Cytol*.1965;9:413–423.
12. Schreiber H, Saccomanno G, Martin DH, et al. Sequential cytological changes during development of respiratory tract tumors induced in hamsters by benzopyrene-ferric oxide. *Cancer Res*. 1974;34:689–698.
13. Fontana RS, Sanderson DR, Miller WE, et al. The Mayo lung project. Preliminary report of "early cancer detection" phase. *Cancer* 1972;30:1373–1382.
14. Woolner LB. Recent advances in pulmonary cytology: Early detection and localization of occult lung cancer in symptomless males. In: *Advances in Clinical Cytology*. London: Butterworths; 1981:95–135.
15. Sayler DC, Eggelstone JC. Bronchial carcinoid tumors. *Cancer*. 1975;36:15.
16. Mark EJ, Ramirez JF. Peripheral small cell carcinoma of the lung resembling carcinoid tumor. A clinical and pathological study of 14 cases. *Arch Pathol Lab Med*. 1985;109:263.
17. Creutzfelt W, Stockman F. Carcinoids and carcinoid syndrome. *Am J Med*. 1987;82 (suppl 5B):4.
18. Kim K, Mah C, Dominquez J. Carcinoid tumors of the lung: Cytologic differential diagnosis in fine-needle aspirates. *Diag. Cytopathol*. 1986;2:343–346.
19. Kim K, Naylor B, Han I. Fine needle aspiration cytology of sarcomas metastatic to the lung. *Acta Cytol*. 1986;30:688–694.
20. LeGolvan, D.P. and Abell, M.R. Thymoma. *Cancer*. 1977;39:2142.
21. Lachman MF, Kim K, Koo BC. Mediastinal teratoma associated with Klinefelter's syndrome. *Arch Pathol Lab Med*. 1986;110:1067–1071.
22. Tao LC. *Guides to Clinical Aspiration Biopsy: Lung, Pleura and Mediastinum*. New York, Tokyo: Igaku-Shoin; 1988:287.

7

Cytopathology of Pleural, Peritoneal, and Pericardial Fluids

Cytologic examination of spontaneously occurring serous effusions is widely performed, especially with a view to detecting cancer cells in the fluid. The finding of cancer cells in such a fluid is of the gravest prognostic significance, denoting that the patient has cancer that is not only advanced but which is almost certainly incurable. Apart from cancer cells, examination of a serous fluid may reveal inflammatory changes, usually nonspecific, but which may be specific for certain diseases. Cytologic examination of serous fluids may also reveal infection with bacteria, fungi, parasites, or viruses. It may also reveal the presence of a fistulous connection with a serous cavity.

The Serous Cavities

The serous cavities, pleural, pericardial, and peritoneal, are derived from the embryonic celomic cavity. The term "serous" refers to the small amount of serumlike fluid that each cavity contains. The serous cavity surrounding each testis is formed by an embryonic extension of the peritoneal cavity. The membranous lining of a serous cavity is the serosa, which, on its aspect facing the serous cavity, is covered by a monolayer of cells, the mesothelium.

Normally each serous cavity is a collapsed sac invaginated by the organ it surrounds. Except for the peritoneal cavity where it receives the fimbriated end of each fallopian tube, each serous cavity is completely closed. The serous cavities contain a small amount of fluid, which is clinically and radiologically undetectable.

Each serous cavity has two layers, the outer parietal and the inner visceral layer. The visceral layer envelops the organ that invaginates the cavity. Under normal conditions the two mesothelial layers are separated by only a thin film of fluid, which enables them to glide over each other. Thus, each serous cavity is only a potential cavity. When fluid accumulates in a serous cavity the two surfaces become separated and the potential cavity becomes an actual cavity. Beneath the monolayer of mesothelial cells are lymphatics and blood vessels. The proximity of these vessels may account for the ready spread of neoplastic cells through the mesothelium into a serous cavity.

Types of Effusions

Serous effusions are generally classified as transudates or exudates. Transudates are characterized by a low protein content, usually less than 3 g dL, and have a low specific gravity, usually less than 1.015. These fluids accumulate by filtration of serum across intact capillaries in situations where fluid outflow exceeds the resorption of fluid through the serous membrane. Such transudation takes place in conditions of high venous pressure, as in congestive heart failure or hepatic cirrhosis, or associated with hypoproteinemia as in renal failure. Transudates usually have a lower cell content than exudates, with the cells consisting mainly of mesothelial cells and macrophages.

Exudates are characterized by a high protein content, 3.0 g dL or more, and a specific gravity that exceeds 1.015. Exudates are a result of damage to the capillary walls in the subserosal connective tissue, which allows escape of protein and various cellular constituents of the blood into the serous cavity. The cellular content of exudates is generally higher than that of transudates and may contain many inflammatory cells if the exudate is caused by inflammation. If an exudate is caused by neoplastic invasion of the serosa, it may contain many neoplastic cells. However, serous effusions caused by neoplasm may be transudates, resulting from failure of resorption of serous fluid due to mechanical blockage of lymphatics by the neoplasm, or they may be exudates caused by neoplasm damaging submesothelial capillaries.

Collecting Serous Fluids

Serous fluids are collected by inserting a wide-bore needle into the serous cavity and allowing the fluid to drain spontaneously into a clean, dry, although not necessarily sterile, receptacle. The receptacle need not contain anticoagulant; however, if anticoagulant is required by the laboratory, heparin should be used. Nor should the receptacle contain any fixative. The specimen should be sent to the laboratory as soon as possible. If it cannot be sent right away it should be kept in a refrigerator at 4°C and not allowed to freeze. Cells in such cooled fluids remain well preserved for many days.

Specimens may also be obtained by instilling physiologic saline solution into a serous cavity. Such specimens are referred to as "washings." Obtaining peritoneal washings is now part of standard gynecologic practice on patients being operated on for gynecologic pelvic neoplasms. Occasionally peritoneal dialysate is submitted for cytologic examination.

Naked Eye Appearance of Serous Fluids

About 50% of pleural and 25% of peritoneal fluids will be visibly blood stained, a term used for fluids whose color ranges from light orange to deep red. Blood-stained fluids are not necessarily caused by cancer, and even if cancer is the underlying cause of the effusion such fluids do not necessarily contain cancer cells. Of the heavily blood-stained serous fluids of all types received in our laboratory, only 22% contained cancer cells. Furthermore, only 50% of serous fluids containing cancer cells were blood-stained, denoting that fluids containing cancer cells are just as likely to be as not to be blood stained.

Fluids that contain numerous cancer cells may sediment spontaneously to produce a thick yellow-white layer of cancer cells at the bottom of the container. Occasionally, cancer cells may grow in the serous fluids to produce cellular clusters visible to the naked eye (Fig. 7.1). Such cancer particles may have an ovoid shape, similar to a sesame seed.

Fluids containing numerous pigmented melanoma cells may be a chocolate brown color. Fluids from jaundiced patients acquire an olive-yellow color, and fluids into which hemorrhage has taken place may have a brown cast due to hemoglobin having become converted into hemosiderin.

Long-standing serous effusions may contain numerous cholesterol crystals. They impart a yellow appearance to the fluid, which shimmers like gold paint, especially when agitated. Because of their content of emulsified lipid, chylous effusions have a milky white appearance with a creamy topmost layer.

Serous effusions caused by diffuse malignant mesothelioma of epithelial type generally contain a high concentration of hyaluronic acid. When the concentration is extremely high, the fluid acquires a viscous, honeylike consistency. To the practiced eye, even fluids with a lower but abnormally high concentration of hyaluronic acid may be perceived as hyperviscous. The most viscous serous fluids are those of pseudomyxoma peritonei because of their high content of mucin.

Cytopreparatory Technique

If a serous fluid contains a clot, it should be removed, compressed to a small size, and then cut into small pieces which are fixed in formalin for 30 min. These pieces are then treated like fragments of tissue to form what is known as a cell block.

The remaining fluid is centrifuged and the supernatant is decanted. Sediment smears are made by placing a loopful of sediment in the center of a glass slide and spreading it with the loop in a longitudinal and crisscross manner. Before any drying of the smear takes place it is fixed with a spray fixative or by immersing it in 95% ethanol. The smear is then stained by the Papanicolaou method. In addition, we routinely prepare a toluidine blue-stained wet film by adding a drop of toluidine blue stain to a loopful of cellular deposit in the center of the slide, mixing the two together with the corner of a coverslip, and immediately examining the film. The toluidine blue-stained wet film is extremely useful for making a rapid cytologic assessment of a serous fluid.

Finally, after preparing the permanent smears, the sediment obtained by centrifugation is solidified by adding a few drops of plasma followed by a few drops of thrombin solution. Clotting takes place immediately, and this newly formed clot is added to any clot that occurred spontaneously to become part of the cell block preparation. Cell blocks sometimes reveal morphologic features about cancers in serous fluids that would not be revealed in the wet film or the permanent smears. Furthermore, cell block preparations can be replicated many times, thereby providing cellular material for special stains and immunocytochemistry. Use of all three cytopreparatory techniques enables the maximum cytologic information to be obtained from each specimen.

Non-Neoplastic Cells in Serous Effusions

Every pleural, peritoneal, and pericardial fluid contains cells. The non-neoplastic cells found in serous fluids are derived mainly from the mesothelium lining the serous cavity and from blood (leukocytes and erythrocytes). The proportions of the different types of cells in a serous fluid depend on the cause and duration of the effusion and the presence of inflammation.

Some cells, although normal, are found rarely in serous fluids. Such cells are megakaryocytes, hepatocytes introduced by a paracentesis needle traversing the liver en route to the peritoneal cavity, and cells derived from the respiratory and alimentary tracts via a fistula. Cells derived from the fimbriated end of the fallopian tube occasionally may be found in specimens obtained by culdocentesis, laparotomy, laparoscopy, or dialysis catheter.

It is difficult to know exactly the range of normal cells in serous fluids. That one is able to withdraw fluid from a serous cavity denotes an abnormal accumulation of the fluid. Despite this uncertainty regarding the normal range, it is common practice for clinicians to send specimens of serous fluid to the hematology laboratory for a total and differential cell count. Such counts can be performed only on fluids that have been anticoagulated immediately after they are withdrawn from the body. Only a few distinctive, but not specifically diagnostic, cytologic pictures emerge from total and differential cells counts: purulent effusions, lymphocytic effusions, and eosinophilic effusions. Ascertaining that the cytologic picture in a serous fluid is one of these types needs neither a total nor a differential cell count; just glancing at the prepared smears by an experienced eye reveals the cytologic picture.

Apart from the nonspecific inflammatory pictures mentioned above, the cytologic pictures of systemic lupus erythematosus and rheumatoid pleuritis or pericarditis may be identified in serous fluids. Apart from these specific inflammatory pictures and those of infection with certain microorganisms, the only specific cytologic picture of any consequence is the presence of neoplastic cells.

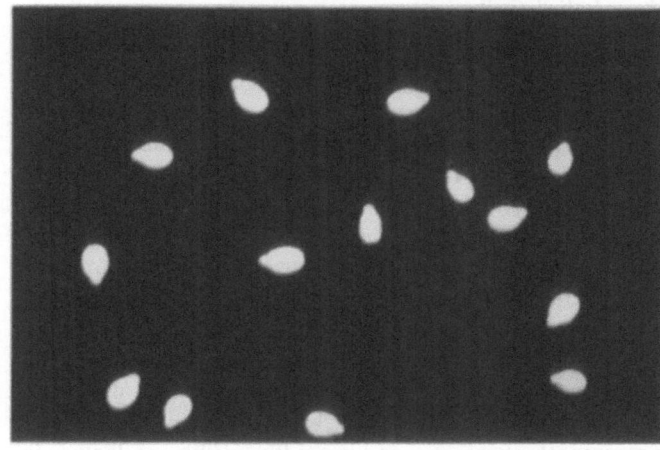

FIGURE 7.1 **Pleural fluid.** Particles of metastatic squamous cell carcinoma visible to the naked eye. They are about the size and shape of sesame seeds.

Mesothelial Cells

Most serous effusions contain readily identifiable mesothelial cells that exfoliate, often in large numbers, either as discrete cells or as clusters of cells or both (Fig. 7.2A). It is likely that mesothelial cells continue to proliferate in a serous effusion since mitotic figures frequently are seen in these cells. Mesothelial cells readily undergo hypertrophy and hyperplasia in response to a wide variety of stimuli, such as the presence of inflammation on a serous membrane, necrosis or inflammation of underlying parenchyma, or the presence of foreign substances, such as air or blood, in the serous cavity.

The typical mesothelial cell (Fig. 7.2B) is round, about 25 μm in diameter, and has a round or oval, smoothly contoured, centrally positioned or eccentric nucleus that contains smooth chromatin and a readily visible nucleolus. In Papanicolaou-stained preparations the cytoplasm is a dense gray-green, which tends to fade at the periphery of the cell. A mesothelial cell may contain tiny cytoplasmic vacuoles or the cell may be dominated by a large single cytoplasmic vacuole. Such vacuoles are regarded as evidence of cellular degeneration. Mesothelial cells vary considerably in size. In a fluid that contains numerous mesothelial cells it is not uncommon to find giant multinucleated forms (Fig. 7.2C).

Mesothelial cells articulate with each other at flattened apposing surfaces (Fig. 7.2B, D) or they may form flat mosaic sheets. One type of articulation typical of mesothelial cells is seen when the cytoplasm of one cells seems to be grasping another cell (Fig. 7.2D). Mesothelial cells frequently form clusters containing 10 or more cells; such clusters tend to have rather scalloped or knobby contours (Fig. 7.2E), unlike the smoother contours of adenocarcinoma cell clusters.

Because of their tendency to undergo hypertrophy and to cluster, mesothelial cells may be misinterpreted as fragments of carcinoma, particularly adenocarcinoma. This is the most prevalent diagnostic pitfall in the cytology of serous fluids. However, attention to morphologic details, such as the smooth contours of their nuclei and the staining reaction of the cytoplasm, with its tendency to fade at the periphery, should enable a correct interpretation to be made. Such cells are frequently referred to as "atypical" or "reactive," inappropriate designations for mesothelial cells that are merely hypertrophic or hyperplastic, or both. Since these changes are nonspecific and benign they should not be mentioned in reports.

Mesothelial cells in specimens collected by culdocentesis, laparoscopy, or laparotomy present some morphologic features different from those seen in spontaneously occurring peritoneal effusions. Frequently they appear as large flat mosaic sheets (Fig. 7.2F). At first glance the size of these sheets is startling; however, careful attention to morphologic detail will reveal that none of the cells shows indisputable evidence of malignancy. In cell block preparations, detached mesothelium may appear as coiled cell strips (Fig. 7.2G), suggestive of papillary adenocarcinoma but, again, the cells composing these fragments do not look malignant.

Focal hyperplasia of mesothelium readily takes place, especially in the female pelvis (which includes the germinal

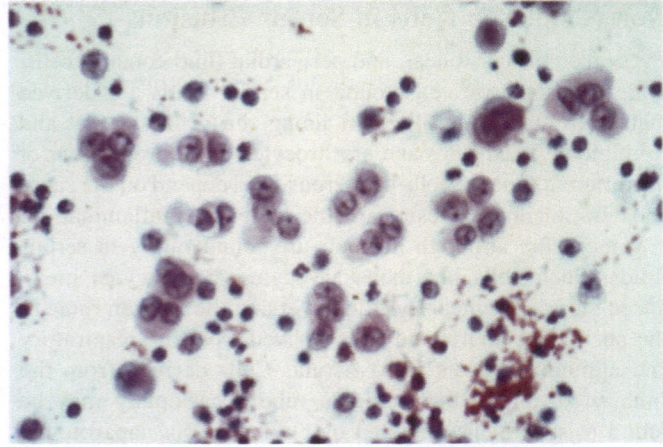

A

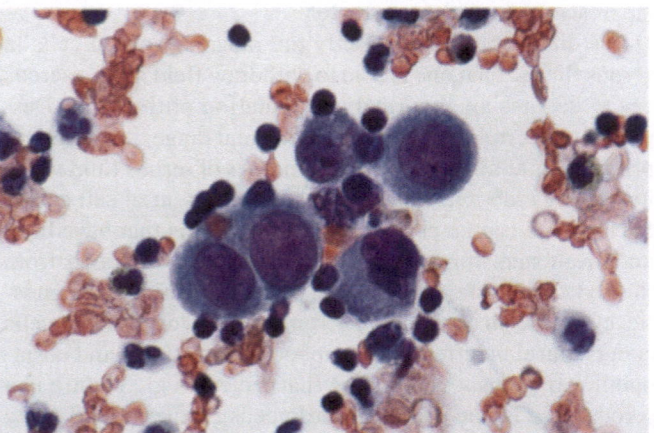

B

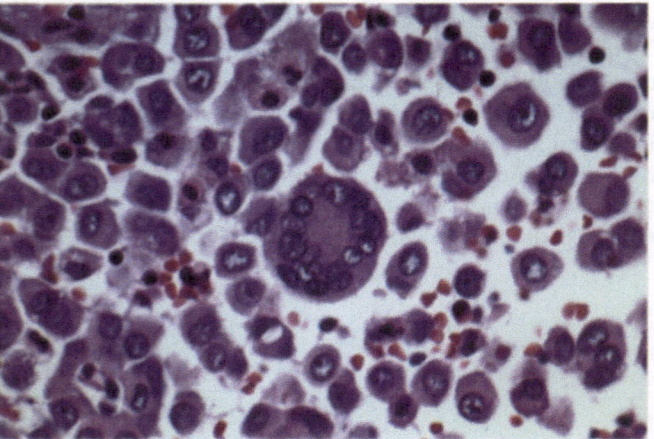

C

Figure 7.2 Mesothelial cells. A: Pleural fluid. Numerous small clusters of mesothelial cells in a background of leukocytes (smears). **B**: Pleural fluid. A group of mesothelial cells illustrating their dense cytoplasm, which tends to fade at the periphery. Their nuclei are central or eccentric, and their nucleoli are easily seen. Two of the cells are joined together at flattened apposing surfaces (smear). **C**: Pleural fluid. A

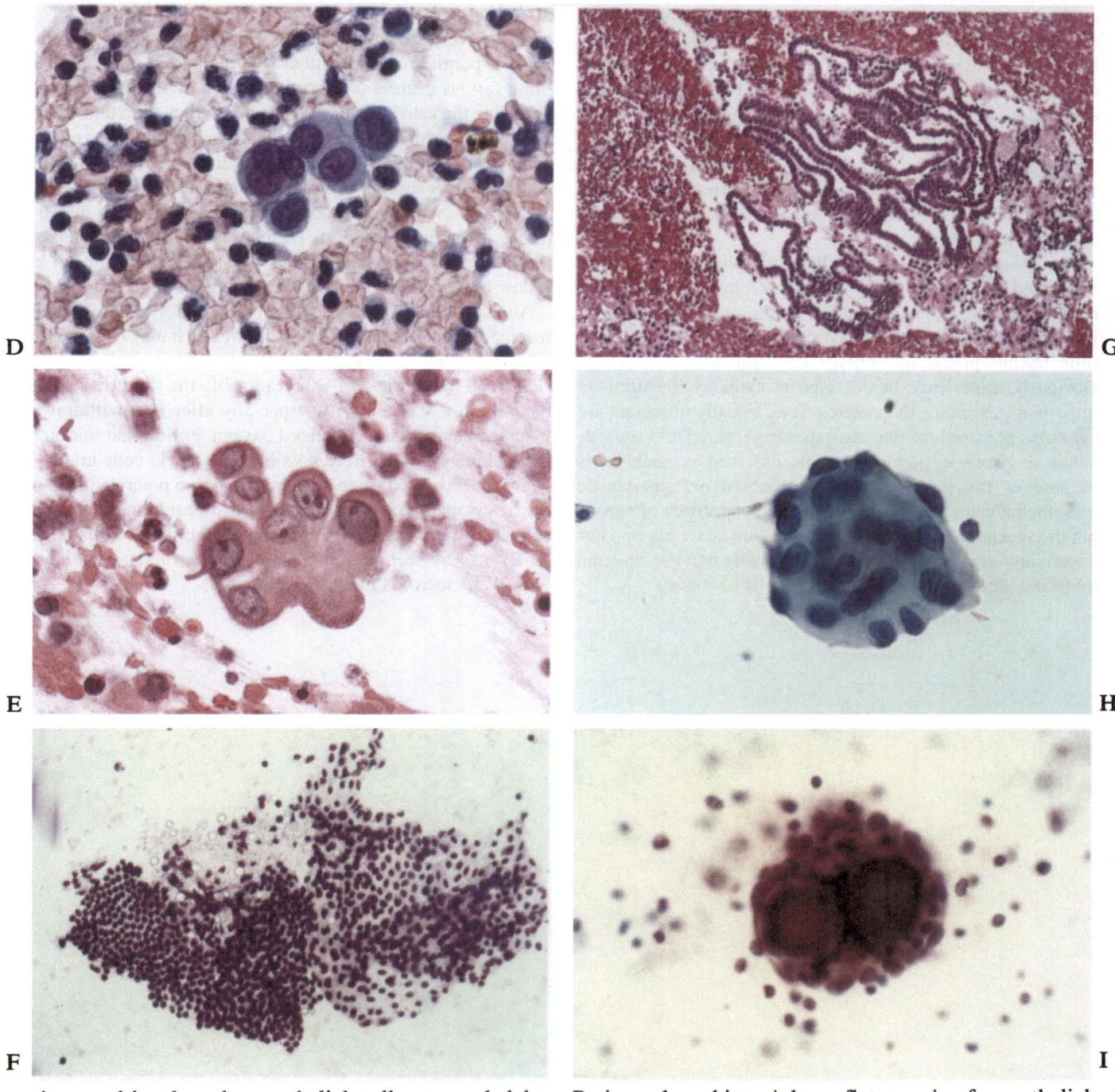

giant multinucleated mesothelial cell surrounded by numerous smaller mesothelial cells (cell block). **D**: Pleural fluid. Mesothelial cells showing the characteristic articulation at flattened apposing surfaces. One mesothelial cell appears to be about to clasp another mesothelial cell (smear). **E**: Pleural fluid. A cluster of mesothelial cells. Note the dense pink cytoplasm and the scalloped contour of the cluster (cell block). **F**: Peritoneal washing. A large flat mosaic of mesothelial cells (stained wet film). **G**: Peritoneal washing. Strips of coiled mesothelium (cell block). **H**: Peritoneal washing. A core of collagen, stained pale green, surrounded by mesothelial cells in different focal planes (smear). **I**: Culdocentesis specimen. Two psammoma bodies surrounded by mesothelial cells (smear).

epithelium of the ovary). When hyperplastic fragments of mesothelium become detached during peritoneal washing, for example, they may present as clusters of cells around a smooth, homogeneous core of collagen (Fig. 7.2H). Such a collagenous core may become calcified to form a psammoma body, suggestive of a papillary ovarian serous neoplasm[1] (Fig. 7.2I). It is important not to mistake such fragments for serous adenocarcinoma. To make such a diagnosis, individual cells composing the fragment must show convincing evidence of malignancy.

The mesothelial cell, with all its morphologic variations associated with hypertrophy and hyperplasia, presents the most important diagnostic pitfall in the cytology of serous fluids. Probably every seasoned cytopathologist has at some time misinterpreted mesothelial cells for adenocarcinoma. Obviously, experience in this type of cytology is extremely important in avoiding diagnostic errors. Equally important are cytologic preparations that are expertly prepared and stained. When a cytologic picture remains unsolved or ambiguous because of the presence of hypertrophied or hyperplastic mesothelial cells, we adopt the pragmatic approach of reporting the specimens as negative for neoplasm or we express our uncertainty in straightforward terms, leaving it to the clinician to decide whether further investigation is necessary.

Red Blood Cells

Virtually every specimen of serous fluid contains red blood cells that, in permanent preparations, appear as red discoids that show various degrees of distortion caused by the technique of spreading the cells. Red blood cells in a serous fluid ultimately disintegrate, with the result that their hemoglobin forms either hemosiderin or hematoidin. Hematoidin is extracellular and may be seen as sheaves of brown crystals. Hemosiderin present as golden-brown granules that undergo phagocytosis by macrophages in the fluid (Fig. 7.3). The presence of a large amount of hematoidin or hemosiderin in a serous fluid may impart a yellow-brown cast to the fluid (xanthochromasia).

Abnormalities of red blood cells are rarely perceived in routinely prepared serous fluids. However, it may be possible to detect sickle cells in persons with sickle cell disease or sickle cell trait[2] (Fig. 7.4A). Presumably the fluid that accumulated in a serous cavity, especially after it is withdrawn from the cavity, has a decreased oxygen tension that initiates the sickling. It is entirely possible that sickle cells are frequently overlooked since it is not a common practice in diagnostic cytopathology to pay too close attention to the shapes of the red blood cells. Rouleau formation of red cells (Fig. 7.4B) may be seen in wet films of serous fluids in patients with Waldenstrom's macroglobulinemia.

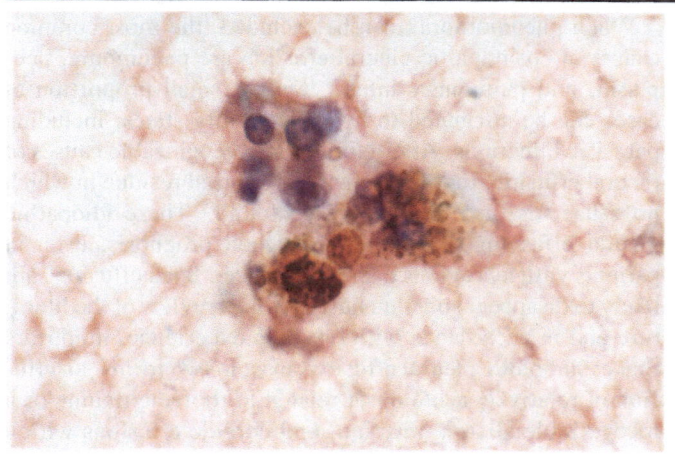

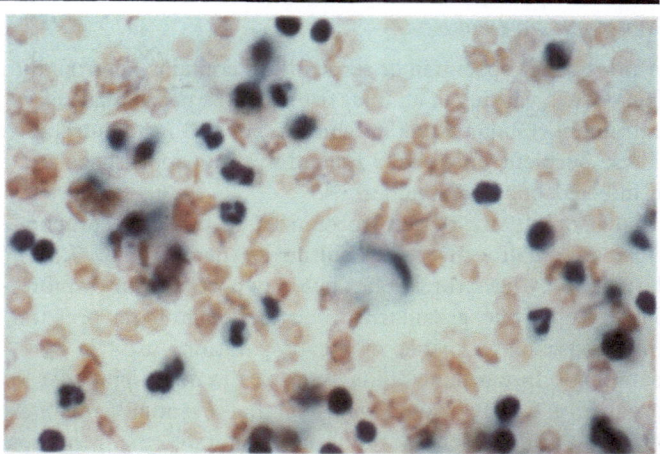

A

FIGURE 7.3 **Pleural fluid.** Macrophages in a bloody effusion that have ingested golden brown granules of hemosiderin (smear).

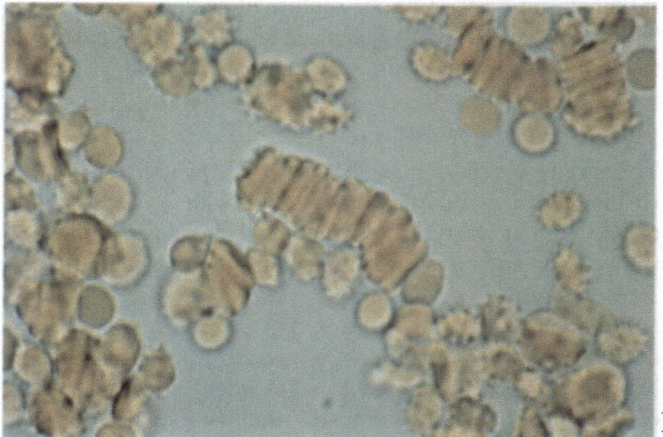

B

FIGURE 7.4 **Red blood cells. A**: Pleural fluid. Sickle cell (smear). **B**: Pleural fluid. Rouleau formation in red blood cells (unstained wet film). The patient had Waldenstrom's macroglobulinemia.

Neutrophilic Leukocytes

Almost every specimen of serous fluid contains neutrophilic leukocytes, varying in number from just the occasional cell to extremely cellular fluids in which every cell is a neutrophil. These purulent fluids have a cloudy yellow appearance and, if infected, may be malodorous.

Neutrophils are readily recognized in cytologic preparations as small cells with multilobed nuclei (Fig. 7.5A). Usually they have three lobes but may possess four or more. The cytoplasmic granularity seen in hematologic preparations is scarcely visible in the preparations used in cytopathology. In purulent fluids many of the neutrophils die to produce a faintly stained particle that eventually disintegrates. Purulent serous fluids are generally the result of inflammation, infarction, or rupture of an underlying organ. Their presence is easily recognized and does not depend on a total and differential white cell count of the fluid.

Eosinophilic Effusions

The arbitrary criterion of designating a pleural effusion as eosinophilic has varied from a fluid with as few as five to one with at least 50% of the cells being eosinophils. For the sake of argument, we have adopted a concentration of 10% or more.

Eosinophilic pleural effusion has been associated with a wide variety of conditions. However, a substantial number, 27% to 64%, have been associated with some form of thoracic trauma, not only the trauma[3,4] related to accidents but also that associated with therapeutic pneumothorax, thoracotomy, and repeated aspiration of pleural fluid. As might be expected, many of these examples of thoracic trauma were associated with some degree of hemothorax, suggesting that blood in the pleural cavity is a stimulus to eosinophilia. However, since many examples of hemothorax are also associated with pneumothorax, it is entirely possible that allergens in the air provide the stimulus to pleural eosinophilia. Even if blood or air does stimulate the eosinophilia, it is important to remember that a high proportion of eosinophilic pleural effusions are associated with neither hemothorax nor pneumothorax.

When pneumothorax can be excluded, the most common causes of eosinophilic pleural effusion are pneumonia, neoplasm, and pulmonary infarct. Only a small proportion of cases can be attributed to hypersensitivity states, including parasitic infections. After eliminating recognizable causes of pleural effusion, there remains a substantial residue in which no cause for the effusion can be found.[3] These idiopathic pleural effusions seem to have a good prognosis, even in patients with a previous history or cancer. Such effusions are likely to disappear spontaneously. From a review of the literature and in accordance with our own experience, it appears that eosinophilic pleural effusions exist in two forms: an effusion of relatively acute onset related to thoracic trauma or a recognizable allergic reaction, and chronic effusions with a longer clinical course and, possibly, no recognizable etiologic background.

Eosinophilic peritoneal effusions are rare. They have been reported in association with malignant neoplasm, allergic states, parasitic infections, eosinophilic gastroenteritis, and chronic peritoneal dialysis. It is possible that various agents used in peritoneal dialysis, such as kelp, particles of tubing, and peritoneal catheters, may provoke a hypersensitivity reaction resulting in peritoneal eosinophilia. Eosinophilic pericardial effusion is even rarer than eosinophilic peritoneal effusion. A few examples have been reported in association with pulmonary eosinophilia, the use of the drug cromolyn sodium, and malignant lymphoma.

Most serous fluids contain at least the occasional eosinophil, which is recognizable in all types of cytologic preparation. Eosinophils are slightly larger than neutrophils and their nuclei are generally bilobed (Fig. 7.5B). Their eosinophilic cytoplasmic granules may be visible, especially in stained wet films and cell block preparations. In Papanicolaou-stained smears their staining reaction tends to be weak.

Basophil Leukocytes and Mast Cells

Basophil leukocytes and mast cells are small, round cells that contain cytoplasmic granules that stain with basophilic dyes. The granules often stain a shade different from that of the dye, the phenomenon of metachromasia. Mast cells are believed to originate in connective tissues of the body, whereas basophils originate with other leukocytes in bone marrow from where they enter the blood stream. In the routinely prepared wet films it is not uncommon to see the occasional basophil or mast cell, recognizable by its delicate purple-pink cytoplasmic granules, quite different in color from the deep blue of the stain itself.

Macrophages

Macrophages (histiocytes) are found in various proportions in almost every serous fluid. They vary in diameter from about 15 to 100 μm with most in the range of 20 to 40 μm, about the size of a mesothelial cell. The typical macrophage is readily recognized by its eccentric round or bean-shaped nucleus and lightly stained foamy cytoplasm (Fig. 7.6). Because of their phagocytic property, they may contain ingested pigment, such as melanin or hemosiderin (Fig. 7.3), nuclear particles (Fig. 7.6), red blood cells, carbon particles or lipid droplets.

Macrophages are characteristically discrete, although they may coalesce, presumably because of their long microvilli becoming entangled. Such coalescent macrophages have a sheetlike arrangement, somewhat similar to sheets of mesothelial cells. However, the overall loose quality of the group and the lacy cytoplasm of the individual cells indicate their true nature.

Occasional macrophages may contain a large solitary or loculated cytoplasmic vacuole. Such cells, with their signet ring appearance, simulate metastatic adenocarcinoma; however, their nuclear features are not those of malignancy. Such cytoplasmic hypervacuolization, seen not only in macrophages but also in mesothelial cells, is believed to be a form of degeneration.

Macrophages in serous fluids are usually uninucleate, although binucleation is not uncommon. Giant multinucleated macrophages, commonly seen in granulomatous inflammatory reactions, are a rare finding in serous fluid. They are almost exclusively associated with the granulomatous form of pleuritis or pericarditis associated with rheumatoid disease (see below).

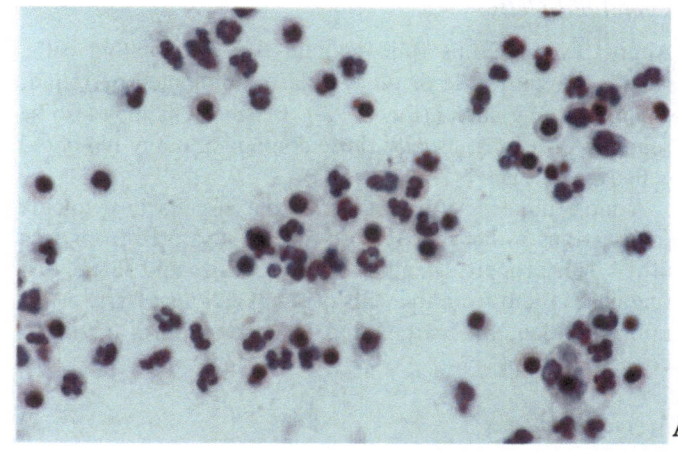

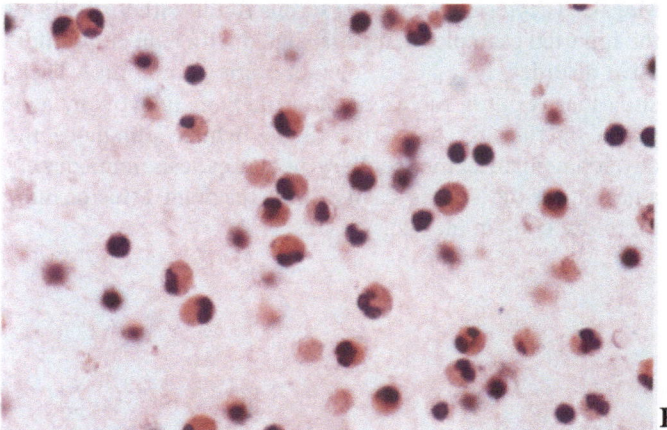

FIGURE 7.5 **Granular leukocytes. A**: Pleural fluid. Neutrophilic leukocytes (smear). The patient had pneumonia. **B**: Pleural fluid. Eosinophil leukocytes in pleural fluid (cell block). The patient had an idiopathic eosinophilic effusion.

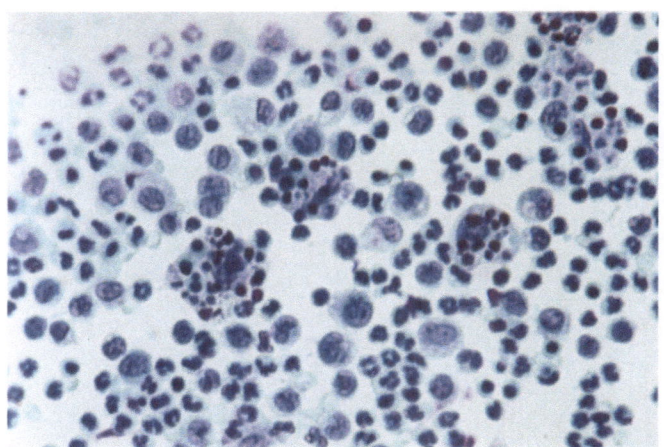

FIGURE 7.6 **Macrophages (histiocytes).** Pleural fluid. Numerous macrophages. The small macrophages have eccentric nuclei and foamy cytoplasm. The large macrophages have ingested nuclear material of cells that have undergone necrosis (smear).

Lymphoid Cells

Almost every serous fluid contains some lymphoid cells, small cells with little or no cytoplasm dominated by round, deeply staining nuclei (Fig. 7.7A). Plasma cells may also be found in effusions, usually those containing many lymphoid cells (Fig. 7.7B).

A most important feature of lymphoid cells in cytologic preparations is that they tend to remain separated from each other. This property, in addition to their size and shape, distinguishes them from the cells of small cell anaplastic carcinomas, which, like carcinomas in general, form distinctly cohesive groups.

Megakaryocytes

Megakaryocytes are a rarity in serous fluids with virtually all the reported examples being associated with a myeloproliferative disorder, lymphoma, or metastatic carcinoma.[5] These situations result in replacement of the bone marrow by neoplasm or fibrous connective tissue, which stimulates the development of extramedullary hematopoiesis immediately adjacent to the serous cavity. Any resultant effusion may therefore contain megakaryocytes.

Detached Ciliary Tufts

Fluid obtained from the peritoneal cavity by laparotomy, laparoscopy, or culdocentesis or as peritoneal dialysate may occasionally contain anucleate, ciliated cellular fragments (Fig. 7.8), which in their fresh state may be seen to be quite motile.[6] These fragments, referred to as detached ciliary tufts (DCT), have never been reported in spontaneously occurring peritoneal effusion. Furthermore, they have been described only in women who have not had their fallopian tubes removed.[7] Therefore, it is concluded that DCTs are derived from "pinched off" ends of the epithelium lining the fallopian tubes. It is important for anyone who examines fluid from the peritoneal cavity under the microscope to know about motile DCT because they have been misinterpreted as parasites.

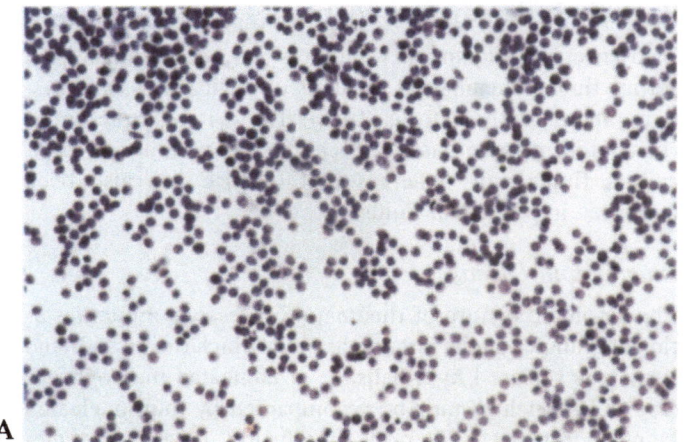

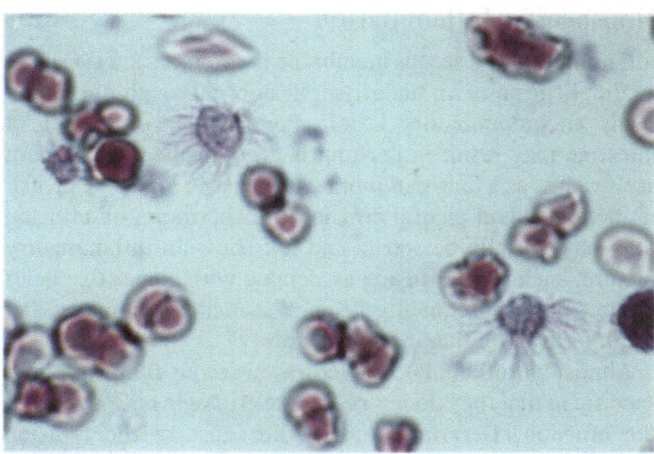

FIGURE 7.8 Culdocentesis specimen. Two detached ciliary tufts that were motile (stained wet film). The patient had a ruptured hydrosalpinx.

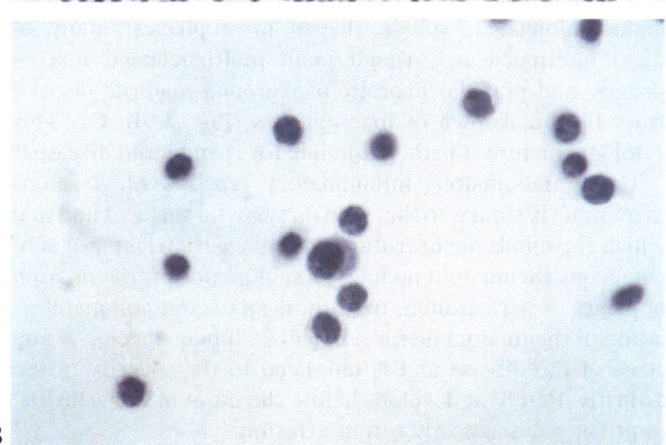

FIGURE 7.7 Lymphocytes and plasma cells. A: Pleural effusion. Numerous mature lymphocytes (smear). The effusion was caused by pulmonary tuberculosis. Well differentiated lymphocytic lymphoma or chronic lymphocytic leukemia could give an identical morphologic picture. **B:** Pleural fluid. Lymphocytes and a plasma cell. The plasma cell has an eccentric nucleus and visible cytoplasm (smear). The patient had chronic postpneumonic pleuritis.

Nonspecific Inflammation

Inflammation of a serous membrane is common and is usually a complication of an underlying lesion, although not necessarily an inflammatory lesion. For example, infarction of intestine may result in peritonitis accompanied by purulent ascites, just as a lung carcinoma may cause secondary pleuritis with purulent pleural effusion. Furthermore, an effusion that may initially be sterile and not show an inflammatory picture, such as an effusion associated with congestive heart failure, may subsequently become secondarily infected and exhibit a frank inflammatory picture.

Almost all inflammatory pictures in serous fluids are nonspecific in that they do not reveal the etiologic background of the effusion. Determination of the cause of the effusion usually has to depend on the knowledge of the clinical background supplemented by ancillary findings.

Nonspecific inflammatory effusions may show two cytologic extremes, that of acute purulent inflammation, with virtually all of the cells being neutrophilic leukocytes, or that of chronic inflammation with virtually every cell being a lymphocyte. Most inflammatory effusions, however, belong to neither of these extremes in that they contain a variety of inflammatory cells. In many examples of inflammation of serous membranes, mesothelial cells are frequently stimulated to undergo hypertrophy and hyperplasia and may become a prominent component of the cytologic picture.

Most frankly purulent effusions are pleural (pleural empyema) and are caused by primary bacterial pneumonia, with the second most common cause being pneumonia secondary to neoplasm in the lung. Other causes are tuberculosis in which secondary bacterial infection of an initially nonpurulent effusion has taken place, thoracic surgery, pulmonary infarct, esophageal carcinoma, and fistula. Purulent pericardial effusion is usually related to carcinoma metastatic to the pericardium, and the uncommon purulent peritoneal effusion is most likely related to infarct of the small intestine.

The cytologic picture of chronic inflammation, consisting mainly of lymphoid cells, may also be secondary to a variety of underlying causes. Most lymphocytic effusions are pleural, with the underlying cause being neoplasm in the lung, either primary or metastatic. The next most frequent cause is pulmonary tuberculosis in which the tuberculous process in the pulmonary parenchyma is presumed to have extended to the pleura. This is followed by a group of lymphocytic effusions whose cause remains unknown, and finally, there is a small group of lymphocytic effusions of miscellaneous underlying causes.

A population of small, mature-appearing lymphocytes in an effusion may be caused by chronic lymphocytic leukemia or malignant lymphoma of small cell type, as well as by a chronic inflammatory process. In the case of lymphoma and leukemia, the lymphoid cells are more likely to be of B rather than T cell type. Therefore, enumeration of the two types of lymphocytes in a lymphocytic effusion might aid in distinguishing between a non-neoplastic and a neoplastic effusion.[8,9]

Specific Inflammatory Pictures

Two specific inflammatory pictures may be manifested in serous fluids: rheumatoid pleuritis or pericarditis, and systemic lupus erythematosus (SLE). The cytologic picture of rheumatoid disease has been recorded in pleural and pericardial fluids only, whereas that of SLE has also been described in peritoneal fluids.

Rheumatoid Disease

The cytologic picture of rheumatoid disease is a manifestation of granulomatous inflammation in which the mesothelial surface is replaced by a palisade of elongated macrophages (Fig. 7.9A), which may be accompanied by multinucleated giant macrophages. The resultant effusion contains three elements: elongated, spindle-shaped macrophages, many of them multinucleated, round giant multinucleated macrophages, and granular necrotic background material derived from the breakdown of macrophages (Fig. 7.9B, C). This cytologic picture is pathognomonic for rheumatoid disease.[10]

The granulomatous inflammatory reaction on a serous membrane is similar to that seen on synovial surfaces and that which surrounds the necrotic center of a periarticular or subcutaneous rheumatoid nodule. Granulomatous inflammation of pleura or pericardium, or both, is an uncommon manifestation of rheumatoid disease; however, it may develop at any stage of the disease and is unrelated to the severity of the arthritis. Rarely, it develops before the onset of the arthritis, to produce a diagnostic serous effusion.

Systemic Lupus Erythematosus

Tissues from patients with SLE show various inflammatory and degenerative changes accompanied by the presence of small, round, cyanophilic bodies about the size of a neutrophil. These are hematoxylin bodies, long recognized as characteristic of SLE. Hematoxylin bodies consist of altered nuclear material.

The effusions of patients with SLE may contain hematoxylin bodies. When a hematoxylin body is phagocytosed the phagocytic cell with its contents is referred to as an LE cell. Such cells may be found in serous fluids[11] (Fig. 7.10). LE cell formation undoubtedly can take place after the fluid has been aspirated; it probably occurs even before the fluid is collected.

A review of the various manifestations of SLE in 962 patients revealed that at some stage of the disease pleural effusion developed in 29% and peritoneal effusion in 11%. Pericarditis, with or without effusion, developed in 33%.[12] Development of a serous effusion may be the first clinical manifestation of the disease.

LE cells may form in pleural and peritoneal fluid from patients who develop an SLE-like syndrome because they have taken certain drugs, such as hydralazine and procainamide. In these cases, the LE cells are morphologically indistinguishable from those seen in fluids from patients with SLE. However, this is a rare occurrence, and the finding of LE cells in a serous fluid should be regarded as strong evidence of SLE.

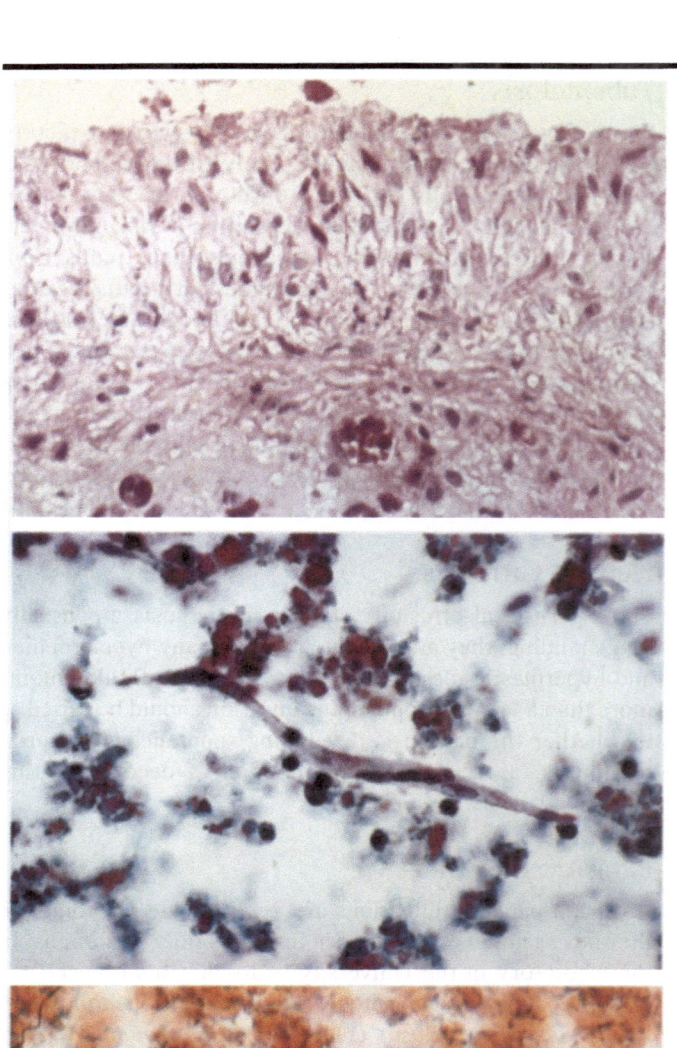

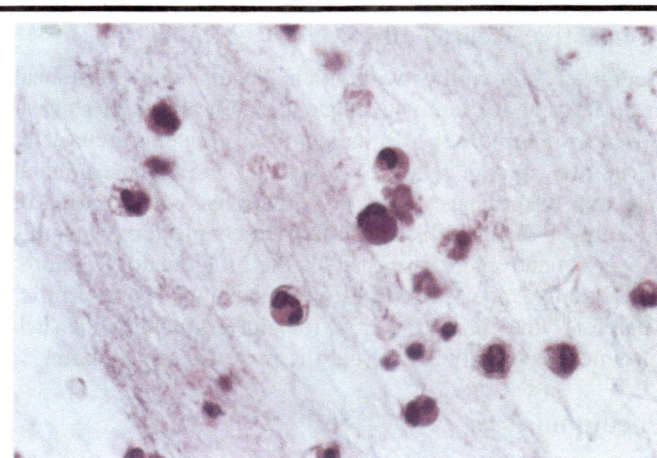

FIGURE 7.10 Pericardial fluid. An LE cell (cell block). The cell has a large intracytoplasmic eosinophilic inclusion.

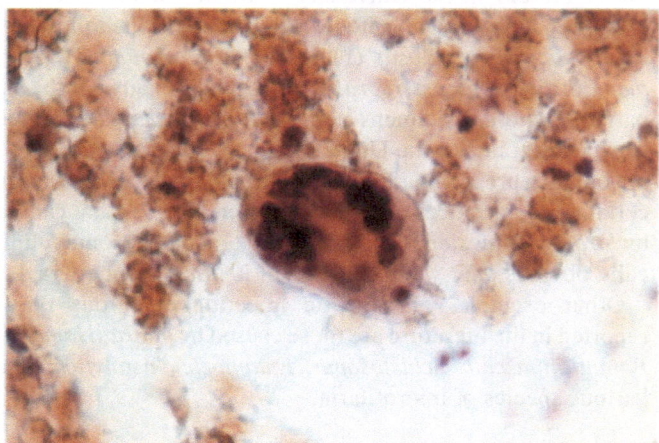

FIGURE 7.9 Rheumatoid pleuritis. A: Pleura. A palisade of elongated macrophages, characteristic of rheumatoid pleuritis (needle biopsy). **B**: Pleural fluid. Elongated multinucleated macrophage in a background of granular material (smear). This cell and the one illustrated in **C** are from the patient whose biopsy specimen of pleura is illustrated above. With permission from J.S. Nosanchuk and B. Naylor, "A Unique Cytologic Picture in Pleural Fluid From Patients with Rheumatoid Arthritis," American Journal of Clinical Pathology 50:330-335, © by Williams & Wilkins, 1968. **C**: Pleural fluid. Multinucleated giant macrophage in a background of granular material (smear).

Congestive Heart Failure

Pleural effusion with or without an accompanying peritoneal or pericardial effusion is a frequent manifestation of congestive heart failure. In the beginning, these effusions are usually sterile and contain relatively few cells, usually mesothelial cells and macrophages. However, the longer the duration of the effusion the more likely it is to become infected; when this happens, neutrophils form part of the inflammatory picture. The cytologic picture of congestive heart failure is nonspecific. Therefore, the main role of cytologic examination of such specimens is usually to rule out the presence of neoplasm.

Pneumonia

Should the inflammatory process of pneumonia extend to the pleural surface, it may result in effusion. In bacterial pneumonias the inflammatory picture in the effusion is typically neutrophilic; with viral pneumonias in the cytologic picture it is typically lymphocytic. However, the cytologic picture in a bacterial pneumonia may develop into a lymphocytic picture, and should secondary bacterial infection take place in the lymphocytic effusion of a viral pneumonia, neutrophils may replace the lymphocytes. Overall, the cytologic picture is nonspecific, merely denoting that the pleural surface is inflamed.

Infarct

The pleural surface over a pulmonary infarct may allow leakage of red blood cells from the hemorrhagic infarcted tissue into the pleural cavity and may also exhibit an inflammatory response as a reaction to the necrotic pulmonary parenchyma. In such a case, an effusion may develop containing numerous red blood cells accompanied by neutrophils. Similarly, with infarcts of other organs, such as the small intestine or liver, an effusion may ensue with a cytologic picture varying from the neutrophilic to the lymphocytic.

Pneumothorax

Patients with pneumothorax often develop pleural effusion to give the condition of hydropneumothorax. An interesting feature of such effusion is that they frequently contain a high concentration of eosinophil leukocytes, possibly a reaction to impurities in the air in the pleural cavity. The presence of air may also stimulate mesothelial cells to undergo hypertrophy and hyperplasia, and these form part of cytologic picture.

Tuberculosis

In tuberculous pleuritis and pericarditis the cytologic picture in any accompanying effusion is likely to be lymphocytic, with mesothelial cells being few or absent. The absence of mesothelial cells is attributed to deposition of fibrin over the serous surface, which prevents the mesothelial cells from gaining access to the fluid. In tuberculous peritonitis the effusion is also likely to be lymphocytic, although other inflammatory cells and mesothelial cells may also be present. When lymphocytic tuberculous effusions become secondarily infected, the cytologic picture changes to include neutrophils. It should be emphasized that even though a lymphocytic effusion is characteristic of tuberculous serositis, it is not diagnostic of the condition.

Hepatic Cirrhosis

Since peritoneal effusions of hepatic cirrhosis are usually long-standing, they are likely to contain many hypertrophied and hyperplastic mesothelial cells. When the fluid contains more than a few neutrophils, the question should be raised as to whether the patient is developing spontaneous bacterial peritonitis, a recognized complication of decompensating hepatic cirrhosis.

Parasitic Infections

Although parasitic infections are a worldwide phenomenon they have seldom been recorded in serous fluid specimens. In the laboratory in the University of Michigan we have seen examples of pleural or peritoneal fluid contains the following: *Echinococcus granulosus* (Fig. 7.11), *Paragonimus westermani*, *Strongyloides stercoralis*, and trichomonads. Of the six patients whose specimens contained these parasites, three were immigrants to the United States, a consequence of this era of widespread and rapid international travel. However, in certain circumstances parasitic infection, such as that caused by *Strongyloides stercoralis*, may be latent and becomes clinically obvious only when the patient is immunosuppressed.

Other examples of parasitic infection of serous fluids reported in the literature are those caused by *Giardia lamblia*, *Balantidium coli*, *Schistosoma*, *Entamoeba histolytica*, and various species of microfilaria.

Fungal Infection

In this age of therapeutic immunosuppression and the latter-day scourge of the acquired immunodeficiency syndrome, most examples of fungal infections in serous fluid occur in patients who are immunosuppressed. However, serous fluids containing fungi are not common. We have seen examples of serous fluids showing opportunistic infections with *Candida* species, *Cryptococus* species, *Coccidioides immitis*, *Blastomyces dermatididis*, and *Aspergillus niger*. Except for the patients with blastomycosis and aspergillosis, the fungal infections were confined to patients whose immunologic defenses were diminished by cancer, anticancer drugs, or therapeutic immunosuppression. Occasional examples of the presumed fungus *Pneumocystis carinii* in pleural fluid have been described in immunosuppressed patients who developed pneumonia because of the organism.

Viral Infection

To diagnose a viral infection of a serous cavity, it is essential to find virocytes, cells showing the morphologic changes typical of a particular viral infection. The finding of virocytes in a serous fluid is a rare event. We have seen only three examples in our laboratory, two associated with herpes simplex and one with cytomegaloviral infection. One of the patients with herpes simplex had an esophagopleural fistula and, presumably, esophageal herpetic infection, and the other had cutaneous herpes simplex in the region on the thoracotomy drainage tube. Both of these patients were severely debilitated. One patient had the virocytes of cytomegaloviral infection in peritoneal dialysate; the patient was immunosuppressed, having undergone renal transplantation.

Fistula

A fistulous connection with a serous cavity may result in an effusion containing nonhuman cells, such as vegetable cells. This may give a bizarre cytologic picture that can be explained only by an abnormal connection between the serous cavity and the alimentary tract (Fig. 7.12). The finding of such cells in a serous fluid may be an important clue that a patient has developed a fistula or ruptured a viscus, or that a surgical anastomosis is leaking.

Endometriosis

Since endometriosis may occur on the surface of the ovaries, on the peritoneum, and rarely on a pleural surface, it is theoretically possible to find endometriotic cells in a serous effusion. However, the diagnosis of endometriosis from cells in spontaneously occurring effusions, peritoneal washings, or culdocentesis specimens is fraught with difficulty because individual endometrial stromal cells may simulate lymphoid cells or may closely resemble macrophages or small mesothelial cells. Probably the only reliable method for detecting endometriosis in a serous fluid is by using a cell block preparation, which can demonstrate both the epithelial and the stromal components of endometriotic tissue.

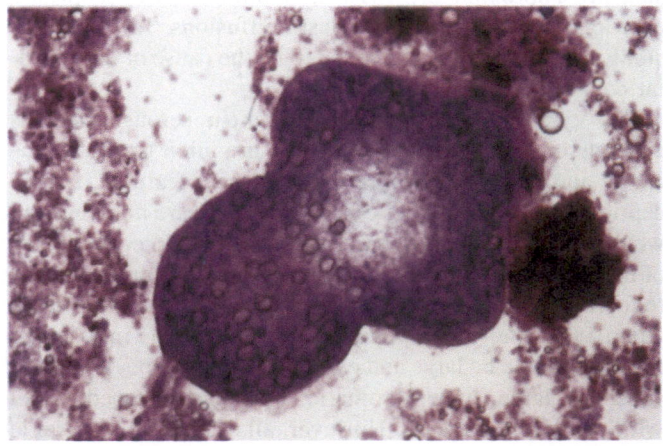

FIGURE 7.11 Pleural fluid. Scolex of *Echinococcus granulosus* (smear).

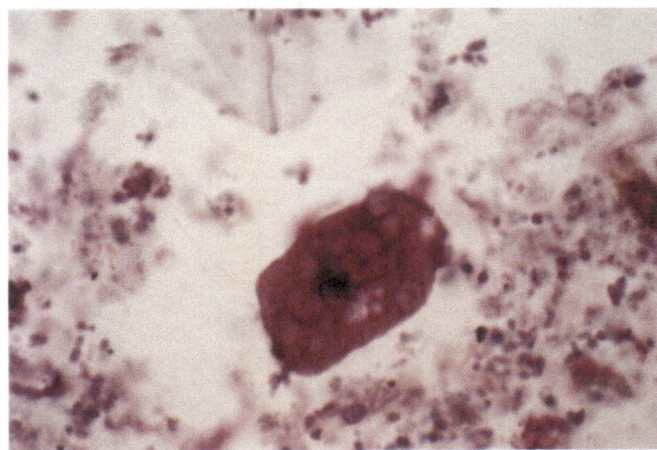

FIGURE 7.12 Pleural fluid. The patient had a gastropleural fistula caused by lymphoma. This illustrates a large vegetable cell in a background of amorphous material (smear).

Neoplastic Effusions

Many of the effusions associated with cancer are caused by an indirect mechanism such as venous obstruction by the neoplasm or parenchymal inflammation induced by the presence of neoplasm. Such situations are extremely common, and in such effusions neoplastic cells may not be found. When neoplastic cells are found in an effusion they may be numerous or few. When numerous, they dominate the cytologic picture, possibly because the neoplasm has penetrated the mesothelium in many areas; they may be few when the neoplasm has penetrated only a small area of the mesothelium.

Effusions that contain neoplastic cells virtually always contain other cells that are non-neoplastic, such as mesothelial cells and various inflammatory cells. Hemorrhagic effusions, the result of vascular congestion of subserosal connective tissue, are approximately twice as common with neoplastic effusions than with non-neoplastic effusions. In such effusions, the neoplasm is presumed to be the cause of the vascular congestion.

The cytologic diagnosis of cancer in serous effusions depends on the finding of cells that are alien to the serous cavity and that exhibit morphologic cancer features. An exception to this is mesothelioma, whose cells are not alien and which may not exhibit the distinctive morphologic attributes of malignancy. Also, some ovarian carcinomas produce cells that are morphologically similar to benign mesothelial cells. Apart from their alien appearance, cancer cells in a serous effusion should be large and exhibit a high nucleocytoplasmic ratio and large, hyperchromatic, irregularly shaped nuclei with prominent nucleoli. However, all of these morphologic features are not always present in cancer cells. For example, the cells of oat cell carcinoma and some adenocarcinomas are frequently quite small, and the cells of some adenocarcinomas and mesotheliomas frequently have a low nucleocytoplasmic ratio. Therefore, in making a diagnosis of neoplastic cells in a serous effusion the observer employs, perhaps subconsciously, many criteria to arrive at a correct diagnosis. Essentially, one is attempting to recognize cells that are alien to the serous cavity (except with mesotheliomas), a finding that virtually always denotes metastatic neoplasm.

Almost all examples of cancer cells in serous fluids are recognizable on routine preparations. Supplementary methods may sometimes be employed, not to make the decision as to whether cells are cancerous but to demonstrate certain characteristics of neoplastic cells. Immunocytochemistry has its most useful application in discriminating between adenocarcinoma and malignant mesothelioma and in confirming a suspected diagnosis of melanoma when the neoplastic cells are amelanotic. Histochemistry is more or less confined to the demonstration of melanin, hemosiderin, mucin, hyaluronic acid, or glycogen; however, it is rarely of any real practical value. Electron microscopy does not enable one to discriminate between benign and malignant cells; it may have some use in demonstrating, for example, dense core granules in neuroendrocrine neoplasms and melanin in the cells of amelanotic melanoma, and in discriminating between adenocarcinoma and mesothelioma. Cytogenetic analysis is too laborious and expensive for routine use.

Most neoplasms in serous fluids can be readily classified as to their type, such as adenocarcinoma, oat cell carcinoma, keratinizing squamous cell carcinoma, melanoma, and lymphoma. The most common type of neoplastic cell in a serous effusion is the adenocarcinoma cell followed by cells of lymphomas and leukemias. Cells of anaplastic carcinomas, such as oat cell carcinoma, are much less frequently seen, and the cells of squamous cell carcinomas are quite uncommon. With experience it may be possible to suggest the primary site of origin of neoplastic cells in a serous fluid; however, such divination is seldom needed since the background to the case usually provides all the clues necessary to know where the primary neoplasm is.

Adenocarcinoma

Most adenocarcinomas in serous fluids originate in breast, lung, or ovary. They may show the classic features of adenocarcinoma: cohesive clusters of large cells that have eccentric, malignant-appearing nuclei, prominent nucleoli, and vacuolated cytoplasm (Fig. 7.13). However, adenocarcinoma cells in serous fluids, while generally conforming to the above description, show great morphologic variation, not only in individual cells but also in the manner in which they are organized.

Generally, adenocarcinoma cells form cohesive clusters that may be small or large. These clusters are amorphous, papillary, or spheroidal and may comprise hundreds of cells. On the other hand, some adenocarcinoma cells in serous fluids are almost all isolated, forming only the occasional small cohesive cluster.

Squamous Cell Carcinoma

The finding of cells of squamous cell carcinoma in a serous fluid is an uncommon event. In a series of 7389 patients whose serous fluids were examined cytologically, squamous carcinoma cells were found in only 46 patients (pleural 34, peritoneal 8, pericardial 4), with most of the cells originating in primary neoplasms of the lung, female genital tract, or larynx.[13]

All of the recognized types of squamous carcinoma cells may be found in serous fluids, with the most common being round, nonkeratinizing carcinoma cells; keratinizing fiber and tadpole cells are seen much less frequently. In contrast to the cells of adenocarcinomas, the cells of squamous carcinomas in serous fluids tend to be discrete and nonvacuolated, and their nuclei are in the center of the cell. Cell blocks can be most helpful in determining that carcinoma cells in a serous fluid are of squamous cell type (Fig. 7.14).

Since the incidence of squamous carcinoma cells in serous fluids is not high, it is easy to overlook their squamous origin if they do not show distinct evidence of keratinization. However, one can expect that in virtually every example of squamous cell carcinoma in a serous fluid the patient will be known to have or have had a squamous cell carcinoma. Such was the situation in the series referred to above.

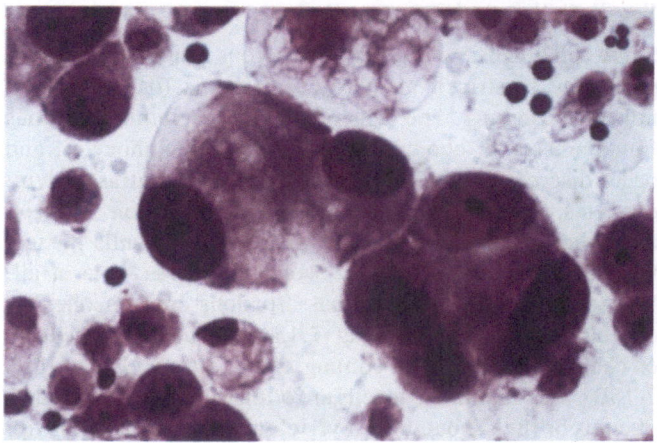

FIGURE 7.13 **Pleural fluid.** Adenocarcinoma cells, metastatic from a primary lung carcinoma (stained wet film). The cells are large with vacuolated cytoplasm and eccentric, malignant-appearing nuclei containing prominent nucleoli.

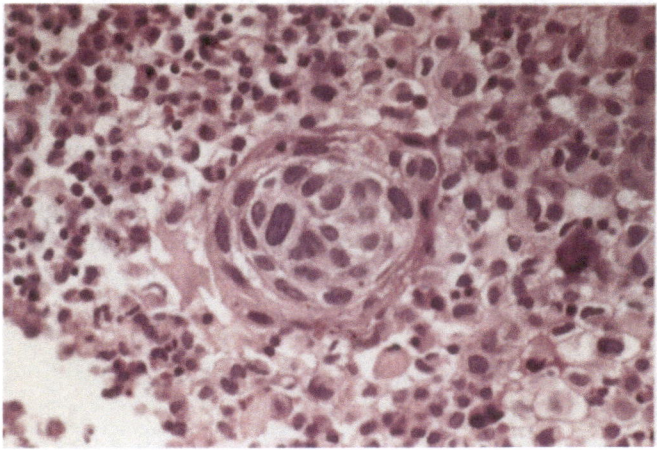

FIGURE 7.14 **Peritoneal fluid.** Fragment of squamous cell carcinoma (cell block). The primary neoplasm was in the uterine cervix.

Small Cell Anaplastic Carcinoma

Small cell anaplastic carcinoma in serous fluids is best exemplified by small cell anaplastic carcinoma (oat cell carcinoma) of the lung. The cells of oat cell carcinoma in serous fluids are small, about twice the size of lymphocytes, and occur discretely or in small clusters.[4,14,15] In contrast to lymphocytes, they show a degree of nuclear angulation. Nucleoli are either invisible or barely visible, and the cells possess very little cytoplasm or may seem to possess none at all. Whereas lymphocytes in serous effusions are noncohesive, oat cells form tiny groups (Fig. 7.15A) frequently in the form of chains with branches coming off at various angles (Fig. 7.15B). The chains of oat cells are often reminiscent of a stack of coins or the silhouette of a vertebral column. Oat cells frequently exhibit a characteristic type of articulation where one cell seems to cap another in a quarter moon manner (Fig. 7.15C). Such configurations and the cells composing them are virtually diagnostic of metastatic oat cell carcinoma of the lung.

Urothelial Carcinoma

The cells of urothelial (transitional cell) carcinomas are seldom found in serous fluids, accounting for no more than one percent of all serous fluids containing cancer cells. The cells of these carcinomas in serous fluids do not have any distinctive features, occurring in clusters or singly. They may be vacuolated, probably because of degeneration, or nonvacuolated, in which they may resemble mesothelial cells, except that their nuclei show features of malignancy. It is unimaginable to find cells of urothelial carcinoma in a serous fluid without the knowledge that the patient has or has had a urothelial carcinoma.

Melanoma

Patients with advanced melanoma frequently develop a serous effusion. Most melanoma cells in serous fluids are derived from a cutaneous melanoma. Such effusions may be the first manifestation of metastatic melanoma several years after treatment of the primary neoplasm. Only rarely is a serous fluid containing melanoma cells a distinctive brown color (Fig. 7.16A). In such a fluid, the cells are heavily pigmented. The typical cytologic picture of melanoma in a serous fluid is that of a fluid containing numerous obviously malignant cells that tend to be discrete, although small clusters may be present.[4,16,17] The cells are round, with abundant cytoplasm, and the nuclei are eccentric with prominent nucleoli. The cytoplasm may contain melanin (Fig. 7.16B), although many melanoma cells are amelanotic.

In some serous fluids, all of the melanoma cells are amelanotic. Attention to nuclear morphology may enable one to decide that the cells are neoplastic; however, further characterization to illustrate their melanomatous origin may require the use of immunoperoxidase staining, using monoclonal antibodies S-100 and HMB 45.[18,19] S-100 protein is not a melanoma-specific marker; on the other hand, the monoclonal antibody HMB-45 has been shown to have specificity for melanoma cells.

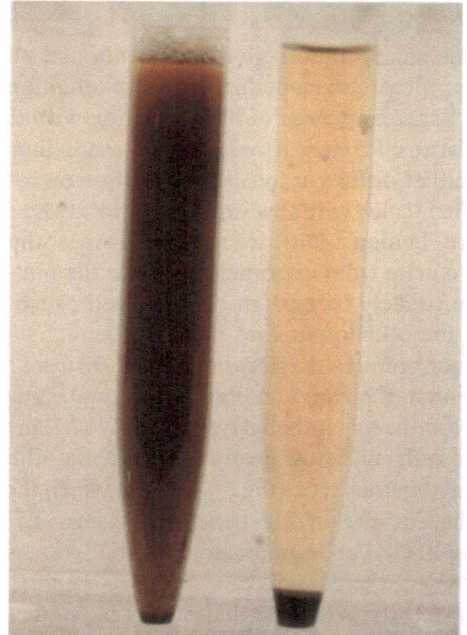

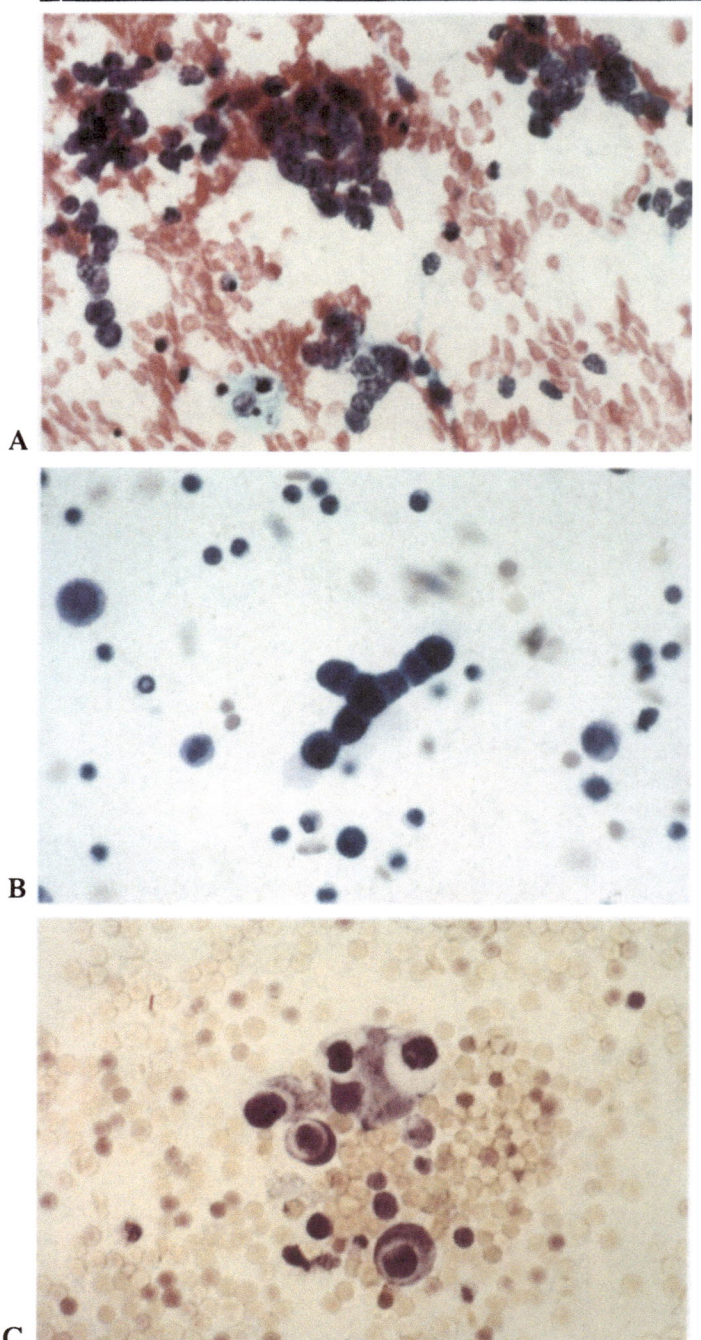

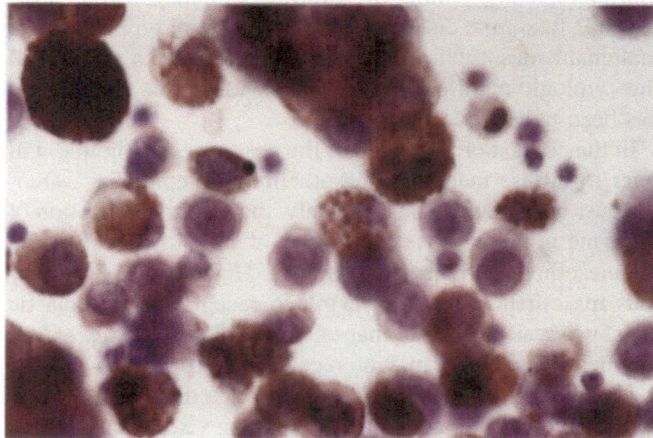

FIGURE 7.16   Malignant melanoma. A: Pleural fluid containing melanoma cells. The tube on the left has not been centrifuged; the tube on the right, containing fluid from the same specimen, has been centrifuged. The patient had metastatic malignant melanoma of the skin. **B:** Pleural fluid illustrated in **A**. Numerous pigmented melanoma cells (smear).

FIGURE 7.15   Oat cell carcinoma. A: Pleural fluid. Fragments of oat cell carcinoma (smear). Some fragments are amorphous and others consist of tiny chains of cells. **B:** Pleural fluid. A branching chain of oat cells (stained wet film). **C:** Pleural fluid. Pairs of oat cells where one nucleus seems to be capping another in a quarter moon manner (stained wet film).

Mesothelioma

Despite malignant mesothelioma of pleura and peritoneum being rare, it has attracted a great deal of attention over the last three decades because of its association with the inhalation of asbestos. Primary neoplasms of mesothelium are classified as either diffuse or localized.[20] Diffuse mesotheliomas are malignant and, with few exceptions, localized mesotheliomas are benign. Diffuse malignant mesothelioma is believed to arise from mesothelial cells or the mesenchymal tissue immediately beneath mesothelial cells, or both. Most localized mesotheliomas are, perhaps, better classified as fibromas or, rarely, as fibrosarcomas. Diffuse malignant mesothelioma of pleura and peritoneum, and rarely of pericardium, is either of epithelial type (Fig. 7.17A), in which the neoplastic cells morphologically resemble mesothelial cells, or is of sarcomatous type (Fig. 7.17B), in which the cells are spindle-shaped. Frequently these neoplasms are biphasic, being of epithelial and sarcomatous type.

In addition, there is a rare primary papillary serous neoplasm of the peritoneum that occurs in women which is morphologically similar to ovarian papillary serous neoplasm.[21] It is quite distinct from the epithelial type of diffuse malignant mesothelioma of peritoneum, and no account of the cytologic manifestation of this condition in ascitic fluid has been published.

In the context of this chapter, the term "mesothelioma" will refer to diffuse malignant mesothelioma of epithelial, sarcomatous, or biphasic type. Typically, the first manifestation of these mesotheliomas is development of an effusion into which the mesothelioma cells may exfoliate. However, the sarcomatous mesotheliomas rarely exfoliate recognizable neoplastic cells, whereas mesotheliomas of epithelial type readily exfoliate their cells, which may be recognizable as such.

In the early stages of development of a diffuse malignant mesothelioma both mesothelial surfaces, visceral and parietal, are studded with inumerable tiny neoplastic nodules. Later, as the nodules become larger, they coalesce to produce a diffusely thickened mesothelium. With further advancement of the mesothelioma, the mesothelial surfaces fuse, thereby partly or completely obliterating the serous cavity, which may then eliminate any effusion. At this stage of pleural mesothelioma the lung is covered by a thick rind of neoplasm (Fig. 7.17C) that may be several centimeters thick.

Usually the first specimen sent to the laboratory from a patient with a mesothelioma is serous fluid. The serous fluid from a patient with mesothelioma may exhibit increased viscosity, observable to the naked eye, due to an increased concentration of hyaluronic acid.[22] Typically, such fluids contain numerous mesothelioma cells that, in their morphologic features, simulate benign mesothelial cells. In contrast to benign mesothelial cells, the cells of mesotheliomas are generally more abundant and tend to form numerous large cohesive clusters (Fig. 7.17D, E); they are larger and their nucleocytoplasmic ratio is low (Fig. 7.17F).[4,23-25] Paradoxically, their nuclei do not show the classic morphologic features of malignancy.

(Discussion continued on p. 116)

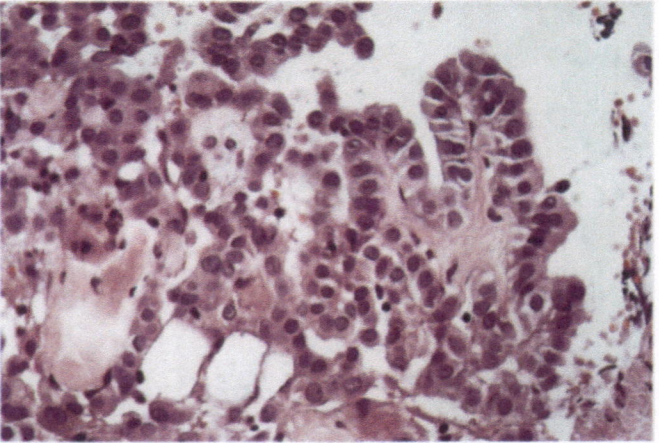

A

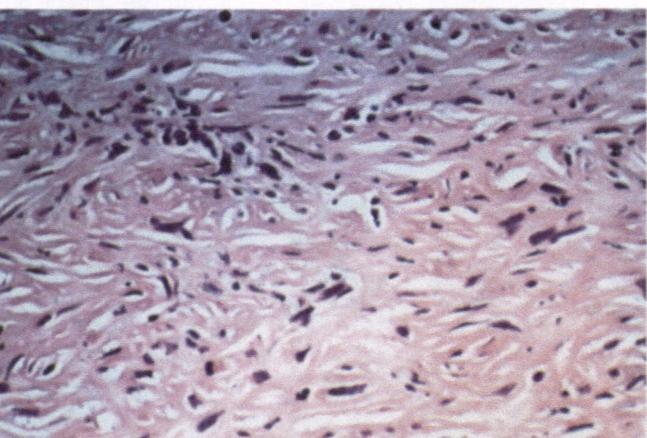

B

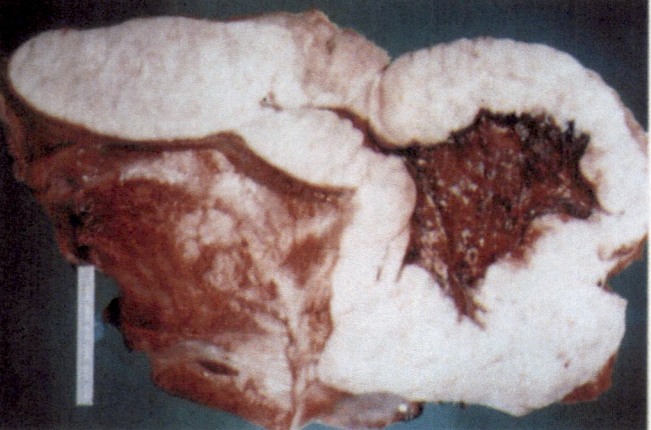

C

FIGURE 7.17 **Diffuse malignant mesothelioma. A:** Papillary diffuse malignant mesothelioma (biopsy). The cells resemble mesothelial cells and do not exhibit frank cytologic evidence of malignancy. **B:** Pleura. Diffuse malignant mesothelioma of sarcomatous type illustrating spindle-shaped nuclei (biopsy). The neoplasm is producing much collagen. **C:** Diffuse malig-

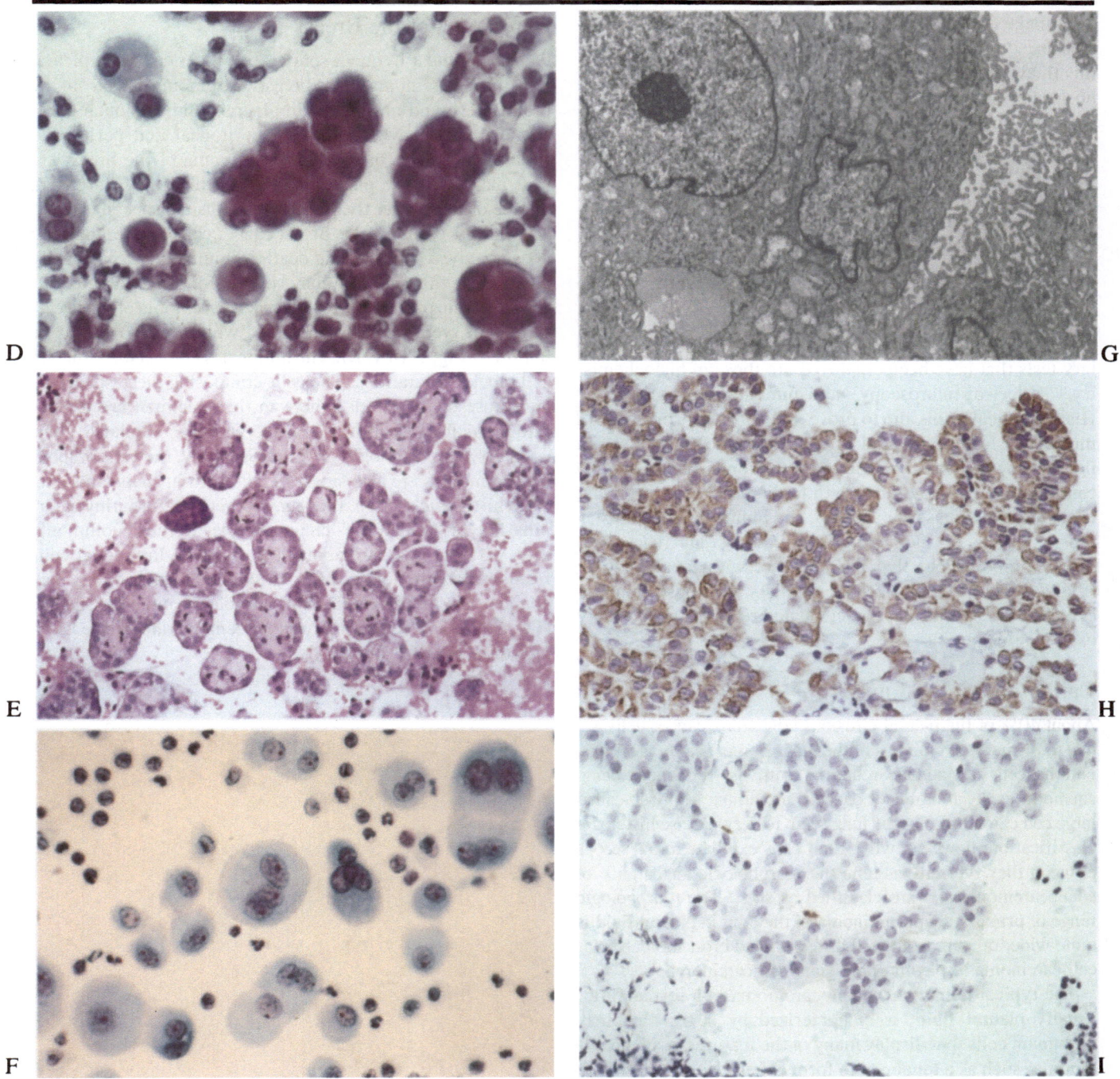

D
E
F
G
H
I

nant mesothelioma of epithelial type surrounding compressed lung (necropsy). Sarcomatous mesothelioma has an identical gross appearance. **D**: Pleural fluid. Many cell clusters of diffuse malignant mesothelioma of epithelial type (smear). **E**: Pleural fluid. Numerous exfoliated fragments of mesothelioma (cell block). The fragments have a collagenous core surrounded by mesothelioma cells. Courtesy Dr. J.D. Schaldenbrand, Ann Arbor, Mich. **F**: Pleural fluid. Mesothelioma cells, which resemble normal mesothelial cells, except that they are much larger and their nucleocytoplasmic ratio is low (smear). **G**: Pleural fluid. Electron micro-graph of malignant mesothelioma cells of epithelial type (cell block). The microvilli are long and undulating ("bushy microvilli"). The microvilli of adenocarcinoma are typically much shorter and straight. **H**: Diffuse malignant mesothelioma of epithelial type illustrating a positive reaction for cytokeratin by the immunoperoxidase method (biopsy). **I**: Diffuse malignant mesothelioma of epithelial type illustrating a negative reaction for carcinoembryonic antigen by the immunoperoxidase method (biopsy).

To make a definite diagnosis of mesothelioma from exfoliated mesothelioma cells usually needs much experience in this field of cytology; however, in most cases a definite diagnosis of mesothelioma can be made. Furthermore, it is desirable that such a diagnosis be made without surgical intervention because mesothelioma tends to grow beneath thoracotomy or laparotomy wounds. It may even grow into thoracentesis or paracentesis needle tracts.

In histologic or cytologic preparations of mesothelioma it may be necessary to apply ancillary techniques to discriminate between mesothelioma and adenocarcinoma, since both of these neoplasms have morphologic features in common. In most cases, such ancillary tests are not needed; the diagnosis may be obvious in routinely prepared specimens. The ancillary tests that have been employed are those of histochemistry,[20,26] electron microscopy,[27] and immunocytochemistry.[28,29] Histochemical stains aim to prove or disprove the presence of mucin and hyaluronic acid in the neoplastic cells, electron microscopy demonstrates that mesotheliomas have a significantly greater microvillus length to diameter ratio than that of adenocarcinomas (Fig. 7.17G), and immunocytochemistry uses a series of monoclonal antibodies that react with adenocarcinoma but that do not react with mesothelioma (Fig. 7.17H, I). Of all of these ancillary methods, immunocytochemistry is the most practical and reliable and is widely used for this purpose.

Carcinoma of the Lung

About 40% of the pleural effusions containing cancer cells are due to primary carcinomas of the lung. In most cases these carcinoma cells are adenocarcinoma, with the remainder being squamous cell carcinoma or oat cell carcinoma. Many so-called large cell carcinomas of the lung seem to defy precise histologic classification; however, when their cells exfoliate into a serous effusion they typically assume the morphologic appearance of adenocarcinoma and are classified as such. The morphologic range of primary adenocarcinoma of the lung in pleural fluid is quite wide, ranging from well differentiated bronchioloalveolar cell carcinoma to pleomorphic giant cell carcinoma.

The typical pulmonary adenocarcinoma in a serous fluid, usually pleural fluid, is characterized by large, obviously malignant cells that display many of the features of adenocarcinoma, such as a tendency to form cohesive clusters (which may be papillary), eccentric malignant-appearing nuclei, and vacuolated cytoplasm (Fig. 7.13).

Carcinoma of the Breast

One of the most frequent sources of cancer cells in a pleural effusion is carcinoma of the breast. Carcinoma cells from the breast are found most often in pleural fluid, although occasionally they may be found in peritoneal and pericardial fluid. Many cases of recurrent carcinoma of the breast are first manifested by pleural effusion, which may develop a decade or more after the primary neoplasm has been treated. The finding of metastatic breast cancer cells in a serous fluid does not always denote that death is imminent. Occasionally a patient in this situation may survive for 2 or more years.

The classic presentation of duct cell carcinoma of the breast is that of well defined spheroids, which may be solid or hollow[30] (Fig. 7.18A, B). The hollowness is best discerned in cell block preparations. The cells composing these spheroids and those dispersed elsewhere in the specimen are usually rather small and uniform in shape and size, similar to their counterpart in histologic sections. Similarly, the cells of lobular carcinomas are also small and uniform in shape and size. As in histologic section, they may sometimes form tiny caterpillarlike or "Indian file" chains, similar to those commonly seen with oat cell carcinoma (Fig. 7.18C). Individual cells from breast carcinomas, especially lobular carcinomas, may contain tiny intracytoplasmic vacuoles containing mucus (Fig. 7.18D). Electron microscopy demonstrates these vacuoles to be lined by microvilli.[31]

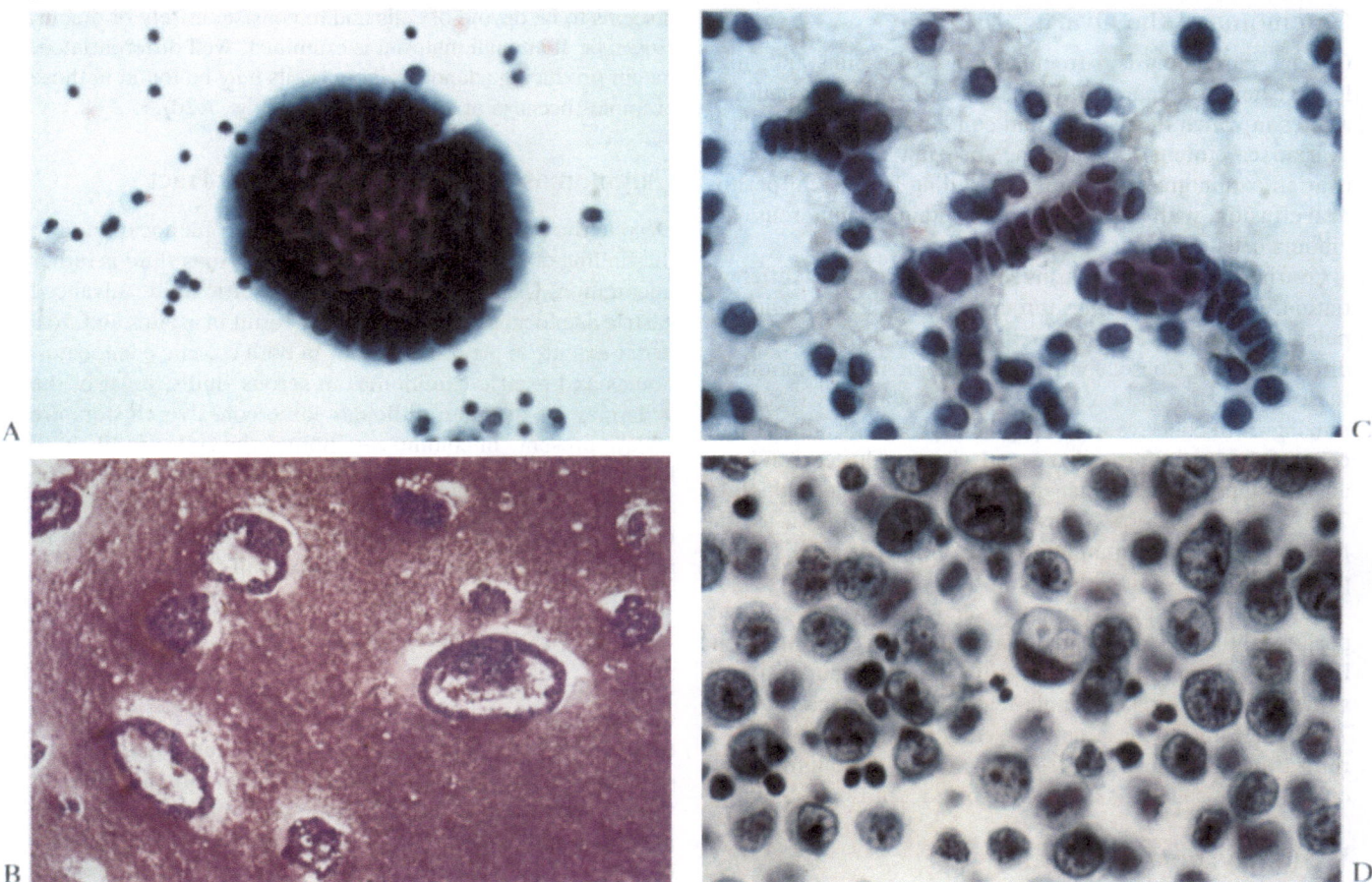

FIGURE 7.18 Carcinoma of the breast. A: Pleural fluid. A dense spheroid of metastatic duct cell carcinoma (smear). **B**: Pleural fluid. Hollow spheroids of metastatic duct cell carcinoma (cell block). **C**: Pericardial fluid. Metastatic lobular carcinoma (smear). The cells are small and some form characteristic chains. **D**: Pleural fluid. Cells of metastatic lobular carcinoma (membrane filter preparation). One cell contains two intracytoplasmic vacuoles, each containing a central dark spot of mucin.

Carcinoma of the Ovary

Ovarian carcinoma is a frequent cause of ascites and, to a lesser extent, of pleural effusion. The most common cause of ascites in which the ascitic fluid contains carcinoma cells is ovarian carcinoma. Frequently, the first manifestation of ovarian carcinoma is abdominal swelling because of peritoneal effusion, with the ascitic fluid containing numerous carcinoma cells.

Ovarian glandular neoplasms show a wide range of differentiation, from cystadenomas through tumors of low malignant potential to invasive adenocarcinomas of various degrees of differentiation. Consequently, the cytologic manifestations of these neoplasms show considerable morphologic variation, ranging from cohesive, often papillary groups of rather small cells of fairly uniform shape and size to clusters of large adenocarcinoma cells that may be hypervacuolated (Fig. 7.19A). Fragments of serous cystadenocarcinoma in ascitic fluid may contain psammoma bodies, best seen in cell block preparations and stained wet films (Fig. 7.19B).

Some serous adenocarcinomas of the ovary present in a peritoneal fluid as rather small, fairly uniform cells that show little or no cytoplasmic vacuolization and whose nuclei do not show the readily recognizable features of malignancy (Fig. 7.19C). Many of these cells resemble mesothelial cells, a reflection of their origin from germinal epithelium of the ovary, which shares its embryonic origin with mesothelium.

Pseudomyxoma Peritonei

Pseudomyxoma peritonei is an uncommon condition that is manifested by a large accumulation of ascitic fluid that has a distinctly mucoid consistency. This type of ascites is caused by well differentiated mucin-producing adenocarcinoma or cystadenoma, usually originating in an ovary or in the large intestine, particularly the appendix. The ascitic fluid is extremely difficult to aspirate, and when examined under the microscope it seems to be devoid of cells and to consist entirely of mucin. However, if enough material is examined, well differentiated, mucin-producing adenocarcinoma cells may be found in those examples because of adenocarcinoma (Fig. 7.20).[32]

Carcinomas of the Gastrointestinal Tract

Despite the many deaths caused by colonic adenocarcinoma, the finding of cells of this neoplasm in a serous fluid is rather uncommon. Usually they are found in ascitic fluid. Advanced gastric adenocarcinomas frequently result in ascites and, to a lesser extent, in pleural effusion. In both colonic adenocarcinomas and gastric carcinomas in serous fluids, most of the cells may be discrete, although some cohesive clusters are always present. In colonic carcinomas the cells are likely to be few, whereas in gastric carcinomas the cells are likely to be abundant with many of signet ring type (Fig. 7.21A). The background to the smears containing colonic or gastric or adenocarcinoma cells may contain mucin (Fig. 7.21B).

Miscellaneous Carcinomas

Most carcinomas in serous fluids are caused by primary neoplasms of breast, lung, or ovary. Excluding carcinomas of these sites, there is a residue of serous fluids that contains carcinomas from a wide variety of other organs. Usually these carcinomas are adenocarcinomas, particularly of the pancreas and biliary tract. Adenocarcinomas from other organs such as endometrium, prostate gland, uterine cervix, thyroid gland, kidney, and liver are much less frequently seen. On the whole the cells of this heterogeneous group of carcinomas bear no distinguishing features that enable one to determine their site of origin. Such a determination has to rely on the overall clinical background of each patient together with a review of any previously obtained histopathologic material.

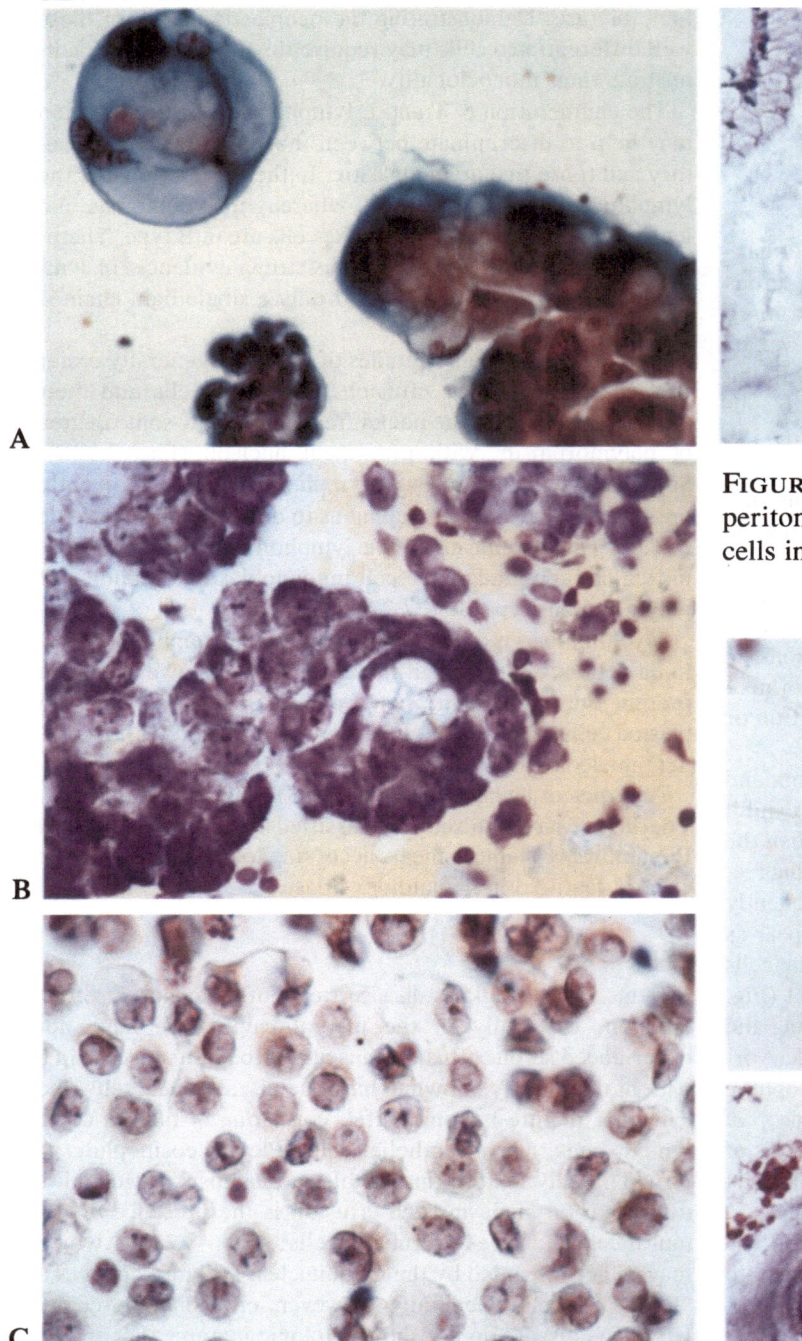

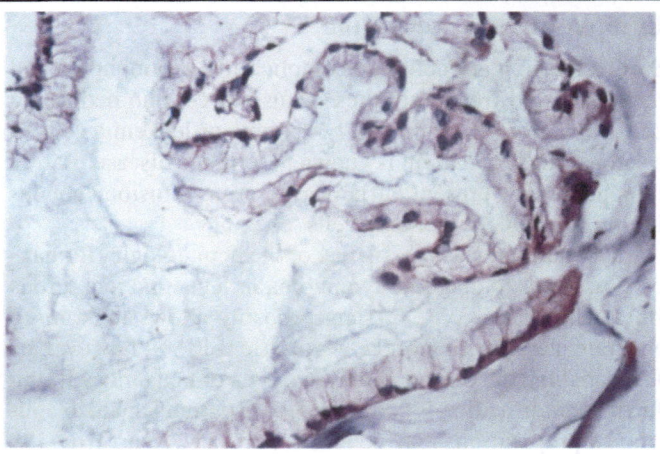

FIGURE 7.20 **Peritoneal fluid.** Pseudomyxoma peritonii. Strips of well differentiated adenocarcinoma cells in a background of mucin (smear).

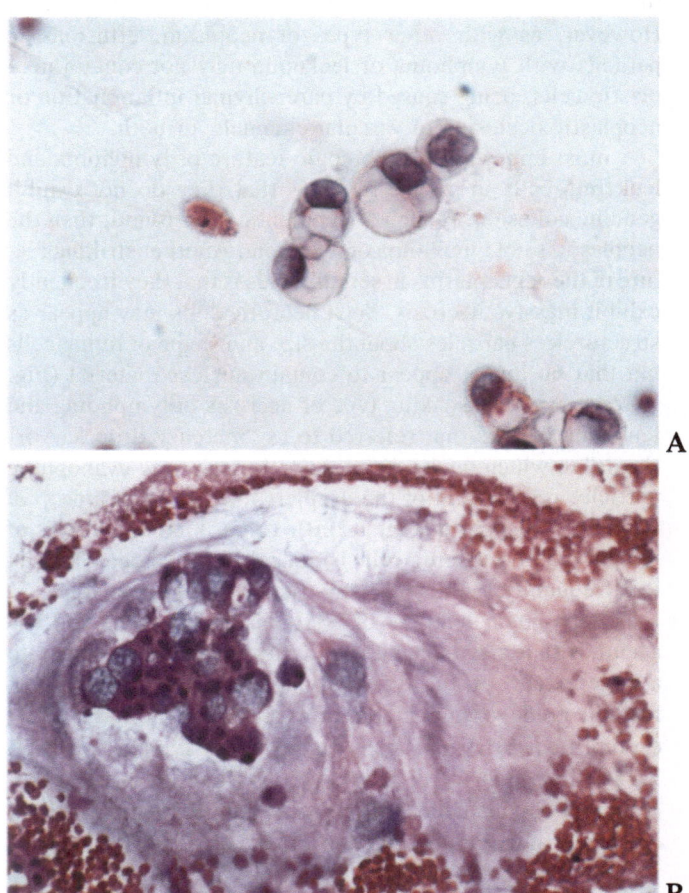

FIGURE 7.19 **Carcinoma of ovary. A**: Peritoneal fluid. A large, hypervacuolated adenocarcinoma cell accompanied by a portion of a papillary fragment of adenocarcinoma (smear). **B**: Pleural fluid. Papillary fragment of ovarian adenocarcinoma (stained wet film). In the center of field is a psammoma body, which does not take up the toluidine blue stain. **C**: Peritoneal fluid. Numerous small ovarian adenocarcinoma cells (smear). Many of the cells resemble mesothelial cells; however, their neoplastic nature is depicted by the hypervacuolization of some of the cells.

FIGURE 7.21 **Gastric and colonic carcinoma. A**: Peritoneal fluid. Gastric adenocarcinoma (smear). Clusters of signet ring adenocarcinoma cells. **B**: Peritoneal fluid. Fragment of colonic adenocarcinoma in a background of blue-gray mucin (smear).

Lymphoma and Leukemia

Serous effusion is a common complication of lymphoma and leukemia, and frequently these effusions contain neoplastic cells. In almost every case of lymphoma or leukemia cells in a serous fluid the patient is known to have the disease. Rarely lymphoma may present initially as a serous effusion containing recognizable lymphoma cells.

Many laboratories rely on one of the hematologic (Romanowsky) stains to diagnose lymphoma or leukemia in a serous fluid. Use of this type of stain probably allows for a more accurate classification of the neoplastic cells[4,33]; however, as far as making the diagnosis of lymphoma or leukemia without further classification is concerned, the routine Papanicolaou-stained preparations may be just as accurate. Apart from the routine morphologic examination of a serous fluid, immunologic and cytometric methods can be applied with some success to the diagnosis and typing of non-Hodgkin's lymphoma (NHL).[34]

When an effusion contains lymphoma or leukemia cells, the cytologic picture may well be dominated by these cells. However, as with other types of neoplasm, effusions in patients with lymphoma or leukemia may not contain neoplastic cells, being caused by parenchymal inflammation or neoplastic occlusion of vascular channels, or both.

A most important morphologic feature of lymphoma and leukemia cells in serous fluids is that they do not exhibit genuine cohesion. If such attachment can be found, then the neoplasm is not lymphoma or leukemia. Another striking feature of these neoplasms in serous fluids is that they frequently exhibit massive necrosis. Such necrotic cells may appear as structureless particles about the size and shape of living cells but that no longer appear to contain nuclear material (Fig. 7.22A). Another striking type of necrosis in lymphoma and leukemia cells is that referred to as "mercury drop karyorrhexis" in which nuclei disintegrate to form tiny cyanophilic particles reminiscent of the droplets formed when a drop of mercury is dispersed (Fig. 7.22B). Either kind of necrosis of lymphoma or leukemia cells is not related to chemotherapy; it is frequently seen before any therapy has been given.

The cytologic features of NHL in serous fluids and the accuracy that may be achieved in their diagnosis depends, to a large extent, on the type of lymphoma: low grade, intermediate grade, or high grade. Low-grade lymphomas are best exemplified by small cell lymphocytic lymphoma (Fig. 7.22C) in which the cells in a serous fluid are morphologically indistinguishable from those of mature benign lymphocytes. Chronic lymphocytic leukemia also gives such a cyto-

logic picture. Demonstrating the neoplastic nature of these well differentiated cells may require flow cytometry to demonstrate their monoclonality.[35]

The enumeration of T and B lymphocytes in such effusion may help to discriminate between those that are inflammatory and those that are neoplastic. In the former, most of the lymphoid cells are of T type, whereas in lymphomas and leukemias a high proportion of the cells are of B type. Therefore, a high proportion of B cells is strong evidence for lymphoma or leukemia, especially if only a single light chain is present.[36]

The cells of the higher grades of NHL are generally easier to recognize in serous effusions. Both the cells and their nuclei are larger and the nuclei frequently show some degree of polymorphism, with prominent nucleoli (Fig. 7.22B). Some degree of necrosis of lymphoma cells is frequently present and may be so abundant as to dominate the cytologic picture. The extreme end of the lymphoma spectrum is exemplified by high-grade large cell immunoblastic lymphoma of polymorphous type (Fig. 7.22D).

Myelomatosis is classified as a low-grade lymphoma. Myeloma cells are rarely seen in serous fluids. However, when present they are usually numerous and appear as enlarged plasma cells, many with two or more nuclei and with prominent nucleoli (Fig. 7.22E).

All types of leukemic cells may be found in serous fluids. They are best recognized and classified by the use of air-dried Romanowsky-stained smears according to usual morphologic criteria featured in hematology atlases.

Hodgkin's Disease

Patients with Hodgkin's disease frequently develop a serous effusion, especially in the pleural cavity. We have not experienced serous effusion caused by Hodgkin's disease in a patient not already known to have the disease. Generally, the cytologic picture is nonspecific, consisting of plasma cells, lymphocytes, and mesothelial cells. Pleural eosinophilia is rare. The only feature that enables a diagnosis of Hodgkin's disease to be made in such effusion is the presence of the multinucleated Reed-Sternberg cells[4] (Fig. 7.22F), which may be accompanied by the mononuclear variant known as a "Hodgkin's cell." Generally, however, effusions caused by Hodgkin's disease do not show cytologic features that enable the diagnosis of Hodgkin's disease to be made on the fluid alone. If Reed-Sternberg cells are present, they are likely to be present in small numbers, and a prolonged search may be required to find more than one or two.

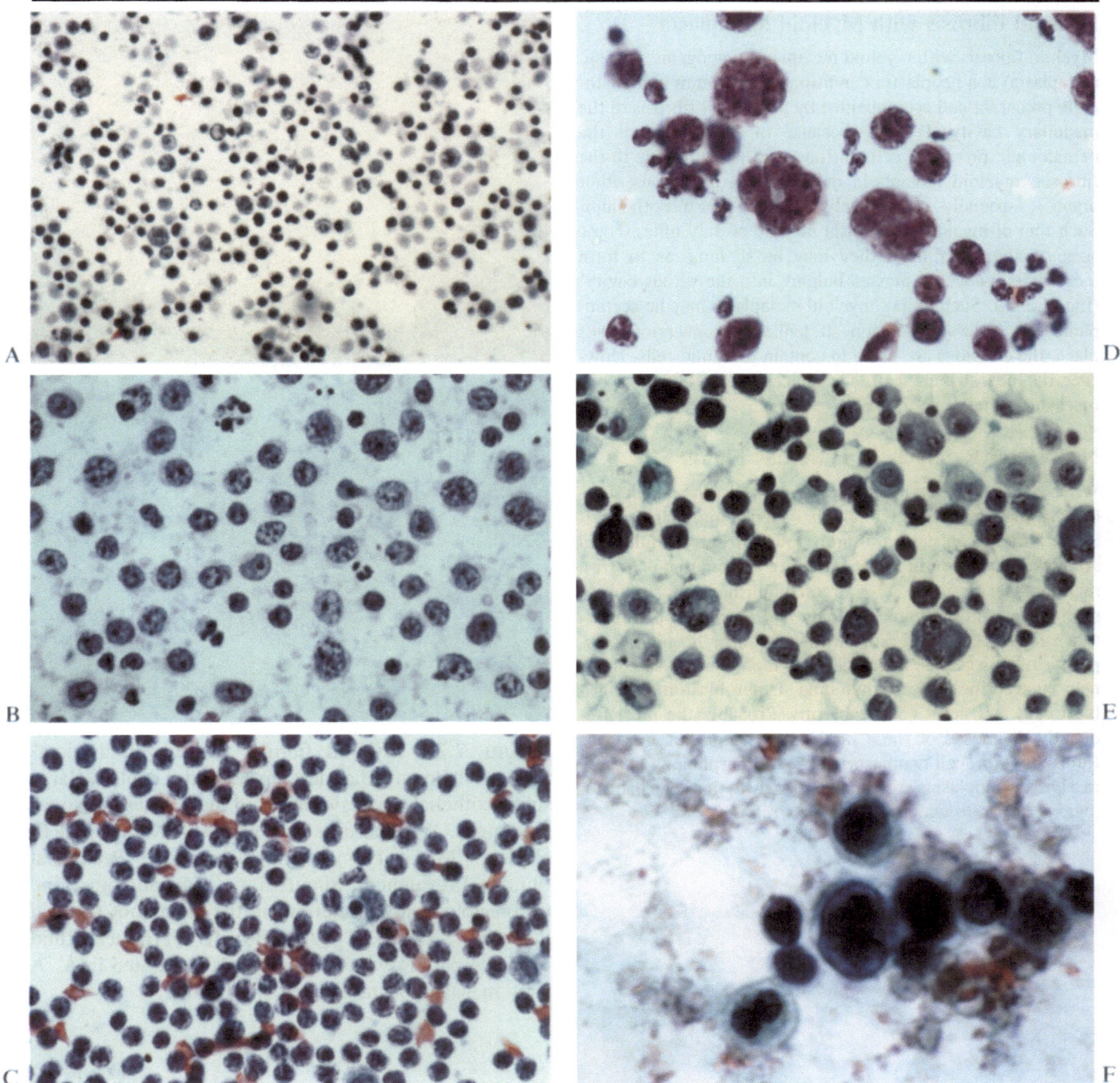

FIGURE 7.22   Leukemia and lymphoma. A: Pleural fluid. Acute myeloblastic leukemia. A high proportion of the cells are necrotic, as evidenced by the presence of numerous gray cells whose nuclei have disappeared (smear). **B**: Pleural fluid. High-grade lymphoma (smear). Notice how the cells are separated from each other. Nucleoli are prominent. In between the cells is a granular background of necrotic cells. A few cells show mercury drop karyorrhexis, in the form of tiny, dense, cyanophilic particles in the cytoplasm. **C**: Pleural fluid. Low-grade lymphocytic lymphoma (smear). These cells were monoclonal. In routine preparations these cells cannot be distinguished from those of an inflammatory exudate. **D**: Pleural fluid. Large cell immunoblastic lymphoma of polymorphous type (smear). **E**: Pleural fluid. Numerous myeloma cells (smear). These cells resemble plasma cells except that they are much larger and many are multinucleate. Notice their tendency to be separated from each other. **F**: Pleural fluid. Hodgkin's disease. In the center of the field is a binucleate Reed-Sternberg cell (smear).

Myeloid Fibrosis with Myeloid Metaplasia

Myeloid fibrosis with myeloid metaplasia (agnogenic myeloid metaplasia) is a neoplastic condition of the common hematologic precursor cell accompanied by prominent fibrosis of the medullary cavity. Possibly because of effacement of the hematologic precursor cells in the marrow cavity due to the fibrosis, myeloid metaplasia may develop in various other organs, especially immediately beneath the mesothelium. Such foci of myeloid metaplasia may be of only microscopic size; on the other hand they may be so large as to form mesothelium-covered masses bulging into the serous cavity[5] (Fig. 7.23A). Such foci of myeloid metaplasia may be accompanied by a serous effusion. If leukemic conversion takes place, the effusions are likely to contain leukemic cells. However, the most striking feature of such effusions is the presence megakaryocytes (Fig. 7.23B).

Neoplasms Rarely Seen in Serous Fluids

When a serous fluid contains neoplastic cells, the neoplasm is likely to be carcinoma, lymphoma or leukemia, or mesothelioma. Other neoplasms are rarely found in serous fluids and are most likely seen in larger reference centers that deal with many cancer patients. The largest published description of such cases is in the book of Hajdu and Hajdu,[37] which illustrates material derived from a major cancer hospital. Neoplasms of this category include nonlymphomatous sarcomas, neuroendrocrine tumors, thymoma, nephroblastoma, neuroblastoma, and germ cell neoplasms. Probably the most frequently diagnosed of these rarely seen neoplasms in serous fluids are germ cell neoplasms. The cytomorphology of these rarely seen neoplasms corresponds closely to that seen in histologic sections, to which the reader is referred.

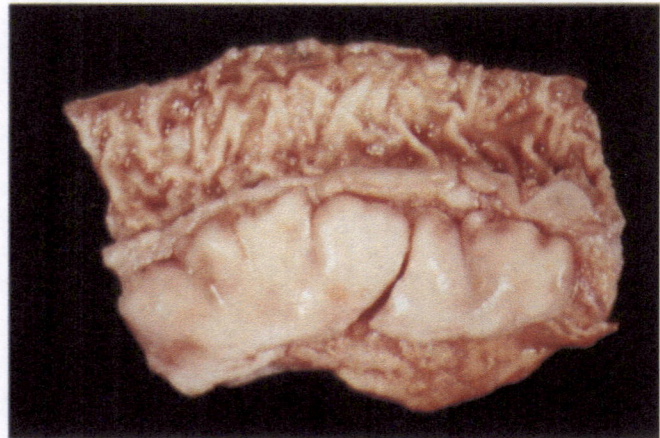

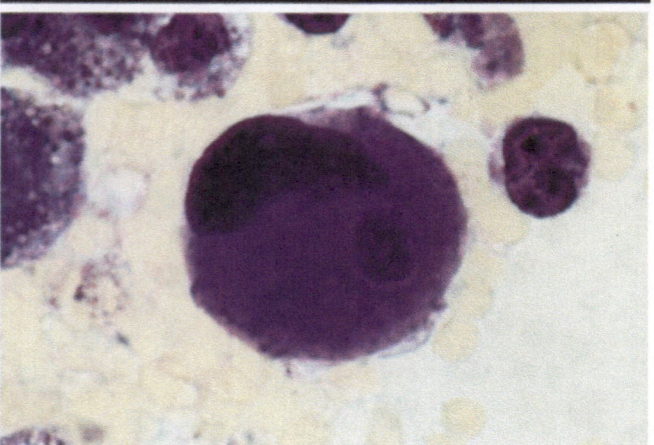

FIGURE 7.23 **Myeloid fibrosis with myeloid metaplasia. A**: Ileum. The mesenteric border contains large submesothelial masses of myeloid metaplasia (necropsy specimen). With permission from N.B. Kumar and B. Naylor, "Megakaryocytes in Pleural and Peritoneal Fluids: Prevalence, Significance, Morphology, and Cytohistological Correlation" in the Journal of Clinical Pathology. 33:1153-1159, 1980. **B**: Peritoneal fluid from the patient whose specimen is illustrated in **A**. A large megakaryocyte (stained wet film).

References

1. Kern WH. Benign papillary structures with psammoma bodies in culdocentesis fluid. *Acta Cytol.* 1969;13:178–180.

2. Dekker A, Graham T, Bupp PA. The occurrence of sickle cells in pleural fluid: Report of a patient with sickle cell disease. *Acta Cytol.* 1975;19:251–254.

3. Veress JF, Koss LG, Schreiber K. Eosinophilic pleural effusions. *Acta Cytol.* 1979;23:40–44.

4. Spriggs AI, Boddington MM. *Atlas of Serous Fluid Cytopathology. A Guide to the Cells of Pleural, Pericardial, Peritoneal and Hydrocele Fluids*, Vol. 14, *Current Histopathology Series*, Gresham GA, ed. Dordrecht: Kluwer Academic Publishers; 1989.

5. Kumar NB, Naylor B. Megakaryocytes in pleural and peritoneal fluids: Prevalence, significance, morphology, and cytohistological correlation. *J Clin Pathol.* 1980;33:1153–1159.

6. Ashfaq-Drewett R, Allen C, Harrison RL. Detached ciliary tufts. Comparison with intestinal protozoa and a review of the literature. *Am J Clin Pathol.* 1990;93:541–545.

7. Sidawy MK, Chandra P, Oertel YC. Detached ciliary tufts in female peritoneal washings. A common finding. *Acta Cytol.* 1987;31:841–844.

8. Domagala W, Emerson EE, Koss LG. T and B lymphocyte enumeration in the diagnosis of lymphocyte-rich pleural fluids. *Acta Cytol.* 1981;25:108–110.

9. Ghosh AK, Spriggs AI, Mason DY. Immunocytochemical staining of T and B lymphocytes in serous effusions. *J Clin Pathol.* 1985;38:608–612.

10. Naylor B. The pathognomonic cytologic picture of rheumatoid pleuritis. *Acta Cytol.* 1990;34:465–473.

11. Osamura RY, Shioya S, Handa K, Shimizu K. Lupus erythematosus cells in pleural fluid. Cytologic diagnosis in two patients. *Acta Cytol.* 1977;21:215–217.

12. Dubois EL. *Lupus Erythematosus.* 2nd ed. Los Angeles: University of Southern California Press; 1974.

13. Smith-Purslow MJ, Kini SR, Naylor B. Cells of squamous cell carcinoma in pleural, peritoneal and pericardial fluids. Origin and morphology. *Acta Cytol.* 1989;29:245–253.

14. Salhadian A, Nasiell M, Nasiell K, et al. The unique cytologic picture of oat cell carcinoma in effusions. *Acta Cytol.* 1976;20:298–302.

15. Spriggs AI, Boddington MM. Oat-cell bronchial carcinoma. Identification of cells in pleural fluid. *Acta Cytol.* 1976;20:525–529.

16. Hajdu SI, Savino A. Cytologic diagnosis of malignant melanoma. *Acta Cytol.* 1973;17:320–327.

17. Yamada T, Itou U, Watanabe Y, Ohashi S. Cytologic diagnosis of malignant melanoma. *Acta Cytol.* 1972;16:70–76.

18. Ordóñez NG, Sneige N, Hickey RC, Brooks TE. Use of monoclonal antibody HMB-45 in the cytologic diagnosis of melanoma. *Acta Cytol.* 1988;32:684–688.

19. Pinto MM. An immunoperoxidase study of S-100 protein in neoplastic cells in serous effusions. Use as a marker for melanoma. *Acta Cytol.* 1986;30:240–244.

20. McCaughey WTE, Kannerstein M, Churg J. *Tumors and Pseudotumors of the Serous Membranes. Atlas of Tumor Pathology, Second series, fascicle 20.* Washington, DC: Armed Forces Institute of Pathology; 1985.

21. Bell DA, Scully RE. Benign and borderline serous lesions of the peritoneum in women. In Rosen PP, Fechner RE, eds. *Pathology Annual, 1989: Part 2.* East Norwalk: Appleton and Lange; 1989:1–21.

22. Castor WC, Naylor B. Acid mucopolysaccharide composition of serous effusions. Study of 100 patients with neoplastic and non-neoplastic conditions. *Cancer.* 1967;20:462–466.

23. Koss LG. *Diagnostic Cytology and Its Histopathologic Bases.* 3rd ed. Philadelphia: JB Lippincott; 1979.

24. Naylor B. The exfoliative cytology of diffuse malignant mesothelioma. *J Pathol Bacteriol.* 1963;86:293–298.

25. Whitaker D, Shilkin KB. Diagnosis of pleural malignant mesothelioma in life—a practical approach. *J Pathol.* 1984;143:147–175.

26. Kannerstein M, Churg J, Magner D. Histochemistry in the diagnosis of malignant mesothelioma. *Ann Clin Lab Sci.* 1973;3:207–211.

27. Kobzik L, Antman KH, Warhol MJ. The distinction of mesothelioma from adenocarcinoma in malignant effusions by electron microscopy. *Acta Cytol.* 1985;29:219–225.

28. Ordonez NG. The immunohistochemical diagnosis of mesothelioma: Differentiation of mesothelioma and lung adenocarcinoma. *Am J Surg Pathol.* 1989;13:276–291.

29. Johnston WW, Szpak CA, Thor A, Simpson J, Schlom J. Antibodies to tumor-associated antigens: Applications in clinical cytology. In: Wied GL, Keebler CM, Koss LG, Reagan JW, eds. *Compendium on Diagnostic Cytology.* 6th ed. Chicago: Tutorials of Cytology; 1988:567–578.

30. Ashton PR, Hollingsworth AS, Johnston WW. The cytopathology of metastatic breast cancer. *Acta Cytol.* 1975;19:1–6.

31. Spriggs AI, Jerrome DW. Intracellular mucous inclusions. A feature of malignant cells in effusions in the serous cavities, particularly due to carcinoma of the breast. *J Clin Pathol.* 1975;28:929–936.

32. Costa M, Oertel Y. Cytology of pseudomyxoma peritonei: Report of two cases arising from appendiceal cystadenomas. *Diagn Cytopathol.* 1989;6:201–203.

33. Spriggs AI, Vanhegan RI. Cytological diagnosis of lymphoma in serous effusions. *J Clin Pathol.* 1981;34:1311–1325.

34. Katz RL, Raval P, Manning JT, McLaughlin P, Barlogie B. A morphologic, immunologic, and cytometric approach to the classification of non-Hodgkin's lymphoma in effusions. *Diagn Cytopathol.* 1987;3:91–101.

35. Martin SE, Zhang H-Z, Magyarosy E, Jaffe ES, Hsu S-M, Chu EW. Immunologic methods in cytology: Definitive diagnosis of non-Hodgkin's lymphomas using immunologic markers for T and B-cells. *Am J Clin Pathol.* 1984;82:666–673.

36. Yam LT, Lin DG, Janckila AJ, Li C-Y. Immunocytochemical diagnosis of lymphoma in serous effusions. *Acta Cytol.* 1985;29:833–841.

37. Hajdu SI, Hajdu EO. *Cytopathology of Sarcomas and Other Nonepithelial Malignant Tumors.* Philadelphia: WB Saunders; 1976.

8
Liver

Anatomy and Histology

The normal adult liver weighs 1400 to 1600 g and is nonpalpable under the costal edge. The anatomic division divides the liver into right and left lobes. The right lobe is divided by the right segmental fissure into an anterior and posterior segment, whereas the left lobe is divided by the left segmental fissure into a medial and lateral segment. The four segmental biliary ducts from each of the four segments of the liver join to form the right and left hepatic ducts, which in turn unite to form the common hepatic duct. The main arterial branch to the liver is via the hepatic propria branch of the common hepatic artery from the celiac.

Three major hepatic veins (the right, middle, and left) are formed in the liver and empty into the suprahepatic inferior vena cava. The portal vein ascends in the hepatoduodenal ligament posterior to the common bile duct and hepatic artery. As it reaches the porta hepatis, it terminates in line with the main lobar fissure by dividing into a right and left portal vein.

Hepatic lobules are the basic histological and functional units of the liver. The hepatic lobule is hexagonal, 1 to 2 mm in diameter, oriented about a central vein (a tributary of the hepatic vein).

Hepatocytes are radially disposed about the central vein in anastomosing sheets or plates, "hepatic cell cords." Interposed between the radial hepatic cell cords are vascular sinusoids receiving blood from both the portal and the arterial systems, and draining into the central veins. The sinusoids are lined by discontinuous endothelial cells, attached to which are scattered Kupffer cells of the monocyte phagocyte system. In the periphery of the lobules are portal triads containing hepatic arterioles, portal veins, and bile ducts (Fig. 8.1A). Although the acinar model of Rappaport better describes the functional units of the liver, the classic lobule is more useful in pathologic descriptions.

Between the sinusoids and liver cell cords are Disse's spaces. The interhepatocytic biliary canaliculi are channels, 1 to 2 μm in diameter, formed merely by grooves along the external surfaces of abutting liver cells (Fig. 8.1B). An elaborate network of biliary canaliculi progressively joins toward the periphery of the lobules eventually into the interlobular bile ducts within the portal triads.

In fine needle aspiration (FNA) smears, the hepatocytes are large polygonal cells with abundant eosinophilic granular cytoplasm. The nuclei are round, but variable in size and often contain a prominent nucleolus. Binucleated hepatocytes are common (Fig. 8.1C).

The cells of the bile duct epithelium occur in sheets. They are rather uniform in shape with round or cuboidal cells and have scanty cytoplasm and round nuclei with inconspicuous nucleoli.

Techniques and Indications for Fine Needle Aspiration of the Liver

Fine needle aspiration of the liver can be performed safely in most space-occupying lesions, such as primary or metastatic cancers, liver abscesses, and hepatic cysts. It is performed under computed tomography (CT) or ultrasound guidance. Aspiration techniques are described in the introductory chapter. Aspiration should be performed with extreme care in cases with abnormal blood clotting, hemangiomas of the liver, or hydatid cysts caused by *Echinococcus*.

Complications related to FNA procedures occasionally occur. They include hemoperitoneum, bile peritonitis, and anaphylactic shock as a result of rupture of an *Echinococcal* cyst.

Liver biopsy with large cutting needles is the preferred and more reliable procedure in diffuse, non-neoplastic liver diseases such as hepatitis, cirrhosis, or metabolic diseases of the liver.

In this chapter, viral hepatitis, cirrhosis, some non-neoplastic lesions, and primary and metastatic tumors will be discussed.

Viral Hepatitis

Although a number of systemic viral infections may cause mild or transient hepatitis, the term "viral hepatitis" is considered to be infection of the liver caused by hepatotropic viruses. They are hepatitis A virus (HAV), hepatitis B virus (HBV), hepatitis delta virus (HDV) and non-A, non-B viruses (NANBV). In the past year, an RNA virus designated hepatitis C has been shown to cause more than 80% of cases on non-A, non-B hepatitis. Viral hepatitis caused by these hepatotropic viruses show the same clinicopathologic patterns with distinct difference in virologic or serologic markers and prognosis.

Hepatitis A Virus

Hepatitis A is a benign, self-limited disease with short incubation period (14–45 days) and overt or transient febrile course. HAV is a nonenveloped, single-stranded RNA virus. Its RNA genome has been transcribed into complementary DNA (cDNA), which can be identified in liver cells by molecular hybridization techniques. The viral agents spread by oral ingestion of contaminated foods and water or close personal contact during the incubation period. Hepatitis A virus does not cause chronic hepatitis, hepatocellular carcinoma, or carrier state and rarely results in fulminant hepatitis.[1] Hepatitis A virus is identified by HAV markers with elevation of immunoglobulin M (IgM) type antibody in the acute phase and depression of the antibody in the convalescent phase. Immunoglobulin G (IgG) HAV antibody titer increases steadily throughout the acute and convalescent phases and provides long-lasting immunity.

Hepatitis B Virus

Hepatitis B is caused by a DNA virus and evolves into more serious clinicopathologic consequences. It can produce acute hepatitis, fulminant hepatitis with massive or submassive necrosis, chronic hepatitis progressing to cirrhosis, and an asymptomatic carrier state. Hepatitis B virus plays an important role in the development of hepatocellular carcinoma. It has a longer incubation period, ranging from 30 to 180 days. Hepatitis B virus is spread by parenteral routes such as blood transfusion and intravenous drug addicts using common needles in nonendemic regions. In endemic regions, spread from an infected mother to a neonate during birth (vertical transmission) is more common. The natural course of the disease can be followed by the serologic markers.

Hepatitis B surface antigen (HB$_s$Ag) is an indicator of active HBV infection and appears before the onset of symptoms, peaks during the overt disease, and then declines to undetectable levels in 3 to 6 months. Anti-HB$_s$ appears several months after the disappearance of the HB$_s$Ag and long after the convalescent phase; it persists in most cases for life, and is considered protective against subsequent infection.

HB$_e$Ag, HBV-DNA, and DNA polymerase appear in the serum soon after HB$_s$Ag is detectable, and they are evidence of active viral replication. Persistence of HB$_e$Ag is an important clinical indication of probable progression to chronic hepatitis. Immunoglobulin M anti-HB$_c$ appears before the onset of symptoms and is replaced by IgG anti-HB$_c$ over several months, so an elevated IgM anti-HB$_c$ level indicates a recent acute infection.

A third type of viral hepatitis that is found only in individuals who have or have had hepatitis B is designated delta (D) viral hepatitis. The agent is an RNA virus that requires the hepatitis B virus as a "helper" virus. Delta virus is particularly likely to cause serious hepatitis and to lead to chronic active hepatitis.

Non-A, Non-B Hepatitis Viruses

Non-A, Non-B (NANB) hepatitis represents the cases of hepatitis with no virologic or serologic markers to identify any of the well-defined viral etiologies. It spreads mostly by blood transfusion and rarely by the water-borne route. Its clinicopathological features are similar to those of hepatitis B save that it has no implication in hepatocellular carcinoma.[2]

Hepatitis C Virus

The recent development of a specific assay for a blood-borne NANBV has identified hepatitis C virus (HCV). The data of the recent studies indicate that HCV is a major cause of NANBH throughout the world[3,4]. It appears to be a single-stranded RNA virus, and marker tests are rapidly becoming available. Currently NANBV accounts for 90% of posttransfusional hepatitis, but with the institution of effective blood screening with these markers, this should change dramatically in the near future.

Clinicopathologic Features of Hepatitis

There are no satisfactory data on carrier state of the prevalence of the HDV, HAV, and NANBV. Only the HBV carrier state is associated with distinctive morphologic changes. The liver biopsy in the "healthy" HBV carrier shows more or less normal morphology except for evidence of the viral infection in isolated cells or clusters of hepatocytes. The cells have "ground-glass," finely granular, eosinophilic cytoplasms that are more conspicuous with orcein or aldehyde fuchsin staining (Fig. 8.2).

Acute Viral Hepatitis

Whatever the causative agent, clinicopathological features of acute hepatitis are more or less similar. Clinically, the preicteric phase of acute hepatitis is marked by nonspecific constitutional symptoms. Later, the preicteric phase is followed by jaundice and dark urine due to conjugated hyperbilirubinemia. Itching caused by retention of bile salts may be present. The liver may be enlarged and tender to palpation. In a few weeks to months, the jaundice and most of the systemic symptoms clear as convalescence begins. The diagnosis of acute hepatitis requires the presence of antigens or antibodies in the serum. Elevation of aminotransferase in the serum is indicative of hepatocytic injury. Other abnormal liver function tests include prolonged prothrombin time, hyperglobulinemia, and hyperbilirubinemia.

Pathology

Grossly, the liver is greenish yellow and slightly enlarged. Histologically, acute hepatitis shows disarray of hepatic lobules, diffuse hepatocytic injury, necrosis of isolated liver cells or clusters, Councilmanlike bodies, Kupffer cell hyperplasia, and inflammatory infiltrate in the portal tracts (Fig. 8.3). (*Discussion continued on p. 128*)

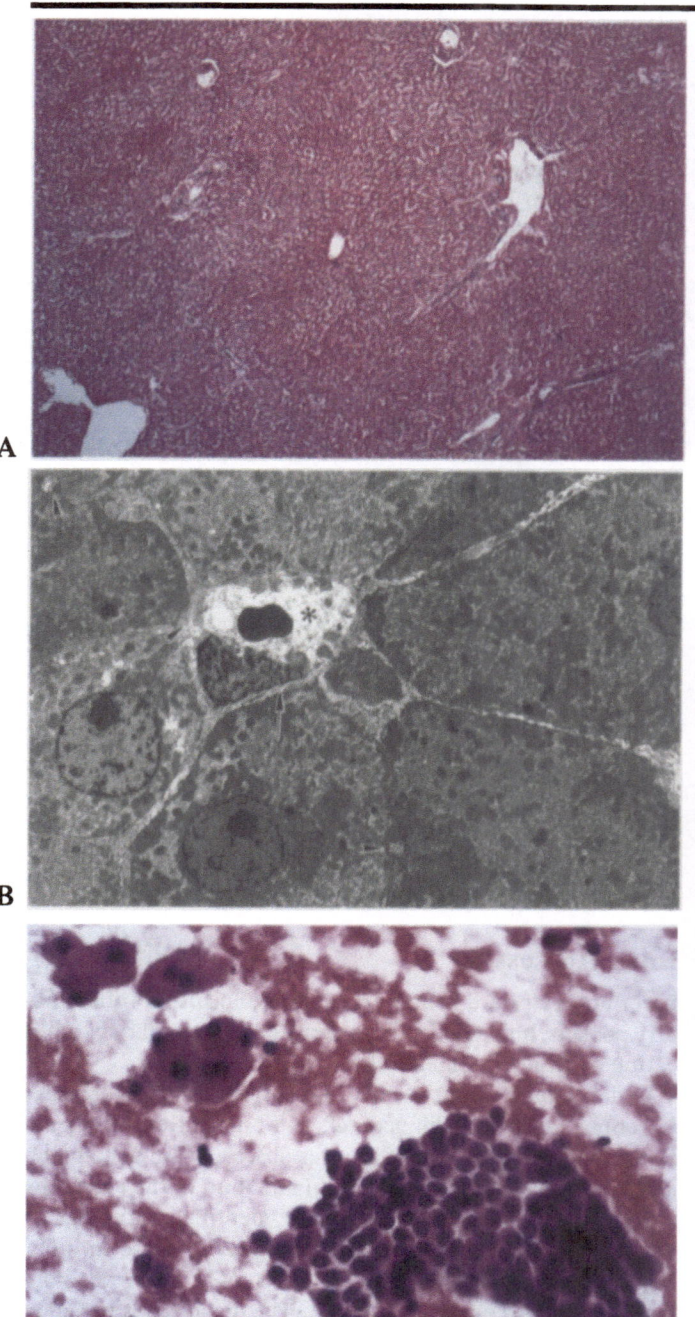

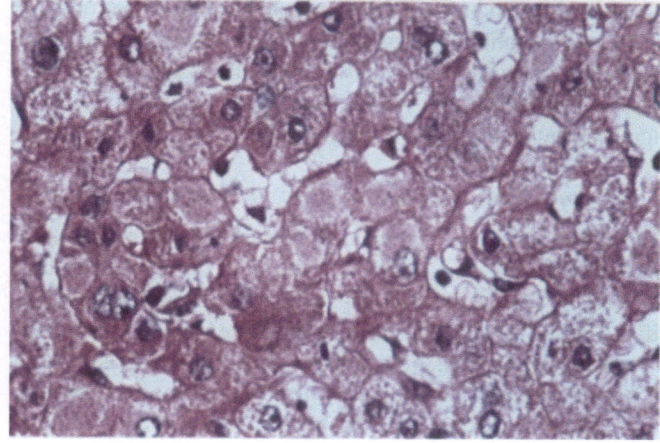

FIGURE 8.2   Hepatocytes with "ground-glass" appearance due to HBV infection in carrier state.

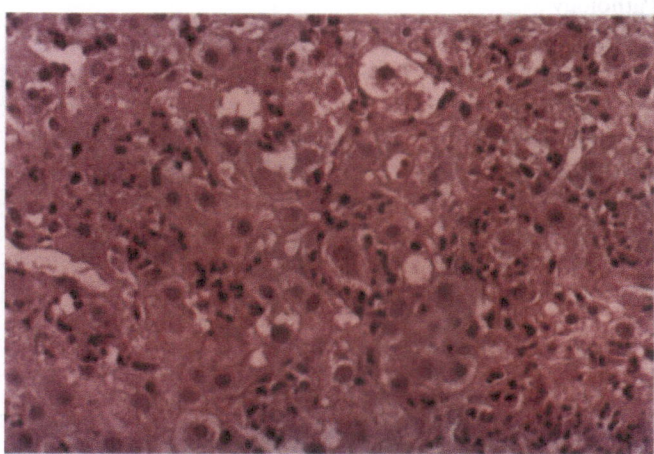

FIGURE 8.3   Acute viral hepatitis. Disarray of hepatic lobules with hepatocytic injury, "piecemeal" necrosis, Councilman's bodies, and inflammatory infiltrate in the portal tract.

FIGURE 8.1   Histology of normal liver. A: Hepatic lobules with central vein in the center and portal triads in the periphery. **B**: Hepatocytes with sinusoids (*asterisk*), Disse's spaces (*arrows*), and bile canaliculi (*arrowheads*). (Courtesy of William Gunning, Ph.D., Medical College of Oh.) **C**: FNA smear showing aggregates of hepatocytes with abundant cytoplasm (*upper portion*) and sheets of bile duct epithelial cells with scanty cytoplasm and uniform round nuclei (*right lower portion*).

Councilman's bodies are cells or cell fragments that are intensely eosinophilic because of extrusion of nuclear material through a process of necrosis called apoptosis. In recovery phase, bi-nucleate and trinucleate liver cells and mitotic figures provide evidence of regeneration.

Fulminant Hepatitis (Submassive to Massive Necrosis)

About 1% of acute hepatitis progresses to submassive to massive necrosis of the liver. More than 50% of fulminant hepatitis cases are of viral origin (HBV and NANBV). Hepatitis A virus rarely causes fulminant hepatitis. Drugs and chemicals are responsible for about 30%. The clinical course of fulminant hepatitis requires a few weeks to a few months from onset to death, which occurs in a very high percentage of cases. Ironically, recovery, when it occurs, is likely to be complete and fulminant hepatitis is not thought to be the antecedent of cirrhosis.

Pathology

Grossly, the liver is soft, pale, and small (Fig. 8.4). The necrosis may involve multifocal, random, or patchy large areas (submassive) or the entire liver (massive). Histologically, the necrosis may involve the lobules or portions of them sparing the periphery of the lobule. The hepatocytes are almost liquefied, which results in collapsed lobules. The reticulin framework and portal tracts become condensed. Regenerative activity may occur in the periphery and shows disarray of the lobular pattern.

Chronic Hepatitis

Chronic hepatitis is defined as continuing inflammatory hepatic disease for more than 6 months. Most cases of chronic hepatitis are caused by HBV and NANBV, and rarely by Wilson's disease, drug reactions, chronic alcoholism, alpha$_1$-antitrypsin deficiency, and autoimmunity. Hepatitis A virus does not produce chronic hepatitis. There are two principal subtypes, with distinct clinical implications.

Chronic Persistent Hepatitis

Chronic persistent hepatitis (CPH) is a mild smoldering infection with a relapsing and recovering condition after acute hepatitis. The patients may be symptom-free or considered as delayed recovery from the acute episode. Most patients have an elevated serum level of aminotransferase. Hepatitis B surface antigen is found in the serum of 20% to 60% of these patients.

Histologically, the hepatic architecture is fairly well preserved but there is a remarkable inflammatory infiltrate of lymphocytes, macrophages, and plasma cells in the portal tracts (Fig. 8.5). Occasionally, "ground-glass" hepatocytes may be observed.

Chronic Active Hepatitis

In contrast to CPH, chronic active hepatitis (CAH) is a chronic necrotizing and fibrosing hepatic disease of varied etiology. Most cases of CAH are caused by HBV and NANBV, and rarely by chemicals and autoimmune reaction (chronic autoimmune hepatitis).

Histologically, CAH is characterized by piecemeal and bridging necrosis of hepatocytes, inflammatory infiltrate involving the portal areas with breaking parenchymal limiting plates, and progressive fibrosis (Fig. 8.6). The clinical features of CAH are variable, and range from asymptomatic to the full-blown pattern of hepatic failure. Laboratory findings in CAH are an elevated serum aminotransferase level and prolongation of the prothrombin time. Clinical course is unpredictable and the 5-year mortality is about 25% to 50%.

Liver Abscess

Liver abscesses are solitary or multiple localized inflammatory pockets, and most of them represent a secondary complication of an infection elsewhere.

In developing countries, liver abscesses represent parasitic infections (amebic, echinococcal, and other protozoal organisms). In developed countries, liver abscesses are uncommon and most are bacterial in origin. In one third of the cases, the sources of the abscesses cannot be identified (cryptogenic abscesses). Pathologic changes are similar to those in other organ sites. Clinical features are fever, right upper quadrant pain, and tender liver on palpation. The diagnosis is based on ultrasonography, CT, or magnetic resonance imaging (MRI). Treatment of liver abscesses is drainage and antibiotic therapy.

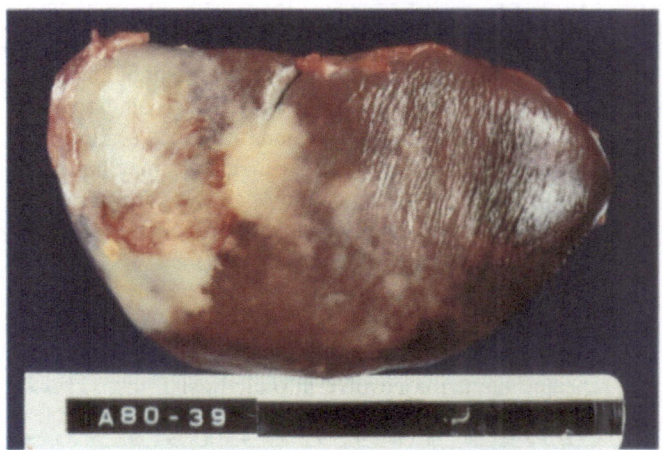

FIGURE 8.4   Fulminant hepatitis with massive necrosis. Small, pale and soft liver with wrinkled capsule.

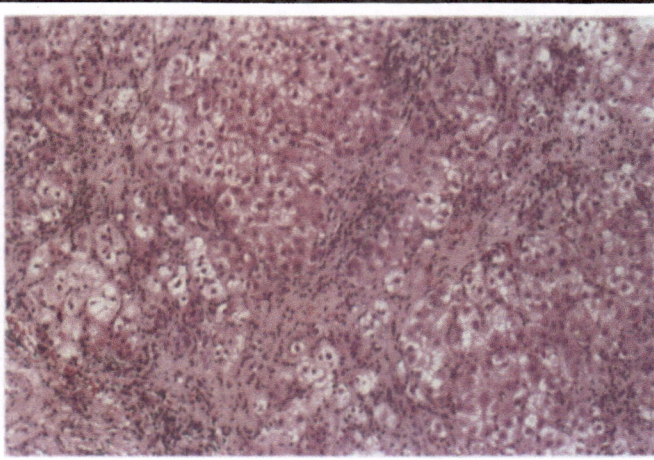

FIGURE 8.6   Chronic active hepatitis. Disarray of lobular architecture with early fibrosis and piecemeal and bridging necrosis of hepatocytes.

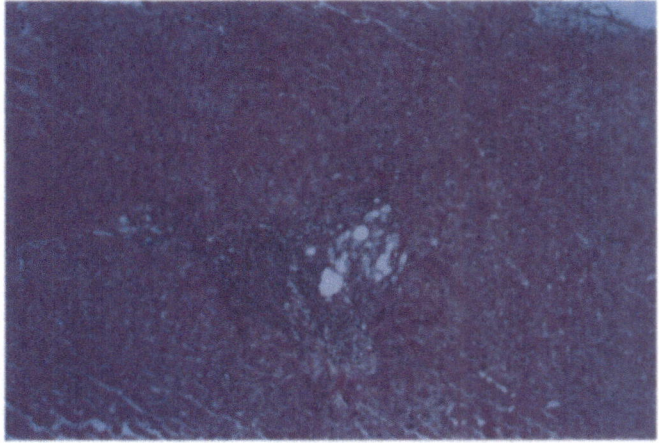

FIGURE 8.5   Chronic persistent hepatitis. Fairly well preserved hepatic lobular architecture with dense mononuclear cell infiltrate in the portal triads.

Cirrhosis

Cirrhosis is a hepatic disease of varied etiology characterized by disorganized architecture of the total liver with fibrosis, regenerative nodules, and vascular architectural reorganization.

Cirrhosis of the liver is divided into two large categories on the basis of gross morphologic features: 1) macronodular cirrhosis with irregular nodules exceeding 3 mm in diameter; 2) micronodular cirrhosis with smaller parenchymal nodules less than 3 mm in diameter. However, this classification does not provide a clear-cut etiologic relationship, pathogenesis, or guidelines for clinical management. Therefore, the following classification as shown in Table 8.1 will be applied on the basis of probable etiologies and presumed pathogenesis.[5]

Table 8.1. Approximate frequency of each category of cirrhosis in Western countries.

Alcoholic cirrhosis	60–70%
Postnecrotic cirrhosis	10%
Biliary cirrhosis (primary and secondary)	5–10%
Pigment cirrhosis (in hemochromatosis)	5%
Cryptogenic cirrhosis	10–15%
Cirrhosis associated with Wilson's disease	Rare
Cirrhosis associated with alpha$_1$-antitrypsin deficiency	Rare

Alcoholic Liver Disease and Cirrhosis

Fatty Metamorphosis of Liver (Alcoholic Steatosis)

Accumulation of fat in the hepatocytes is probably an ethanol-induced injury. The origin of the fat is an increased synthesis of triglycerides, decreased fatty acid oxidation, and decreased formation and release of lipoproteins. In the early phase, lipid accumulates in fat droplet form in the cytoplasm of the hepatocytes around centrilobular zone. Subsequently, the fat droplets coalesce to form large fat vesicles involving entire hepatic lobules (Fig. 8.7A). Grossly, the liver is enlarged with a soft, yellow, greasy cut surface (Fig. 8.7B). Fatty liver is reversible to normal unless there is perivenular and pericellular fibrosis.

Alcoholic Hepatitis

Alcoholic hepatitis is characterized by acute liver cell necrosis usually occurring in fatty or cirrhotic livers. It usually occurs after a bout of heavy drinking in patients with other manifestations of alcoholic liver disease. Liver cell necrosis occurs in scattered foci usually around the perivenular region, and shows eosinophilic cytoplasmic inclusions in lytic or coagulative necrotic cells (Fig. 8.7C). These inclusions are called Mallory bodies or alcoholic hyalin. Since similar inclusions may be seen in other liver diseases, this designation of alcoholic hyalin is misleading. Neutrophils and mononuclear leukocytes are commonly found around the necrotic liver cell foci.

Alcoholic hepatitis may produce malaise, anorexia, weight loss, upper abdominal discomfort, or jaundice with elevated aminotransferase levels. Each bout of hepatitis may be fatal, and repeated bouts may evolve into cirrhosis.

Alcoholic Cirrhosis

Alcohol is the most common cause of cirrhosis in the Western world. About 10% to 15% of the people with daily excess alcohol consumption for more than 10 years will develop cirrhosis. Although there is some concept of the interrelationship among alcohol-induced steatosis, hepatitis, and cirrhosis, the pathogenesis of alcoholic cirrhosis remains unknown.

Alcohol-induced cirrhosis begins as alcoholic steatosis, followed by perivenular fibrosis, which extends from central veins to portal regions as well as from portal region to portal region. Hepatic lobules are irregularly separated by fibrous bands to form new irregular lobules and large nodules resulting from regenerative activity (Fig. 8.8A). Liver cell necrosis and bile stasis may or may not be present. Bile duct proliferation and lymphocytic infiltration are usually present in the portal region. In the early phase, the liver is large, with prominent fatty change. With increasing severity of fibrosis, the amount of fat and weight of the liver are reduced. The micronodular pattern in the early phase is converted into a macronodular pattern, resembling postnecrotic cirrhosis (Fig. 8.8B).

Clinically, most patients present with malaise, weakness, weight loss, loss of appetite, and portal hypertension with its sequelae (ascites, esophageal varices with hematemesis, and hemorrhoids) (Fig. 8.8C). Significant laboratory findings are elevated serum transferase levels, hyperbilirubinemia, elevation of serum alkaline phosphatase, anemia, and hypoalbuminemia.

The 5-year survival rate for patients free of jaundice, ascites, and hematemesis is almost 90% if they abstain from alcohol. Development of hepatocellular carcinoma is well below that seen with postnecrotic cirrhosis.

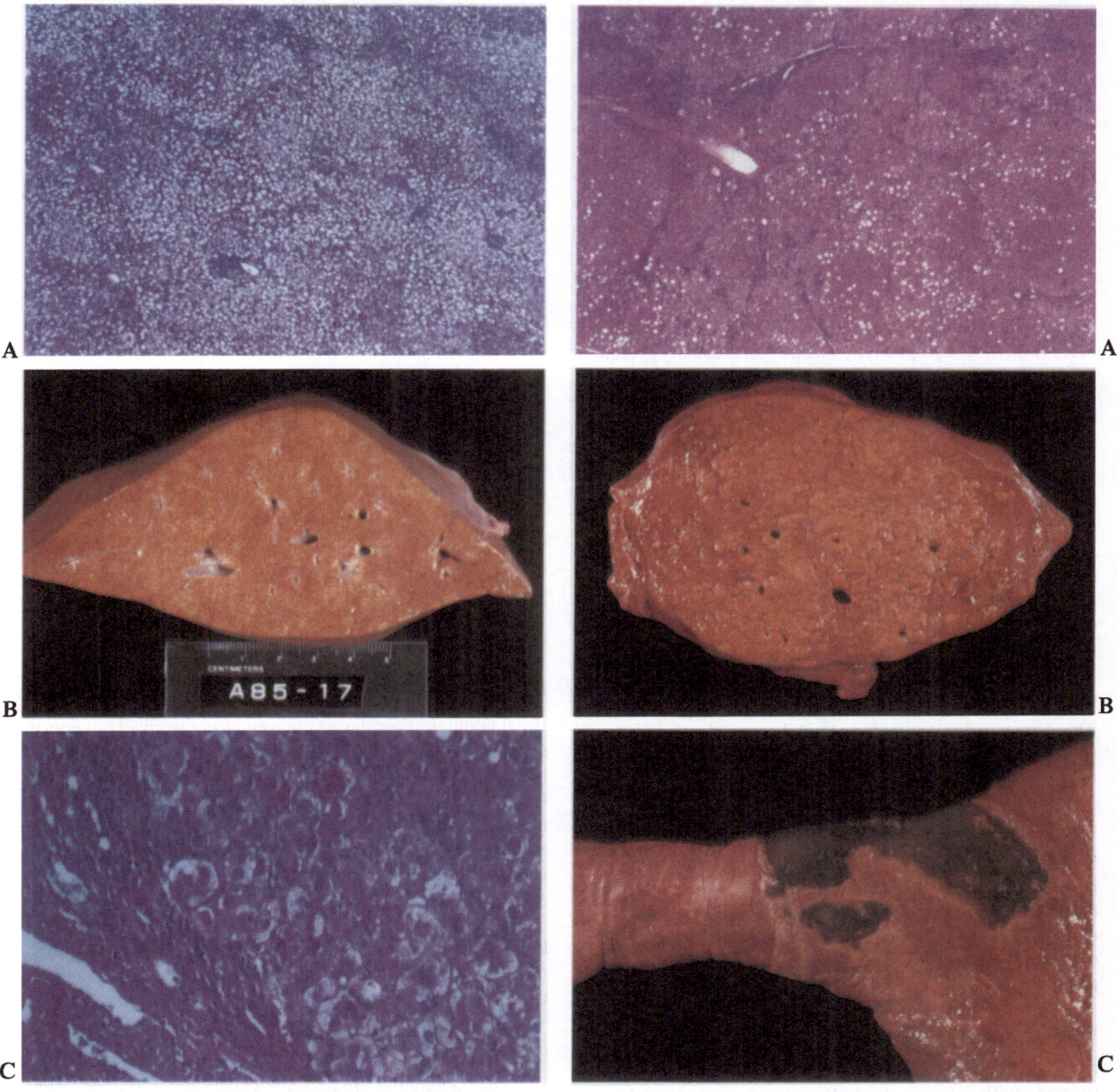

FIGURE 8.7 Alcoholic liver disease. A: Fatty metamorphosis (alcoholic steatosis) of liver. Lipid vacuoles accumulate in the cytoplasm of the hepatocytes in early phase. **B**: Alcoholic steatosis with early cirrhosis showing yellow, greasy, enlarged liver with smooth capsule. **C**: Alcoholic hepatitis. Diffuse hepatocytic injury with alcoholic hyaline (Mallory bodies) in the cytoplasm.

FIGURE 8.8 Alcoholic cirrhosis. A: Small irregular hepatic lobules and pseudolobules separated by fibrous bands. **B**: Cut surface showing small and large nodules separated by irregular fibrous bands. **C**: Esophageal varices showing mucosal ulcers with prominent venous distention in the distal segment of the esophagus (specimen turned inside out).

Postnecrotic Cirrhosis

Postnecrotic cirrhosis is characterized by large irregular nodules separated by broad fibrous scars (macronodular pattern). Most cases have evolved from hepatitis infection (B, non-A-non-B, and delta types), and a small number of cases show a well documented history of acute liver damage caused by some hepatotoxic agent. A significant number of cases are of unknown origin. Grossly, the liver is small and coarsely nodular with broad fibrous bands and scarring. The nodules measure up to several centimeters in diameter.

Histologically, hepatic lobules have been destroyed and collapsed with remnants of strands of hepatocytes and regenerated bile ducts and cholangioles in the irregular fibrous scars (Fig. 8.9). Lymphocytic infiltration is usually present in the scars. Active liver cell necrosis and fat may or may not be present. The diagnosis is based on irregular large nodules separated by coarse scarring and exclusion of other causes for a macronodular cirrhosis. The clinical course is variable, and may be asymptomatic and discovered only at laparotomy or by chance finding of abnormal liver function tests. Sometimes the patients may present with full-blown symptoms and signs of hepatic failure. If it follows a relentless course of chronic active hepatitis, death may occur within a year. If this form of cirrhosis is related to hepatitis B virus infection in early life, it leads to hepatocellular carcinoma in 15% to 30% of cases.[6]

Biliary Cirrhosis

There are two distinctive forms of biliary cirrhosis in terms of their pathogenesis and clinical basis. Both forms are characterized by a micronodular cirrhosis.

Secondary Biliary Cirrhosis

Secondary biliary cirrhosis results from prolonged extrahepatic obstruction. The extrahepatic duct obstruction produces bile stasis throughout the entire biliary tree leading to damage of the interlobular bile ducts and cholangioles. A secondary inflammation and bacterial infection may contribute to the damage.

Primary Biliary Cirrhosis

Primary biliary cirrhosis (PBC) is largely a disease of women, with a female to male ratio of approximately 9:1, and average age of onset at 50 to 55 years of age. It is a progressive, often fatal cholestatic and cirrhotic condition of unknown etiology.[7] Histologically, it begins with random destruction of the bile ducts, dense mononuclear cell infiltration, and cholestasis. This has led to the suggestion that "nonsuppurative destructive cholangitis" be used to describe this disorder. Granulomas within the lymphoid infiltrates may be present. As normal bile ducts reduce in number, ductal cell proliferation increases, resulting in bizarre-shaped ducts, and the inflammatory infiltrate extends beyond the portal triads with destruction of some cells in the limiting plates (Fig. 8.10). In advanced stages, fibrosis is more prominent and encircles hepatic lobules with a micronodular cirrhotic pattern. Inflammatory infiltrates are less prominent. Primary biliary cirrhosis is an autoimmune disease, and patients with this condition have an increased incidence of other autoimmune diathesis. The prominent immunologic abnormalities are 1) increased serum IgM level, 2) circulating antimitochondrial antibodies in 95% of patients, 3) increased levels of circulating immune complexes, 4) decreased number of T cells, and 5) rapid turnover of complement components. The clinical course of primary biliary cirrhosis is insidious in onset, and eventually progresses to the common hepatic symptoms and signs of chronic liver failure. Prognosis for patients who are asymptomatic at the time of diagnosis is excellent. The average length of survival from the onset of symptoms to death is approximately 12 years.

Tumorlike Lesions and Benign Tumors

Hepatic Cysts

Congenital hepatic cysts vary greatly in size and may be solitary or multiple. Grossly, the cyst wall is smooth and glistening (Fig. 8.11). Histologically, the cystic wall is lined by a single layer of cuboidal epithelium. The fluid aspirated from the cysts is clear and acellular and rarely contains cuboidal epithelial cells.

Hydatid cyst of the liver caused by *Echinococcus* is one of the contraindications for FNA.

Focal Nodular Hyperplasia

Focal nodular hyperplasias are well circumscribed but poorly encapsulated hepatic lesions measuring up to many centimeters in diameter. They are tan to pale yellow on cross section. Pale gray central radiating scars are frequently observed. Histologically, the lesions consist of liver parenchyma intersected by fibrous septa containing large, thick-walled arteries and bile ducts, which may lack lobular organization (Fig. 8.12).

In aspirate smears, the hepatocytes appear normal. These lesions may represent a hamartomatous malformation, reparative nodule after acinar injury, or possibly lesions induced by oral contraceptives.

Liver Cell Adenoma (Hepatic Adenoma)

Liver cell adenomas are partially encapsulated lesions, ranging from several to up to 30 cm in diameter. Liver cell adenomas tend to occur in young women who have used oral contraceptives. Histologically, the tumors consist of liver parenchyma without portal tracts or bile ducts. There are abundant small arteries within the tumor (Fig. 8.13). Subcapsular liver cell adenomas tend to rupture during pregnancy and cause severe intraperitoneal hemorrhage. In aspirate smears, the cells appear to be normal hepatocytes.

Hemangioma and Bile Duct Adenoma

Hemangiomas and bile duct adenomas are benign tumors that are found incidentally and rarely present as clinical diagnostic problems.

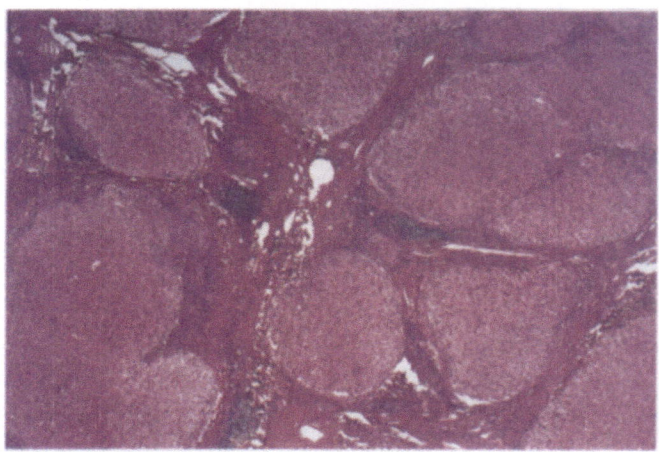

FIGURE 8.9 Postnecrotic cirrhosis. The liver is partly replaced by broad scarring with remnants of strands of hepatocytes, segmented bile ducts, and lymphocytic infiltration.

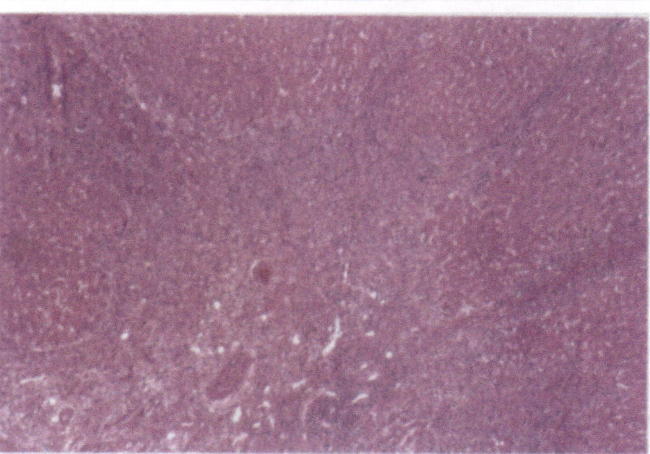

FIGURE 8.12 Focal nodular hyperplasia of liver. Liver parenchyme is intersected by fibrous septa with thick-walled arteries and bile ducts.

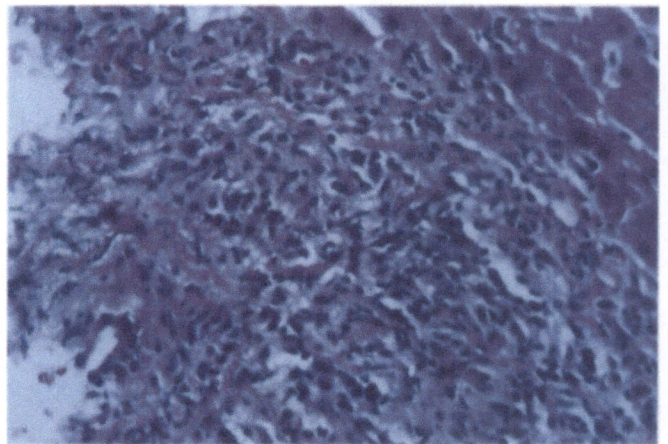

FIGURE 8.10 Primary biliary cirrhosis. Widening of the portal triad and bile duct cell proliferation with bizarre clustering and inflammatory infiltration. (Courtesy of William M. Murphy, M.D., Memphis, Tenn.)

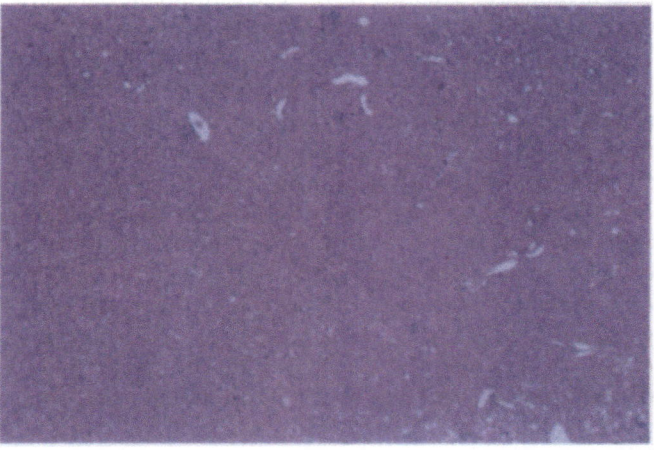

FIGURE 8.13 Liver cell adenoma. The tumor consists of uniform normal-appearing hepatocytes arranged compactly without portal tracts or bile ducts.

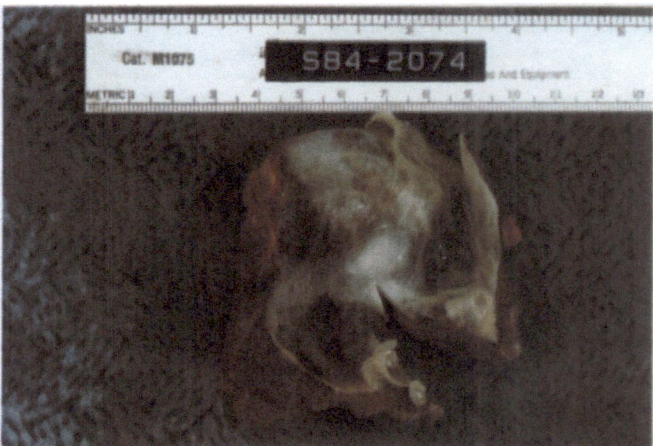

FIGURE 8.11 Hepatic cyst. Cystic wall is lined by smooth, thin, glistening membrane.

Primary Tumors of Liver

Hepatocellular Carcinoma (Hepatoma)

Hepatocellular carcinoma (HCC) is the most common type of primary cancer of the liver, accounting for more than 90% of primary liver cancers. The tumors are closely linked to hepatitis B virus infection. The incidence rate of the tumors is proportional to that of hepatitis B virus infection or carrier. In the United States and Western Europe, HBV carriers are less than 1%, and HCC represents only 2% to 3% of all cancers, whereas in Africa and some Asian countries the HBV carrier rate is tenfold higher and HCCs constitute almost 40% of all cancers.[8] In endemic areas, HBV carriage usually begins soon after birth, and HCC tends to occur in younger individuals.[9] In Taiwan, where maternal-infant spread of infection is common, the relative risk of developing HCC is more than 200 times greater among carriers than among noncarriers.[10]

Direct pathogenetic evidence includes the documentation of integration of HBV-DNA into the genome of HCC tumor cells in humans.[11] Another possible hepatocarcinogen is aflatoxin B_1 produced by the fungus *Aspergillus flavus*.

Grossly, HCCs may be focal, multifocal, or diffusely infiltrative cancers, and cause liver enlargement with discrete nodular masses. A cirrhotic background and bile staining are frequently observed (Fig. 8.14A). HCC has a strong propensity for invasion of vascular channels.

Clinically, the liver is palpable beneath the costal margin as a discrete nodular feeling. Valuable laboratory studies are an elevated serum alpha-fetoprotein, and positive des-gamma-carboxyprothrombin, precursor of prothrombin. Ultrasonography, CT, MRI scan, or angiography are valuable for diagnostic work-up (Fig. 8.14B). Conclusive diagnosis is based on FNA biopsy under an imaging guide or an open biopsy.

Histology

The well differentiated forms of HCC consist of trabecular or acinar patterns. The trabeculae comprise several layers of tumor cells, recognizable as hepatocytic in origin, separated by vascular channels resembling sinusoids (Fig. 8.14C). In the acinar structures, the tumor cells form lumina, which may contain bile droplets (Fig. 8.14D).

Poorly differentiated forms consist of pleomorphic giant cells, undifferentiated cells, or spindle cells arranged in haphazard sheets (Fig. 8.14E). The tumor cells lose cytologic characteristics of hepatocytic origin.

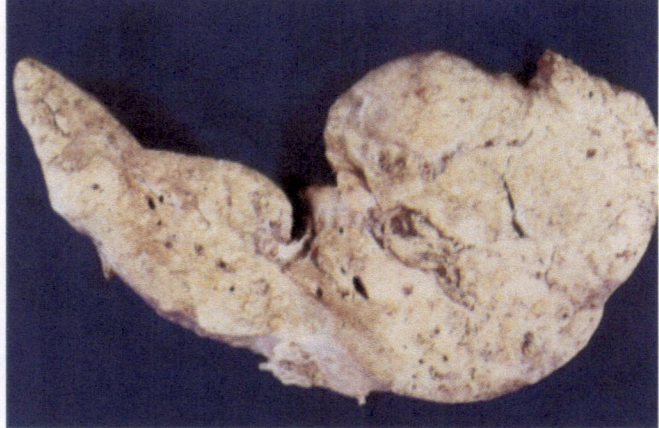

A

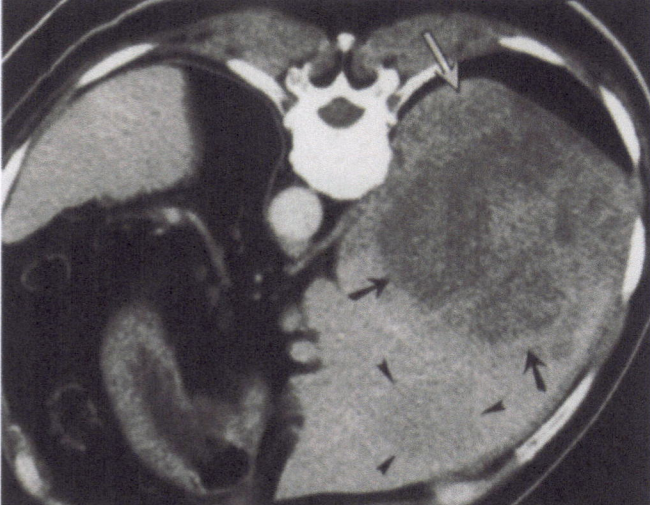

B

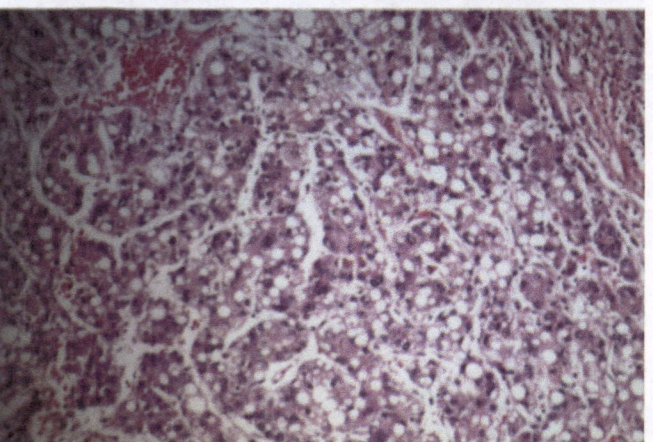

C

FIGURE 8.14 **Hepatocellular carcinoma. A**: Enlarged liver with multiple discrete nodular masses in cirrhotic background. **B**: A CT scan of the liver showing two large, discrete, low density masses (*arrows and arrowheads*) representing hepatocellular carcinoma. **C**: Histologic section of well differentiated tumor showing tumor cells arranged in trabeculae and clusters with dis-

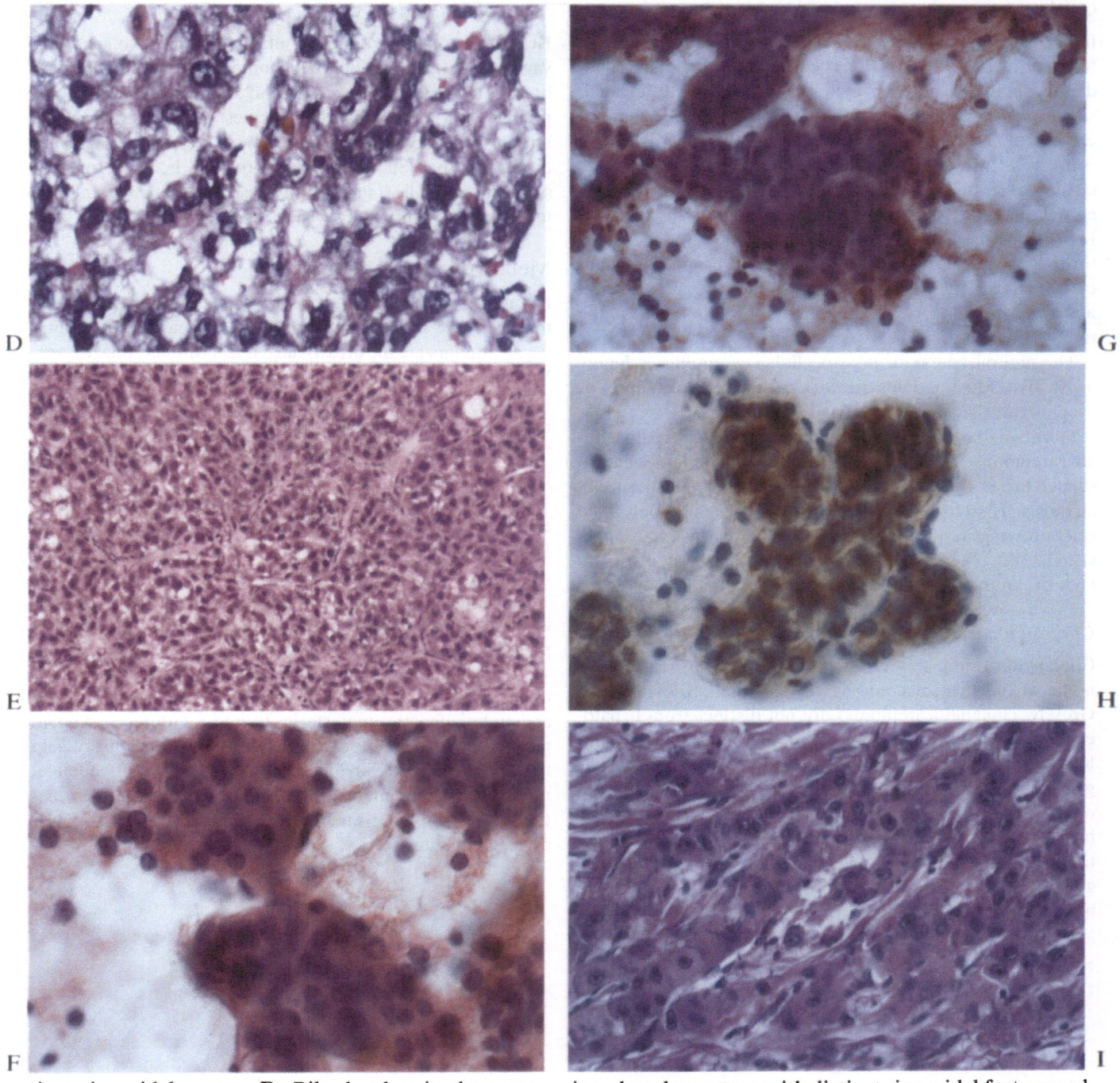

tinct sinusoidal spaces. **D**: Bile droplets in the tumor cells. **E**: Poorly differentiated hepatocellular carcinoma comprising large, pleomorphic tumor cells arranged in sheets. **F**: FNA smears showing clusters of tumor cells with abundant eosinophilic cytoplasm and large hyperchromatic nuclei and macronucleoli. **G**: FNA smears of well differentiated tumor showing tumor cells arranged in trabecular pattern with distinct sinusoidal feature and intranuclear cytoplasmic inclusion (center field). **H**: Immunostain of FNA smear showing a strong positive reaction to alpha-fetoprotein. **I**: Hepatocellular carcinoma, fibrolamellular type, showing eosinophilic polygonal cells arranged in cords separated by hyaline fibrous stroma.

Cytology

In FNA smears, the cells of HCC occur in clusters, trabecular form, or loose aggregates. The cells are large and have abundant eosinophilic granular cytoplasm and centrally located, single or double nuclei. The nuclei have coarsely clumped chromatin and prominent macronucleoli (Fig. 8.14F).

In well differentiated forms, trabecular clusters with sinusoidal features are well preserved in smears. Intranuclear cytoplasmic inclusions are frequently observed (Fig. 8.14G). In poorly differentiated forms, the tumor cells are so anaplastic that they lack features of hepatocytic origin. Immunocytochemical staining can demonstrate the presence of alpha$_1$-antitrypsin (A$_1$AT) or alpha-fetoprotein (AFP) in the tumor cells in 60% to 80% of the cases (Fig. 8.14H).

The natural course of hepatocellular carcinoma is highly aggressive. Most patients die with cachexia, liver failure, or esophageal varices and bleeding.

Fibrolamellar carcinoma is a unique variant of hepatocellular carcinoma.[12] Grossly, the tumor is a single, large, encapsulated mass. This variant arises more often in the absence of cirrhosis. Histologically, it comprises acidophilic polygonal cells growing in nests or cords separated by hyaline fibrous stroma (Fig. 8.14I). Prognosis of this variant is distinctly better than the usual type of hepatocellular carcinoma.

Cholangiocarcinoma

Cholangiocarcinoma is a less common type of primary carcinoma of the liver, accounting for less than 10% of them. Grossly, cholangiocarcinomas are not distinct from hepatocellular carcinomas, but they are rarely bile stained. Histologically, cholangiocarcinomas consist of cuboidal cells growing in glandular or papillary patterns in dense collagenous stroma (Fig. 8.15A, B). Since the tumors arise from the bile duct epithelium, bile droplets are not identified in the tumor cells. Usually, cholangiocarcinoma cannot be distinguished from a metastatic adenocarcinoma on cytologic basis.

Hepatoblastoma

Hepatoblastoma is a tumor of infancy and has two anatomic variants: 1) the epithelial type, comprising small embryonal or fetal hepatocytes (Fig. 8.16) and 2) the mixed type, comprising fetal embryonal hepatocytes admixed with more mature hepatocytes, interspersed with foci of mesenchymal differentiation. Successful resection can be performed in some cases. Unless successfully resected, both variants are usually fatal within a few years.

Metastatic Tumors of Liver

Metastatic tumors are the most common neoplasms involving the liver. The most common primaries among the metastatic hepatic tumors are the breast, lung, and gastrointestinal organs. Virtually any neoplasm in any site may spread to the liver.

Grossly, the liver is markedly enlarged and shows multiple metastatic nodular masses (Fig. 8.17A). Metastatic neoplastic nodules may outgrow their blood supply and produce central tumor necrosis.

Clinically, the liver is palpable with some nodularity in the edge. Jaundice and abnormal liver function tests may appear. Diagnosis can be established by FNA biopsy under CT guidance (Fig. 8.17B).

Although FNA cytology provides the tumor type such as adenocarcinoma, squamous cell carcinoma, sarcoma, or lymphoma, identification of the primary site is often difficult without clinical information and review of prior histologic or cytologic material. Unfortunately, it is not uncommon to encounter hepatic metastatic tumors without a known primary. In searching for the primary tumor, it may be of help to study the cellular material by immunocytochemical methods, electron microscopy, and thorough clinical information. The following are representative examples of FNA cytology diagnosis.

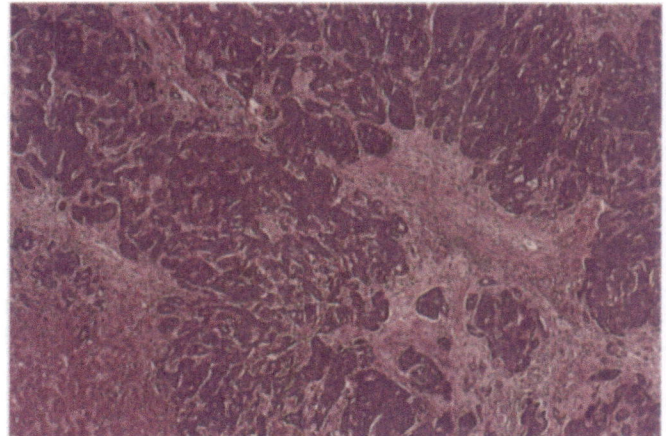

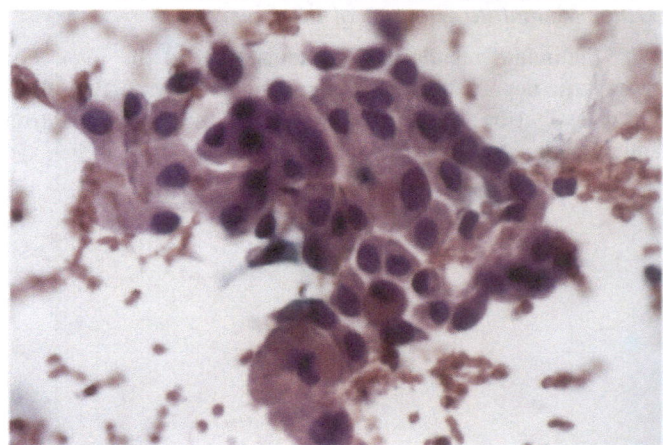

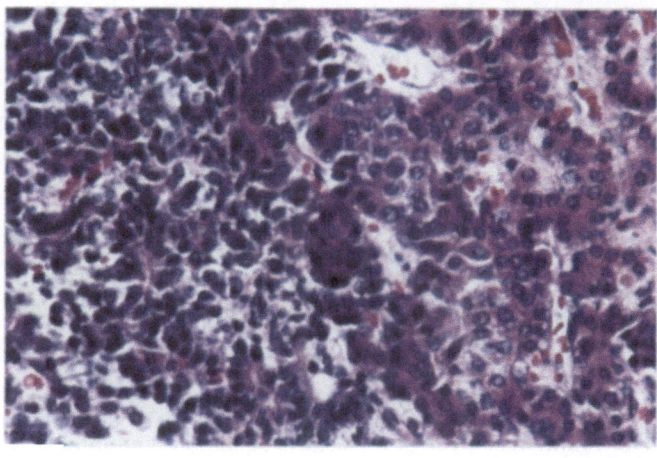

FIGURE 8.16 Hepatoblastoma. Tumor cells resembling embryonal hepatocytes (*left*) and solid cords of fetal hepatocytes (*right*).

FIGURE 8.15 Cholangiocarcinoma. A: The neoplasm consists of poorly formed glands separated by fibrous stroma. Non-neoplastic liver parenchyma is seen in the left lower portion. **B**: FNA smear showing cuboidal neoplastic cells arranged in glands with abundant cytoplasm and large, oval-shaped nuclei.

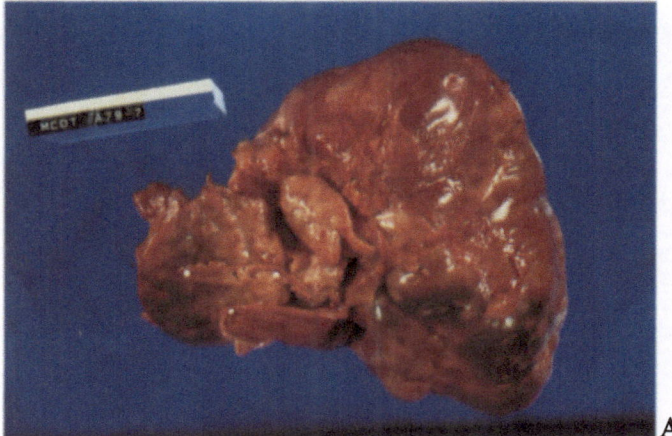

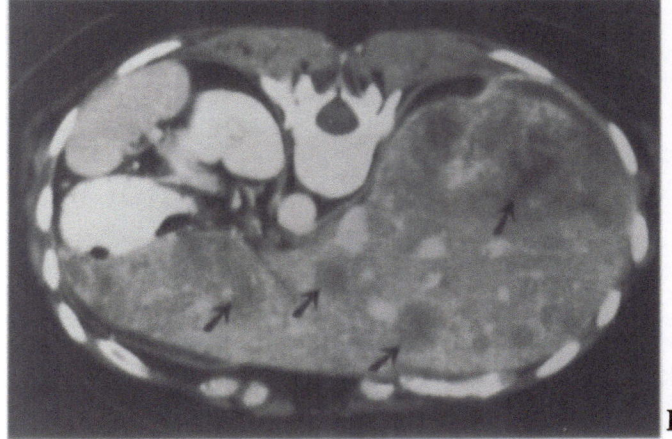

FIGURE 8.17 Metastatic carcinoma of liver. A: The liver is studded with small and large metastatic neoplastic nodules. **B**: A CT scan showing multiple low density nodules (*arrows*).

Adenocarcinoma

Adenocarcinomas are the most common type of metastatic hepatic tumors. In FNA aspirates the cells occur in clusters, sheets, and singly. The cells have scanty to moderate amounts of granular cytoplasm and round to oval hyperchromatic nuclei. Macronucleoli are frequently observed (Fig. 8.18A).

There are commercially available immunocytochemical markers for some tumors, such as alphalactoalbumin (breast), CA19.9 (pancreas), insulin (insulinoma), prostate-specific antigen (prostate), prostate acid phosphatase (prostate), and thyroglobulin (thyroid).

Squamous Cell Carcinoma

The common sources of metastatic squamous carcinomas of the liver are the lung, larynx, and uterine cervix. Cytologic features are similar to those of squamous cell carcinomas of other organs (Fig. 8.18B).

Small Cell Carcinoma

Metastatic small cell carcinomas of the liver arise most often from the lung. In aspirates, the cells occur in clusters and in loose aggregates with characteristic nuclear molding. They have scanty cytoplasm and round, spindle-shaped hyperchromatic nuclei (Fig. 8.18C). Small cell carcinomas may be distinguished from lymphoma and other undifferentiated malignant neoplasms on cytologic and immunocytochemical basis. The cells arising from lymphomas almost always occur singly.

Immunocytochemical studies may be of help. The cells of lymphoma are positive for leukocyte common antigen. Small cell carcinomas and other neuroendocrine tumors are positive for neuron-specific antigen and chromogranin.

Other Metastatic Tumors of the Liver

Any malignant neoplasm can metastasize to the liver. For metastatic hepatic tumors of unknown primary, further clinical investigation, immunocytochemical studies, and electron microscopic studies are of help (Fig. 8.18D–F).

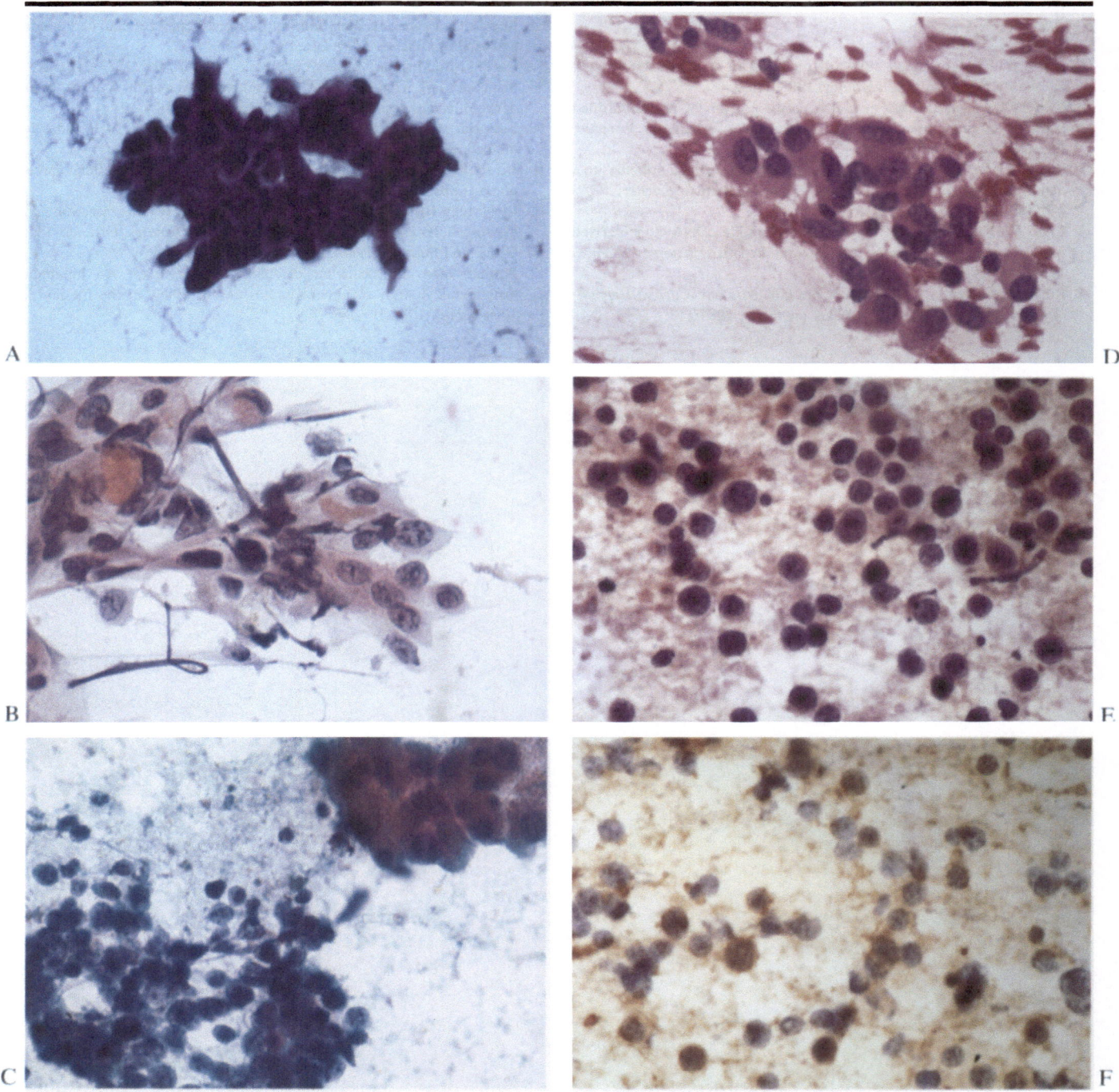

FIGURE 8.18 Metastatic neoplasms involving liver. A: Metastatic adenocarcinoma. FNA smear showing cluster of neoplastic cells with columnar configuration. **B:** Metastatic squamous cell carcinoma. FNA smear showing loose aggregates of pleomorphic cells with evidence of keratinization and pleomorphic hyperchromatic nuclei. **C:** Metastatic small cell carcinoma. FNA smear showing aggregates of small anaplastic cells with scanty cytoplasm and hyperchromatic nuclei (*left lower portion*) and normal liver cells (*right upper portion*). **D:** Metastatic leiomyosarcoma. FNA smear showing loose aggregates of spindle-shaped cells with abundant acidophilic cytoplasm and cigar-shaped nuclei. **E:** Large cell lymphoma. FNA smear showing monomorphic neoplastic cells occurring singly. **F:** Immunostain of the same smear showing a strong reactivity to leukocyte common antigen.

References

1. Lesnicar G. A prospective study of viral hepatitis A and the question of chronicity. *Hepatogastroenterology*. 1988;35:69.

2. Shih JWK, et al. Non-A, non-B hepatitis: Advances and unfulfilled expectations of the first decade. In: *Progress in Liver Diseases*. Orlando, Fla: Grune and Stratton, 1986:433.

3. Kuo G, Choo QL, Alter J, et al. An assay for circulating antibodies to a major etiologic virus of human non-A, non-B hepatitis. *Science*. 1989; 244:362–364.

4. Choo JL, Kuo G, Weiner AJ, et al. Isolation of a cDNA clone derived from a blood-borne non-A, non-B viral hepatitis genome. *Science*. 1989;244:359–362.

5. Riepe SP, Galambos JT. Cirrhosis. In: Gianik G, ed. *Current Hepatology*, Vol. IV. New York: John Wiley and Sons, 1984:117.

6. Kew MC, Popper H. Relationship between hepatocellular carcinoma and cirrhosis. *Semin Liver Dis*. 1984;4:136.

7. Kaplan MM. Primary biliary cirrhosis. *N Engl J Med*. 1987;316:521.

8. Szumuness W. Hepatocellular carcinoma and hepatitis B virus. Evidence of causal association. *Prog Med Virol*. 1978;24:40.

9. Editorial. Hepatocellular cancer: Differences between high and low incidence regions. *Lancet*. 1987;2:1183.

10. Beasly RP. Hepatitis B virus. The major etiology of hepatocellular carcinoma. *Cancer*. 1988;61:1942.

11. Lieberman HM, Schafritz D. Persistent hepatitis B virus infection and hepatocellular carcinoma. In: *Progress in Liver Diseases*. Orlando, Fla: Grune and Stratton, 1986:395.

12. Berman MM. Fibrolamellar carcinoma of the liver: An immuno-histochemical study of nineteen cases and a review of the literature. *Hum Pathol*. 1988;19:784.

9

Pancreas and Biliary Tract

Malignant Neoplasms of the Pancreas

In this chapter neoplasms will be discussed, with particular emphasis on fine needle aspiration (FNA). Epidemiologic data indicate that incidence and mortality rates of carcinoma of the pancreas steadily increased until 1970, and has since then plateaued.[1] The epidemiology of pancreatic cancer has been controversial. Most consistently documented etiologic factors are cigarette smoking, a high fat diet, diabetes mellitus, and an industrial carcinogenic exposure.[2-5] Most pancreatic cancers are duct cell adenocarcinoma and 65% occur in the head of the pancreas, resulting in jaundice. The remaining cases occur in the body and tail and are at an advanced stage at the time of diagnosis.

Unfortunately, no early detection method or tumor markers are available. Ultrasound or computed tomography (CT) is the most common initial diagnostic technique. Traditionally, abnormal lesions detected by imaging methods were confirmed by open biopsy at the time of exploratory laparotomy. Since the early 1970s, the introduction of the FNA has made a significant contribution to the diagnosis of pancreatic cancer, largely eliminating the need for laparotomy and open biopsy.[6] In cases that do come to laparotomy, intraoperative FNA may be used.

Indications for Fine Needle Aspiration Biopsy

Fine needle aspiration is applied to space-occupying or cystic lesions of the pancreas detected by CT, ultrasonography, or angiography. Lesions that are clinically diagnosed acute pancreatitis are not suitable for FNA.

Technique

1. *Percutaneous Transabdominal FNA*
   Recommended needle is a long needle of 22 gauge with a cutting edge (West-Cot)

   a. The needle is inserted directly into the lesion under radiologic guidance.
   b. When the needle tip is in the lesion, aspirate cellular material while moving the needle back and forth and in different directions to get an optimal sample from multiple areas of the lesion.
   c. Release the suction to prevent sucking the cellular material into the syringe.
   d. Withdraw the needle, detach it from the syringe, draw air into the syringe, and reattach the needle.
   e. With the needle tip in contact with the slide expel a drop of the aspirate.
   f. Make thin, evenly dispersed smears by placing another glass slide on top of the expelled material and pulling apart the slides.
   g. Fix the slides in 95% ethanol or with spray fixative (or air-dry for staining with Wright stain).
   h. The smears may be stained by the Diff-Quik procedure, with hematoxylin and eosin, or with the Papanicolaou stain.

2. *Intraoperative FNA*
   Intraoperative FNA is applied if percutaneous FNA failed or the pancreatic lesion is detected incidentally at the time of exploratory laparotomy. Fine needle aspiration is applied directly to the lesion or transduodenally. The advantages of FNA in such situations are that it minimizes leakage of pancreatic enzymes and allows rapid diagnosis.

Normal pancreas consists of innumerable lobules comprising acini connected to draining ductules, reminiscent of a bunch of grapes. The intralobular ducts drain into interlobular ducts that terminate in the main pancreatic duct. The islets of Langerhans are randomly distributed throughout the lobules (Fig. 9.1). In terms of cell origin, three distinct types of neoplasm arise from the pancreas.

Adenocarcinoma of Duct Cell Origin

About 90% of all pancreatic cancers are adenocarcinomas of duct cell origin. They vary in differentiation, ranging from well differentiated to poorly differentiated forms.

Histologically, well differentiated adenocarcinomas show fairly well formed glands lined by rather uniform cuboidal to polygonal cells. Fibrous stroma varies in amount (Fig. 9.2A, B). Cells aspirated from well differentiated adenocarcinomas occur in clusters and sheets. The cells have granular cytoplasm and enlarged, round to oval nuclei with finely granular chromatin and prominent nucleoli (Fig. 9.2C). Poorly differentiated adenocarcinomas show nests and sheets of pleomorphic cells separated by various amounts of fibrous stroma (Fig. 9.3A).

Cells of poorly differentiated adenocarcinoma occur in clusters and singly. The cells have granular cytoplasm and enlarged pleomorphic nuclei with irregularly dispersed chromatin clumps and prominent macronucleoli (Fig. 9.3B). (*Discussion continued on p. 144*)

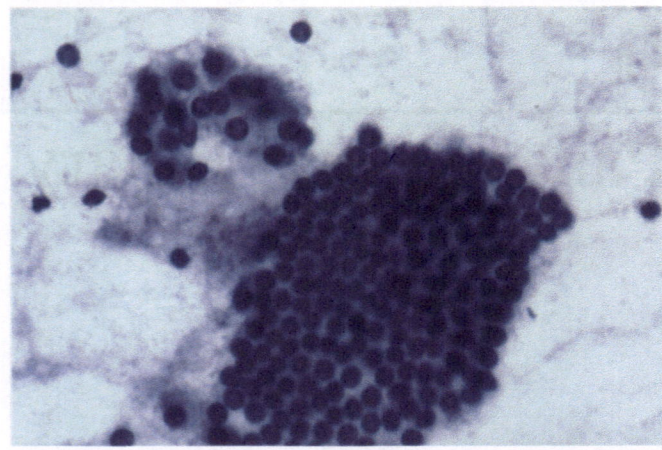

A

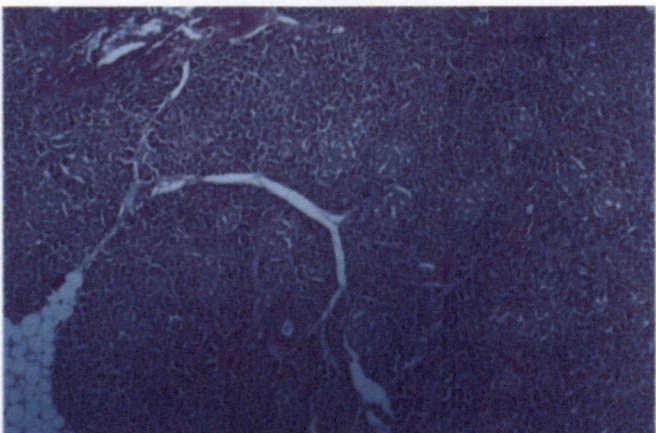

B

FIGURE 9.1   A: Normal pancreatic acinar cells (*left upper portion*) and sheets of duct cells (*lower portion*). B: Normal pancreatic lobules separated by thin delicate stroma.

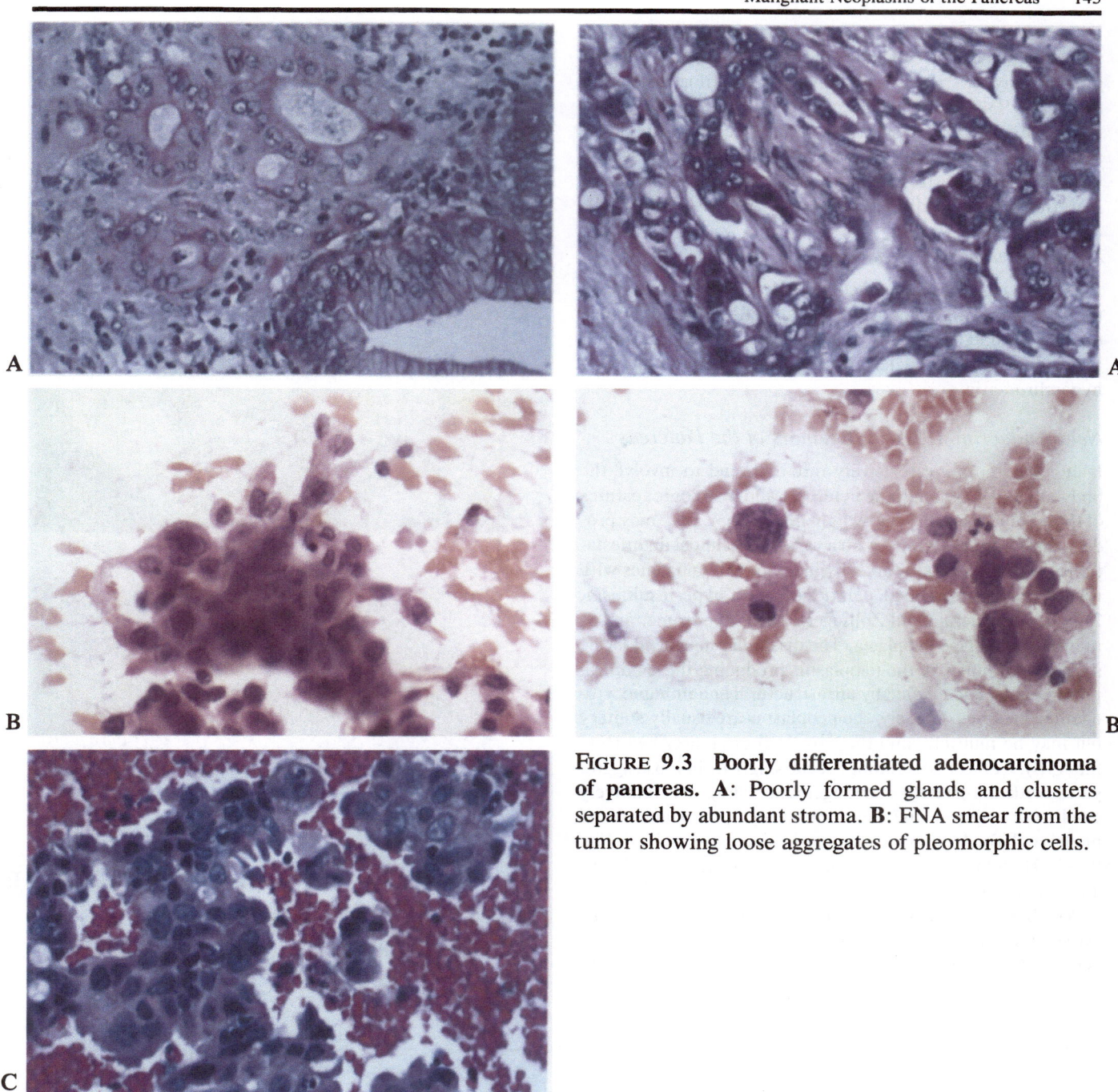

FIGURE 9.3 **Poorly differentiated adenocarcinoma of pancreas. A**: Poorly formed glands and clusters separated by abundant stroma. **B**: FNA smear from the tumor showing loose aggregates of pleomorphic cells.

FIGURE 9.2 **Well differentiated adenocarcinoma of pancreas. A**: Well formed neoplastic glands (*upper portion*) and non-neoplastic pancreatic duct (*right lower portion*). **B**: FNA smears from the tumor showing cluster of relatively uniform polygonal to cuboidal cells. **C**: Cell block section prepared from a washing of the syringe fluid used for FNA.

Cystadenocarcinomas of the pancreas are an uncommon variant of pancreatic cancer and are probably of duct cell origin. Grossly, cystadenocarcinoma is a multilocular, cystic mass (Fig. 9.4A). In FNA smears the cells are relatively uniform columnar cells occurring in papillary clusters and loose aggregates (Fig. 9.4B). Histologically, the tumor consists of well formed cystic structures lined by a single layer of mucin-secreting cuboidal cells and papillary structures (Fig. 9.4C).

Adenocarcinoma of Acinic Cell Origin

Acinic cell carcinoma, an uncommon variant of carcinoma of the pancreas, originates from acinar cells. This carcinoma consists of solid nests of polygonal cells with abundant granular cytoplasm. The nuclei are relatively small, round, and hyperchromatic.

Neuroendocrine (Islet cell) Tumors of the Pancreas

Islet cell tumors are relatively rare and tend to involve the body and tail. Although the cytologic and histologic features of these tumors are similar by light microscopy, they may produce dissimilar hormones with a variety of clinical manifestations. Among these are three distinct clinical syndromes with related hormones: 1) beta cell tumors with hyperinsulinism, 2) hypergastrinemia and Zollinger-Ellison syndrome, and 3) multiple endocrine neoplasia. The dissimilar neuroendocrine secretory granules of the neoplasms producing these clinical pictures can be identified by ultrastructural and immunocytochemical studies. Grossly, the neoplasms are usually solitary but may be multiple, and they are well circumscribed (Fig. 9.5A, B). Cells of islet tumors occur singly or in loose aggregates with a rosettelike arrangement. They are relatively small and uniform and have scanty cytoplasm and round nuclei with finely granular chromatin and micronucleoli (Fig. 9.5C). Histologically, the tumors consist of clusters, islands, and cords separated by vascular stroma (Fig. 9.5D, E).

Whether they are benign or malignant cannot be evaluated by cytology and histology. Establishment of malignancy requires clear evidence of invasion either by contiguity or by metastasis.

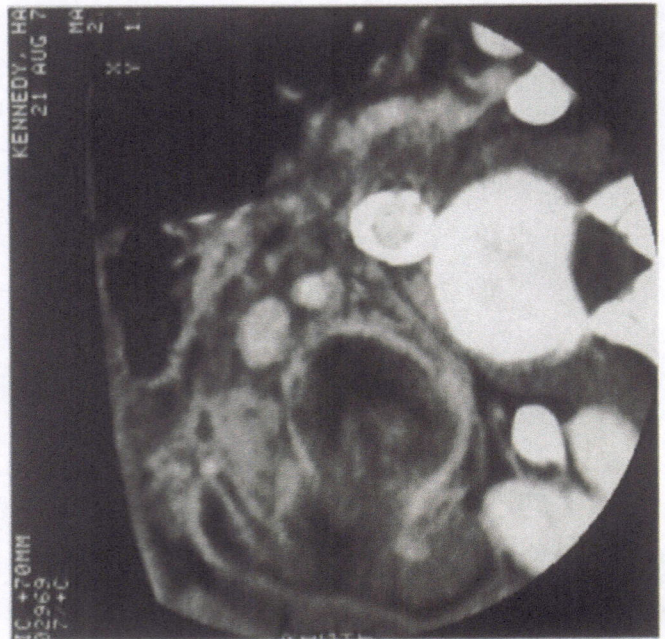

A

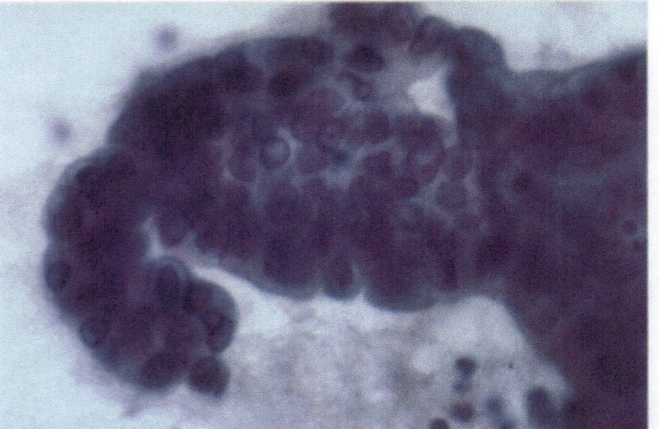

B

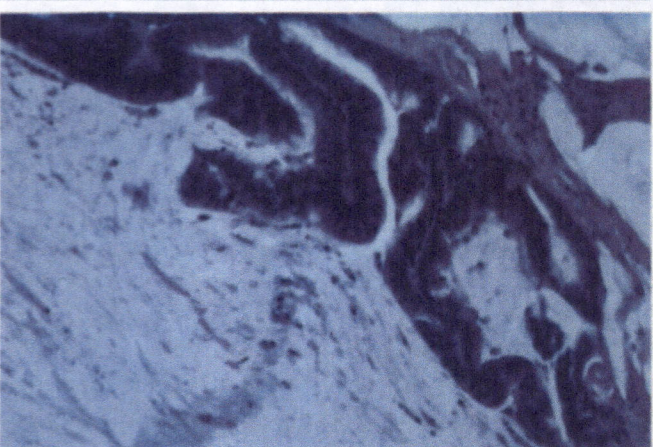

C

FIGURE 9.4 **Cystadenocarcinoma of pancreas (CT).** **A**: Well delineated cystic mass in the pancreas (CT). **B**: FNA smears from the cystic mass showing a papillary cluster of columnar cells. **C**: Histologic section of the tumor showing cystic spaces lined by papillary structures.

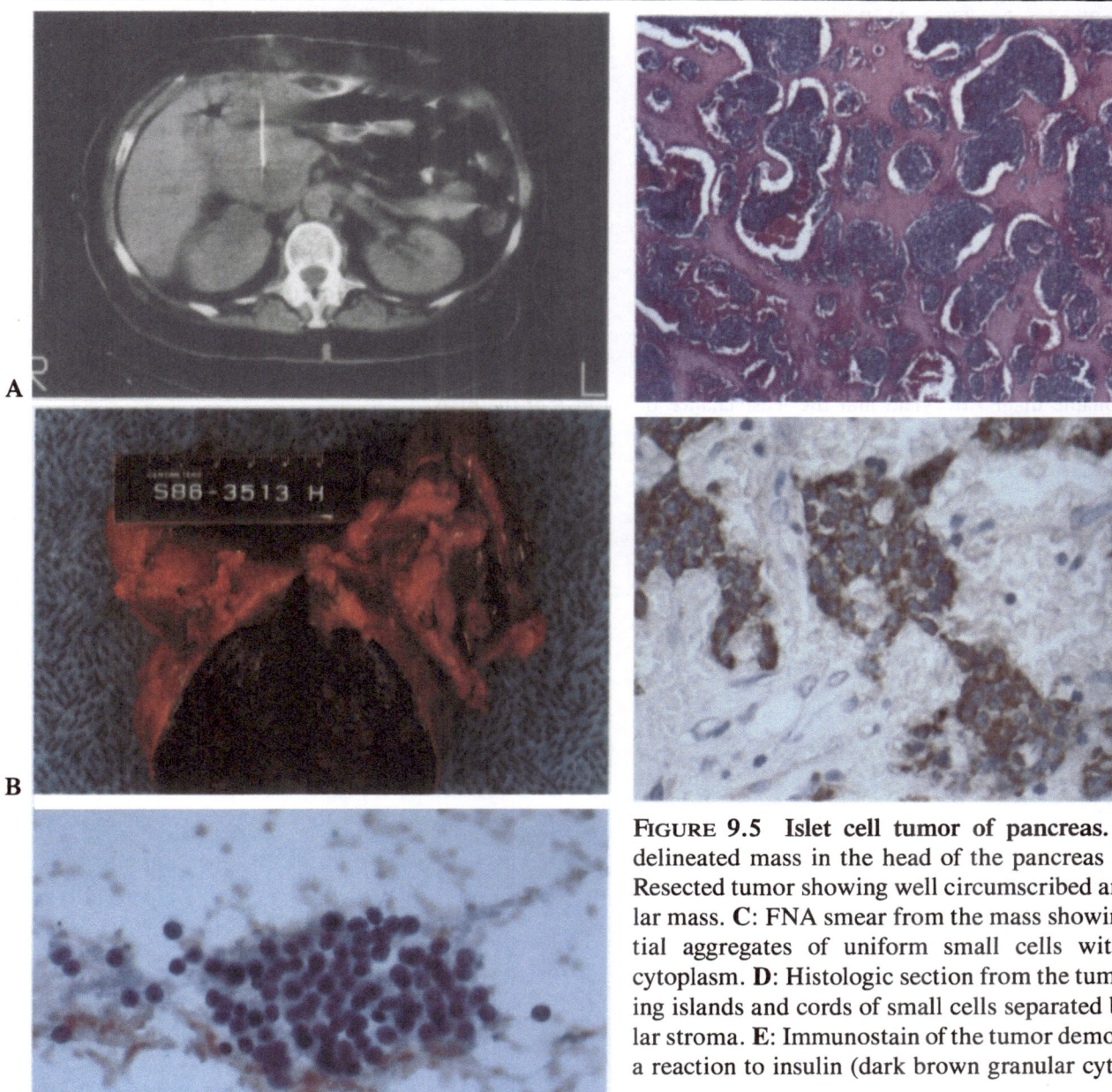

FIGURE 9.5 Islet cell tumor of pancreas. **A**: Well delineated mass in the head of the pancreas (CT). **B**: Resected tumor showing well circumscribed and vascular mass. **C**: FNA smear from the mass showing syncytial aggregates of uniform small cells with scanty cytoplasm. **D**: Histologic section from the tumor showing islands and cords of small cells separated by vascular stroma. **E**: Immunostain of the tumor demonstrating a reaction to insulin (dark brown granular cytoplasm).

Metastatic Tumors Involving the Pancreas

Neoplasms may spread to the pancreas either by contiguity or by metastasis. The common primary sites of such neoplasms are the stomach, breast, lung, kidney, prostate, and lymphoreticular system (lymphoma) (Figs. 9.6, 9.7, and 9.8).

Comments

Fine needle aspiration cytology of pancreatic tumors is of great value because of its diagnostic sensitivity and specificity, and cost containment by eliminating the need for exploratory laparotomy in inoperable cases. Intraoperative FNA is performed directly in the lesion or transduodenally and provides reasonable diagnostic yield and the least chance of enzyme leakage. The technique is simple when used in conjunction with radiologic imaging to delineate the lesion.

The diagnostic accuracy of pancreatic percutaneous aspiration in cases of pancreatic cancer is about 85% and is closely related to the experience of the radiologist carrying out the aspiration.[7]

Most false negative cases have been mainly a result of inadequate samples or samples obtained from outside the lesion. In most studies complications related to FNA are negligible. We have had one case complicated by septicemia, resulting in death 3 days after the aspiration. The patient underwent endoscopic retrograde choledochopancreatography (ERCP) and FNA on the same day; consequently, we were not sure whether the complication was related to the ERCP or the FNA.

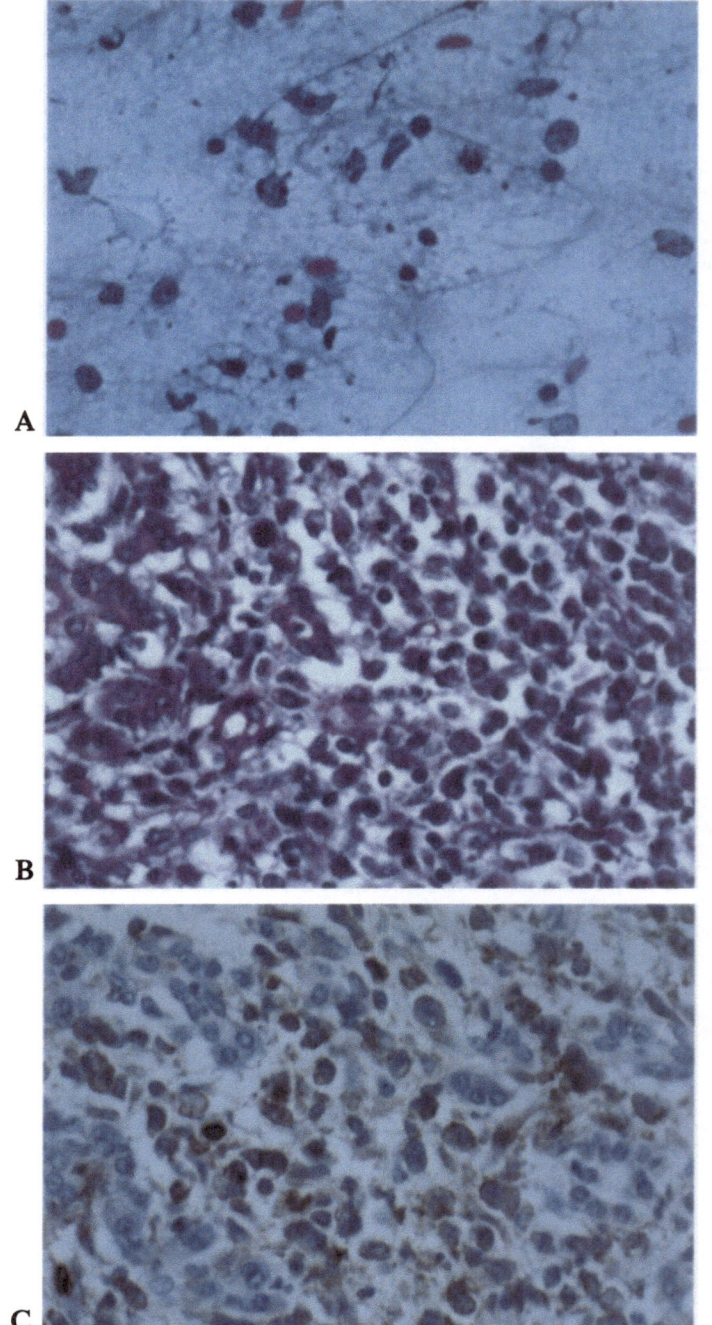

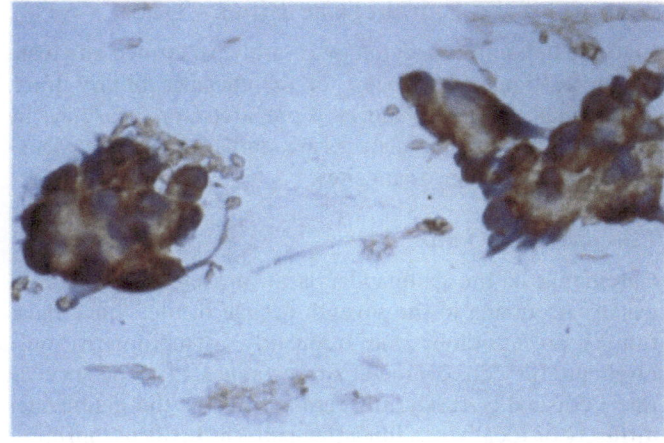

FIGURE 9.7 Metastatic breast carcinoma involving the pancreas showing aspirated tumor cells reactive to alpha-lactoalbumin.

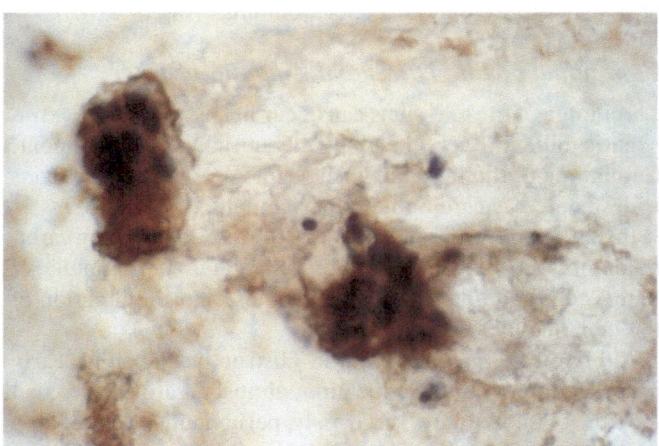

FIGURE 9.8 Metastatic melanoma involving the pancreas showing the aspirated tumor cells reactive to S-100 protein.

FIGURE 9.6 Large cell lymphoma of pancreas. A: Large lymphoid cells occurring singly (FNA). B: Biopsy specimen showing diffuse infiltration of large neoplastic lymphoid cells. C: Immunostain of the tumor showing the cells reactive to leukocyte common antigen.

Tumors of the Extrahepatic Biliary Tract

Fine needle aspiration cytology is rarely performed and technically difficult for cancers of extrahepatic biliary tract. Occasionally, cellular material is prepared from brushings by ERCP. Their cytologic features are similar to those of adenocarcinomas of other organ sites.

Carcinoma of Gallbladder

Carcinoma of the gallbladder is an uncommon neoplasm, usually occurring in the seventh decade of life. Since these tumors are insidious and frequently asymptomatic, only rarely are they discovered at a resectable stage. The survival rate is dismal. Grossly, the tumors involve the gallbladder diffusely or focally in a fungating pattern. In diffuse infiltrating forms, the gallbladder is thickened and firm (Fig. 9.9A). In both forms, the tumors invade the liver bed, metastasize to the porta hepatis lymph nodes, and spread directly through the bile ducts.

Histologically, almost all of these neoplasms are papillary or poorly differentiated adenocarcinomas (Fig. 9.9B).

Carcinoma of Bile Ducts and Ampulla of Vater

Carcinoma of the bile ducts can occur in any part of the extrahepatic biliary tract including the intraduodenal segment. Carcinoma of the intraduodenal segment of the biliary ducts is designated as carcinoma of periampulla of Vater.

In descending order of frequency the sites of primary carcinomas of the biliary tract are gallbladder, periampulla of Vater, common bile duct, hepatic ducts, and the junction of the hepatic and common ducts.[8]

Although these tumors cause obstructive jaundice early because of their strategic location, almost all are advanced at the time of their discovery. Grossly, periampullary carcinoma appears as a protruding hemispheric submucosal nodule, 2 to 3 cm in diameter in the area of the papilla of Vater (Fig. 9.10A). The orifice of the ampulla is narrowed or obstructed and marked dilatation of the proximal segment. A cholangiogram may demonstrate enlargement and dilatation of the bile ducts (Fig. 9.10B). Among the imaging methods, ultrasonography is said to be 95% accurate in diagnosis.[9] Histologically, these lesions usually are adenocarcinomas and rarely mixed adenosquamous carcinomas (Fig. 9.10C, D).

Most of the biliary tract cancers are unresectable and have a dismal prognosis. Their diagnosis can be established by transhepatic or retrograde cholangiography and ultrasonography (Fig. 9.11). Periampullary carcinomas, however, offer a better prognosis. The 5-year survival rate after surgical resection for early localized lesions is 85%; the overall 5-year survival rate is about 25% and about 50% for patients with negative lymph nodes.[10,11]

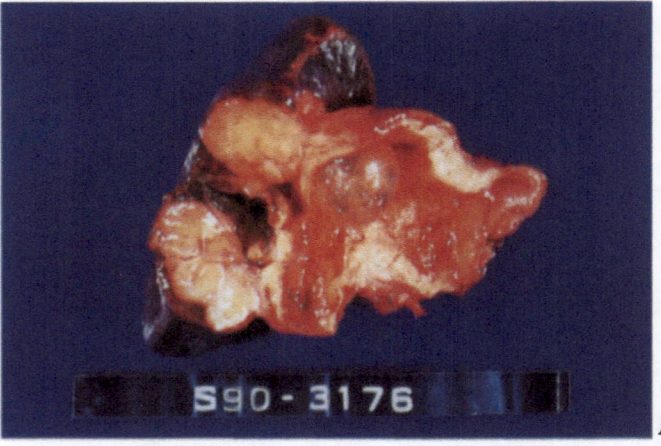

A

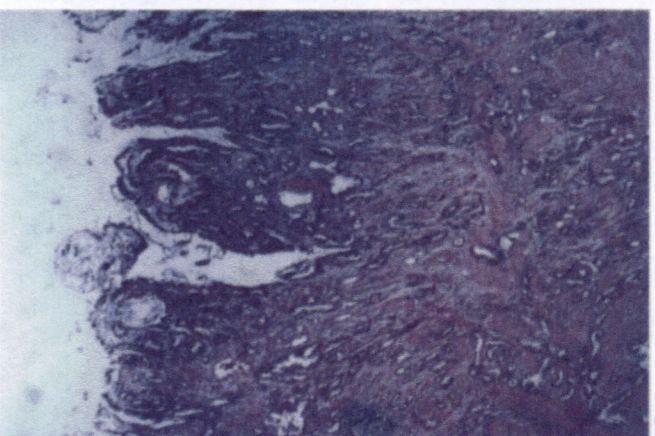

B

FIGURE 9.9 **Adenocarcinoma of gallbladder. A:** Neoplastic infiltration of the gallbladder with thickening of the wall and extending to the underlying hepatic bed (gross). **B:** Histologic section showing adenocarcinoma infiltrating through the muscularis and serosa.

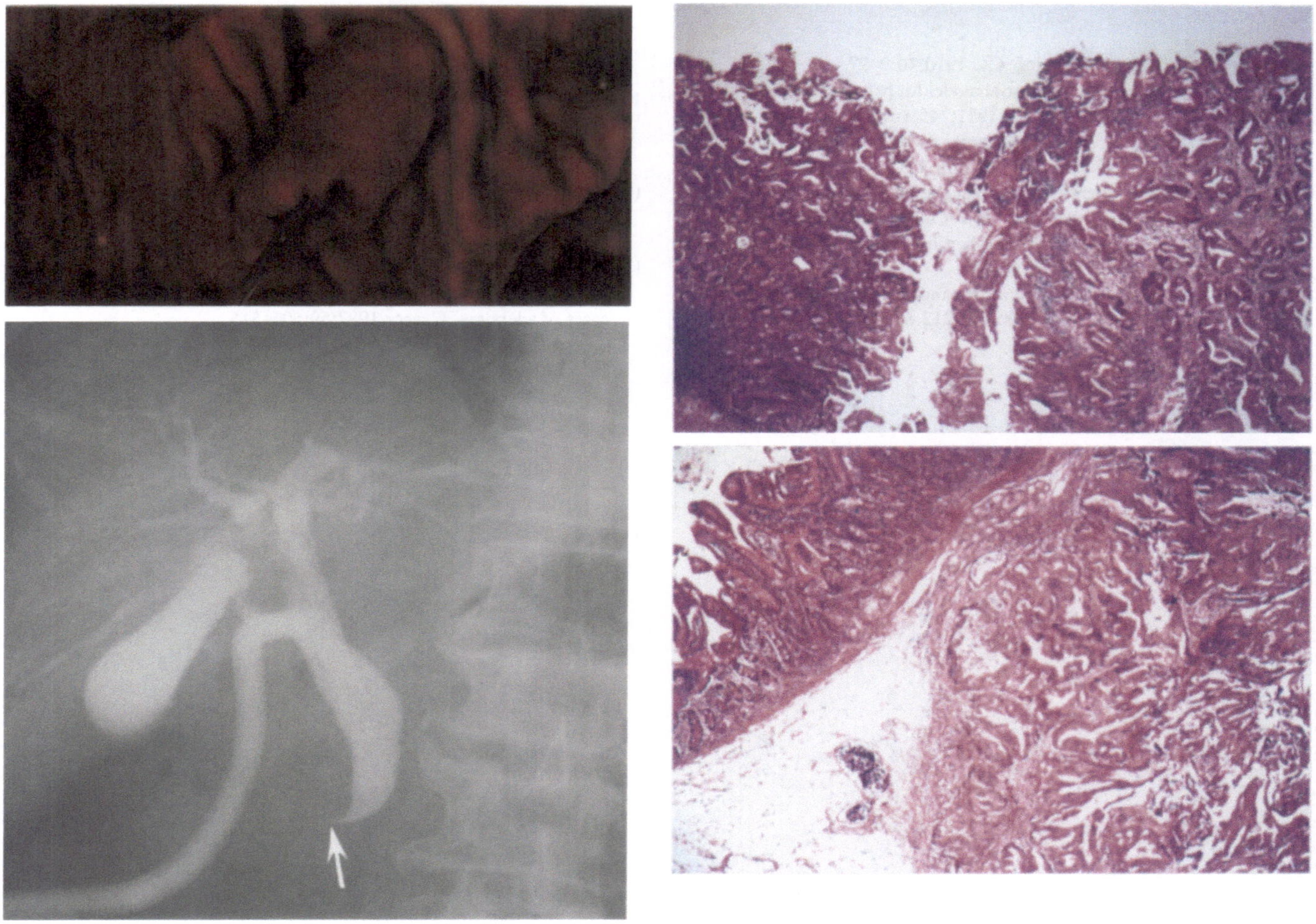

FIGURE 9.10   Periampullary carcinoma (ampulla of Vater). A: Submucosal tumor with central necrosis. **B**: Cholangiogram showing neoplasm obstructing the distal common bile duct lumen with dilatation of the bile duct. **C**: Histologic section through the center of the ampulla. **D**: Histologic section at the outer margin showing the tumor infiltrating the duodenal submucosa (*right portion of the picture*).

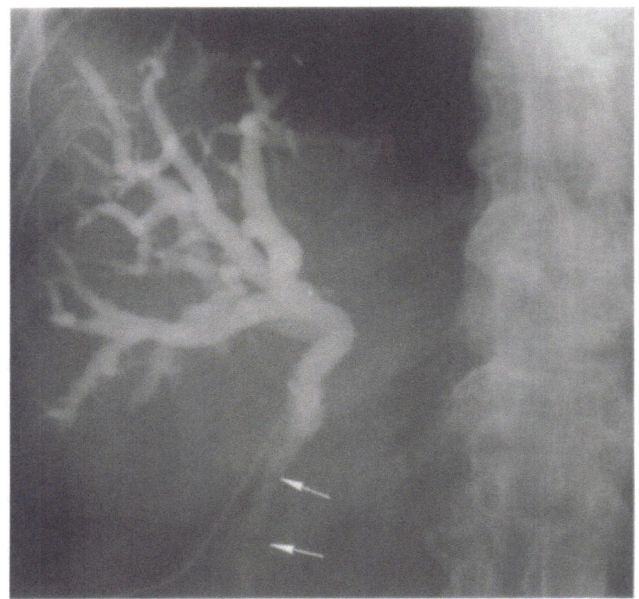

◄

FIGURE 9.11   Adenocarcinoma of the common bile duct. Cholangiogram showing nodular masses (*arrows*) obstructing the common bile duct.

References

1. Silverburg E. Cancer statistics. *CA*. 1990;40:9–27.
2. Lin RS, Kessler II. A multifactorial model for pancreatic cancer in man. Epidemiologic evidence. *JAMA*. 1981;245:147.
3. Fraumeni JF, Jr. Cancers of the pancreas and biliary tract: Epidemiological considerations. *Cancer Res*. 1975;35:3437.
4. Malagelada JR. Pancreatic cancer. An overview of epidemiology, clinical presentation, and diagnosis. *Mayo Clin Proc*. 1979;54:459.
5. Wynder EL. An epidemiological evaluation of the causes of cancer in the pancreas. *Cancer Res*. 1975;35:2228.
6. Christoffersen P, Poll P. Preoperative pancreas aspiration biopsies. *Acta Pathol Microbiol Scand*. 1970;(suppl):212:82–92.
7. Kim K, Booth R, Myles J. Percutaneous fine needle aspiration biopsy of cancer of the pancreas. *Int J Pancreatol*. In press.
8. Sons HU, Barchard F. Carcinoma of the extra-hepatic bile ducts: A post mortem study of 65 cases and review of the literature. *J Surg Oncol*. 1987;34:6.
9. Bruggen JT, et al. Primary adenocarcinoma of the bile ducts: Clinical characteristics and natural history. *Dig Dis Sci*. 1986;31:840.
10. Wise L, Pizzimbono C, Dehner LP. Periampullary cancer. A clinicopathologic study of sixty two patients. *Am J Surg*. 1976;131: 141–148.
11. Yamaguchi K, Enjoji M. Carcinoma of the ampulla of the Vater. A clinicopathologic study pathologic staging of 109 cases of carcinoma and 5 cases of adenoma. Cancer 1987;59:506–515.

10
Esophagus and Stomach

Esophagus

Many widely different esophageal lesions are clinically manifested by dysphagia, heartburn, or hematemesis. Inflammatory disease and carcinoma of the esophagus will be reviewed.

Esophagitis

Esophagitis, acute or chronic, occurs more often in terminally ill patients or immunoincompetent patients. The inflammation is usually associated with nonspecific bacterial, candidal, or herpetic infection (Fig. 10.1). In Western countries, recurrent reflux of gastric juice in association with hiatal hernia can be a cause of esophagitis in otherwise healthy persons. The most common symptoms of esophagitis are dysphagia or heartburn.

Barrett's esophagus is a specific variant of esophagitis that is characterized by epithelial metaplasia of intestinal type of the lower or mid segments (or both) of the esophageal mucosa. This condition is associated with an increased risk of developing primary esophageal adenocarcinoma.[1] Diagnosis is made by esophagoscopy with biopsy and esophageal brushing cytology (Fig. 10.2).

Carcinoma of the Esophagus

Squamous cell carcinoma is by far the most common type of esophageal cancer. The incidence of esophageal carcinoma is quite variable, depending on different geographic areas, ranging from 2 to 5 per 100,000 in North America and most Western countries to more than 100 per 100,000 in Northern China and Iran. The most common established causes of the cancer are alcoholism, heavy cigarette smoking, and esophagitis.

The geographic difference in incidence rates is highly suggestive of other environmental factors, for example dietary carcinogens (nitrosamines), malnutrition, or vitamin deficiency.

Grossly, the tumors develop most often in the mid and lower one third of the esophagus, and grow in polypoid, ulcerating, or diffuse infiltrative patterns (Fig. 10.3A–C).

In the high-risk regions of China, where cytologic screening is routinely performed, about half of the cases are intraepithelial neoplasms at the time of esophagectomy. During the developmental phase of the neoplasm, the patient may be asymptomatic for an uncertain length of time. When symptoms appear, dysphagia is almost always the first clinical manifestation of esophageal carcinoma, and at this stage the tumor is likely to extend at least halfway of the wall. With more advanced tumors, intractable hiccough or hoarseness may develop, caused by neoplastic involvement of the phrenic or recurrent laryngeal nerve. The overall 5-year survival rate is about 5% to 10%.

Cytology and Histology

The cytologic features of esophageal dysplasia and carcinoma in situ have been well documented in the high-risk regions in Northern China. At the symptomatic stage of esophageal cancer, biopsy and brushing cytology using fiberoptic esophagoscopy is one of the most rewarding of diagnostic tests, with up to 90% to 95% accuracy.[2]

Our own study, using the same methods, showed 95% accuracy in diagnosis. It is not uncommon to have positive cytologic findings and a negative biopsy. Combined biopsy and brushing cytology, using fiberoptic esophagoscopy, are highly recommended to establish a diagnosis. Radiographic examination, used for the initial diagnostic approach, is usually not suitable for detecting the early or developmental phase of the neoplasms.

In cytologic smears, the cells of squamous cell carcinoma occur in syncytia and as isolated cells. The cells are large and pleomorphic, with abundant cytoplasm. The nuclei are large, pleomorphic, generally centrally positioned, and hyperchromatic (Fig. 10.3D).

The histologic and cytologic features of squamous cell carcinoma of the esophagus are similar to those of other organs (Fig. 10.3E). Adenocarcinomas of the esophagus occur almost always in the esophagogastric junction. Cells of adenocarcinoma occur in clusters and syncytia, and have a small amount of granular cytoplasm. The nuclei are round to oval, tend to be eccentric, and have prominent macronucleoli (Fig. 10.4).

Clinical Course

Esophageal carcinoma is insidious in onset and eventually produces severe dysphagia. At the time of diagnosis, resection is possible in less than half the cases. Esophageal carcinomas have a strong propensity to infiltrate locally, which may result in esophagotracheal fistula and aspiration pneumonia (Fig. 10.4D).

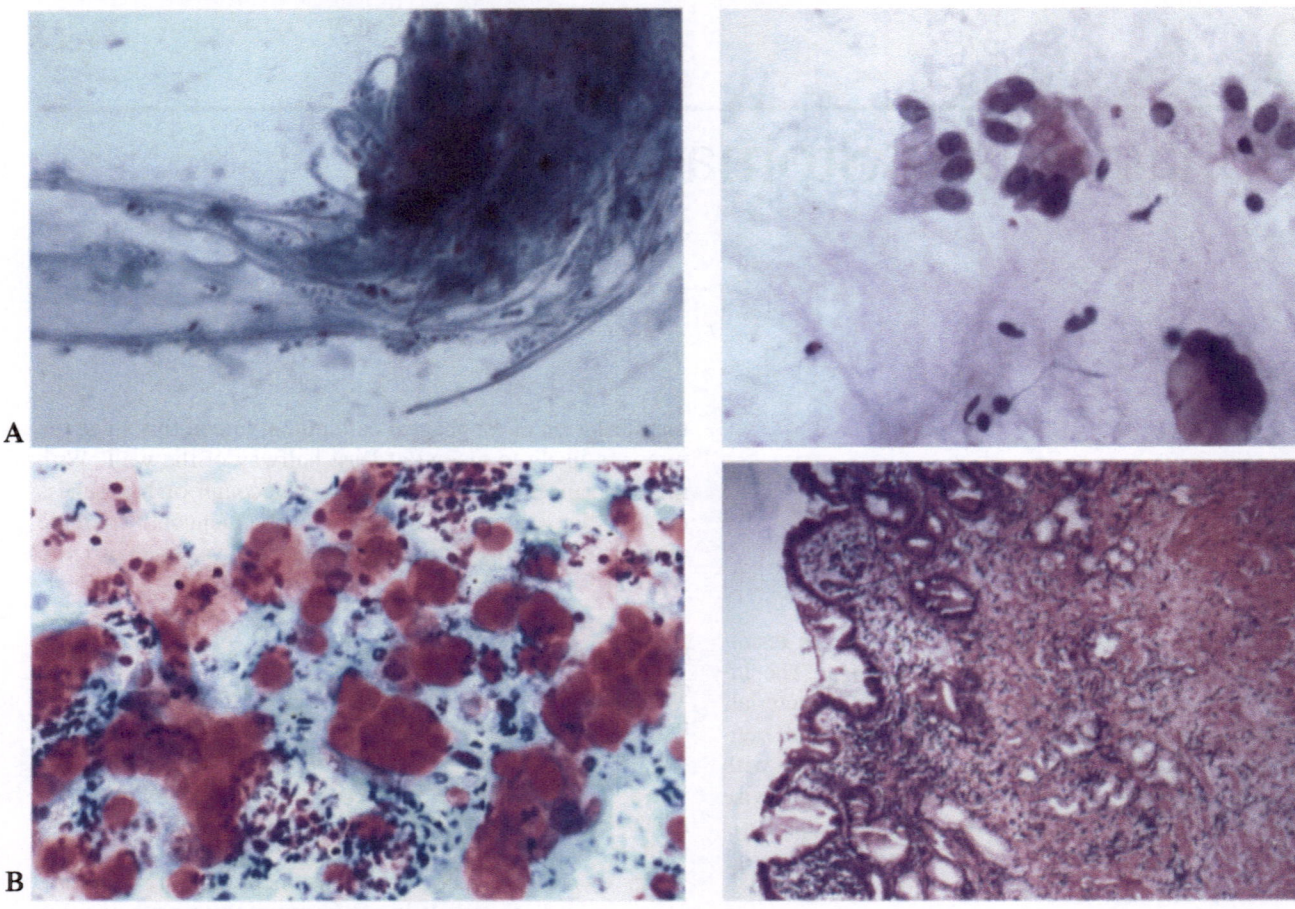

FIGURE 10.1 Cytology of esophagitis. A: *Candida* species showing pseudohyphae and yeast forms (esophageal brushing smear). B: Herpetic esophagitis showing multinucleated herpetic giant cells (esophageal brushing smear).

FIGURE 10.2 Barrett's esophagus. A: Esophageal endoscopic brushing smear showing sheets and strips of columnar cells. B: Biopsy section from the lesion showing colonic type mucosa.

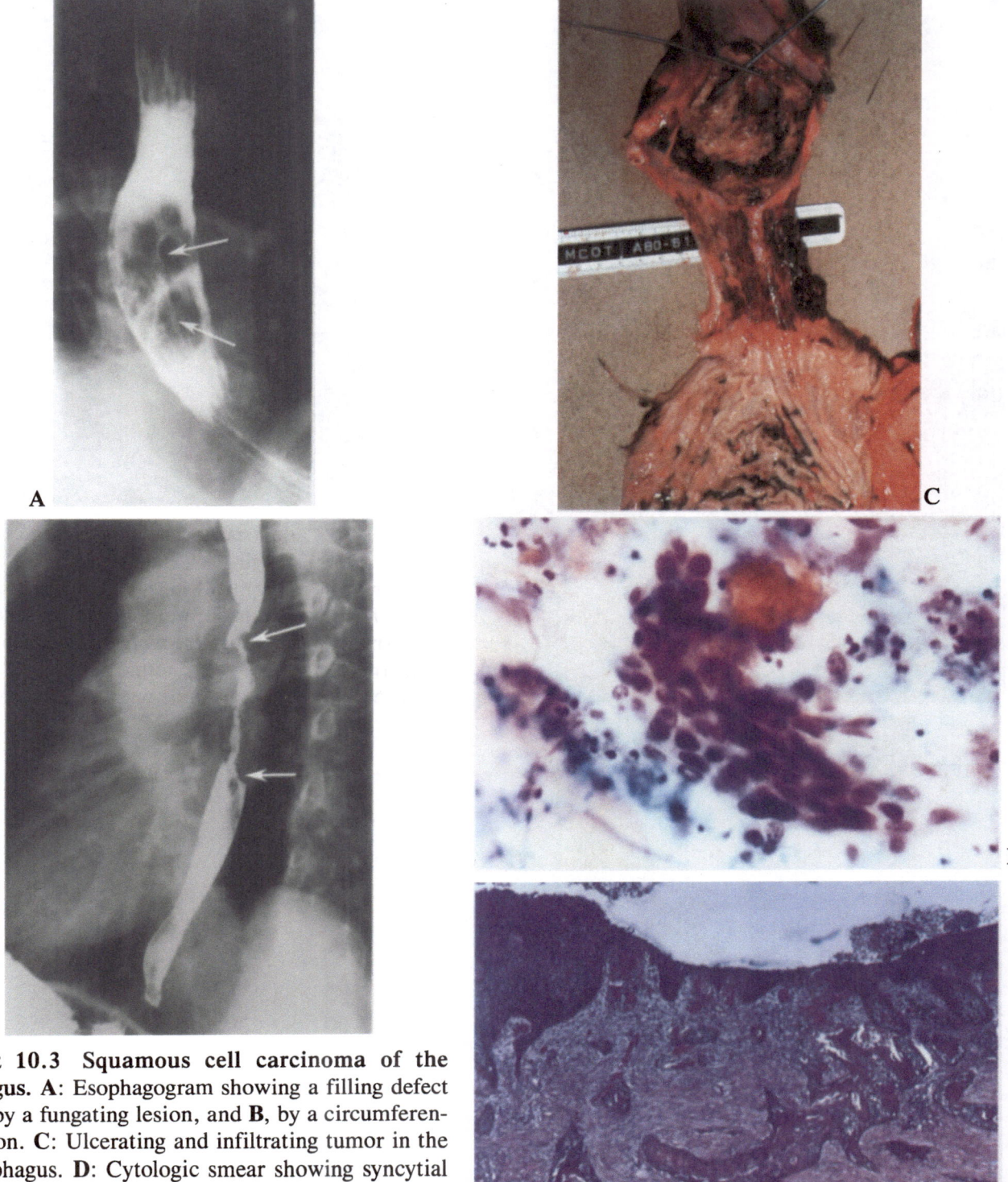

FIGURE 10.3 **Squamous cell carcinoma of the esophagus. A**: Esophagogram showing a filling defect caused by a fungating lesion, and **B**, by a circumferential lesion. **C**: Ulcerating and infiltrating tumor in the midesophagus. **D**: Cytologic smear showing syncytial aggregates of pleomorphic cells (esophageal brushing). **E**: Biopsy of the same lesion showing cords and islands of infiltrating neoplastic cells.

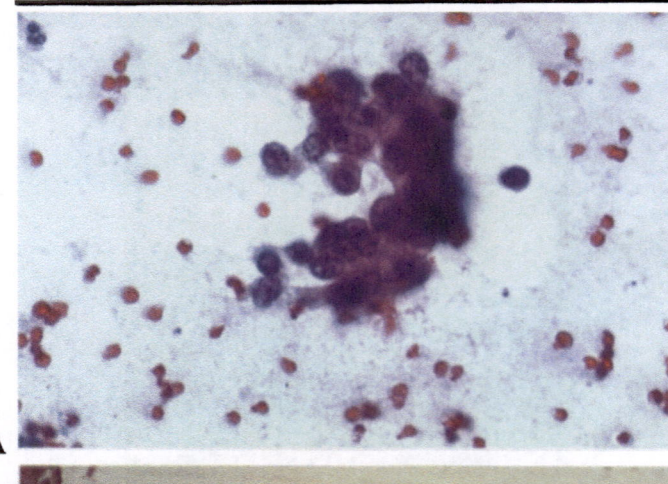

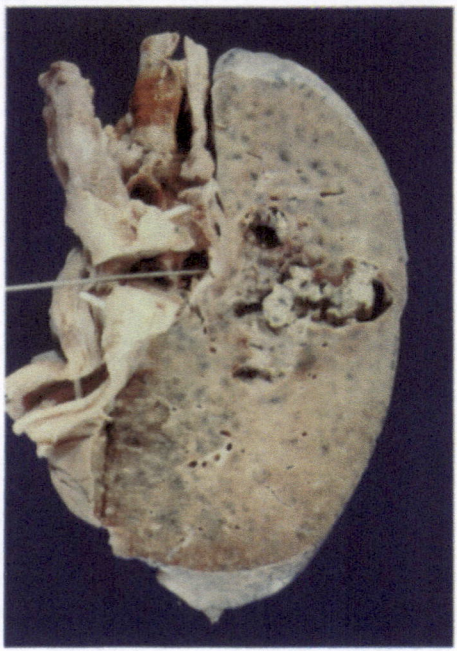

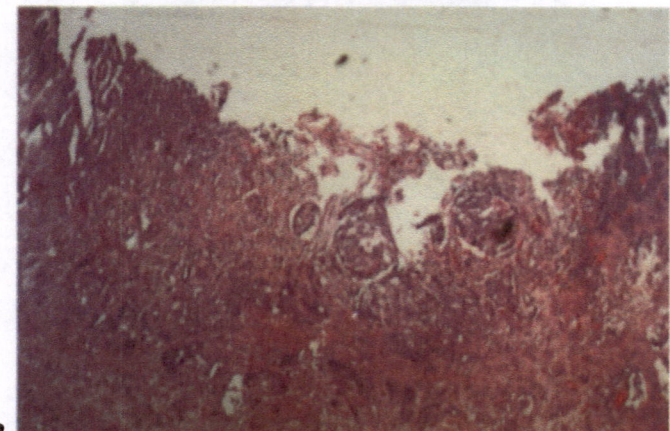

FIGURE 10.4 **Adenocarcinoma of esophagus.** **A**: Cytologic smear showing clusters of neoplastic cells (esophageal brushing). **B**: Biopsy of the lesion showing poorly formed glands infiltrating the wall. **C**: The neoplasm extends through the wall and extraesophageal tissue (necropsy). **D**: Carcinoma of esophagus with tracheoesophageal fistula and consequent pneumonia.

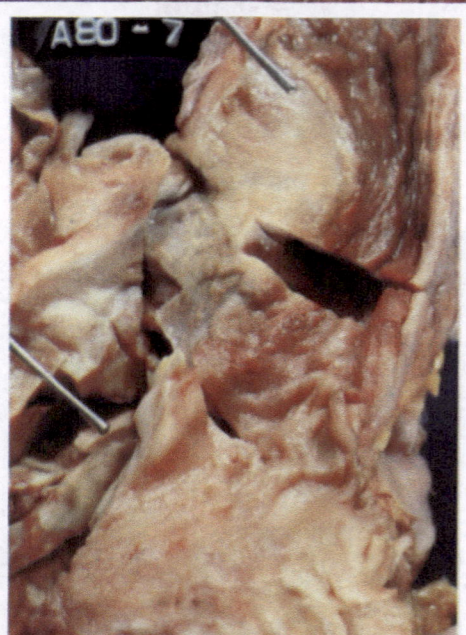

Stomach

This section will cover only neoplastic disease.

The most common and important malignant neoplasm is carcinoma. Carcinoid tumor can occur in the stomach and will be discussed in the section of small intestine. However, nonepithelial neoplasms may occur in the gastrointestinal tract. Among these are leiomyomas, leiomyoblastomas, leiomyosarcomas, lipomas, neurofibromas, and lymphomas.

Gastric Polyps

Gastric polyps are rare and are usually found incidentally. Most gastric polyps are of hyperplastic type; adenomatous polyps are less common and are true benign neoplasms.

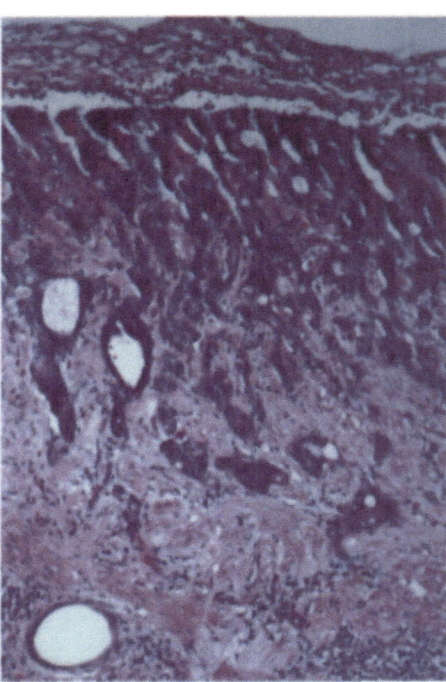

FIGURE 10.5 Early carcinoma of stomach (gross). Poorly demarcated flat granular mucosa in the gastric antrum.

Malignant Neoplasms

Adenocarcinoma

The incidence of gastric adenocarcinoma in the United States has declined from 33 per 100,000 in 1930 to 6 per 100,000 at the present time. However, it is still one of the top 10 leading causes of deaths from cancer in the United States. In contrast, gastric carcinoma is one of the most common causes of cancer death in Japan, Korea, Finland, and Iceland.[3] Dietary factors are strong in gastric carcinogenesis with the most culpable dietary factor being nitrites. Genetic influence may play a weak role.

Grossly, early gastric carcinoma may be slightly elevated, depressed, or flat (Fig. 10.5). Japanese studies, using gastric brushing cytology, demonstrated early asymptomatic gastric carcinomas in routine screening of the population at risk.[4,5] Early gastric carcinomas are regarded as those carcinomas limited to the mucosa and submucosa.

As the tumors advance, they infiltrate deeper into the muscularis propria and spread to lymph nodes, liver, and other organs. The growth pattern may be fungating, ulcerative, polypoid, or diffusely infiltrative (Fig. 10.6A, B). The tumors at this stage are usually delineated by radiologic examination or gastroscopy. Endoscopic brushing cytology and biopsy are the most reliable diagnostic methods, with more than 95% diagnostic accuracy. This method is also highly recommended for routine screening in asymptomatic high-risk populations.

Gastric washing cytology is time-consuming and gives less accurate results.

Cytology and Histology

In brushing smears, the cells occur in clusters, syncytial aggregates, and as isolated cells. The cells are enlarged and have scanty granular cytoplasm. The nuclei are large and hyperchromatic, with irregularly dispersed chromatin and prominent single macronucleoli. The nuclei often are indented (Fig. 10.6C, D).

In signet-ring cell carcinoma (diffuse, infiltrating), the cells occur usually as isolated cells and have abundant mucinous secretion pushing the nuclei eccentrically.

In benign gastric ulcers, the cells occur in sheets with well preserved polarity and a columnar configuration. The nuclei are rather uniform and round and have a bland chromatin pattern. Histologically, gastric carcinoma comprises well formed to poorly formed acini arranged compactly. The acini are lined by a single layer of large pleomorphic cells (Fig. 10.6E, F). Patients with gastric carcinoma usually have vague symptoms for about 6 months to 1 year. At the time of the full blown symptomatic stage, the neoplasms usually have already metastasized to regional lymph nodes, liver, pancreas, and peritoneum to cause ascites. It is not unusual to detect metastasis to supraclavicular lymph nodes (Virchow's nodes) and the rectal shelf.

The overall 5-year survival rate of gastric carcinomas in the United States, 5% to 15%, has not changed over the last several decades. This is in striking contrast to the 80% to 95% 5-year survival rates for early gastric carcinomas in Japan.[6]

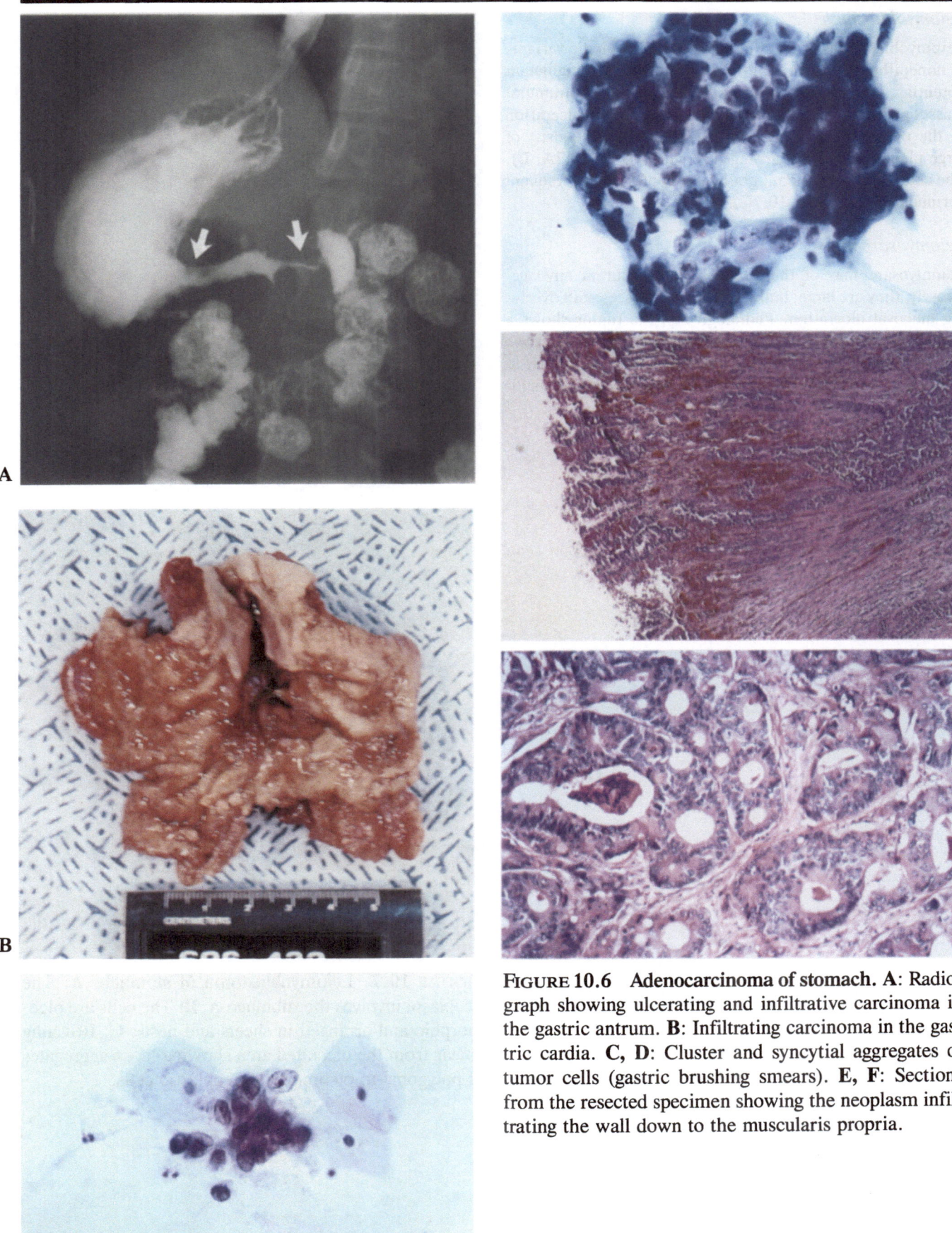

FIGURE **10.6**   **Adenocarcinoma of stomach. A**: Radiograph showing ulcerating and infiltrative carcinoma in the gastric antrum. **B**: Infiltrating carcinoma in the gastric cardia. **C, D**: Cluster and syncytial aggregates of tumor cells (gastric brushing smears). **E, F**: Sections from the resected specimen showing the neoplasm infiltrating the wall down to the muscularis propria.

Leiomyoblastoma

Leiomyoblastomas of the stomach are rare histologic variants of nonepithelial gastric tumors with intermediate malignant potential. Grossly, they are well circumscribed intramural masses protruding into the lumen, sometimes with ulceration of the overlying mucosa. Microscopically, they consist of large pleomorphic cells arranged in sheets (Fig. 10.7A, B). The cells have an abundant granular cytoplasm with frequent perinuclear halos (Fig. 10.7C).

Leiomyosarcoma

Leiomyosarcomas of the stomach may occur at any age. Grossly, they are large, bulky, intramural masses with overlying mucosal ulceration. Radiologically, the tumor shows a well delineated submucosal mass without diffuse infiltrative characteristics (Fig. 10.8). Histologically, they are similar to those found elsewhere. Most are surgically resectable, yielding a 50% to 60% 5-year survival rate.

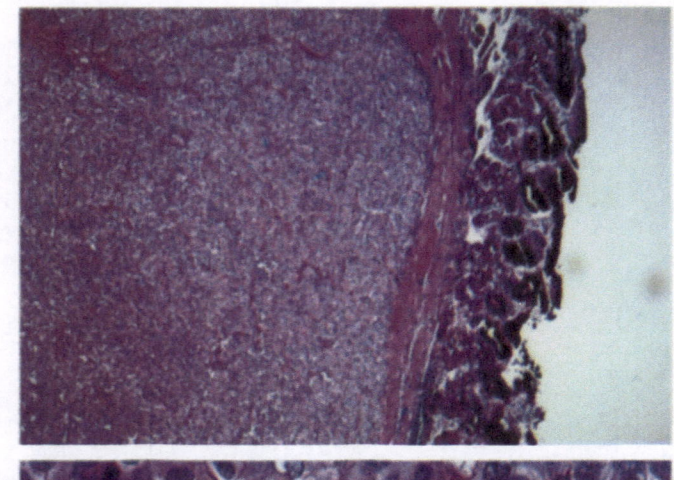

A

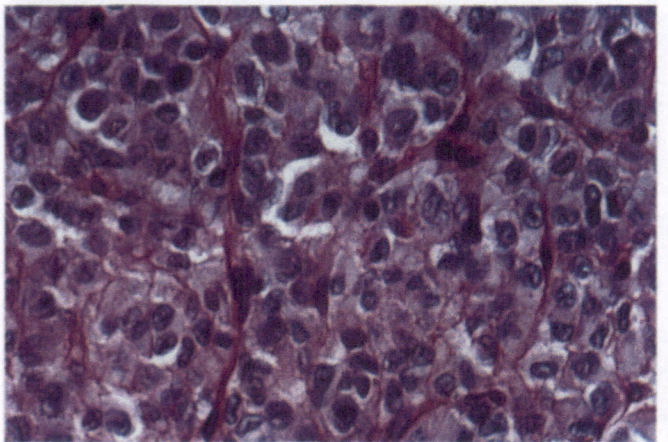

B

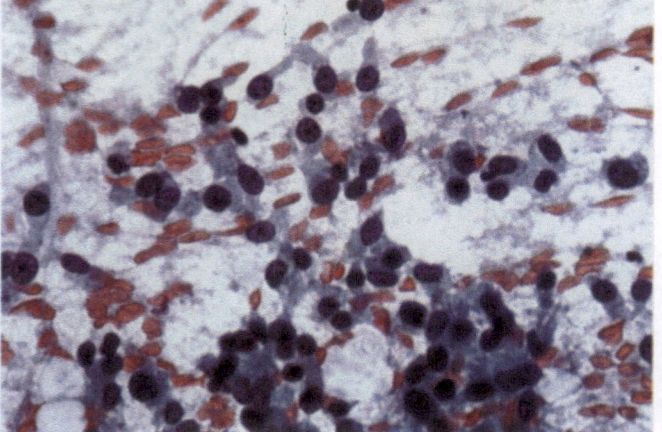

C

FIGURE 10.7 **Leiomyoblastoma of stomach. A:** The neoplasm involves the submucosa. **B:** The cells are pleomorphic and arranged in sheets and nests. **C:** Brushing smear from the ulcerated area showing loose aggregates of polygonal to pleomorphic neoplastic cells.

References

1. Cameron AJ, et al. The incidence of adenocarcinoma in columnar-lined (Barrett's) esophagus. *N Engl J Med*. 1985;313:857.
2. Prolla JC, Reilly RW, Kirsner JB, Cockerham L. Direct vision endoscopic cytology and biopsy in the diagnosis of esophageal and gastric tumors: Current experience. *Acta Cytol*. 1977;21:399–402.
3. Silverburg E. Cancer statistics. *CA*. 1989;39:5.
4. Grundmann E. Early gastric cancer—Today. *Pathol Res Pract*. 1978; 162:347.
5. Kobayashi S, Suriura H, Kasuga T. Reliability of endoscopic observation in diagnosis of early carcinoma of the stomach. *Endoscopy*. 1972; 4:61–65.
6. Hirota T, et al. Clinicopathologic study of minute and small early gastric cancers. *Pathol Annu*. 1980;15(2):1.

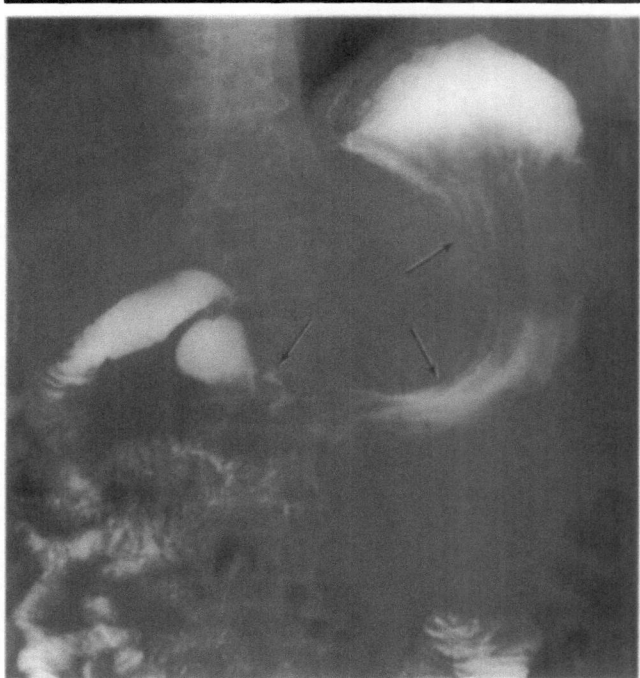

FIGURE **10.8 Leiomyosarcoma of stomach.** Radiograph showing displacement of the lesser curve of the stomach.

11
Small and Large Intestine

Small Intestine

Only neoplasms of the small intestine will be reviewed in this chapter. Approximately 5% of all gastrointestinal neoplasms arise in the small intestine. In descending order of frequency, the common benign neoplasms arising in the small intestine are leiomyoma, lipoma, adenoma, adenomatous polyp, angioma, and fibroma.[1]

Malignant neoplasms arising in the small intestine, in descending order of frequency, are adenocarcinoma, lymphoma, carcinoid tumor, and leiomyosarcoma.[2]

Adenocarcinoma

Adenocarcinomas of the small intestine are rare and occur after the age of 40 years. They grow in a napkin ring, encircling pattern. Because obstruction may occur late as a result of the fluid intestinal contents, these neoplasms produce symptoms late. At the time of diagnosis the neoplasms are usually advanced. The 5-year survival rate is 15% to 20%.[3]

Gastrointestinal Lymphoma

Lymphomas may arise in the gastrointestinal tract or they may spread to the gastrointestinal tract from other origins. The term "primary" is used for any lymphoma if the initial manifestation of the disease is gastrointestinal.

Grossly, lymphomas involve the intestinal wall as a diffuse infiltrate resulting in marked thickening, polypoid masses projecting into the lumen or elevated plaquelike lesions. They may be limited to the gut, but more often they are accompanied by involvement of the regional lymph nodes and sometimes of other organs, such as liver and spleen.

Cytology and Histology

Cytologic smears are obtained by endoscopic brushing of the stomach or the rectosigmoid colon if there is mucosal ulceration. The cytologic features of lymphomas are a monomorphic population of singly occurring lymphoid cells. They may be large cleaved or noncleaved cells, small cleaved cells, or small noncleaved cells. The most common variant is diffuse, large cell lymphoma, but any histologic variant can occur in the gastrointestinal tract.[3,4] Histologically, lymphomas involve the submucosa and extend to the overlying mucosa and underlying muscularis propria (Fig. 11.1). Most gastrointestinal lymphomas are of B-cell origin. One unique type of intestinal lymphoma is Burkitt's lymphoma (American Burkitt's), comprising small, noncleaved B cells (Fig. 11.2). American Burkitt's lymphomas usually arise in the small intestine in children in contrast to the head and neck involvement in African Burkitt's. Their histological features are similar.

Carcinoid (Endocrine Cell Tumor, Argentaffinoma)

Carcinoid tumors are capable of secreting bioactive amines and polypeptides by virtue of their cells, which are part of the amine precursor uptake and decarboxylation (APUD) system.[5] This property is shared by cells in the adrenal medulla and by hypothalamic neurons. All APUD cells are considered to be neuroectodermal origin, and thus they are called neuroendocrine cells. Carcinoid tumors have an affinity for soluble silver salts, hence their designation as "argentaffinomas." Carcinoid tumors arise usually in the gastrointestinal and respiratory tracts and may arise rarely in the pancreas, female genital tract, or thyroid.

In descending order of frequency, carcinoid tumors are distributed as follows: appendix, small intestine, rectosigmoid colon, lungs and bronchi, esophagus, and stomach.[6] Grossly, intestinal carcinoids tend to be small, ranging from 1.0 to 4.0 cm in greatest dimensions. They involve the mucosa and submucosa. They are pale gray to pale yellow and may permeate the serosa and overlying mucosa with ulceration. Carcinoids grow slowly and may metastasize to regional lymph nodes and liver.

Carcinoids of the appendix are usually localized, rarely spreading beyond the organ.

Histology and Cytology

The histologic features of all carcinoids at all sites of origin are similar. The tumors involve the submucosa and extend into muscularis propria and mucosa. The cells that are cuboidal to polygonal show little variation in size and have uniform, round nuclei and a moderate amount of granular cytoplasm. The cells are arranged in trabecular, insular, acinar, or rosette formations separated by fibrous stroma (Fig. 11.3A). Nuclear atypia or mitotic figures are rare. Neurosecretory granules ranging from 70 to 250 nm in diameter can be identified by electron microscopy (Fig. 11.3B). The granules in carcinoids have an affinity for silver turning black with silver salts in solution (argentaffine-positive), and in others an exogenous reducing agent is needed (argyrophil-positive). The neurosecretory granules can be identified by immunocytochemistry.

Cytologic samples are not available from small intestinal carcinoids. However, they are remarkably similar to those from other sites.

Clinical Course

Carcinoid tumors of the small intestine are found more often incidentally at necropsy than during surgical exploration of the abdomen. Patients with carcinoid tumors appear to have an increased incidence of other malignant neoplasms of the gastrointestinal tract.

Carcinoid tumors of the small intestine (foregut) may or may not produce symptoms. Most carcinoid tumors grow slowly and are rarely detected by clinical or radiologic examination. However, they may come to clinical attention because of 1) hepatomegaly due to metastasis, 2) crampy abdominal pain, or 3) the carcinoid syndrome.

Although the diagnosis of the carcinoid syndrome may be obvious clinically, it usually requires confirmation by a serum concentration of 5-hydroxy-indol acetic acid (5 HIAA) or other metabolites of 5-hydroxytryptamine (5-HT). In cases without hepatic metastasis, the 5-year survival rate is 80% to 90%.[7]

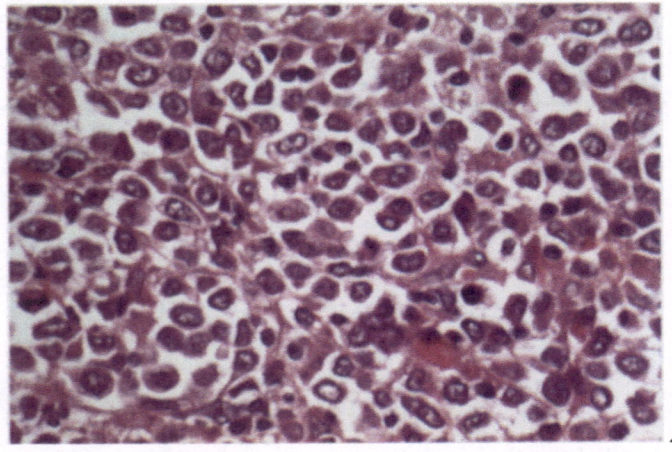

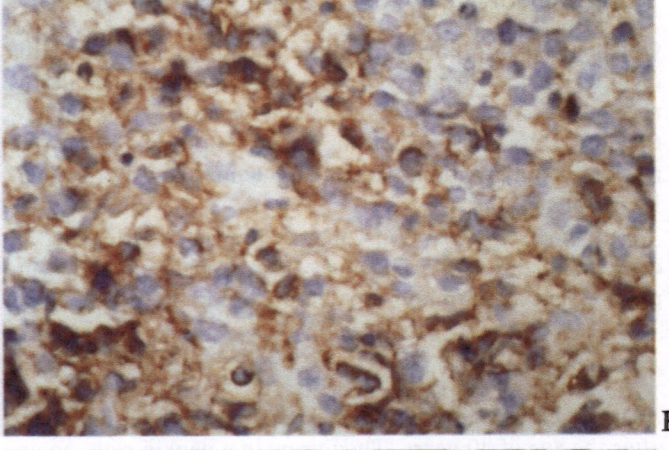

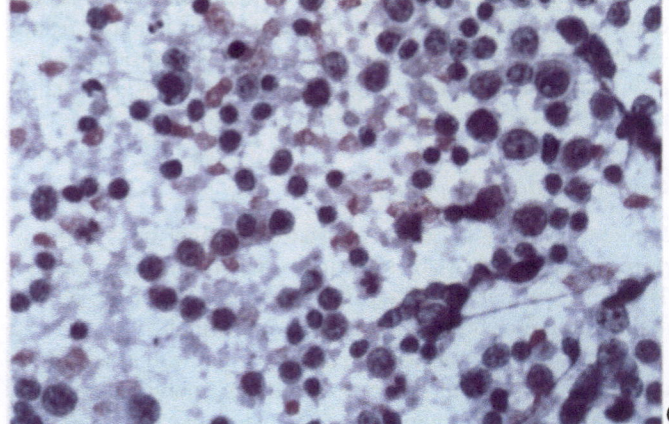

FIGURE 11.1 "Histiocytic" lymphoma of stomach. **A**: Sheets of monomorphic large neoplastic lymphoid cells. **B**: Immunostain of the same neoplasm, using leukocyte common antigen. **C**: Large, noncleaved neoplastic lymphocytes occurring singly (gastric brushing, Papanicolaou stain).

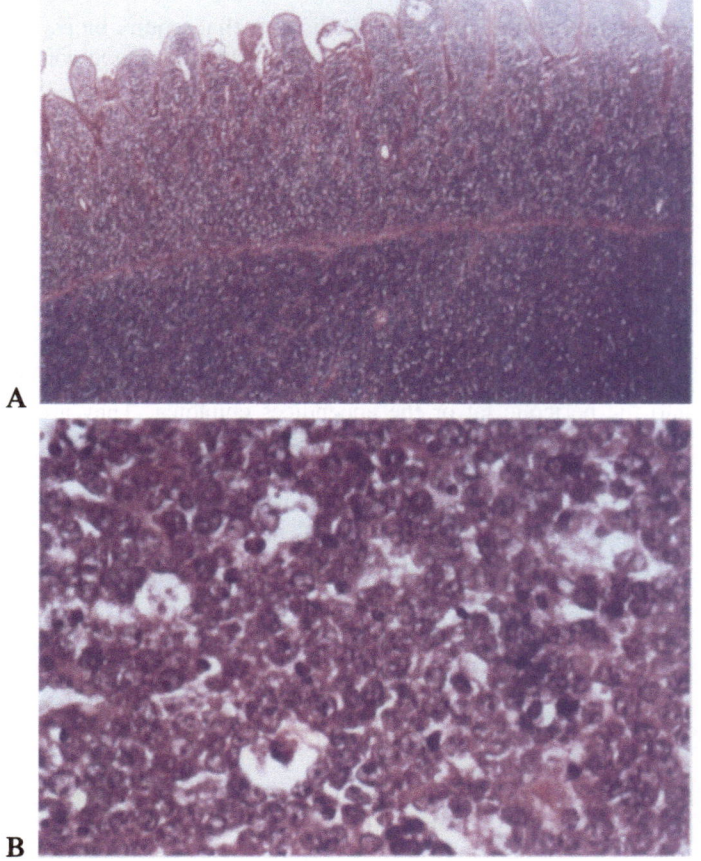

FIGURE 11.2   Burkitt's lymphoma (small, noncleaved cell) of small intestine. A: Small, noncleaved neoplastic lymphocytes infiltrate throughout the wall. B: The same neoplasm showing tingible body macrophages.

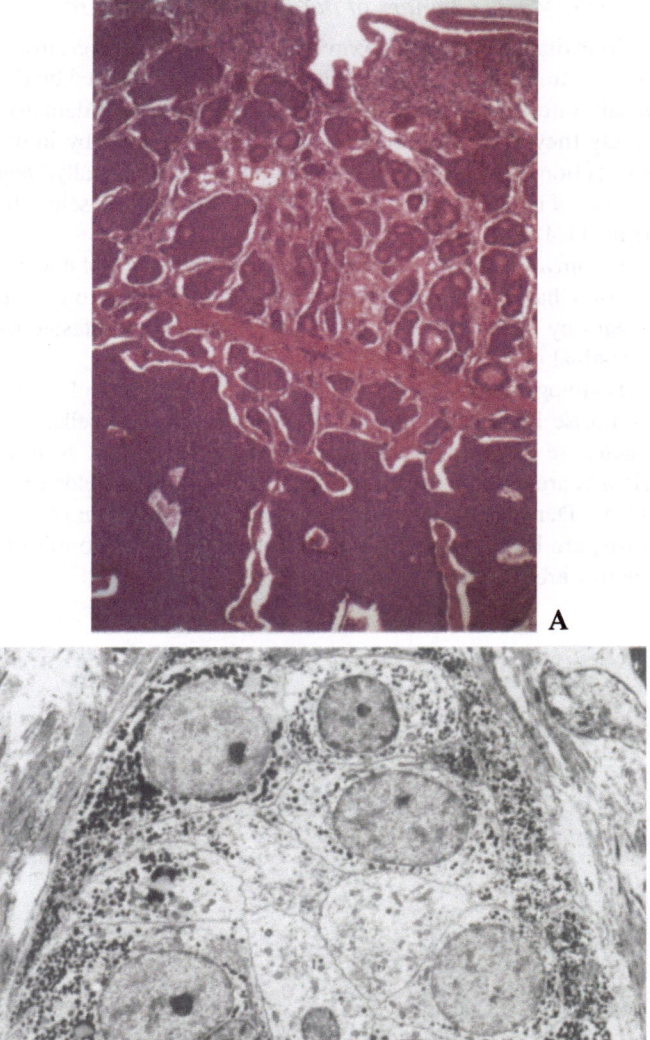

FIGURE 11.3   Carcinoid tumor of small intestine. A: Islets and cords of neoplastic cells infiltrate the submucosa. B: Neurosecretory dense core granules in the neoplastic cells. (EM)

Smooth Muscle Tumors of the Gastrointestinal Tract

Leiomyomas and leiomyosarcomas arising in the gastrointestinal tract occur most often in the stomach, followed by the small intestine. Most leiomyomas are found incidentally; rarely they cause bleeding or intestinal obstruction by intussusception. They grow as solitary nodules. Histologically, they consist of interlacing bundles of elongated smooth muscle cells (Fig. 11.4).

Leiomyosarcomas tend to be large and at the time of diagnosis they have usually spread to adjacent organs and to distant organs by metastasis. Sometimes they are first manifested by intestinal obstruction.

Histologically, leiomyosarcomas are highly cellular and comprise interlacing bundles of atypical elongated cells. The nuclei are often oval to elongated, with blunted ends. Mitotic figures are usually 10 or more per 10 high power fields (Fig. 11.5). Dense cellularity, with nuclear atypia and foci of necrosis, are highly suggestive of malignancy, even if no mitotic figures are present.

Colon

This section will review only the diseases that require biopsy or cytology for diagnostic confirmation. Other common colonic disease will be briefly mentioned.

Diverticular Disease

Colonic diverticula are found in 30% to 50% of human necropsy patients older than 60 years in the United States. In contrast, diverticular disease is rare in African and Asian countries.[8] Only about 10% to 15% of individuals having diverticula are symptomatic. In 95% of patients, the diverticula are limited to the sigmoid colon.

Diverticulosis refers to the presence of mucosal outpouching into the pericolic fat or the appendices epiploica. They are usually found between the mesenteric and antimesenteric taenia. Histologically, the wall of the outpouching comprises only the mucosa and submucosa without any supporting muscular layer (Fig. 11.6).

The usual symptoms are vague lower abdominal pain and change of bowel habit. The major complications are rectal bleeding, infection with abscess or perforation, and bowel narrowing.

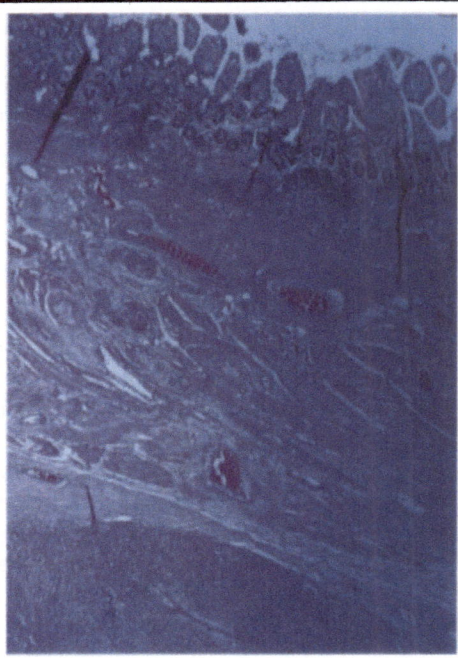

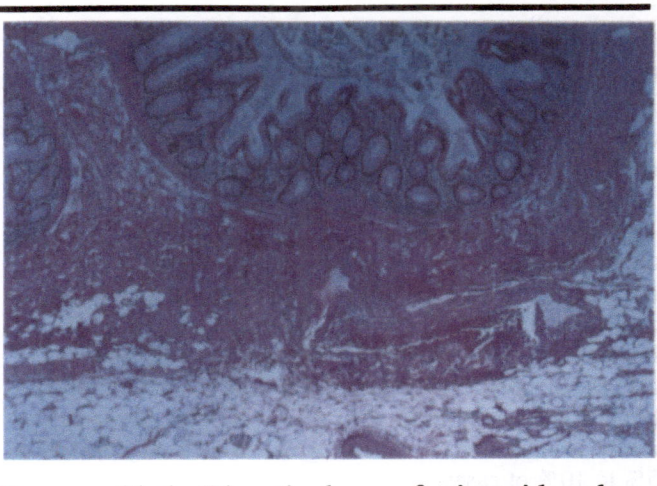

FIGURE 11.6 Diverticulum of sigmoid colon. Mucosal outpouching to the serosa.

FIGURE 11.4 Leiomyoma of small intestine. The neoplasm arises in the muscular layer and consists of a well circumscribed mass of interlacing bundles of elongated cells. (arrows)

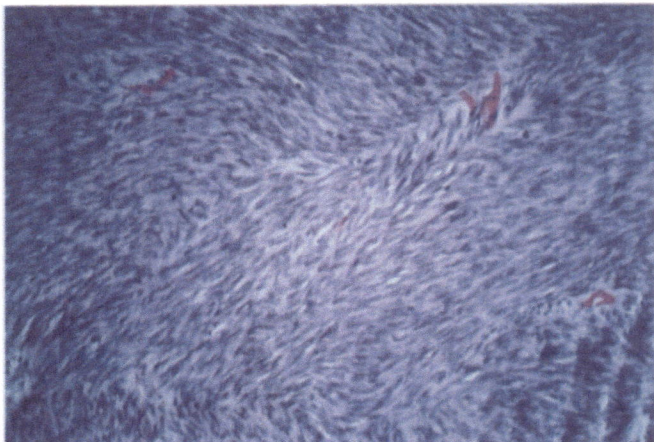

FIGURE 11.5 Leiomyosarcoma of small intestine. Histologic section showing interlacing bundles of elongated neoplastic cells with mitotic figures.

Idiopathic Ulcerative Colitis

Idiopathic ulcerative colitis refers to colonic mucosal ulceration and chronic recurrent diarrhea without known cause. Ulcerative colitis begins most often in the second to fourth decades of life. It begins in the rectosigmoid and spreads proximally without the "skip" lesions that may be seen in Crohn's disease.

In the early stage of the disease, the mucosa shows small ulcers in a background of hyperemic and edematous and friable mucosa. With progression, the ulcers become large and coalescent and extend down to the submucosa (Fig. 11.7A). Residual edematous hyperplastic islands of mucosa may create "pseudopolyps" (Fig. 11.7B, C). Fibrous induration with luminal stenosis, intestinal fistula, or abscess formation are rarely seen. Perianal or rectovaginal fistulae may be seen in 5% to 10% of cases.

Two serious complications are "toxic" megacolon and perforation of the bowel.

In the acute phase of ulcerative colitis, there are multiple mucosal crypt abscess collections of neutrophils in mucosal crypts. Subsequently they progress to ulceration by mucosal surface necrosis (Fig. 11.7D).

In active colitis, the process of epithelial repair is frequently associated with cellular atypia at the margins of the ulcers. With increasing severity of atypia, the risk of carcinoma increases.

Clinical Course

Ulcerative colitis usually develops insidiously over the course of several months with bloody, mucoid diarrhea. Lower abdominal pain and tenderness are common. Various constitutional signs, including fever and weight loss, are commonly present. The clinical course is characterized by remissions and relapses. The diagnosis is based on rectosigmoid endoscopic biopsy. Specific infectious processes must always be ruled out, and subsequently patients should be closely monitored by endoscopic biopsies.

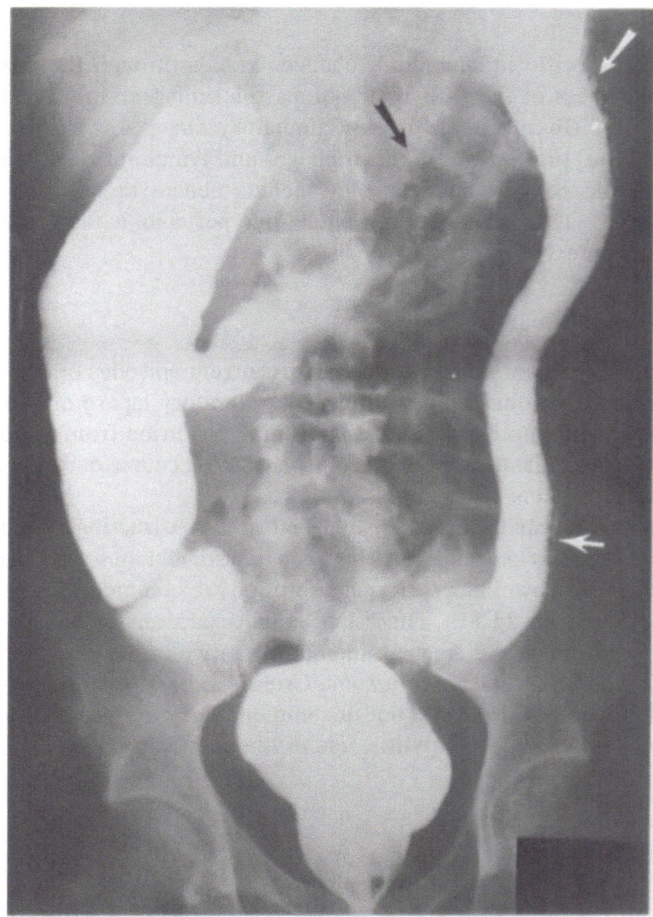

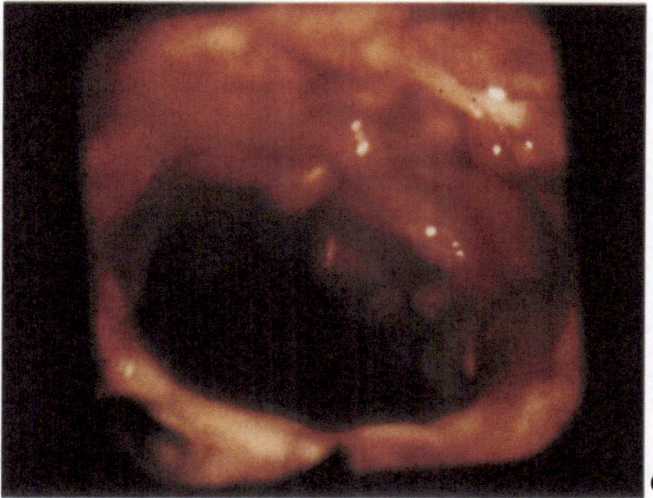

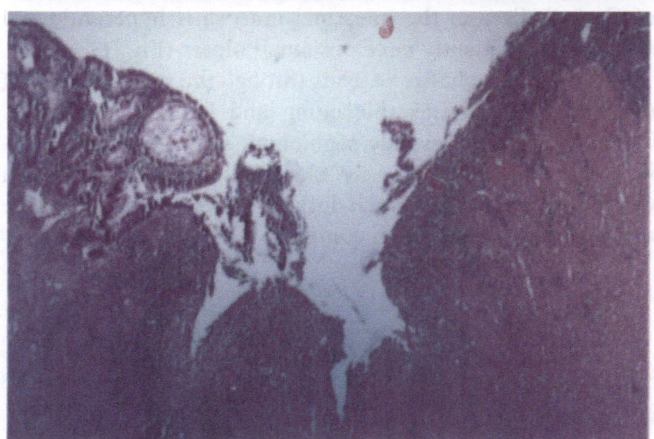

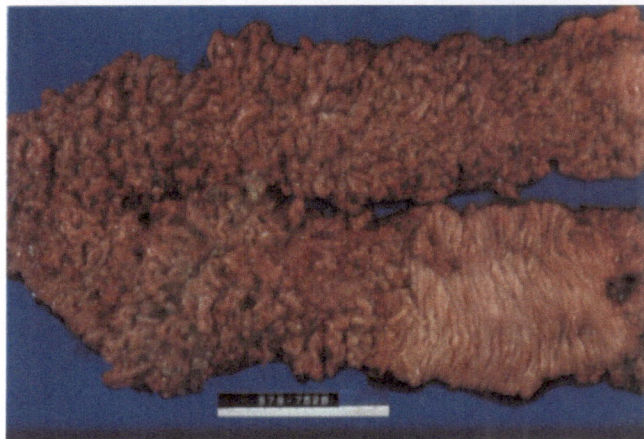

FIGURE 11.7 **Ulcerative colitis. A**: Radiograph after barium enema showing multiple "collar-button" ulcers (*arrows*) and lack of haustral markings. **B**: Almost all of the colonic mucosa is studded with pseudopolyps. **C**: Endoscopic picture showing multiple pseudopolyps (Courtesy of Dr. John Stroehlein, Houston, Tex.). **D**: Mucosal ulcers with inflammation.

Regional Enteritis (Crohn's Disease)

Crohn's disease is a chronic inflammatory bowel disease involving any portion of the gastrointestinal tract from esophagus to anus, but most often the small intestine and colon are affected. Since there are some similarities between Crohn's disease and ulcerative colitis, both are embraced by the term "inflammatory bowel disease." Both are of unknown cause. Although there are distinctive differences in clinicopathological presentation of the two conditions, 10% to 20% of cases cannot be distinguished one from the other.

In most cases, pathologic changes involve both the small intestine and colon. The pattern of involvement of Crohn's disease can be colon alone or small intestine alone. In the absence of total colonic involvement, the rectosigmoid is usually spared, a contrast with ulcerative colitis, in which these segments are almost always involved. In the early stage of Crohn's disease, the intestinal mucosa is hyperemic and soft and subsequently develops small ulcers (Fig. 11.8A).

Inflammatory change extends through the full thickness of the wall with fibrous thickening and luminal narrowing. These changes are usually segmental, with alternating normal segments referred to as "skip" lesions, a contrast with ulcerative colitis, in which inflammatory changes involve mucosa and submucosa in continuity (Fig. 11.8B).

Histology

Nonspecific inflammatory change extends through the full thickness of the wall with fibrous thickening and mucosal ulcers (Fig. 11.8C). The inflammatory changes consist of various proportions of macrophages and lymphoid cells in a fibrous background, and may include noncaseating granulomas. These changes may extend into pericolonic fat or the mesentery (Fig. 11.8D).

Clinical Course

The dominant manifestations are recurrent episodes of diarrhea, abdominal pain, and fever. Exploratory laparotomy is frequently necessary to distinguish the condition from acute appendicitis. Most patients follow a chronic course of repeated remissions and relapses.

Perianal and perirectal fistulae, intestinal obstruction caused by stenosis on adhesions between intestinal loops, fistulae between bowel loops, or malabsorption are common complications (Fig. 11.8E). The risk of colonic cancer in Crohn's disease is much less frequent than in ulcerative colitis.

In both ulcerative colitis and Crohn's disease, extraintestinal manifestations are not uncommon. They are polyarthritis, ankylosing spondylitis, and erythema nodosum.

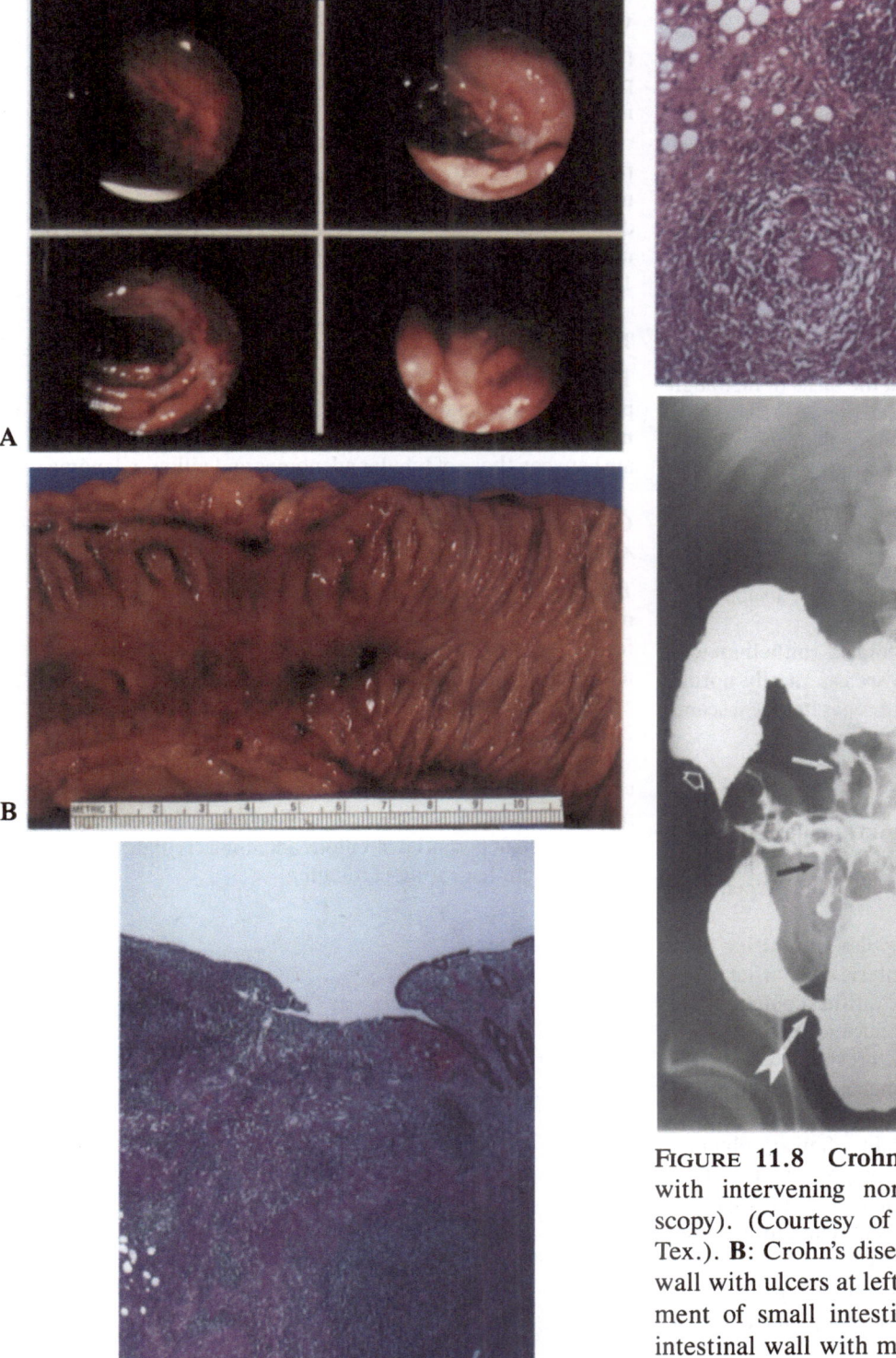

FIGURE 11.8 Crohn's disease. A: Irregular ulcers with intervening normal appearing mucosa (endoscopy). (Courtesy of Dr. John Stroehlein, Houston, Tex.). **B**: Crohn's disease showing a skip lesion. Thick wall with ulcers at left side, and normal appearing segment of small intestine at right side. **C**: Thickened intestinal wall with mucosal ulcer and chronic inflammation. **D**: Noncaseating granuloma involving the serosa in Crohn's disease. **E**: Radiograph after barium enema showing involvement of the cecum (*open arrow*) and multiple fistulae in the terminal ileum (*arrows*).

Tumors

Tumors of the large intestine are among the most common forms of neoplasia and the second most common cause of cancer deaths in the United States and Western countries.

Large intestinal polyps are benign neoplasms, although some forms are considered to be precursors of colon carcinoma. Large intestinal polyps are common in older adults. Mass population screening by testing stool for occult blood will reduce the death rate of colorectal carcinoma by detecting the cancers at an early stage.

Polyps

"Polyp" is a term for a grossly visible mucosal nodule protruding above the mucosal surface. On the basis of histologic architecture, colorectal polyps are divided into 1) hyperplastic polyp and 2) adenomatous polyp, which is further divided into tubular adenoma and villous adenoma.

Hyperplastic Polyps

Hyperplastic polyps are more common in adults. Grossly, they are small, tan-pink, smooth protrusions, usually less than 5 mm in diameter.

Hyperplastic polyps consist of proliferated epithelium with expanded crypts. The epithelial cells are essentially normal and include goblet cells. The crypts are separated by a scanty stroma (Fig. 11.9).

Tubular Adenoma

Ninety percent of adenomatous polyps are tubular adenomas. Tubular adenomas have a raspberrylike head, usually less than 1 cm in diameter, attached to a slender stalk ("pedunculated polyp") (Fig. 11.10A).

Histologically, they are polypoid nodules comprising compact glands and tubules with scanty intervening stroma. The glands and tubules are lined by pseudostratified columnar cells with slightly enlarged hyperchromatic nuclei. Mitotic figures are frequently observed. Goblet cells are not present. The pedicle is covered by normal colonic mucosa (Fig. 11.10B).

Based on our experience, endoscopic brushing cytology of polypoid lesions is of no practical value. Smears obtained from an intact mucosal surface of the polyps may give false negative cytology, and those from an ulcerated surface of the polyp may give spuriously positive results. Therefore, biopsy is the only reliable diagnostic procedure.

The malignant potential of adenomatous polyps increases with size, the degree of villous formation, and a sessile growth pattern.[9]

Villous Adenoma

Villous adenomas are the less common type of adenomatous polyps, tending to be large and to occur in a sessile growth pattern (Fig. 11.11A). They occur most often in the rectosigmoid (Fig. 11.11B).

Histologically, villous adenomas consist of tightly packed papillary structures, comprising more than 50% of the volume of the growth. Papillary structures resemble fingers with delicate fibrovascular cores and are covered by atypical columnar cells. Mitotic figures are frequently observed (Fig. 11.11C).

Tubulovillous Adenoma

Tubulovillous adenoma denotes adenomatous polyps comprising tubuloglandular and villous structures. Their malignant potential and clinicopathologic features are intermediate between those of tubular adenomas and villous adenomas.

Clinical Course and Malignant Potential of Adenomatous Polyps

Tubular adenomas are most often discovered incidentally but may attract attention by bleeding or by positive screening test for occult blood screening. Tubular adenomas have the least malignant potential. Tumors less than 1 cm in diameter have a 1% change of being malignant, whereas 10% of those 1 to 2 cm in diameter are malignant.[10]

Villous adenomas are more frequently symptomatic because of bleeding. Occasionally they produce potassium and protein-rich secretion resulting in diarrhea and hypokalemia. The malignant potential of villous adenomas is high, with one third of them harboring carcinoma.

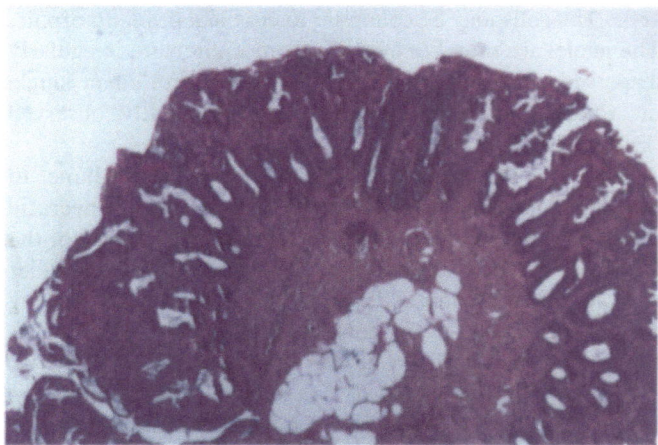

FIGURE 11.9 **Hyperplastic polyp.** Biopsy section showing epithelial hyperplasia with expansion of crypts.

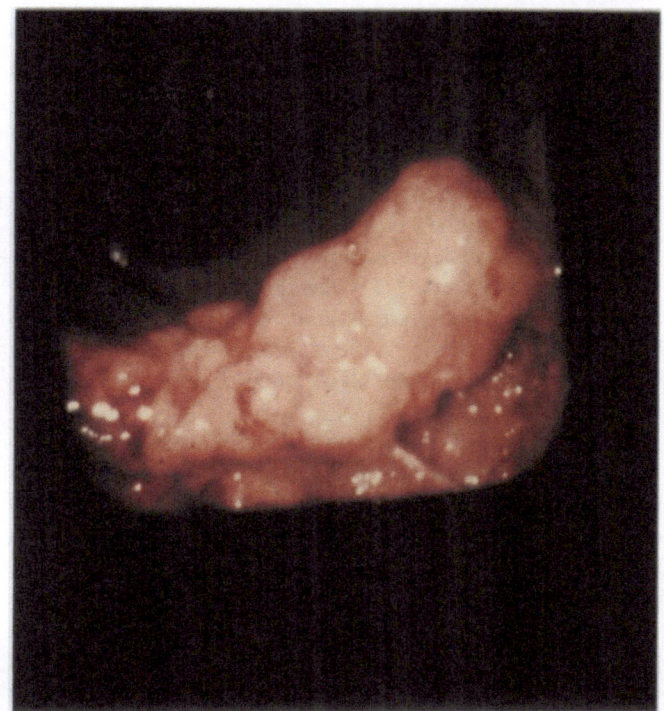

A

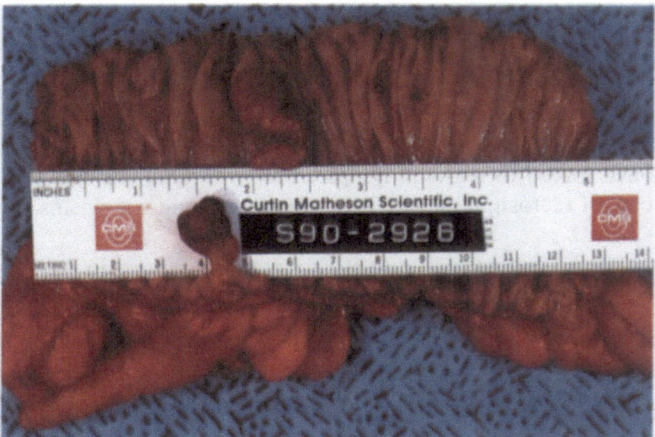

A

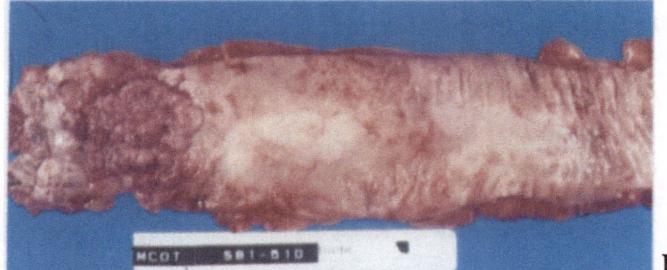

B

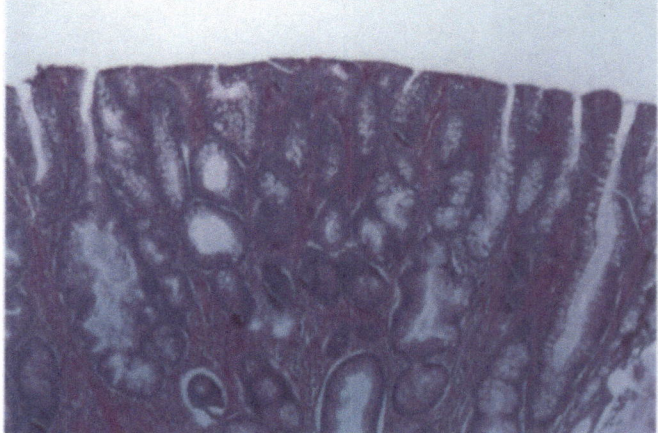

B

FIGURE 11.10 **Tubular adenoma of colon. A**: Pedunculated polyp. **B**: Biopsy of the polyp reveals tubular adenoma showing compactly arranged tubules and glands.

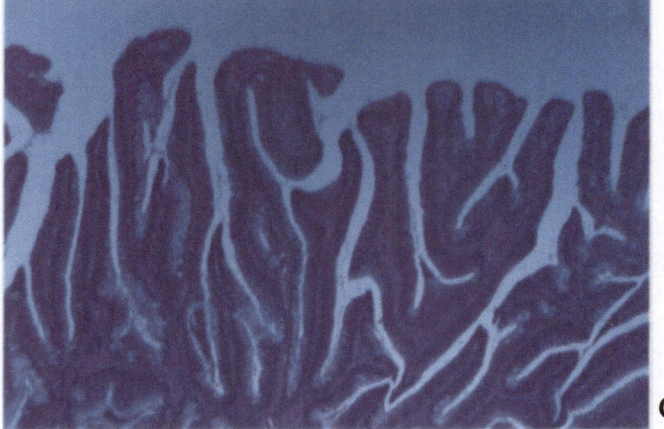

C

FIGURE 11.11 **Villous adenoma. A**: Frondlike multilobulated sessile tumor (endoscopic view). (Courtesy of Dr. John Stroehlein, Houston, Tex.). **B**: Broad sessile velvety mass in the rectum. **C**: Biopsy section of the lesion showing multiple fingerlike projections.

Carcinoma of the Large Intestine

Almost all large intestinal cancers are adenocarcinomas, with the remainder consisting of carcinoids, lymphomas, and sarcomas. Colorectal carcinoma is the second leading cause of cancer death in Western countries, a contrast with gastric cancer, the leading cause of cancer deaths in Asian countries. Epidemiologic studies indicate that environmental factors, notably diet, play a significant role in the causation of gastric and colorectal cancers.[11,12,13] The distribution of these carcinomas is as follows: rectosigmoid 60%, right colon 20% to 25%, and the remainder in the other segment. The prevailing opinion is that most colorectal carcinomas arise in preexisting adenomas.

There are distinct differences in the clinicopathological features of left-sided and right-sided lesions. Most carcinomas of the left side of the colon tend to be annular, encircling the entire circumference of the bowel producing a so-called napkin ring constriction (Fig. 11.12A, B). They tend to cause change of bowel movement, bloody stool, or obstructive symptoms.

Most carcinomas of the right side of the colon tend to be polypoid fungating growths (Fig. 11.12C). Since the right side of the colon is capacious, these fungating lesions rarely cause obstruction. Most right colonic carcinomas are detected at an advanced stage.

Histology and Cytology

The histologic features of the right-sided and left-sided colonic carcinomas are similar, consisting of well to poorly formed glands separated by a small amount of fibrous stroma. The glands are lined by single or multiple layers of atypical cells. The cells may be columnar to cuboidal or pleomorphic. The nuclei are round to oval or pleomorphic with irregularly dispersed chromatin. Most nuclei have a prominent single macronucleolus. Mitotic figures are frequently observed (Fig. 11.12D, E).

Endoscopic brushing cytology is a diagnostic adjunct to biopsy. Occasionally, biopsy samples may consist of necrotic tissue or tissue adjacent to tissue truly representative of the lesion. A brushing can obtain cellular material from a wider area and yield diagnoses in up to 90% of cases. If brushing cytology and biopsy are combined, diagnostic accuracy is better than that of biopsy alone.

The cytologic features of colonic adenocarcinomas are similar to those of other gastrointestinal adenocarcinomas. The cells occur in clusters and loose aggregates. The cells range from columnar to polygonal or pleomorphic. The nuclei are round to oval, with irregularly dispersed clumps of chromatin and have prominent macronucleoli (Fig. 11.12F).

Prognosis

The prognosis depends on the stage of the tumor. A staging system for colorectal carcinomas is based on depth of tumor penetration, the presence or absence of regional lymph nodal metastasis, and the presence or absence of distant metastasis. At the time of resection, 25% to 40% of colorectal cancers have spread to regional lymph nodes (stage C). Fifteen percent of rectosigmoid and 35% of right colonic neoplasms are stage D.

The 5-year survival rate of patients with tumors in stage A and B after therapy is 75% to 80%; this rate falls to about 45% with stage C and 10% with stage D.

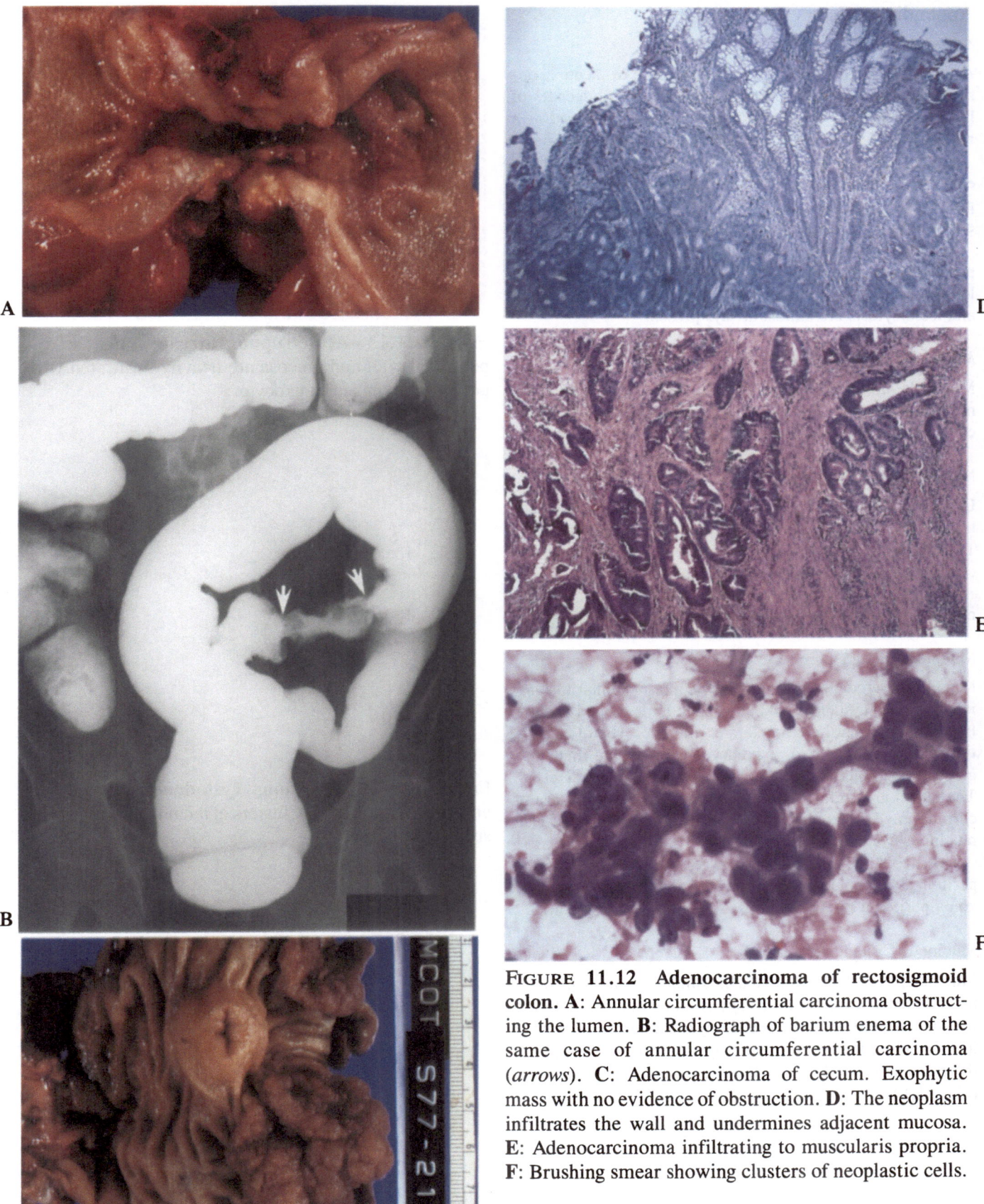

FIGURE 11.12 **Adenocarcinoma of rectosigmoid colon. A**: Annular circumferential carcinoma obstructing the lumen. **B**: Radiograph of barium enema of the same case of annular circumferential carcinoma (*arrows*). **C**: Adenocarcinoma of cecum. Exophytic mass with no evidence of obstruction. **D**: The neoplasm infiltrates the wall and undermines adjacent mucosa. **E**: Adenocarcinoma infiltrating to muscularis propria. **F**: Brushing smear showing clusters of neoplastic cells.

Appendix

Appendicitis

Acute appendicitis, the most common cause of "acute abdomen," occurs most often in the second and third decades of life. The appendix is enlarged, swollen, and dark red as a result of the serosal vessels being congested and prominent.

Acute suppurative inflammatory changes extend partly or entirely through the appendix wall and may progress to gangrene with perforation (Fig. 11.13). The existence of the entity chronic appendicitis is a subject of controversy.

Symptoms and signs of acute appendicitis begin with mild periumbilical pain followed by pain localized to the right lower quadrant, anorexia, nausea, and vomiting. Slight fever and leukocytosis are almost always present.

Mucocele and Pseudomyxoma Peritonei

Mucocele of the appendix is dilatation of the lumen by mucinous material. There are three distinct clinicopathological entities embracing this condition.

Non-Neoplastic Mucocele

Dilatation of the lumen is not associated with mucosal cytologic atypia and does not lead to pseudomyxoma peritonei. This entity does not cause any symptoms and is usually discovered as an incidental finding at laparotomy.

The appendix is dilated with mucinous material, and the mucosa may be hyperplastic or undergo atrophy.

Mucinous Cystadenoma

Mucinous cystodenoma is a benign neoplasm similar to ovarian mucinous cystadenoma. The appendix is dilated and enlarged up to several centimeters in diameter. Histologically, the neoplasm consists of papillary structures and mucinous glands. The cells are tall, columnar, and mucin-secreting. The nuclei are uniformly round and have a bland pattern of chromatin. This neoplasm is histologically similar to ovarian mucinous cystadenoma.

The neoplasm rarely ruptures to spill mucus into the peritoneal cavity. Even when this does happen, pseudomyxoma peritonei rarely develops. Appendectomy is curative.

Mucinous Cystadenocarcinoma

Mucinous cystadenocarcinoma is similar to ovarian mucinous cystadenocarcinoma. It may rupture and spread to the peritoneal cavity to cause pseudomyxoma peritonei consisting of an enormous volume of intraperitoneal mucus in which there are suspended mucin-producing adenocarcinoma cells (Fig. 11.14).

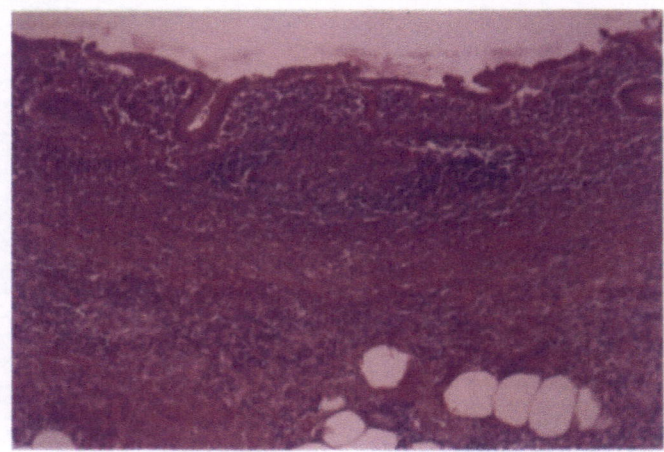

FIGURE 11.13   Acute suppurative appendicitis. Appendiceal wall and mucosa are heavily infiltrated with polymorphonuclear leukocytes.

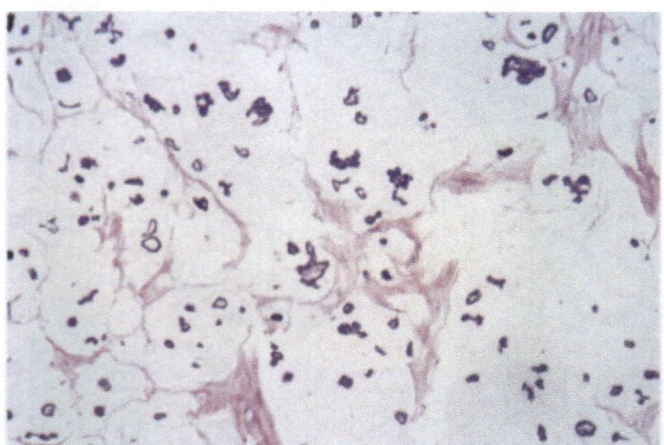

FIGURE 11.14   Mucinous cystadenocarcinoma of vermiform appendix. Clusters of adenocarcinoma cells suspended in mucus.

References

1. Garvin PJ, et al. Benign and malignant tumors of the small intestine. *Curr Probl Cancer.* 1979;3:1.
2. Barclay THC, Shapira DV. Malignant tumors of the small intestine. *Cancer.* 1983;51:878.
3. Williamson RCN, et al. Adenocarcinoma and lymphoma of the small intestine. *Ann Surg.* 1983;197:172.
4. Wiengrad DN, et al. Primary gastrointestinal lymphoma. A thirty-year review. *Cancer.* 1982;49:1258.
5. Pearse AGE. The cytochemistry and ultrastructure of polypeptide hormone-secreting cells of the APUD series and the embryologic, physiologic, and pathologic implication of the concept. *J Histochem Cytochem.* 1969;17:303.
6. DeLellis RA, et al. Carcinoid tumours (editorial). Changing concepts and new perspectives. *Am J Surg Pathol.* 1984;8:295.
7. Martensson H, et al. Carcinoid tumors in the gastrointestinal tract—An analysis of 156 cases. *Acta Chirurg Scand.* 1983;149:607.
8. Painter NS. Lifestyle and disease. Diverticular disease of the colon. *S Afr Med J.* 1982;61:1016.
9. Fenoglio-Preiser CM, Hutter RVP. Colorectal polyps: Pathologic diagnosis and clinical significance. *CA.* 1985;35:332.
10. Coutsoftides T, et al. Malignant polyps of the colon and rectum. A clinicopathologic study. *Dis Colon Rectum.* 1979;22:82.
11. Schlag P, et al. Are nitrate and N-nitroso compounds in gastric juice risk factors for carcinoma in the operated stomach? *Lancet.* 1980;1:727.
12. Joossens JV, Geboers J. Nutrition and gastric cancer. *Proc Nutr Soc.* 1981;40:37.
13. Bresalier RS, Kim YS. Diet and colon cancer. *N Engl J Med.* 1985;313:1413.

12
Adrenal Gland

An adrenal gland lies on the top of each kidney, and each gland in an adult weighs 4 to 5 g. Each gland consists of the steroid-secreting cortex and the catecholamine-secreting medulla. The cortex is mesodermal in origin, derived from the urogenital ridge, and consists of three layers: zona glomerulosa beneath the capsule, comprising round to cuboidal cells arranged in clusters; zona fasciculata constituting the major portion of the cortex, lying beneath the zona glomerulosa and comprising large polyhedral cells arranged in columns; and zona reticularis, the innermost layer of the cortex composed of polyhedral cells arranged in clusters (Fig. 12.1).

The adrenal medulla is derived from the neural crest and is considered to be part of the paraganglionic system (Fig. 12.2). The extraadrenal paraganglionic system is widely distributed such as in the organ of Zuckerkandl and the paravertebral and visceral paraganglia. Paraganglionic cells are typical neuroendocrine cells that synthesize and secrete both catecholamines and a variety of peptides. Only neoplastic disease of the adrenal gland will be reviewed here.

Cortical Adenoma

Cortical adenomas are usually detected as an incidental finding, and almost all of them are nonfunctional. Primary hyperaldosteronism (Conn's syndrome) is caused by a functioning cortical adenoma that secretes an excessive amount of aldosterone, with sodium retention and potassium loss. The loss of renal potassium induces hypokalemia, hypokalemic alkalosis, and muscular weakness.

Secondary hyperaldosteronism refers to secretion of aldosterone in response to increased levels of renin angiotensin. Hypersecretion of renin by the kidneys occurs with renal ischemia, renal edema, renin-producing neoplasm, or hyperplasia. Occasionally adrenal cortical adenomas produce an excessive amount of cortisol to cause Cushing's syndrome. The morphology of functioning or nonfunctioning adenomas is identical. Grossly, a cortical adenoma is usually less than 2 cm in diameter, and a well circumscribed but nonencapsulated yellow nodule (Fig. 12.3A).

Histologically, the adrenal cortical adenoma is characterized by uniform cells arranged in alveoli and compact sheets. The cells have features of both fasciculata and glomerulosa types ("hybrid" cells) (Fig. 12.3B). These small functioning cortical adenomas rarely undergo fine needle aspiration.

Cortical Carcinoma

Adrenal cortical carcinomas occur usually in adults and rarely in children, and half of them are accompanied by hormonal manifestations.[1] Adrenal cortical carcinomas are highly malignant and tend to metastasize to the liver, lymph nodes, and lungs. The neoplasm usually weighs more than 100 gm and sometimes as much as 1000 g. Grossly, the tumors are partly encapsulated, variable in color, and soft and friable, with multifocal hemorrhage and necrosis (Fig. 12.4A).

Histology

Adrenal cortical carcinomas vary greatly in their histologic appearance, with the degree of differentiation ranging from normal-appearing cortical cells to highly anaplastic giant cells and cells with bizarre hyperchromatic nuclei. The cells are arranged in sheets or may reproduce the alveolar or trabecular pattern of normal adrenal gland (Fig. 12.4B, C).

Distinguishing between cortical adenomas and well differentiated cortical carcinomas can be difficult. Carcinomas tend to be large and to exhibit atypical nuclei, mitotic figures, necrosis and vascular and capsular invasion.

Cytology

Aspiration smears show large polygonal cells with scanty or abundant, finely vacuolated, eosinophilic cytoplasm and bizarre hyperchromatic nuclei (Fig. 12.4D, E).

The combined evaluation of clinical features and the size and microscopic features of the neoplasm are necessary for predicting the prognosis.[2,3]

Pheochromocytoma (Intra-Adrenal Paraganglioma)

Pheochromocytoma is a unique neoplasm of chromaffin cells that secrete norepinephrine and epinephrine. As a consequence, the dominant clinical features are hypertension and symptoms resulting from the sudden release of catecholamines such as headache, anxiety, abdominal pain, and visual disturbance.

Similar neoplasms arising elsewhere are referred to as extraadrenal paragangliomas. The common extraadrenal sites are the region of the organ of Zuckerkandl, thoracic paravertebral area, and urinary bladder wall. The neoplasms

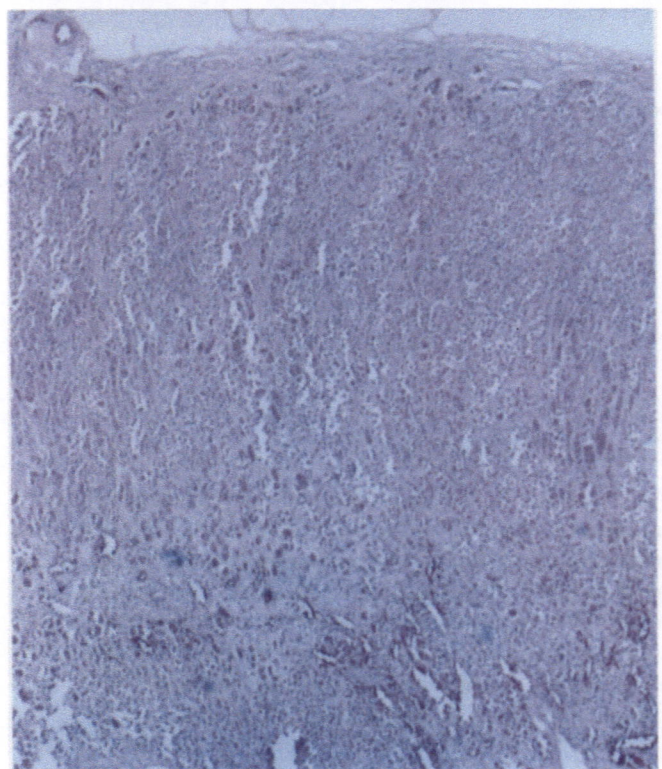

FIGURE 12.1 **Normal adrenal cortex.** From the top to the bottom of the picture, zona glomerulosa, zona fasciculata, and zona reticularis.

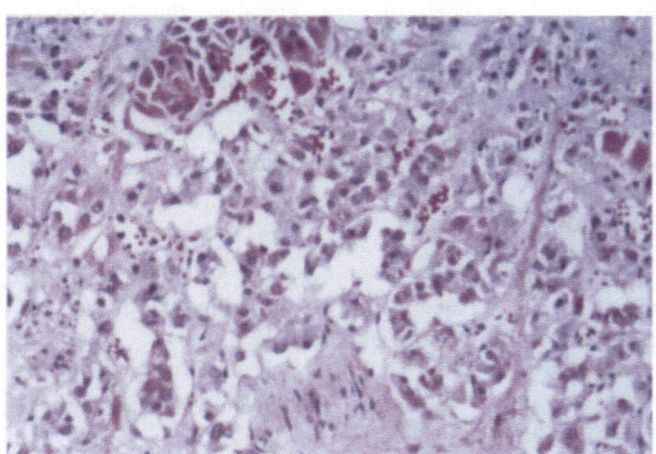

FIGURE 12.2 **Normal adrenal medulla.** Aggregates of paraganglionic cells.

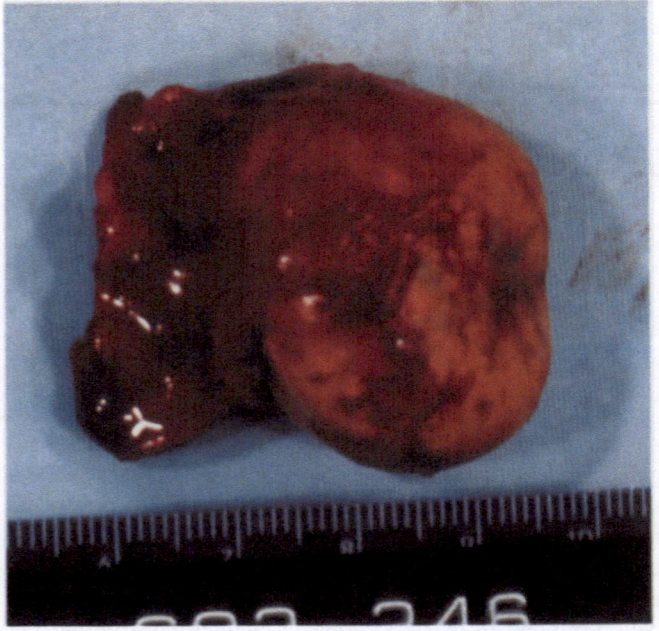

A

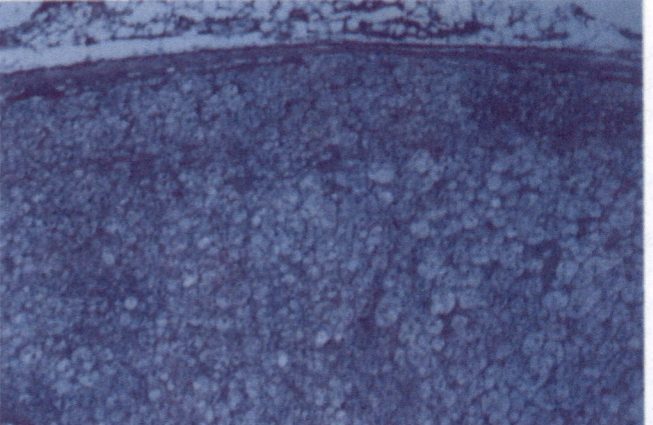

B

FIGURE 12.3 **Adrenal cortical adenoma. A**: Yellow, soft, nodular mass (gross). **B**: Histologic section of the neoplasm showing lipid-laden "clear" cells arranged in compact alveoli.

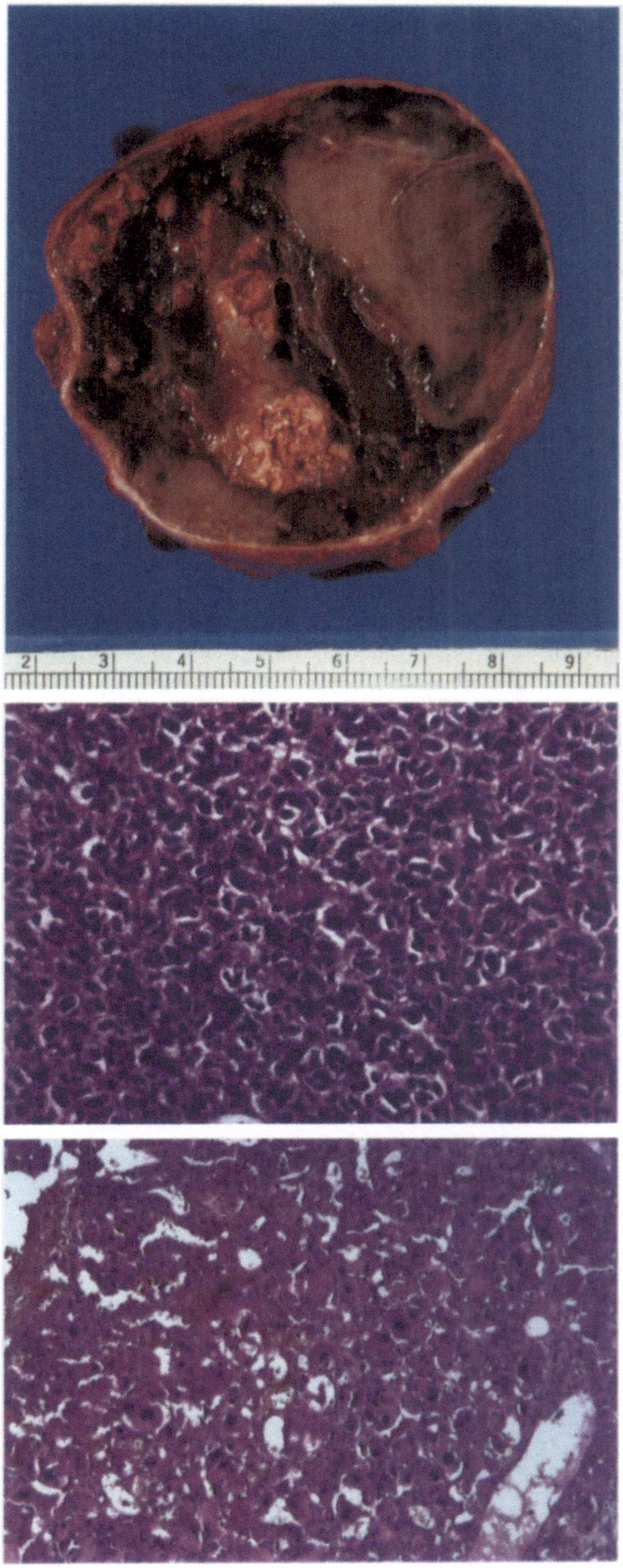

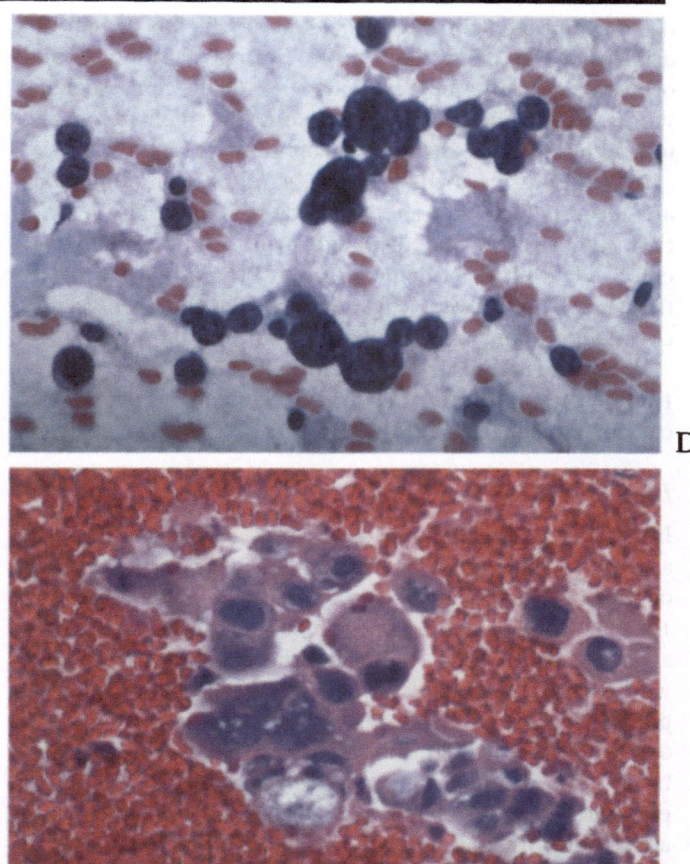

FIGURE 12.4   Adrenal cortical carcinoma. A: Partly encapsulated, soft, friable mass with multifocal hemorrhage and necrosis on section (gross). **B, C**: Histologic sections showing sheets and alveoli of neoplastic cells with variable morphologic features. **D, E**: Aspiration smears showing aggregates of pleomorphic tumor cells with scanty to abundant cytoplasm.

occur at any age, with a peak incidence in the fourth and fifth decades of life. About 80% to 90% of pheochromocytomas occur sporadically; the remaining 10% to 20% are associated with various familial syndromes, some of which are characterized by multiple endocrine neoplasms (MEN).

Grossly, the tumors range from 1 g to 1000 g in weight, and are encapsulated and trabeculated by fibrous bands. On section, they are pale gray or light brown, soft, and richly vascularized. Multifocal hemorrhage, necrosis, or cyst formation can be observed (Fig. 12.5A). They may be partly covered by remnants of the adrenal cortex.

When the tumor is fixed in dichromate fixative (Zenker's or Helly's solution), it turns brown-black owing to oxidation of catecholamines (Fig. 12.5B).

Histology and Cytology

In aspiration smears, the cells occur singly and in loose aggregates. The cells are polygonal and have abundant eosinophilic cytoplasm and hyperchromatic, round nuclei (Fig. 12.5C). Histologically, they comprise large polygonal cells arranged in trabeculae, nests, and sheets punctuated by thin-walled vascular sinusoids. Giant and bizarre cells and nuclear pleomorphism may be observed. Mitotic figures are rarely observed (Fig. 12.5D). Ten percent of pheochromocytomas behave in a malignant manner. Since malignant and benign pheochromocytomas may be identical in their histologic appearance, the diagnosis of malignancy should be based on the presence of metastasis.

Extra-adrenal Paraganglioma

Paraganglionic cells in the carotid, vagal, and jugulotympanic bodies are parasympathetic ganglia responding to variations in oxygen and carbon dioxide tension of the blood. Because of this chemoreceptor property, neoplasms arising from these parasympathetic ganglia have been designated as chemodectomas. However, some of these neoplasms are nonfunctional and currently they are designated as paraganglioma, with the localizing anatomic site being appended (e.g., jugulotympanic paraganglioma).

On the basis of their biochemical, histologic, and clinical similarities to those of the adrenal glands, neoplasms arising from the aorticosympathetic paraganglia are extraadrenal pheochromocytomas. The currently recommended terminology is paraganglioma with the anatomic site (e.g., paraganglioma of organ of Zuckerkandl). Paragangliomas are rare, and occur in adults. They usually occur singly and sporadically and rarely are familial. Ten percent of these neoplasms are malignant, with local recurrence and metastasis.

Grossly, these neoplasms are relatively small, tan-red, and firm. They are encapsulated but are markedly adherent to the adjacent tissue (Fig. 12.6A). Histologically, they are similar to adrenal pheochromocytomas. The paragangliomas of head and neck tend to form clusters of cells (Zellballen) or cords (Fig. 12.6B).

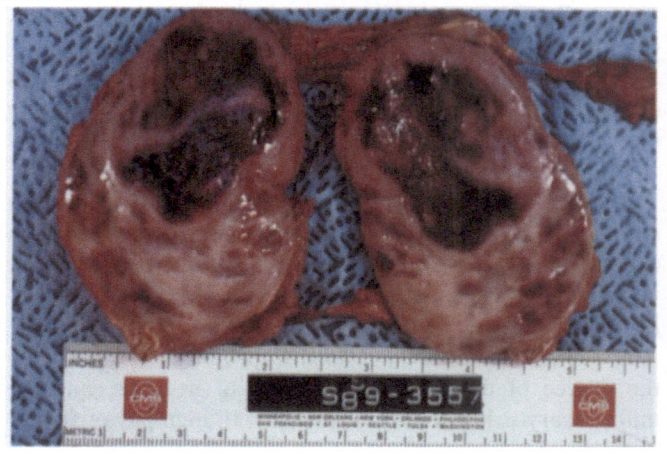
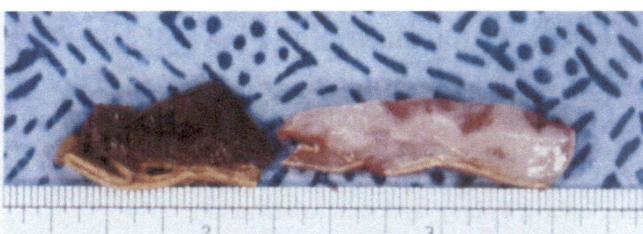
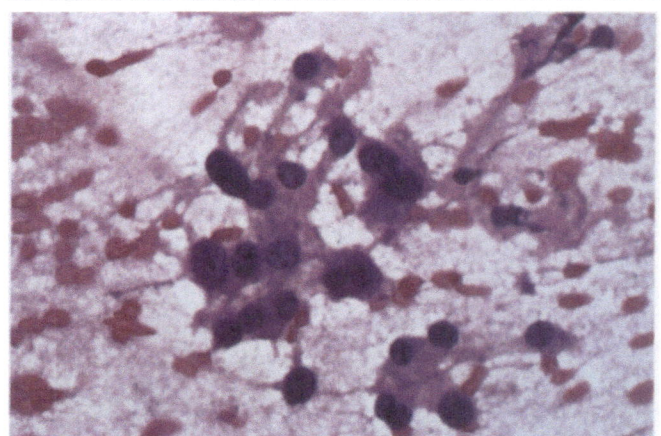
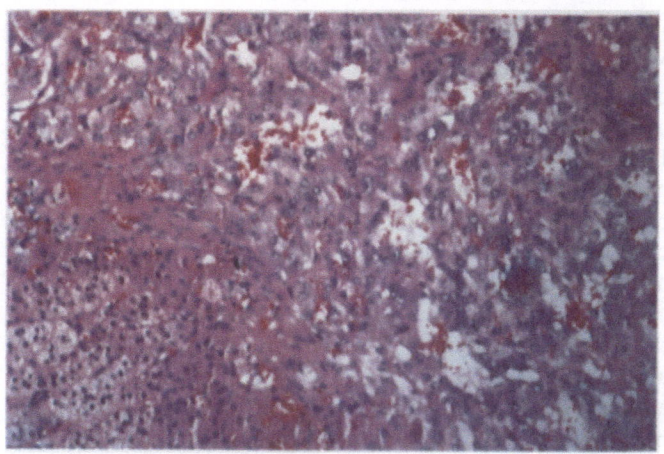

FIGURE 12.5 **Pheochromocytoma. A**: Encapsulated pale gray to brown, soft and focally necrotic neoplasm on cut section (gross). Note a remnant of the adrenal cortex at arrow. **B**: Brown-black discoloration of the pheochromocytoma owing to oxidation of stained catecholamines (potassium dichromate fixation). Note the compressed adrenal cortex at the bottom. **C**: Aspiration smear showing loose aggregates of polygonal cells with abundant eosinophilic cytoplasm. **D**: Histologic section showing sheets and nests of polygonal cells and prominent thin-walled vascular sinusoids. Note a portion of the normal adrenal cortex attached in the left lower corner.

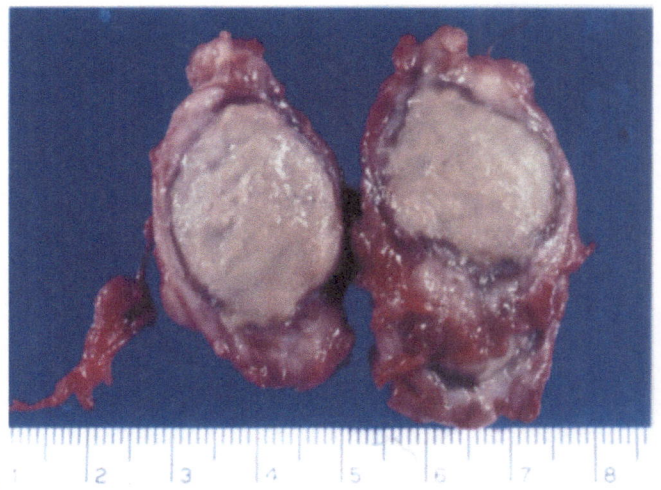
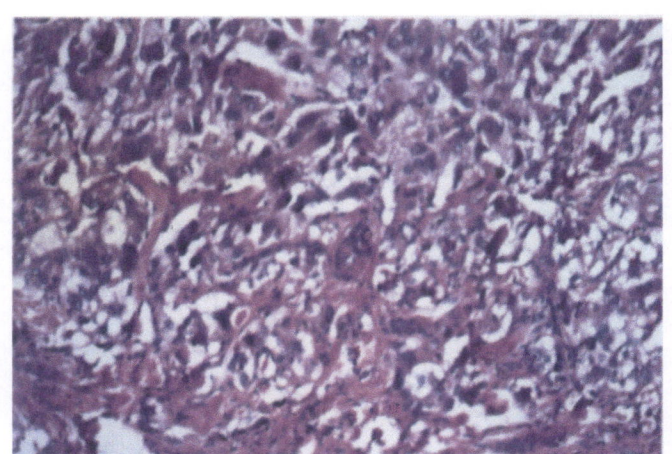

FIGURE 12.6 **Extraadrenal paraganglioma. A**: Encapsulated neoplasm adherent to the adjacent tissue. **B**: Histologic section showing clusters (Zellballen) and cords of tumor cells.

Neuroblastoma and Ganglioneuroma

Neuroblastoma is one of the four most common forms of childhood cancer. More than 80% of these neoplasms occur under the age of 5 years. Clinical manifestations are variable. Loss of weight, weakness, fever, and general malaise are probably a result of rapid tumor growth and resorption of products of necrotic tumor. The neoplasms elaborate catecholamines. In contrast to patients with pheochromocytomas, hypertension is rare.

Neuroblastomas are found in the adrenal medulla and in the retroperitoneal tissue where neural crest cells exist. They also can occur in the cervical and thoracic paravertebral sites and in the lower abdominal sympathetic chain. Grossly, the neoplasms are lobular, pale gray to pale red, and soft. Hemorrhagic and necrotic foci with cystic change are frequently observed (Fig. 12.7A). Calcification is common and of help in radiologic interpretation.

Histology and Cytology

In aspiration smears, the cells occur singly and in loose aggregates with occasional rosettelike structures. The cells are small with scanty cytoplasm and have small, round, hyperchromatic nuclei (Fig. 12.7B).

Histologically, the tumors are arranged in sheets with characteristic rosette formations at the center of which are nerve fibrils (Fig. 12.7C). Metastasis develops rapidly and widely with spread to lymph nodes, liver, lungs, and bones.

Neuroblastomas may differentiate to ganglioneuroma comprising ganglion cells embedded in fibrous and Schwann cell stroma (Fig. 12.8). Ganglioneuroblastomas occupy an intermediate position of differentiation between pure neuroblastoma and ganglioneuroma (Fig. 12.9).

The histologic features related to prognosis are based on the degree of differentiation, extent of necrosis, and the mitotic-karyorrhectic cell number per 10 high power fields.[4]

Metastatic Carcinomas

Metastatic carcinomas to the adrenal glands are common and tend to be bilateral. Fine needle aspiration under computed tomography guidance is the method of choice for their diagnosis. The most common sites of the primary neoplasms are lung, breast, kidney, and skin (melanoma).

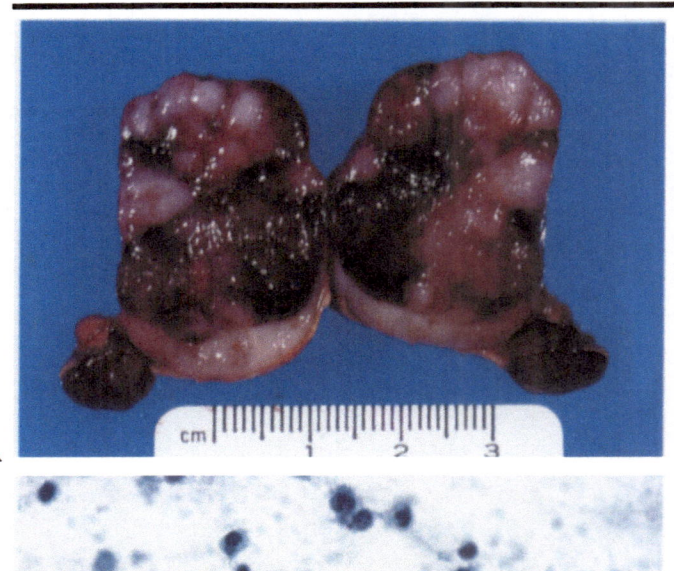

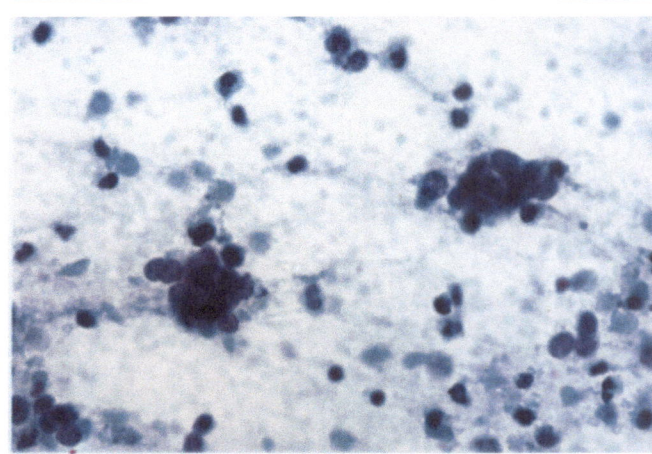

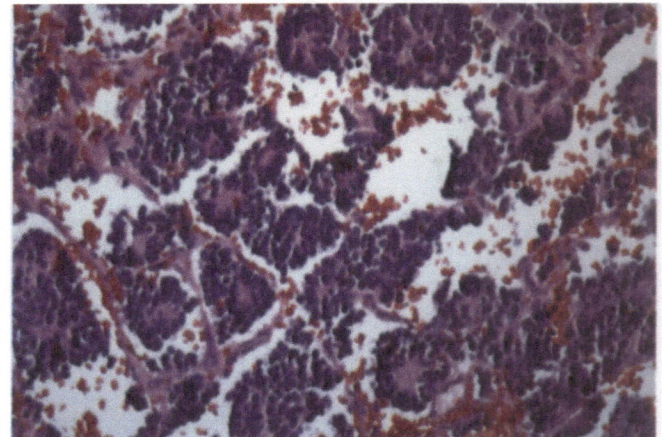

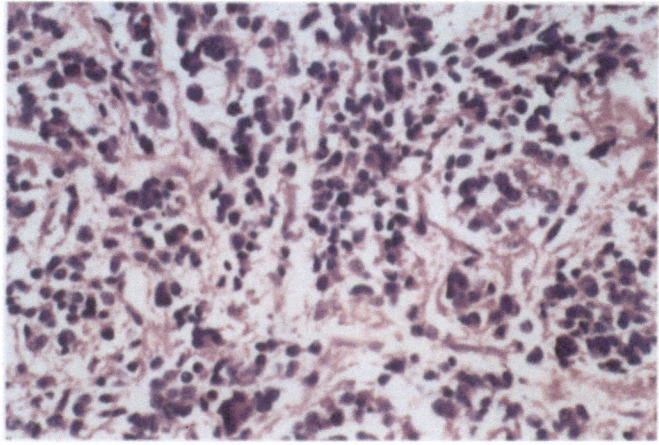

FIGURE 12.8 **Ganglioneuroma**. Ganglion cells embedded in fibrous and Schwann cell stroma.

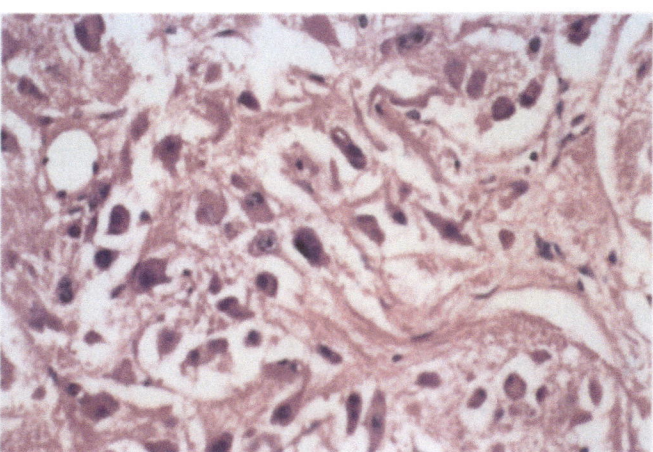

FIGURE 12.9 **Ganglioneuroblastoma**. Neoplasm comprising primitive neuroblasts and ganglion cells.

FIGURE 12.7 **Neuroblastoma**. **A**: Pale red, lobular, soft, and hemorrhagic neoplasm (gross). **B**: Aspiration smear showing clusters and aggregates of neuroblastoma cells with scanty cytoplasm. **C**: Histologic section showing sheets and rosette formation of neuroblastoma cells.

References

1. Samaan NA, Hicky RC. Adrenal cortical carcinoma. *Semi Oncol*. 1987; 14:292–296.
2. Page DL, Hugh AJ, Gray GF. Diagnosis and prognosis of adenocortical neoplasm. *Arch Pathol Lab Med*. 1986;110:993–994.
3. Slooten MV, Schaberg A, Smeenk D, Mollenar AJ. Morphologic characteristics of benign and malignant adrenocortical tumors. *Cancer*. 1985; 55:766–773.
4. Shimada H, et al. Histopathologic prognostic factors in neuroblastic tumors: Definition of subtypes of ganglioneuroblastoma and an age-linked classification of neuroblastomas. *J Natl Cancer Inst*. 1984;73:405.

13
Kidney

Non-Neoplastic Renal Diseases

Although cytology does not contribute to the diagnosis of non-neoplastic renal disease, representative non-neoplastic renal diseases will be briefly reviewed in terms of their clinical significance with particular reference to clinicopathological features. They will be reviewed on the basis of four clinicopathologic features: glomeruli, tubules, interstitium, and blood vessels, and renal diseases associated with other systemic diseases as well as transplantation.

Primary Glomerular Diseases

Introduction and Pathogenesis

The vast majority of glomerular disease is immunologically mediated. The mechanism of glomerular injury depends on the site of the antigen and the pathway of complement activation. Three mechanisms are involved: 1) antiglomerular basement membrane mediated nephritis, 2) immune complex mediated nephritis, and 3) nephritis due to alternate complement pathway activation.

Antiglomerular Basement Membrane

Glomerular injury is a result of antibodies to antigen fixed to the basement membrane, which includes antigenic constituents of the basement membrane and foreign antigen fixed in the basement membrane.

Immune Complex Nephritis

Both antigens and antibodies are involved in circulating immune complexes that deposit in the capillary basement membrane and activate complement. The activated complement stimulates chemotaxis of polymorphonuclear leukocytes that migrate to the glomerulus and release lysosomal enzymes causing local tissue damage and glomerular injury.

Alternate Complement Pathway Activation

Cleavage of C_3 bypassing C_1, C_2, and C_4 is seen. Polymorphonuclear leukocytes and enzymes along with a lytic effect of the complement lead to tissue damage, which leads to glomerulonephritis. There is a dose-dependent relationship between the immune complexes and the glomerular damage.

As a result of the above mechanisms, the following lesions can be seen: 1) crescent formation, 2) mesangial cell proliferation, 3) necrosis and polymorphonuclear leukocyte infiltrates, 4) thickening of the capillary basement membrane, 5) mesangial sclerosis, and 6) hyalinization.

There is a close relationship between the morphologic changes in the glomeruli and the clinical picture. With necrosis and mesangial cell proliferation the patients usually present with hematuria and perhaps azotemia. Along with thickened basement membranes the patients usually have proteinuria and nephrotic syndrome with crescent formation, most of the patients have a very rapidly progressive course. When the glomeruli become hyalinized, the patients go into chronic renal failure. Glomerular diseases are best diagnosed by renal biopsy. Each renal biopsy specimen is split into three. The first part is processed for light microscopy to assess the morphologic changes in the glomeruli, tubules, vessels, and interstitium. The tissue processed for light microscopy is usually stained by a panel of special stains (Fig. 13.1). In addition to the hematoxylin and eosin, each tissue is stained with PAS periodic acid-Schiff (PAS) to assess the mesangial matrix; with silver (Jones stain) to assess the capillary basement membrane; with trichrome to assess sclerosis; with Congo red to assess for the presence of amyloid.

The second part of the tissue is quickly frozen and processed for immunofluorescence and is stained with fluorescein-labeled antisera to assess the presence of immunoglobulins and complement deposits in the glomeruli. The third part is fixed in gluteraldehyde and processed for electron microscopy.

Clinical Picture in Glomerular Diseases

As mentioned above, there are four major clinical presentations for glomerular diseases: 1) nephrotic syndrome with proteinuria of >3 g/24 hr, edema, hypoproteinemia, and hyperlipidemia usually associated with thickened basement membranes, 2) nephritic syndrome with hematuria, red blood cell casts, mild proteinuria, azotemia, and hypertension usually associated with mesangial cell proliferation and necrosis, 3) hematuria syndrome with clinical signs including pure hematuria associated with variable morphologic changes in the glomeruli, and 4) chronic renal failure usually associated with hyalinization of the glomeruli.

Nephrotic Syndromes

The primary causes of nephrotic syndrome are lipoid nephrosis, focal glomerulosclerosis, membranous glomerulonephritis, and membranoproliferative glomerulonephritis.

Clinically, edema, proteinuria, hypoproteinemia, and hyperlipidemia are present. The proteinuria is caused by leaky capillary basement membranes. The hypoproteinemia is caused by spillage of protein into the urine. Edema is caused by decreased oncotic pressure. The cause of hyperlipidemia is unclear but is possibly a result of decreased oncotic pressure and increased lipoprotein synthesis in the liver. There is also excessive loss of plasma proteins in the urine, including factors regulating lipoprotein, synthesis and disposal. These contribute to hyperlipidemia and increased risk of atherosclerosis as well as the presence of oval fat bodies in the urine, which are tubular cells filled with lipid droplets.

Lipoid Nephrosis (NIL Disease)

Primary nephrotic syndrome occurs in children in 80% of cases, and only 20% in adults. The male:female ratio is 2.5:1 in childhood and 1:1 in adults, with a peak incidence from 1 to 5 years of age. Twenty to 30% of the cases follow upper respiratory tract infections and 9% follow immunizations, but in 70% of patients no preceding illnesses are noted. The pathogenesis is unknown.

Serologic tests for autoimmune disease are usually negative and the proteinuria is selective. Only albumin is filled. Light microscopy shows no changes, immunofluorescence is negative, and electron microscopy reveals diffuse podocyte fusion as well as epithelial cell swellings (Fig. 13.2). Approximately 90% to 98% of children respond to steroids, whereas only 66% to 77% of adults respond. About 70% of children go into complete remission. Twelve percent show simple proteinuria. Nephrotic syndrome recurs in about 10% of cases and there is a 7% mortality rate.

Focal Glomerulosclerosis

In addition to the nephrotic syndrome, focal glomerulosclerosis is associated with hematuria, nonselective proteinuria, and no response to steroids.

The proteinuria in focal glomerulosclerosis is nonselective, and 60% to 80% present with pure nephrotic syndrome while 30% have azotemia and 25% have hypertension. There is a tendency for recurrence in renal allografts.

Light microscopy shows focal scarring (sclerosis) starting in the glomeruli at the corticomedullary junction, which spreads toward the glomeruli at the cortical surface as disease progresses. Immunofluorescence shows large focal segmental immunoglobulin M (IgM) deposits in the mesangium. The typical prognosis is for a downhill course leading to renal failure with persistent episodes of proteinuria, hematuria, nephrotic syndrome, and a recurrence in allografts.

Membranous Glomerulonephritis

The proportion of cases of membranous nephritis is 1% to 9% in childhood cases and 10% to 30% in adults with primary nephrotic syndrome. The male to female ratio is 1.5:1, with a mean age of 38 years. Possible preceding illnesses include poison oak dermatitis, chronic hepatitis with persistent hepatitis B antigenemia, syphilis, malaria, and Guillain-Barré syndrome. Extrarenal malignancies including lymphoma and gastrointestinal tumors are commonly associated with membranous nephritis. Prolonged gold therapy can also precipitate membranous glomerulopathy.

The cause of membranous nephropathy is chronic immune complex disease, as mentioned earlier. The antigens include gold, treponemas, tumors, renal tubular antigen (experimental), chronic hepatitis B antigenemia. All the patients have nephrotic syndrome, with 10% to 50% having hypertension and azotemia at the onset. Serum complement level is normal except in patients with systemic lupus erythematous (SLE), who have a decreased serum complement.

Light microscopy shows uniform diffuse thickening of the basement membrane (Fig. 13.3A, B). Immunofluorescence reveals diffuse, peripheral, granular IgG, and complement. Electron microscopy shows four stages: 1) epimembranous electron-dense deposits, 2) intramembranous electron-dense deposits with spikes (Fig. 13.3C), 3) intramembranous electron-dense deposits (Fig. 13.3D), and 4) electron-lucent (clear) areas where the deposits used to be.

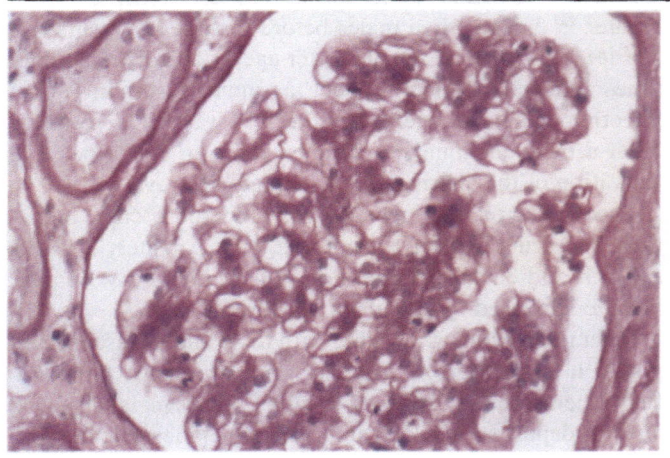

FIGURE 13.1 Normal glomerulus. Note capillary loops with thin wall and mesangium (H&E, ×120).

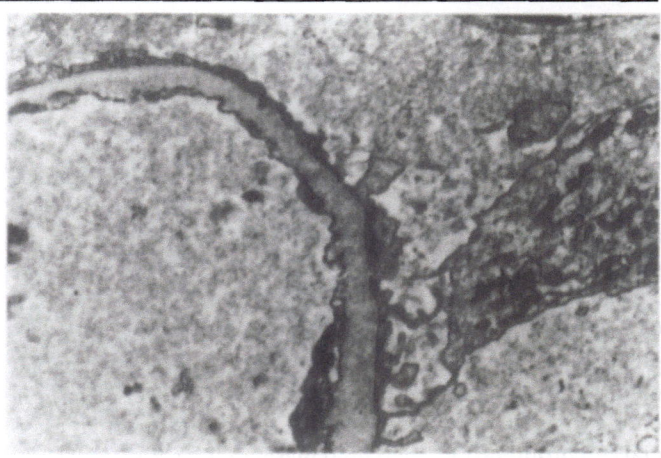

FIGURE 13.2 Electron micrograph of lipoid nephrosis. Podocyte fusion.

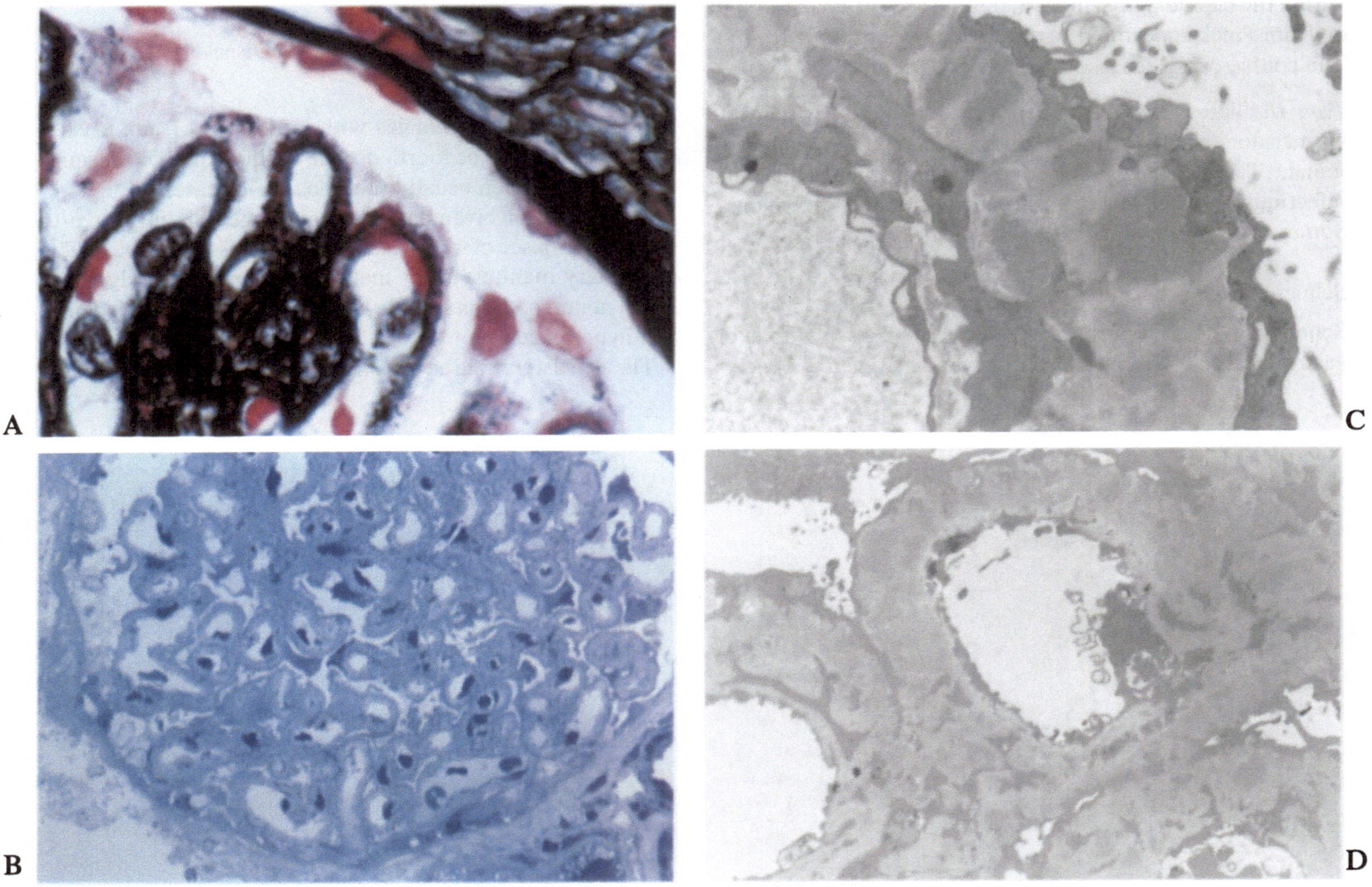

A

B

C

D

FIGURE 13.3 Membranous glomerulonephritis. A: Thickened capillary loops with spikes (Jones silver stain, ×120). **B:** One-micron section. Thick capillary loops. **C:** Stage II. Membranous nephritis with large intramembranous electron dense deposits and spikes. Electron micrograph. **D:** Stage III. Multiple large intramembranous electron-dense deposits. Electron micrograph.

Membranoproliferative Glomerulonephritis

There are three types of membranoproliferative nephritis; Type I (mesangiocapillary), type II (dense deposit disease), and type III (mesangial proliferative disease).

Type I. The incidence of mesangiocapillary nephritis is 5% to 20% of primary nephrotic syndrome with female incidence greater than male incidence. Usually there are no preceding illnesses.

There is activation of the alternate complement pathway. Clinical findings include nephrotic syndrome and hypocomplementemia with decreased serum total hemolytic complement (CH_{50}), decreased C_3, and normal C_4 levels. On light microscopy, there is a lobular glomerular pattern with mesangial cell proliferation, increased mesangial matrix, and thickening of the basement membrane. Silver stain shows a split basement membrane. Immunofluorescence shows properdin and C_3 deposits in a peripheral lobular distribution. Electron microscopy shows mesangialization. Mesangial cells are seen within the capillary basement membrane resulting in the split or Tram Track appearance of the capillary loops (Fig. 13.4A). The course of the disease is slowly progressive.

Type II. The incidence rate is 0.5% to 2.5% of chronic glomerulonephritis with no difference between male and female. The mean age is 16 years. Preceding illnesses include infectious diseases, namely streptococcus and pneumonia. Some cases are familial.

Schoenlein-Henoch Purpura

Schoenlein-Henoch purpura is a systemic disease with skin, gastrointestinal (GI) and renal involvement. The incidence is greater in females than males before the age of 7 years and greater in males than females after age 7. The disease sometimes follows an infection such as upper respiratory tract infection. The pathogenesis is diffuse vasculitis resulting from a transient immune complex reaction and a possible activation of the alternate complement pathway.

The clinical picture includes gross and microscopic hematuria and acute nephritic syndrome, approximately 3 weeks after GI and cutaneous manifestations. Laboratory findings include increased IgA levels in the serum.

Light microscopy is variable with focal and diffuse mesangial cell proliferation, necrosis, and crescents. Immunofluorescence shows diffuse IgA, IgG, C_3, mesangial deposits, and IgA deposits in the skin at the dermal-epidermal junction. Electron microscopy shows mesangial and subendothelial deposits and crescents. Treatment usually involves steroids.

There is recurrence in 20% to 40% of the patients. A delayed recurrence has been reported in transplanted kidneys. There is a 40% to 80% cure.

Antiglomerular Basement Membrane Disease (Goodpasture's Syndrome)

Incidence is higher in males with a ratio of 4:1 and usually occurs in the third or fourth decade of life. An upper respiratory tract infection usually precedes the disease.

Pulmonary involvement occurring concomitantly or preceding the onset of renal manifestations is often seen. The pulmonary manifestations include hemoptysis and dyspnea. Renal manifestations include hematuria, proteinuria, edema, and hypertension.

The disease is caused by circulating antiglomerular basement membrane antibodies. The same antibodies cross react with the alveolar basement membrane giving rise to the pulmonary lesions.

Light microscopy reveals necrotizing lesions, focal proliferation, capillary thrombosis, and crescents. The interstitium shows recent hemorrhage. Immunofluorescence shows diffuse linear IgG deposits along the alveolar septae and glomerular basement membrane. Electron microscopy shows endothelial swelling, capillary thrombi, basement membranes collapsed and compressed by crescents, and electron-lucent widening of the lamina rara interna. The treatment is usually steroids and anticoagulants as well as plasmapheresis. Sometimes a nephrectomy and transplantation can be lifesaving.

The prognosis is very poor with a rapidly progressive course.

Crescentic Glomerulonephritis

Many glomerular diseases are associated with crescent formation. Therefore, crescents are not specific for any given disease. They merely indicate severe glomerular injury and a rapidly progressive course.

Most cases are associated with activation of the alternate complement pathway. Clinically, proteinuria is present in 100% of patients, nephrotic syndrome in 80%, hypertension 60%, hematuria 50%, and serum C_3 is decreased. Light microscopy is the same as in mesangiocapillary nephritis. Immunofluorescence shows there are discontinuous linear deposits of C_3 in the periphery of the lobules. Electron microscopy shows ribbonlike, electron-dense deposits in the lamina densa (Fig. 13.4B).

Type III. Nephrotic syndrome with low C_3 is seen in 50% of the patients. Pathologically, there is a variable morphology including mesangial cell proliferation and mild membrane thickening. Immunofluorescence reveals mesangial C_3 and IgM. Electron microscopy is variable. It is a slowly progressive disease.

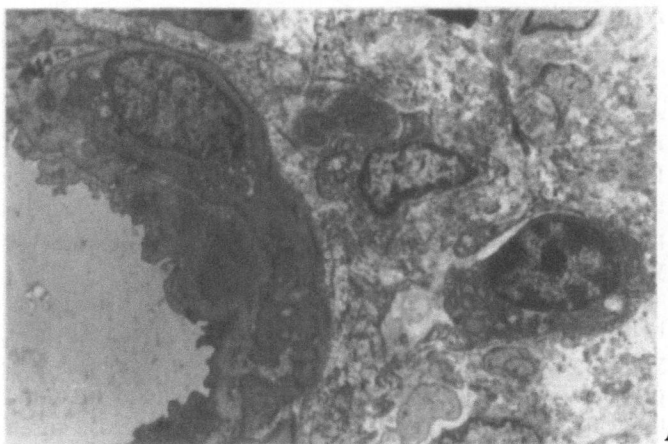

A

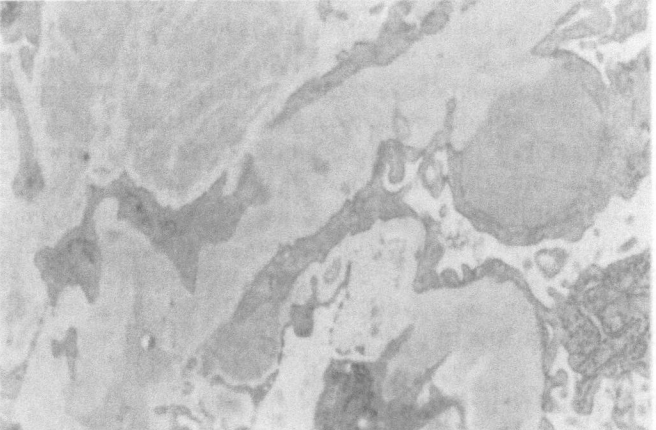

B

FIGURE **13.4 Membranoproliferative glomerulonephritis. A**: Type I. Mesangialization of capillary loops. **B**: Type II. Ribbonlike electron-dense deposits in the lamina densa.

Hematuria and Nephritic Syndromes

Acute Poststreptococcal Glomerulonephritis

Acute poststreptococcal nephritis or acute proliferative nephritis has an incidence rate of 0.2 per 1000 each year. Preceding illnesses include pharyngitis (Strep Type 12) with the onset of nephritis 10 days postpharyngitis. It usually presents in the early school-age years, with a mean age of 8 years. A circulating immune complex is involved.

The clinical findings are periorbital edema, moderate hypertension, dark urine (hematuria), and azotemia. Urinalysis shows red blood cells (RBCs) and RBC casts plus 1-2+ protein. The antistreptolysin ASO titer is elevated with more than 500 Todd units. Serum CH_{50} and C_3 is decreased at onset and returns to normal levels by 12 weeks. There is moderate azotemia and a slight increase in blood urea nitrogen (BUN) and creatinine. Fewer than 5% of the patients are nephrotic.

Light microscopy shows diffuse proliferation of mesangial cells, polymorphonuclear leukocytic infiltration, and focal necrosis (Fig. 13.5A). Occasionally some crescent formation is noted. Immunofluorescence shows lumpy, bumpy (Fig. 13.5B), peripheral granular deposits of immunoglobulin and complement in the glomeruli. Electron microscopy reveals subepithelial electron dense deposits appearing as humps.

The course is good, with an 80% to 95% recovery rate in children and 50% to 70% in adults.

IgA Nephropathy (Berger's Disease)

Twelve to 20% of primary chronic glomerulonephritis patients have IgA nephropathy. The median age is 33 years and the male to female ratio is 2:1 and 3:1. Preceding illness is usually an upper respiratory infection. There are two major theories as to the pathogenesis: immune complexes rich in IgA, or an alternate complement pathway. The clinical findings show recurrent hematuria, both grossly and microscopically, with mild proteinuria.

Light microscopy is variable; immunofluorescence shows diffuse, mesangial IgA deposits (Fig. 13.6). On electron microscopy, multiple intramesangial deposits are seen. The prognosis is benign for children. In adults, 19% develop renal failure and 32% develop hypertension. There is a recurrence in renal allografts.

Light microscopy shows marked proliferation of the epithelial cells lining the Bowman's capsule (Fig. 13.7). Immunofluorescence shows fibrin deposits in these crescents and other deposits vary according to etiology. Electron microscopy is variable depending on the underlying etiology.

Systemic Diseases Associated with Renal Involvement

Nephrotic Syndrome

Diabetes

The development of renal disease is related to the duration of the diabetes, the severity, and whether or not the diabetes is under control. Kimmelstiel-Wilson disease (nodular glomerulosclerosis) and diffuse glomerulonephritis are some of the renal diseases to which diabetes contributes. The incidence of adult onset diabetes is 9% in the general population.

Most juvenile diabetic patients die of renal failure. Renal changes usually develop 13 to 16 years postonset.

The diffuse microangiopathy leads to changes in multiple organs including loss of muscle tone, gangrene, peripheral neuropathy, skin lesions, retinopathy, and renal disease. The etiology of the microangiopathy is not entirely clear. It could be caused by autoimmune, metabolic, or genetic factors. Increasing evidence favors nonenzymatic glycosylation of macromolecules as a major pathogenetic factor.

Light microscopy reveals nodular or diffuse sclerosis of the glomeruli with hyaline droplets (fibrin cap) (Fig. 13.8) in the basement membranes and capsular drops in the Bowman's capsule. Hyalinization of afferent and efferent arterioles is also seen. Vacuoles in tubular epithelium (glycogen), hyalinized arterioles and medium-sized vessels, fibrotic interstitium, and tubular basement membrane thickening are also seen. Immunofluorescence is not specific. Electron microscopy shows microangiopathy (marked thickening of the capillary loops). There is also increased mesangial matrix and insudative lesions.

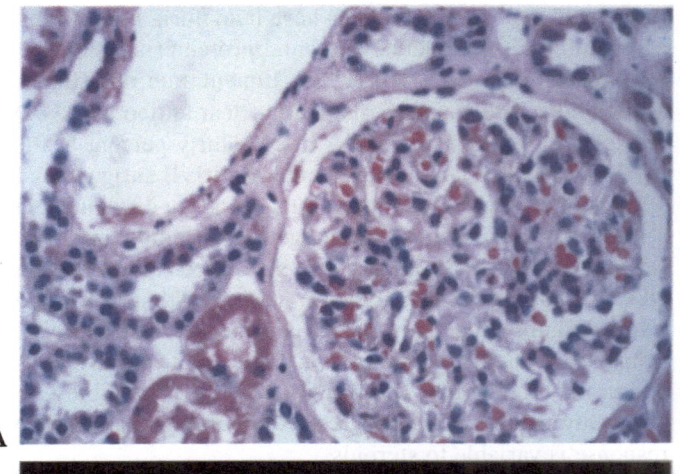

A

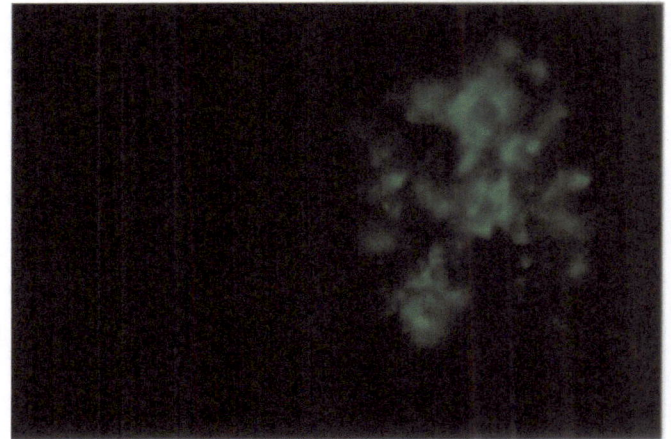

B

FIGURE 13.5   Acute poststreptococcal glomerulonephritis. A: Glomerulus showing diffuse proliferation of mesangial cells (H&E, ×120). **B**: Glomerular lumpy bumpy coarse IgG deposits (immunofluorescence stain, ×120).

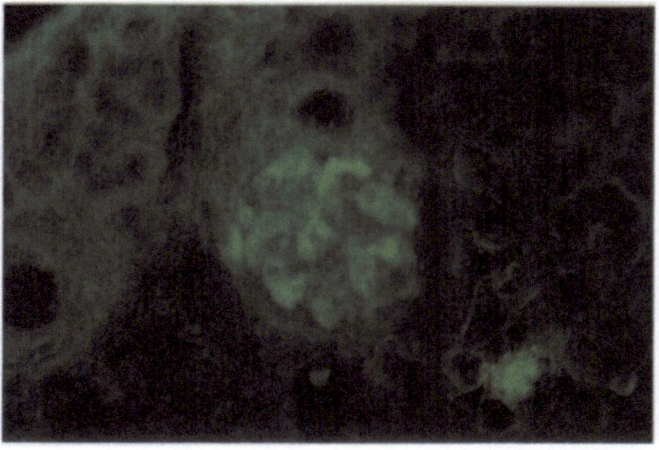

FIGURE 13.6   IgA nephropathy. Diffuse mesangial IgA deposits (immunofluorescence stain, ×120).

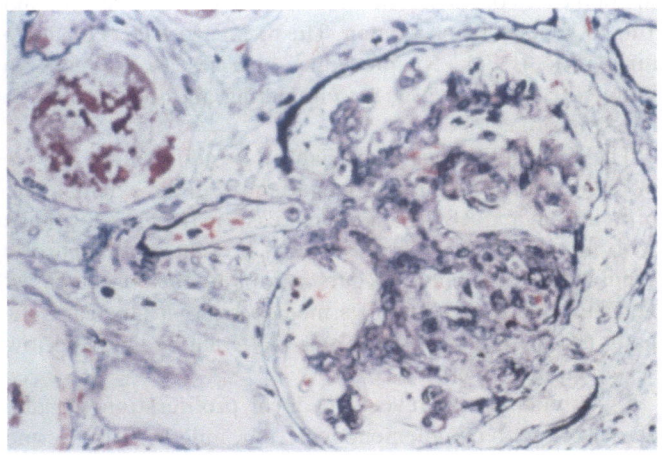

FIGURE 13.7   Crescentic glomerulonephritis. Crescent formation (PAS stain, ×120).

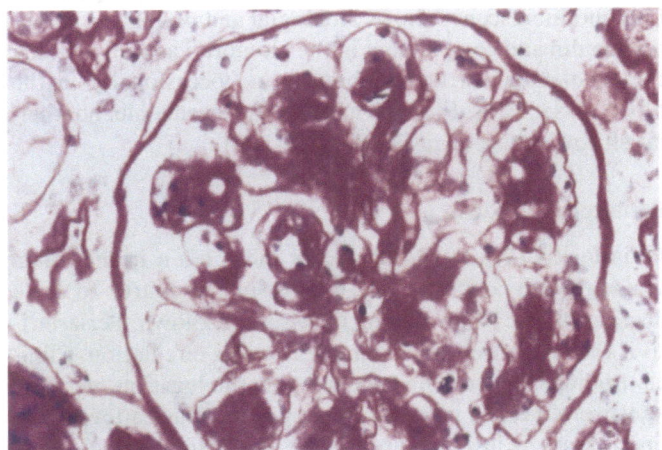

FIGURE 13.8   Diabetic nephropathy. Nodular sclerosis (PAS stain, ×120).

Amyloidosis

Of the cases of diabetes, 75% to 93% also have secondary amyloidosis. It is familial in the third decade, secondary in the fourth decade, and primary in the sixth decade of life. Clinical findings show a nephrotic syndrome. On light microscopy a nodular lesion is seen along with deposits in vessel walls and mesangial matrix and capillary basement membranes which show apple green birefringence with Congo red stain (Fig. 13.9A). Immunofluorescence demonstrates positivity for light chains. Electron microscopy shows fibrils in the basement membranes, mesangium, and vessel walls. The course of the disease is slowly downhill to renal failure with no response to steroids (Fig. 13.9B).

Hematuria Syndromes and Nephritic Syndromes

SLE (Systemic Lupus) Disease

Overall incidence of SLE is 8 per 100,000 population with 1 in 2000 cases occurring in women 15 to 64 years of age, and 1 in 7000 being black women. The mean age is 29. Female to male ratio is 7:1. No preceding illnesses are known. An immune complex caused by circulating antibodies to DNA is responsible.

The clinical findings are variable depending on the degree of renal involvement but most patients will have hematuria, proteinuria, and RBC and granular casts in the urine. Patients with membranous nephropathy will present with nephrotic syndrome. Renal failure occurs in 50% to 60% of the cases. Pertinent laboratory findings include high antinuclear antibody (ANA) titers, positive anti-DNA antibodies, and low serum complement.

Light microscopy reveals 1) focal proliferation, usually associated with complement depletion, mild hematuria, and proteinuria, 2) diffuse proliferation associated with gross hematuria, moderate proteinuria, and casts (Fig. 13.10A), 3) membranous nephritis associated with nephrotic syndrome, and 4) necrosis and crescent formation. Interstitial inflammation and vasculitis are also seen in many of the patients. Immunofluorescence shows mesangial and peripheral immunoglobulin and complement in the glomeruli as well as along the tubular basement membranes and occasionally in the blood vessel walls. Electron microscopy reveals subendothelial electron-dense deposits (Fig. 13.10B).

Periarteritis Nodosa

Periarteritis nodosa (PAN) occurs more often in men than women, with a 15:1 ratio, usually in the fourth to sixth decades of life. No preceding illnesses are known. Periarteritis is the result of chronic immune complex circulation. Clinical findings are variable depending on the location, number, and size of vessels involved. Most patients have a fever. The major systems involved are the renal, gastrointestinal, musculoskeletal, central nervous system, and skin. Because of renal involvement, the patients have hematuria microscopically and mild to moderate casts and proteinuria. Lab findings include elevated erythrocyte sedimentation rate (ESR), eosinophilia, and leukocytosis. Antinuclear antibody (ANA) is negative or reveals very low titers. Thirty percent of the patients have transient or persistent hepatitis B antigenemia.

Light microscopy reveals that the lesions are distributed in a segmental fashion involving large and medium-sized vessels. Glomerular lesions are also seen. Lesions can be seen in all stages of the disease ranging from acute, with necrosis and acute inflammation, to subacute and healed with fibrosis. Immunofluorescence shows fibrin in the wall of the vessels and in the mesangium. Electron microscopy is variable.

A chronically slow progressive course is seen. The response is variable to steroids.

Wegener's Granulomatosis

The age of onset of Wegener's granulomatosis can be from 3 months to 75 years, with the mean age being 44. There is a slight male predominance of 1.5:1. No preceding illnesses are known. The possibility of a hypersensitivity reaction has been suggested. Clinical findings include necrotizing sinusitis, pneumonitis, and glomerulonephritis.

Light microscopy shows focal necrosis of the glomeruli with crescent formation and usually giant cells in the interstitium. Immunofluorescence reveals fibrin deposits in the crescents. The prognosis is poor.

Hemolytic Uremic Syndrome

Hemolytic uremic syndrome occurs either postpartum or in children under 1 year of age. Preceding illnesses include gastroenteritis in 70% to 90%, 15% after upper respiratory infection. In postpartum cases, the onset occurs 6 weeks after labor. Intravascular coagulation, decreased platelets, and increased fibrin split products are seen. The patient presents with oliguria, renal failure, hemolytic anemia, and thrombocytopenia. Necrosis as well as intracapillary thrombi are seen histologically.

Progressive Systemic Sclerosis (Scleroderma)

The incidence of progressive systemic sclerosis is greater in females than males. The renal involvement in scleroderma is secondary to the systemic involvement. Vascular sclerosis associated with the disease is often seen. This is autoimmune in nature. Patients usually have high ANA titers and positive anti-scleroderma$_{70}$ antibodies. Renal manifestations include hypertension and renal failure.

Light microscopy shows the arterioles to be hyalinized. Necrosis as well as intimal thickening occurs as the disease progresses. Vascular sclerosis develops. Immunofluorescence reveals early fibrin deposits in the arteriolar wall but this is negative late in the disease. Electron microscopy is variable. The course is rapidly progressive.

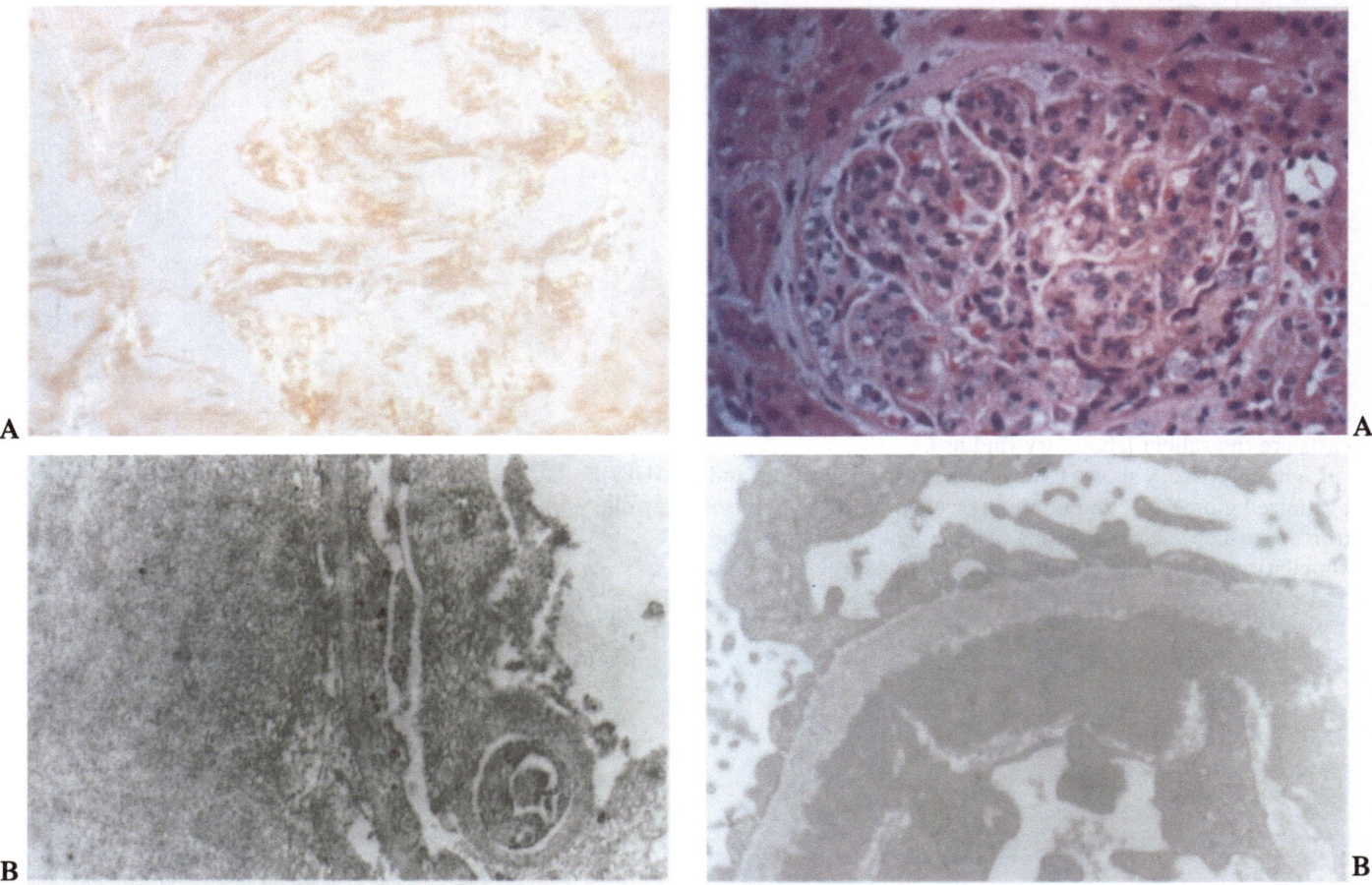

FIGURE 13.9   Amyloidosis. A: Birefringent amyloid deposits under polarized light (Congo red stain, ×120). **B**: Electron micrograph demonstrating amyloid fibrils in the capillary loop and mesangium.

FIGURE 13.10   Lupus nephritis. A: Diffuse proliferative type. Diffuse mesangial cell proliferation (H&E, ×120). **B**: Subendothelial electron-dense deposits.

Hereditary Glomerular Diseases

Benign Recurrent Hematuria

The clinical picture of benign recurrent hematuria shows recurrent episodes of gross hematuria. The incidence in men is greater than in women. Light microscopy shows no changes. Immunofluorescence is negative (Fig. 13.11). Electron microscopy shows a thin basement membrane. The course is benign in the sense that it rarely if ever progresses to renal failure.

Hereditary Nephritis (Alport's Syndrome)

Clinically, both men and women are affected; although the course is more severe in men and is associated with deafness and visual disturbances. Hematuria, proteinuria, and urinary casts are the salient laboratory findings.

Light microscopy shows foamy cells in the interstitium and hyalinized glomeruli. Immunofluorescence is negative. Electron microscopy shows splitting of basement membranes and lamellation of the lamina densa (Figure 13.12).

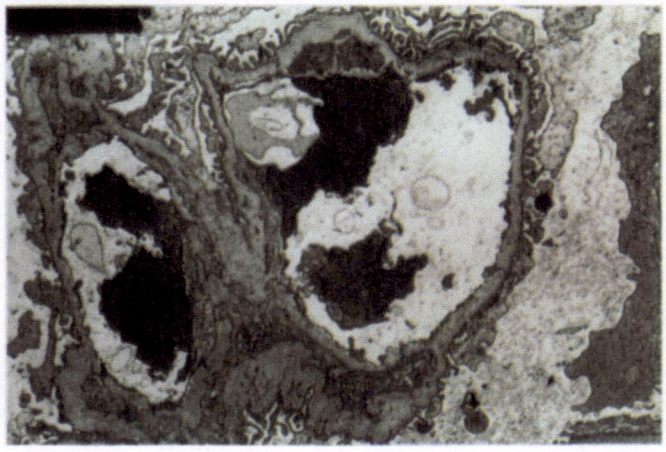

FIGURE **13.11   Benign recurrent hematuria.** Thin capillary basement membrane.

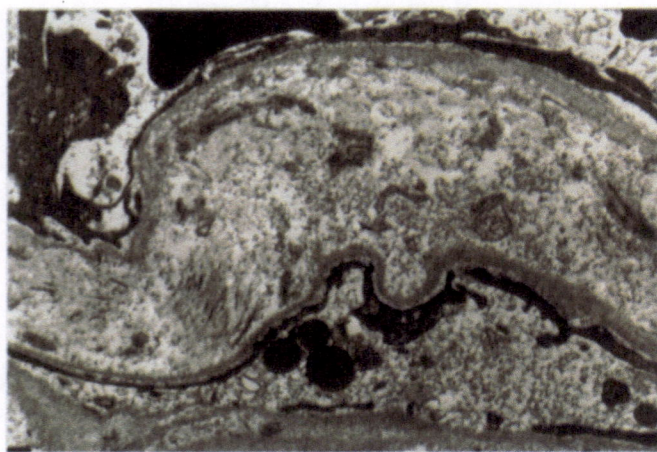

FIGURE **13.12   Alport's syndrome.** Split lamina densa in the capillary basement membrane.

Renal Vascular Disease

The kidney is an end-arterial system that receives approximately 25% of the cardiac output. Moreover, the pressure of the afferent arteriolar end of the glomerular capillary bed is maintained over a wide range of systemic blood pressures (autoregulation) and thus the renal vessels are subjected to high blood flow and high pressure. They are therefore frequent sites of pathologic change such as occlusion by thromboembolic phenomena including atherosclerotic or fibrin-containing emboli. They are also particularly prone to develop intrinsic changes in association with the collagen vascular diseases (see above) and in association with hypertension.

With regard to the latter, there is a strong association between renal vascular disease and primary (essential) hypertension. Of all individuals with high blood pressure, probably 90% suffer from the "essential" type in which the cause of the pressure elevation is unknown. This is an extremely common disorder in the Western world, affecting more than 20% of the adult population in the United States (almost 40 million people). It takes two forms clinically: a rapidly progressive form (malignant) that is almost always accompanied by renal failure (uremia), and a slowly progressive course (benign) in which the patients usually die of complications of cardiovascular disease (heart failure, myocardial infarct, and stroke). In the initial stages these patients, who are the majority of hypertensives by a wide margin, do not show any indication of renal functional impairment. However, after many years a number of these patients develop renal failure, and, in fact the scarred kidneys of benign nephrosclerosis, which is the pathologic concomitant of essential hypertension, is the most frequent cause of chronic renal failure. The association between the large heavy heart and scarred and contracted kidneys was first noted by Richard Bright in London in 1832, and chronic kidney disease has been referred to as Bright's disease since that time.

The two clinical presentations are accompanied by two different pathologic pictures.

Benign Nephrosclerosis (Slowly Progressive Form)

In benign nephrosclerosis the kidneys are usually only slightly smaller than their normal counterparts. Their cortical surfaces, however, have a finely granular or pitted appearance. Each fine depressed scar relates to an altered cortical vessel. On section, the cortex is thinner than normal and the surface is irregular. Microscopically, two types of vascular changes are seen: the larger intrarenal vessels (segmental, interlobar, arcuate) show intimal fibrosis, duplication of the internal elastic lamina, narrowing of the media which also shows hyaline change, and adventitial fibrosis. The smaller vessels (interlobular, afferent arterioles) show marked medial thickening and hyaline change (Fig. 13.13A). The hyaline is mostly due to deposition of type IV collagen (basal lamina) around the medial smooth muscle cells, but also involves plasma protein components.

Malignant Hypertension (Rapidly Progressive Form)

In most patients as well as those of the accelerated phase in whom the malignant hypertension develops after a long course of benign hypertension, there may be gross and microscopic changes of benign nephrosclerosis. When the patient develops the rapid course de novo, the kidneys may be of normal size with a smooth cortex. The cortex shows small punctate hemorrhages ("flea-bitten") that correspond to microscopic changes in the cortical vessels ("fibrinoid necrosis"). Again, larger blood vessels show changes that differ from the smaller blood vessels. The vessels of the size of segmental, interlobar, and arcuate arteries exhibit marked proliferation and reduplication of the endothelial cells and edema of the smooth muscle termed onion-skin change. The small blood vessels show eccentric patches of intense subendothelial and medial hyalin change, which results from leakage of plasma proteins, including fibrin, into the vessel wall (Fig. 13.13B). This "fibrinoid necrosis" is usually not accompanied by inflammatory infiltrate, but may show extravasated red blood cells, corresponding to the "flea bites" on the cortical surfaces.

With antihypertensive therapy these vascular changes have been shown to subside and the larger vessels may show healed vascular lesions with mucopolysaccharide deposition and fibrosis of the intimal layer, titled "mucoid" degeneration.

The vascular changes in the kidney in malignant hypertension resemble changes seen in collagen vascular disease, in particular in scleroderma. The absence of significant inflammation has been used to distinguish these lesions from diseases such as polyarteritis, which also affects arteries and arterioles of the kidney (see above).

Renal Artery Stenosis

Along with the intrarenal vessels, the main renal artery is also frequently affected by vascular changes. Renal artery stenosis is most frequently the result of atherosclerotic narrowing usually near the origin of one or both main renal arteries from the aorta (Fig. 13.13C). This form of renal vascular hypertension occurs in elderly individuals (seventh and eighth decade), whereas the onset of hypertension under the age of 20 years is often associated with a condition known as fibromuscular dysplasia, which has several variants. Therefore, disease of the main renal artery should be suspected when the patient is over the age of 60 years or under the age of 20 years at the time of detection of the raised blood pressure. Essential hypertension is a disease of the middle years. So-called renovascular hypertension appears to be caused by raised circulating renin levels in analogy with the Goldblatt experimental model initiated by constricting the main renal artery. Raised renin levels may also be found frequently in association with malignant hypertension. Renin levels may be high or low, but most frequently are normal or low in benign essential hypertension.

In addition to the vascular changes in hypertension, focal atrophy of the cortical tubules, mild interstitial fibrosis, and slight interstitial lymphocytic infiltration in the cortex are frequently found in benign nephrosclerosis. Glomeruli may show complete hyalinization, which appears to be an ischemic change.

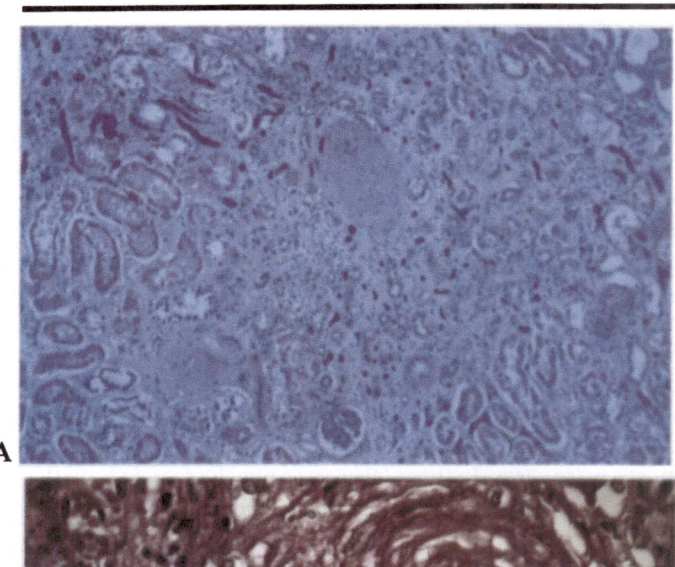

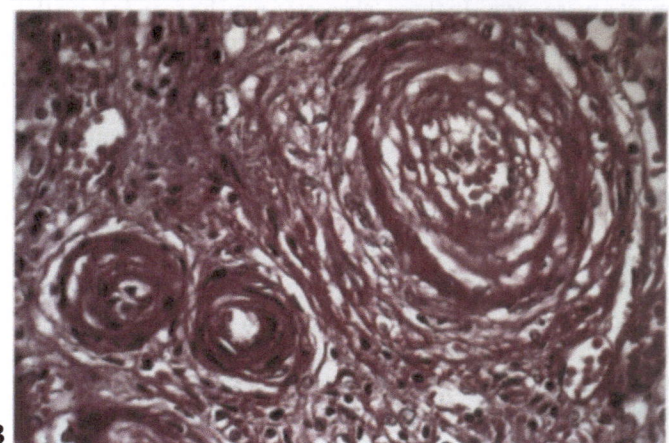

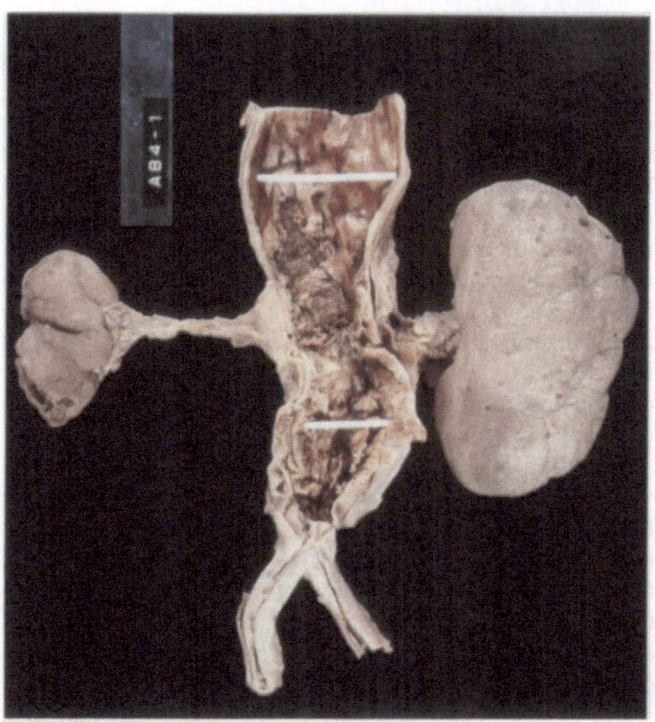

FIGURE 13.13   Renal vascular disease. A: Arteriolar nephrosclerosis (benign hypertensive renal disease). Arterioles and small arteries are narrowed with hyaline thickening of the wall. The glomeruli show hyaline sclerosis. **B**: Rapidly progressive form (malignant hypertension). Necrotizing arteriolitis with fibrinoid degeneration of small arteries and arterioles. Also seen is hyperplastic arteriolitis with concentric layering of collagen and smooth muscle cells ("onion skinning"). With permission from Richard R. Lindquist, M.D. Renal Biopsy. MEDCom Inc., 1970. **C**: Renal artery stenosis. The right renal artery stenosis is a result of atheromatous plaques, causing diffuse ischemic atrophy of the right kidney.

Interstitial Diseases

The term "interstitial nephritis" has been used rather loosely in the past to cover a variety of conditions whose pathologic manifestations appear primarily between the tubules. The renal interstitium consists of a scanty stroma and the basal lamina of the tubules as well as tubular blood and lymphatic capillaries. In the normal kidney inflammatory cells are rarely present in either the cortex or medulla. The interstitium gradually becomes more prominent, especially in the medulla, with age, but even in elderly individuals it is usually represented by acellular eosinophilic (hyalin) deposition comprising increased basal lamina (type IV collagen). Thus, the presence of acute or chronic inflammatory infiltrate in the interstitium, of any degree, probably represents a significant finding.

Interstitial diseases have often been equated in the past with infectious diseases (pyelonephritis). However, it is clear that many of the cases, especially of chronic interstitial disease, are toxic in origin. Indeed, the pathogenesis of so-called chronic pyelonephritis has undergone significant reevaluation over the past few decades, and despite many advances, our understanding of this process remains incomplete. In the discussion that follows, we will first consider infectious interstitial disease (acute and chronic pyelonephritis) and then briefly consider noninfectious interstitial nephritis. Entities such as papillary necrosis will receive only passing mention.

Acute Pyelonephritis

It is clear that in most instances pyelonephritis is associated with some obstruction of the urinary tract. The acute disease is most frequently an ascending infection resulting from gram negative organisms (*E. coli*). Typically, the patient develops symptoms of lower urinary tract infection (frequency, urgency, dysuria) first, followed by flank pain and tenderness over the kidneys and high fever. The urine contains polymorphonuclear leukocytes and red blood cells but also white blood cell casts, indicating parenchymal renal involvement. In most instances the renal pelvis and renal medulla are the only parts of the kidney involved (pyonephrosis, pyelitis), and the infectious process is irradicated with appropriate antibiotic therapy. Thus, the pathologist probably sees only the most severe cases. In these, abscesses may be seen in both the cortex and medulla as circumscribed yellow foci of pus one to several millimeters in diameter. The renal papillae may be pale yellowish grossly if papillary necrosis is also present. The latter is seen most often in association with diabetes mellitus or analgesic abuse. Histologically, the inflammatory process comprises acute inflammatory cells in the interstitium, particularly in the medulla. The epithelium of the renal pelvis may be eroded and inflamed. As the infection progresses, the inflammatory process ruptures into the tubules producing collections of pus cells in tubules, particularly of the distal nephron (large collecting ducts, collecting tubules). These are passed in the urine as casts. Since women are more prone to cystitis than men, they are also more frequently affected by pyelonephritis. Pregnancy, because it frequently produces urinary tract obstruction, also is associated with an increased incidence of acute pyelonephritis.

Chronic Pyelonephritis

The incidence of chronic pyelonephritis has probably been significantly overestimated in the past. This is because the pathologic picture is not specific. Chronic inflammation and fibrosis in the kidney may not be the result of infection but may accompany hypertensive vascular disease or result from toxic insult (see below). Therefore, true chronic pyelonephritis is probably significantly less common at autopsy than was previously estimated. The true incidence at autopsy is probably 0.5% to 1.0% (as opposed to 10–20% as estimated previously).

Grossly, chronic pyelonephritis appears as broad, flat, cortical scars. On section, the papilla may show blunting or atrophy. This is particularly evident if gross obstruction of the urinary tract is present. Even if obstructive uropathy is not seen, the mechanism of the chronic infection is felt to involve vesicoureteral reflux. This has led to the suggestion that chronic pyelonephritis should be called "reflux nephropathy."

Histologically, there is a constellation of changes. Most pathologists insist that there be chronic inflammation of the pelvis and medulla in addition to cortical inflammation and fibrosis to support the concept of an ascending infection. Periglomerular fibrosis also is often present, with the glomerular tuft being relatively spared. Nonetheless, the changes are difficult to separate unequivocally from other conditions, such as ischemia, which produce tubulo-interstitial changes. So-called thyroidization produced by protein casts in the tubular lumina frequently is present, but is nonspecific (Fig. 13.14). Interstitial foam cells in the medulla are more typical of other forms of interstitial nephritis such as the hereditary types.

It must be emphasized that the changes in chronic interstitial nephritis are nonspecific and a careful history is essential in distinguishing one type from another. Interstitial disease is prevalent in some geographic locations (Balkan nephritis), may result from a variety of toxic insults (analgesic abuse), and may be hereditary. Some authors have felt that unilateral disease is more apt to be infectious in origin. The demonstration of overt obstruction such as prostatic hypertrophy also may suggest an infectious origin. Diabetes and analgesic abuse are likely to be associated with frank papillary necrosis in which ischemia probably plays a major pathogenetic role.

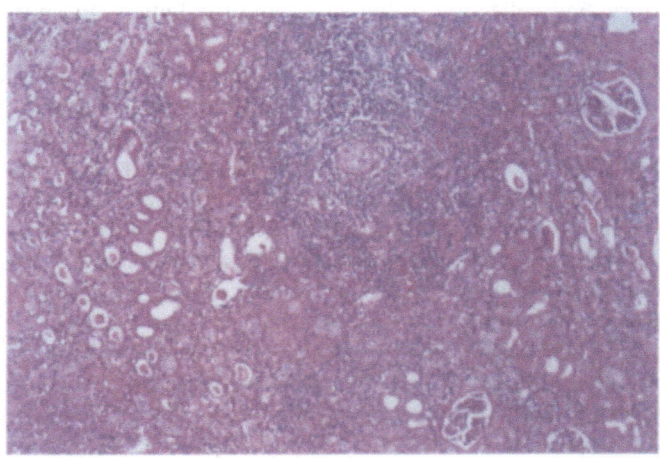

FIGURE 13.14 Chronic pyelonephritis. Tubules filled with colloid casts, "thyroidization," and interstitial fibrosis and inflammation.

Transplantation

Renal transplantation is the most effective rehabilitative therapy for end-stage renal diseases, because the kidney provides not only excretory functions but also a number of metabolic functions such as vitamin D metabolism, erythropoietin production and the extracellular fluid balance of the renin-angiotensin system. Dialysis cannot substitute for the metabolic functions. With a good match the current success rate of renal transplants is very high. However, three main types of complications are of special importance in renal transplantation: 1) *technical*—at surgery there can be leakage from the kidney through the newly implanted ureter, stenosis of the artery, and collection of lymph around the kidney. Prompt corrective surgery can save the graft; 2) *rejection*—the mechanisms involved in rejection are cell mediated or antibody mediated. These mechanisms may become synergistic. Structural components of the kidney vary in their sensitivity to different types of injury. Humoral rejection leads to necrotic changes in the glomeruli and arteries while cellular rejection results in damage to the interstitium, tubules, and capillaries. 3) *recurrence* of original glomerular disease. In addition to the above three major complications, one needs to address a fourth possible complication, which is cyclosporin toxicity. One of the side effects of cyclosporin is nephrotoxicity and often it is difficult clinically to differentiate between cyclosporin effects and acute rejection. Renal biopsy in most cases resolves the dilemma. As in cyclosporin toxicity, one finds tubular necrosis and peritubular inflammation (mixture of lymphocytes and eosinophils), and in long-standing cyclosporin effect, a chronic vasculopathy develops with thickening of the arteriolar walls but without necrosis or perivascular inflammation.

Classification of Rejection

Hyperacute

Recipient has preformed antibodies against the donor antigens. Minutes after transplant the kidney becomes cyanotic and flabby. Fibrin and platelets lead to thrombi along with acute tubular necrosis, cortical necrosis, and damaged vascular endothelium leads to hemorrhagic infarction. Immunofluorescence shows immunoglobulins and complement in the vessel walls.

Acute

Days, months, or years after transplantation cellular and humoral tissue injury plays a part in any patient. Interstitial lymphocytic infiltrates as well as fibrinoid necrosis in the glomeruli and arterioles are seen. Immunoflourence reveals immunoglobulins and fibrin in the vessels and glomeruli.

Chronic Rejection

Intimal hyperplasia and sclerosis in arteries of various sizes, hyalinized glomeruli, and intimal scarring are seen.

Recurrence of the Disease

Systemic diseases such as diabetes and SLE will recur in the allograft. Also some primary diseases like focal sclerosis, antiglomerular basement membranes, membranoproliferative glomerulonephritis and IgA nephropathy tend to recur in allografts.

Kidney Neoplasms

The diagnostic approach of a suspected renal mass begins with intravenous pyelography, and is followed by ultrasonography and computed tomography (CT). Fine needle aspiration biopsy under CT guide may be required as a part of a complete preoperative work-up.

Wilms' Tumor (Nephroblastoma)

Ninety percent of Wilms' tumors occur under the age of 10 years. The classic clinical presentation of Wilms' tumor is an abdominal mass felt by the mother. Ultrasound or intravenous pyelogram shows a renal mass distorting the pelvis. Computer tomography scans can further delineate the mass. Grossly, the tumors are large, well circumscribed, and firm. On section, they are solid and exhibit multifocal necrosis and hemorrhage (Fig. 13.15A).

Microscopically, the tumors comprise undifferentiated blastema, mesenchymal tissue, and epithelial tissue in various proportions. However, some tumors consist of only one or two components. The blastematous areas show small, round to oval primitive cells with scanty cytoplasm (Fig. 13.15B). They are highly cellular and arranged compactly. Mesenchymal elements show spindle-cell configuration or smooth or skeletal muscle type.

The epithelial components show primitive tubuloglomerular structures (Fig. 13.15C).

Mesoblastic Nephroma (Fetal Mesenchymal Hamartoma)

Mesoblastic nephroma is a congenital renal neoplasm that is usually discovered before 6 months of age. Grossly, it is a solid, yellowish gray to tan mass, reminiscent of uterine leiomyoma (Fig. 13.16A). Microscopically, the tumor consists of myofibroblastlike cells arranged in interlacing bundles (Fig. 13.16B). Cytologic atypia is not present. The tumor is benign.

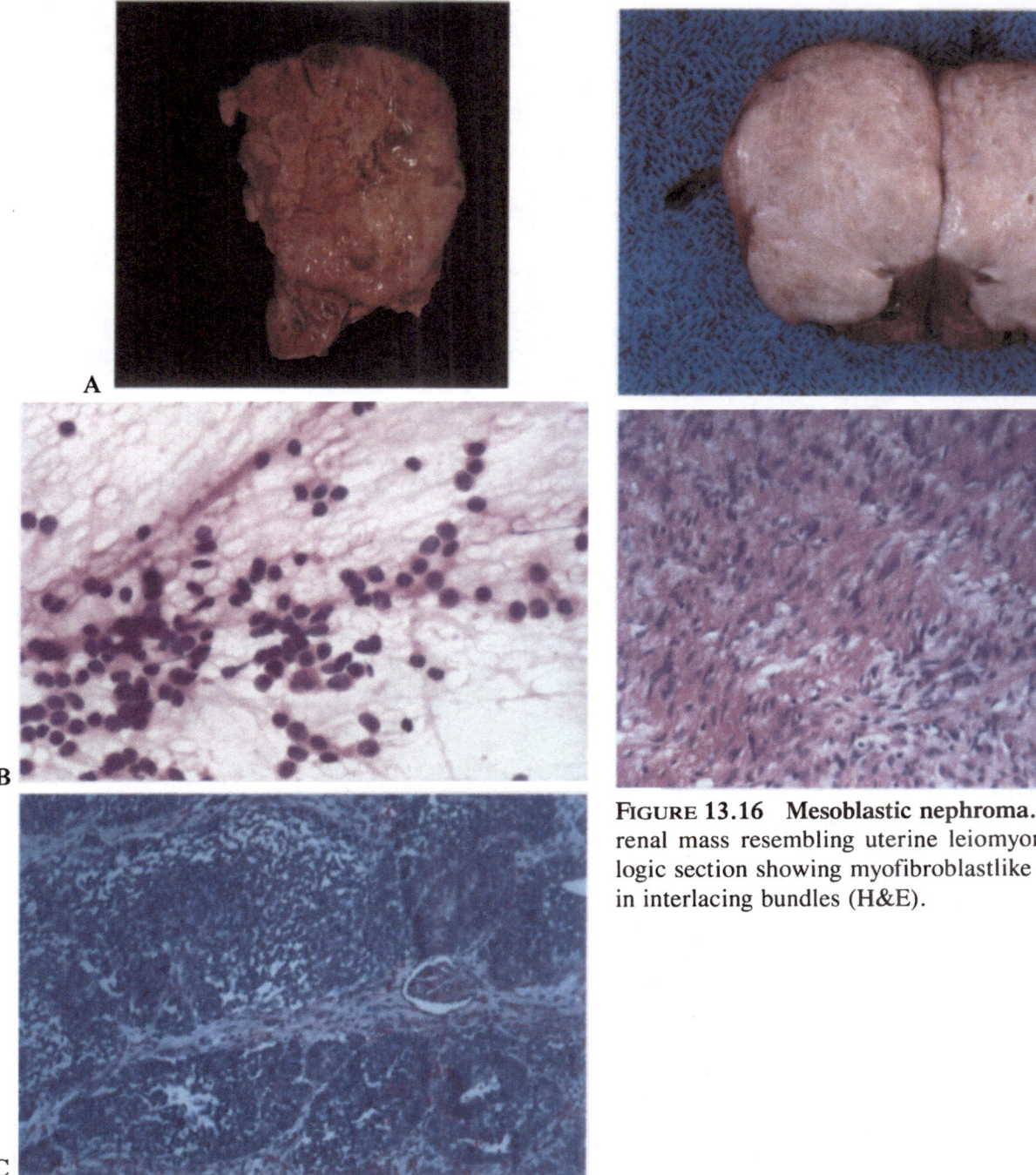

FIGURE 13.16 Mesoblastic nephroma. A: Tan solid, renal mass resembling uterine leiomyoma. B: Histologic section showing myofibroblastlike cells arranged in interlacing bundles (H&E).

FIGURE 13.15 Wilms' tumor. A: Large, circumscribed solid mass in the upper pole of kidney (gross). B: FNA smears showing clusters of embryonal epithelial cells (blastemal element). C: Histologic section showing tubuloglomerular epithelial structures in blastematous background. (H&E).

Renal Adenocarcinoma (Renal Cell Carcinoma)

Renal adenocarcinoma is a tumor of adults. Renal adenocarcinoma usually presents with hematuria, flank pain, and abdominal mass, which are regarded as the diagnostic triads, but occur in fewer than 10% of the patients.

Grossly, renal cell carcinoma is well circumscribed in the cortex. On section, the tumor is pale yellow, soft, and hemorrhagic. The margins of the tumor are thickened with fibrosis (Fig. 13.17A).

Cytology and Histology

Percutaneous fine needle aspiration is a safe and reliably diagnostic procedure. Aspirates show abundant cells in a necrotic and bloody background. The cells occur in loose aggregates and papillary clusters. The cells may be polygonal, round, or pleomorphic and have optically clear cytoplasm and relatively small, round, hyperchromatic nuclei (Fig. 13.17B). Renal adenocarcinoma cells show characteristic lipid droplets in the cytoplasm, which are more distinct in air-dried smears (Fig. 13.17C). Presence of lipid drops in the cytoplasm is a unique feature of renal clear cell adenocarcinoma, and a reliable cytologic feature in the differential diagnosis of other types of adenocarcinomas of the kidney.[7]

Histologically, clear cell adenocarcinoma consists of large clear cells arranged in solid sheets, nests, or papillary structures (Fig. 13.17D). The granular cell type of renal carcinoma consists of large granular cells arranged in papillary structures or solid sheets separated by abundant vascular stroma (Fig. 13.17E).

The sarcomatoid type of renal carcinoma consists of pleomorphic, large bizarre cells arranged in sheets. The cells have abundant eosinophilic cytoplasm and large bizarre pleomorphic nuclei (Fig. 13.17F). Granular cell types and sarcomatoid types of renal carcinoma are more aggressive than clear cell types. Sarcomatoid types of renal carcinoma are less than 2% of all renal carcinomas, and highly aggressive.

Renal Oncocytoma

Renal oncocytoma is a low grade or benign variant of renal cell carcinoma and is a rare type of renal tumor. Grossly, oncocytomas are usually large, solid, well circumscribed masses. On section, they are dark brown and soft. Histologically, oncocytomas consist of polygonal cells arranged in solid sheets. The cells have abundant acidophilic granular cytoplasm and small, round nuclei (Fig. 13.17G). Most oncocytomas behave in a benign fashion, except for the cases with high grade nuclear atypia.

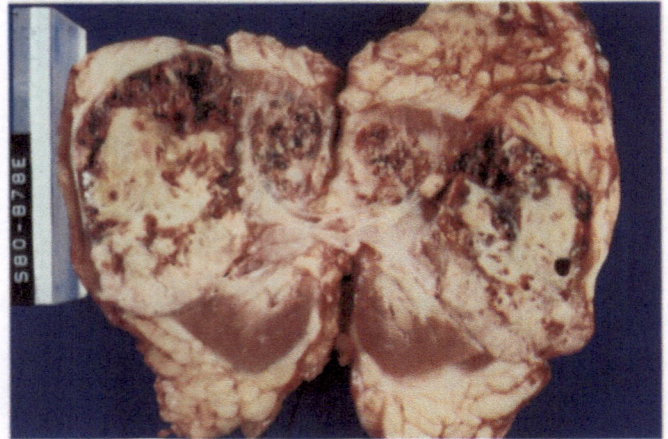

A

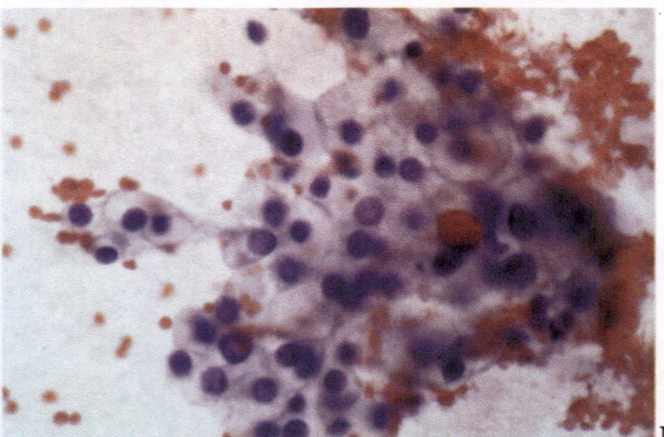

B

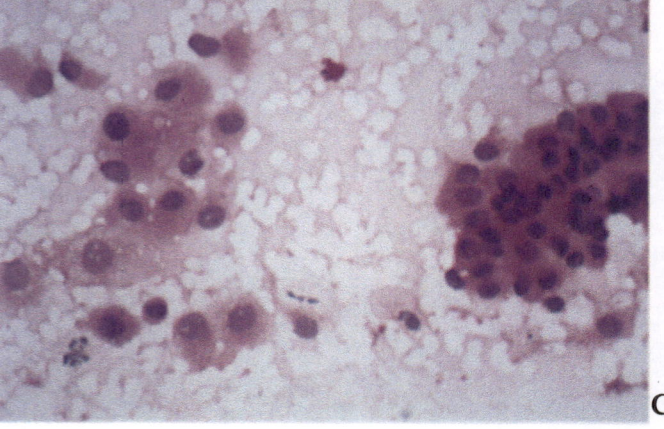

C

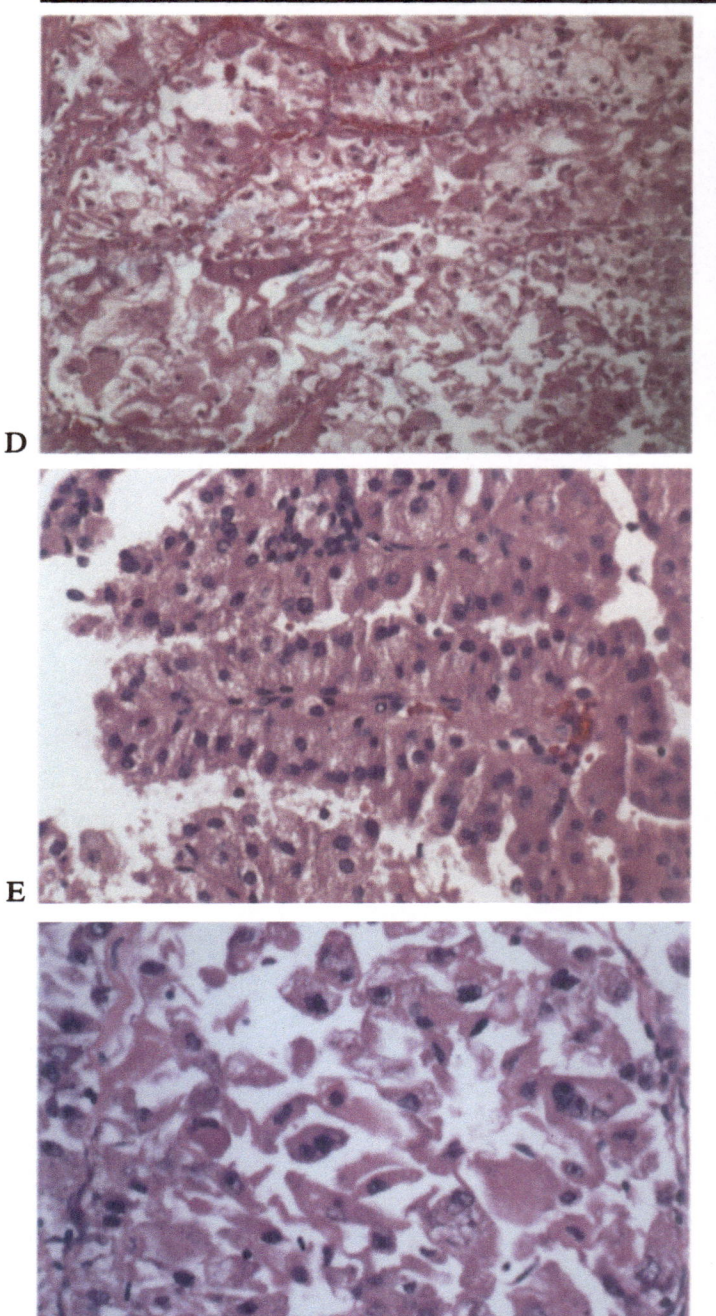

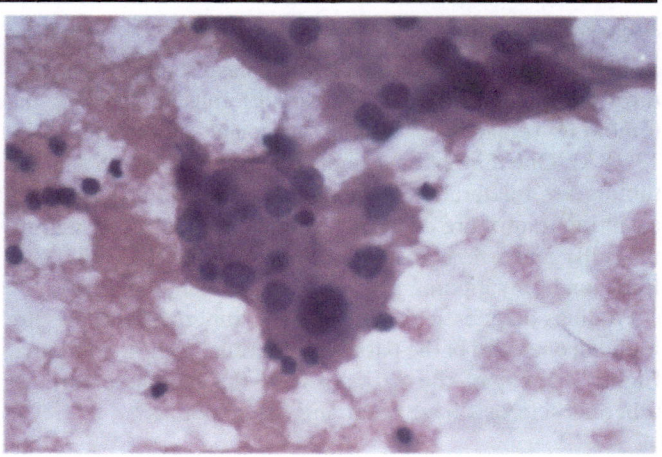

FIGURE 13.17   Renal adenocarcinoma. A: Resected kidney with large yellowish mass extending to the capsule. B: FNA shows sheets of round cells with abundant clear cytoplasm. C: FNA air-dried smear showing lipid droplets in the cytoplasm. D: Histologic section showing sheets and papillary structures of clear cells and prominent vascular stroma. E: Histologic features of granular cell type. F: Sarcomatoid type of renal carcinoma showing sheets of pleomorphic cells. G: Renal oncocytoma showing polygonal cells with abundant eosinophilic cytoplasm and small round nuclei.

Angiomyolipoma

Angiomyolipoma is a rare renal neoplasm comprising mixtures of fat, blood vessels, and smooth muscle. Grossly, the tumor is remarkably similar to renal carcinoma (Fig. 13.18A). One third of the tumors are multiple and 15% of the tumors are bilateral.[4,6] Histologically, the tumor comprises an intimate mixture of large tortuous blood vessels, mature fat cells, and irregular smooth muscle cells (Fig. 13.18B). Renal angiomyolipoma may cause massive hemorrhage.

Findings diagnostic or suggestive of tuberous sclerosis are found in one third of the patients with renal angiomyolipoma. Eighty percent of the patients with the complete form of tuberous sclerosis have renal angiomyolipomas.[5]

Tumors of Renal Pelvis and Ureter

Most renal pelvic and ureteral tumors are transitional cell carcinomas. Adenocarcinoma and squamous cell carcinoma may be observed focally in transitional cell carcinoma.

Synchronous or metachronous tumors elsewhere in the urinary tract are found in almost 40% of the patients.[3] Grossly, these tumors involve the renal pelvis partially or diffusely, and are pale gray, soft, nodular masses (Fig. 13.19A). High grade tumors may extend to the renal parenchyma. Histologically and cytologically, these tumors are identical to those of the urinary bladder (Fig. 13.19B).

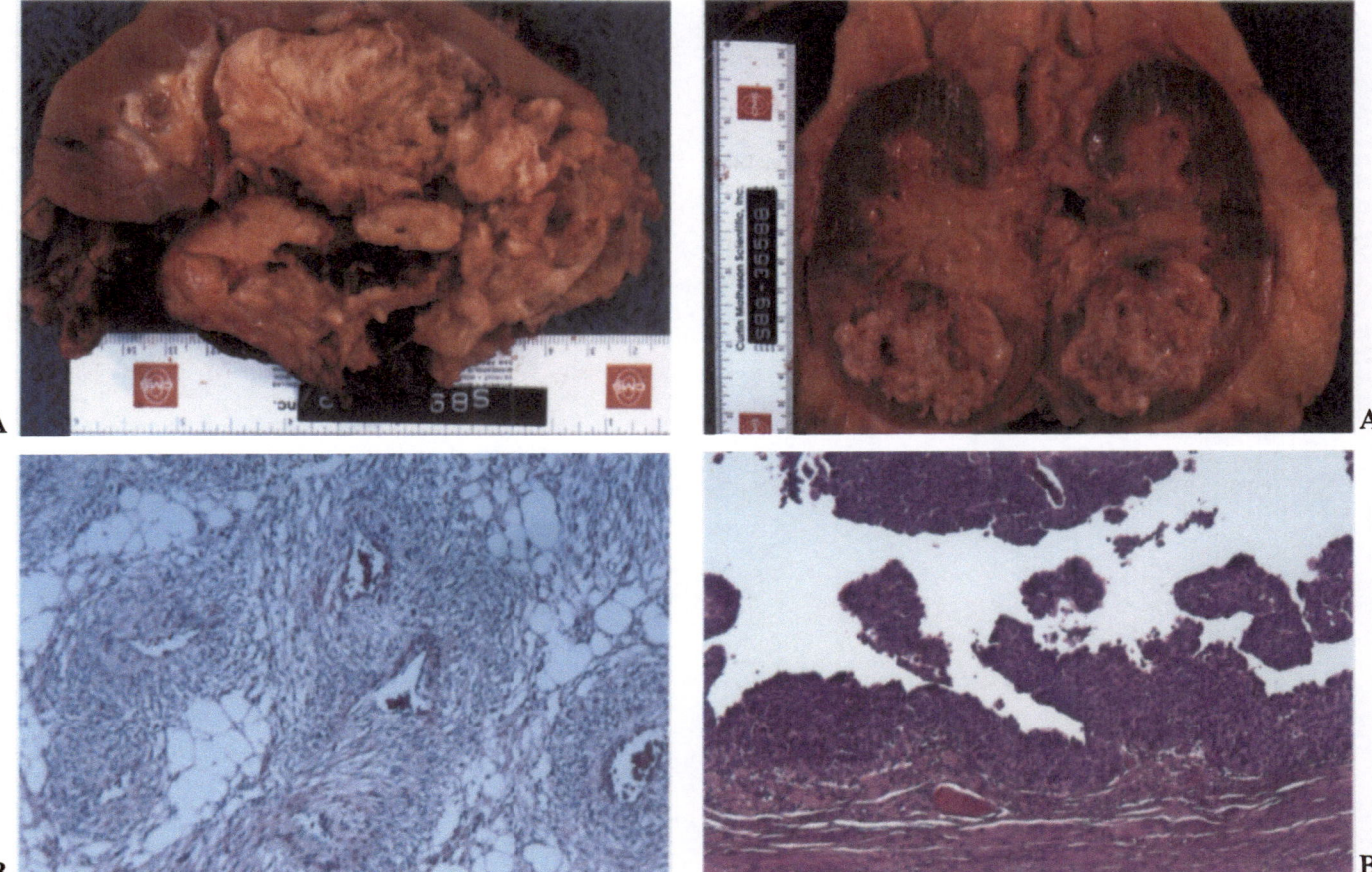

FIGURE 13.18 **Angiolipoma of kidney. A**: Large solid mass expanding and compressing renal parenchyma. **B**: Histologic section showing exuberant vascular structures in adipose tissue background.

FIGURE 13.19 **Carcinoma of renal pelvis. A**: Pale soft nodular mass in the renal pelvis. **B**: Histologic section showing sheets and papillary structures of urothelial cells (transitional carcinoma).

References

1. Tisher CC, Brenner BM. *Renal Pathology with Clinical and Functional Correlations*. Philadelphia: JB Lippincott Company, 1989.

2. Heptinstall RH. *Pathology of the Kidney*. 3rd ed. Boston, Toronto: Little, Brown & Co, 1986:637–724.

3. Gohara A, Goldblatt PJ. Current concepts of glomerular disease. In: Didio J, Motta PM, ed. *Clinical and Surgical Nephrology*. The Hague: Martinus Nijhoff Publishers, 1985.

4. Farrow GM, Harrison EG Jr, Utz DC, Jones DR. Renal angiomyo-lipoma A clinicopathologic study of 32 cases. *Cancer*. 1968;22:564–570.

5. Bernstein J, Robbins TO, Kissane JM. The renal lesions of tuberous sclerosis. *Semin Diagn Pathol*. 1986;3:47–105.

6. Brecher ME, Gill WB, Straus FH II. Angiomyolipoma with regional lymph node involvement and long-term follow-up study. *Hum Pathol*. 1986;17:962–963.

7. Zajicek J. Aspiration biopsy cytology, part 2. Cytology of intradiaphragmatic organs. Basel, Switzerland: *Monographs in Clinical Cytology*, Vol 7. 1979:1–34.

14
Lower Urinary Tract

Diseases of Urinary Bladder

Cystitis

Interstitial (Hunner's) Cystitis

Interstitial cystitis usually occurs in elderly women, who present with lower abdominal or perineal pain and urinary frequency. The lesion can involve anywhere in the bladder. Histologically, the lesion is a mucosal ulceration covered by fibrin and necrotic material. The underlying lamina propria and muscularis show edema, hemorrhage, granulation tissue, and a mononuclear cell infiltrate. Mast cells are frequently observed (Fig. 14.1).

Cystitis Glandularis and Cystitis Cystica

Cystitis glandularis and cystitis cystica result from chronic inflammation or mucosal irritation caused by neurogenic bladder, ureteral reimplantation, or bladder exstrophy. Cystoscopically, the bladder mucosa is nodular, usually in the trigone. Histologically, the lesions begin with focal proliferation of urothelial cells, subsequently extending to the lamina propria. Some of these nodules develop central cystic change (cystitis cystica) or metaplasia of colonic mucosal type (cystitis glandularis) (Fig. 14.2). These disorders usually regress if the underlying causative factors are removed.

Malakoplakia

Malakoplakia is a unique inflammatory change characterized by soft, yellow mucosal plaques, 3 to 4 cm in diameter, usually in the trigone. Malakoplakia occurs more often in immunosuppressed patients.

Histologically, the plaques consist of closely packed large histiocytes in the lamina propria. The histiocytes have abundant foamy acidophilic cytoplasm. Some of these cells contain concentrically laminated intracytoplasmic inclusions known as Michaelis-Guttman (MG) bodies. In cytologic preparations of urine there are scattered histiocytes, some containing round, concentrically laminated MG bodies (Fig. 14.3). The MG bodies are thought to result from the deposition of calcium phosphate and other minerals on overloaded, disintegrating phagosomes.

Benign Tumors

Inverted Papilloma

Inverted papilloma, commonly seen in elderly men, presents with hematuria or urinary obstruction. Cystoscopy reveals a pedunculated polypoid lesion in the trigone, bladder neck, or prostatic urethra. Histologically, the tumor comprises compact, papillary structures in a subepithelial location. No cytologic atypia is present. Exophytic papillae are absent (Fig. 14.4).

Nephrogenic adenoma (Adenomatoid Tumor)

Adenomatoid tumor occurs mainly in adults, but can occur in children and is often associated with chronic inflammation and cystitis glandularis. Grossly, the tumors may be papillary, polypoid, or sessile. Histologically, the tumor comprises papillary and cystic structures, covered or lined by a single layer of cuboidal cells (Fig. 14.5).

Paraganglioma (Extraadrenal Pheochromocytoma)

Paraganglioma can occur in the wall of the urinary bladder. Its histologic appearance and immunohistochemical profile are similar to those in other sites.[1]

Malignant Tumors of Urinary Bladder

Approximately 95% of bladder neoplasms are of urothelial origin. Bladder neoplasms are rather common tumors in the United States. There is substantial evidence that mucosal epithelial hyperplasia and progressive atypia antedates the appearance of these neoplasms. These neoplasms are commonly multiple and tend to recur after resection. With each recurrence, the tumors may show greater atypia and have a worse prognosis. Cytology is of great value for detecting bladder neoplasms.

Since its diagnostic yield for preneoplastic lesions and low grade tumors is not great, urinary cytology is not appropriate for screening in the general population for the detection of early lesions. However, it is extremely valuable with symptomatic patients and for follow up of patients known to have had a bladder tumor.

Transitional Cell Papilloma

Transitional cell papillomas are usually small (0.5–2.0 cm in diameter) and comprise delicate, soft, branching structures attached to the mucosa by a slender stalk. The papillae are covered by normal-appearing urothelial cells, usually less than seven layers in thickness (Fig. 14.6). Since cells of transitional cell papilloma are normal appearing, cytologic identification of these tumors is difficult. Occasionally, portions of the papilla obtained by bladder washing may reveal papilloma. Although transitional cell papillomas are morphologically benign, they predispose to carcinoma and tend to recur.

Transitional Cell Carcinoma

Ninety percent of transitional cell carcinomas are papillary. Most papillary tumors are noninvasive and of low grade. High grade papillary tumors are relatively rare and tend to be invasive. Flat transitional cell carcinomas grow as plaquelike lesions and tend to be invasive and high grade. Grading of transition cell carcinomas is based on the degree of cytologic atypia.[2]

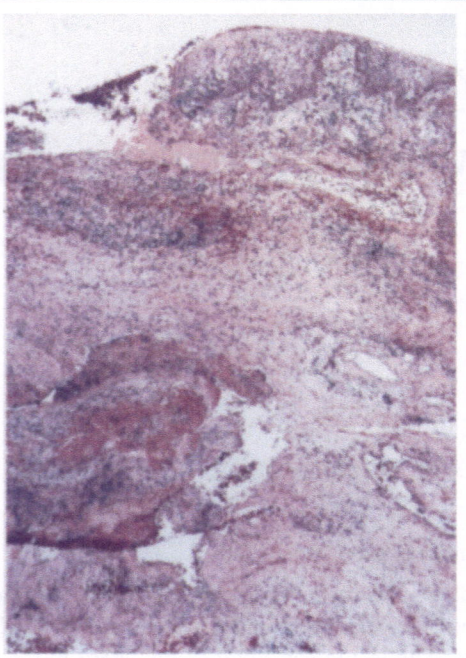

FIGURE 14.1   Interstitial cystitis. Mucosal ulceration and edema, hemorrhage, granulation tissue of the lamina propria (biopsy).

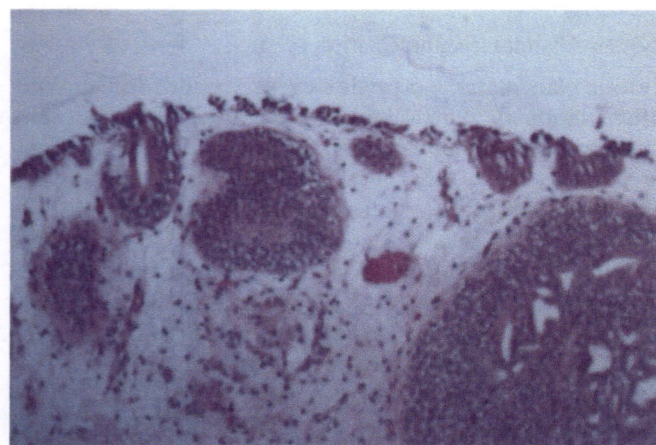

FIGURE 14.2   Cystitis glandularis. Focal proliferation of urothelial cells with cystic change and gland formation (biopsy).

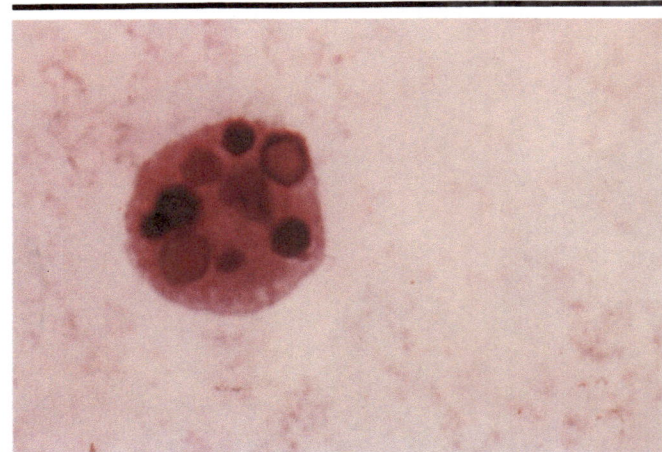

A

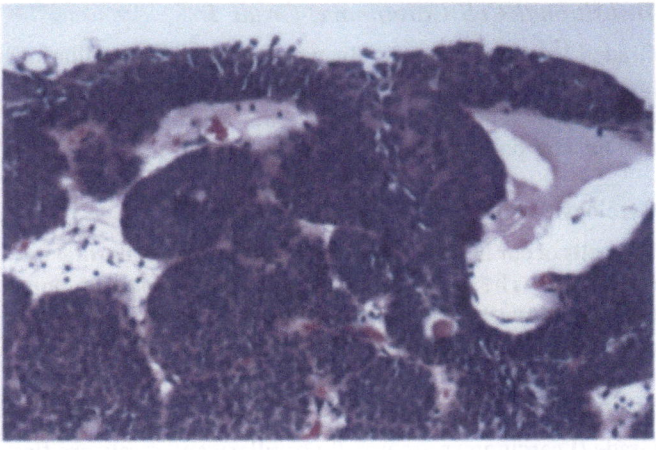

FIGURE 14.4 Inverted papilloma. Compact urothelial papillations in subepithelial tissue.

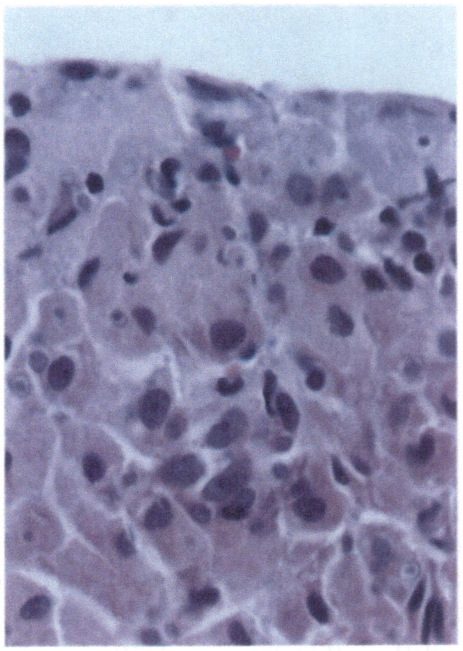

B

FIGURE 14.3 Malakoplakia. A: MG bodies in the foamy macrophages, showing concentrically laminated round inclusion bodies (urinary cytology). (Courtesy of Dr. Nelson Helmquist, ASCP.) B: Cystoscopic biopsy of soft yellow mucosal plaques showing closely packed macrophages with multiple intracytoplasmic MG bodies. (Courtesy of Dr. William M. Murphy, Tenn.).

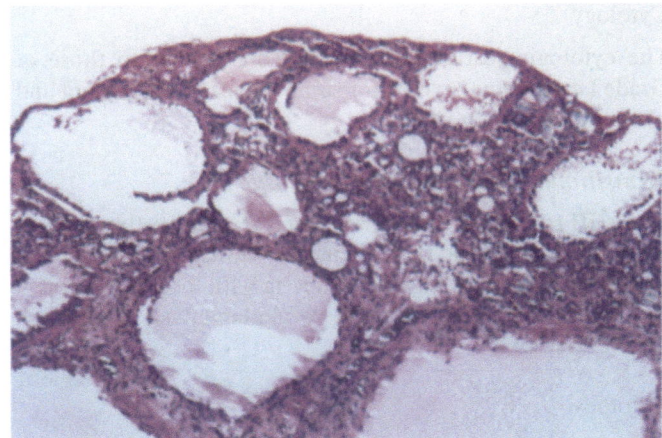

FIGURE 14.5 Nephrogenic adenoma. Polypoid nodule comprising cystic or papillary structures lined or covered by a single layer of cuboidal cells (biopsy).

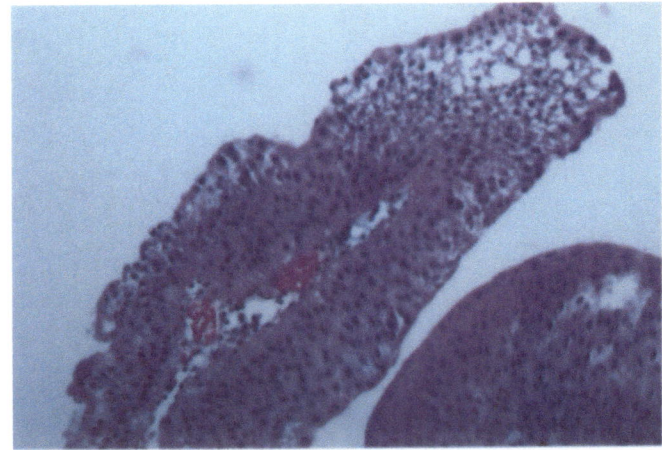

FIGURE 14.6 Transitional cell papilloma. Papillary structures covered by multiple layers (fewer than seven) of normal-appearing urothelial cells.

Transitional Cell Carcinoma, Grade I

Grade I lesions are almost always papillary. The papillations are covered by more than seven layers of cells. The tumor cells resemble normal urothelial cells. There is slight abnormal nuclear polarization but no mitotic figures (Fig. 14.7A).

Cytology

The cells occur in clusters or singly and appear as normal urothelial cells. The nuclei are round to oval with finely granular, bland chromatin. Papillary clustering of cells is a reliable diagnostic feature (Fig. 14.7B).

Transitional Carcinoma, Grade II

Grade II carcinomas are usually papillary and rarely are flat. Cells covering the papillations are slightly enlarged and show some loss of nuclear polarization. Mitotic figures are common (Fig. 14.8A).

Cytology

The cytologic features of Grade II are similar to those of Grade I carcinoma, except for some nuclear enlargement and pleomorphism (Fig. 14.8B).

Transitional Cell Carcinoma, Grade III

Grade III transitional cell carcinomas tend to be flat, fungating, or ulcerative and they are usually invasive. The cells are pleomorphic and arranged in syncytia with loss of cell polarity (Fig. 14.9A). There may be focal glandular or squamous differentiation.

Cytology

The cells are highly pleomorphic and have scanty cytoplasm and hyperchromatic nuclei with prominent macronucleoli (Fig. 14.9B).

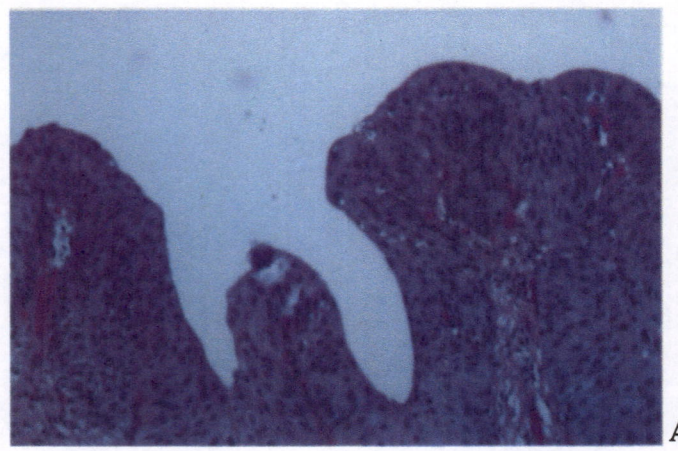

A

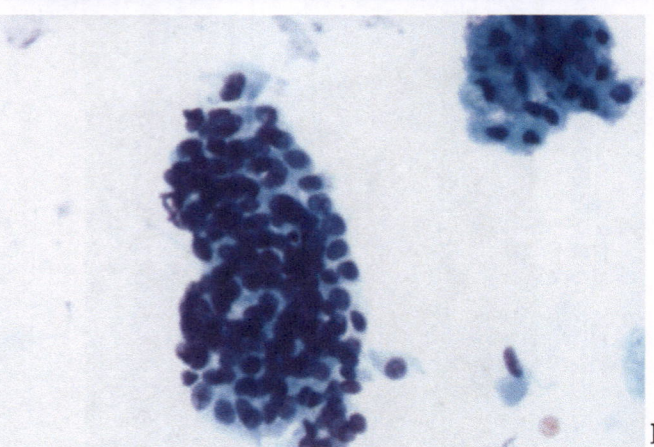

B

FIGURE 14.7 **Papillary transitional cell carcinoma, Grade I. A**: Cystoscopic biopsy showing papillary structures covered by multiple layers of slightly atypical urothelial cells. **B**: Urine cytology showing cluster of neoplastic urothelial cells (centerfield) contrasting with non-neoplastic urothelial cell aggregate (right upper field).

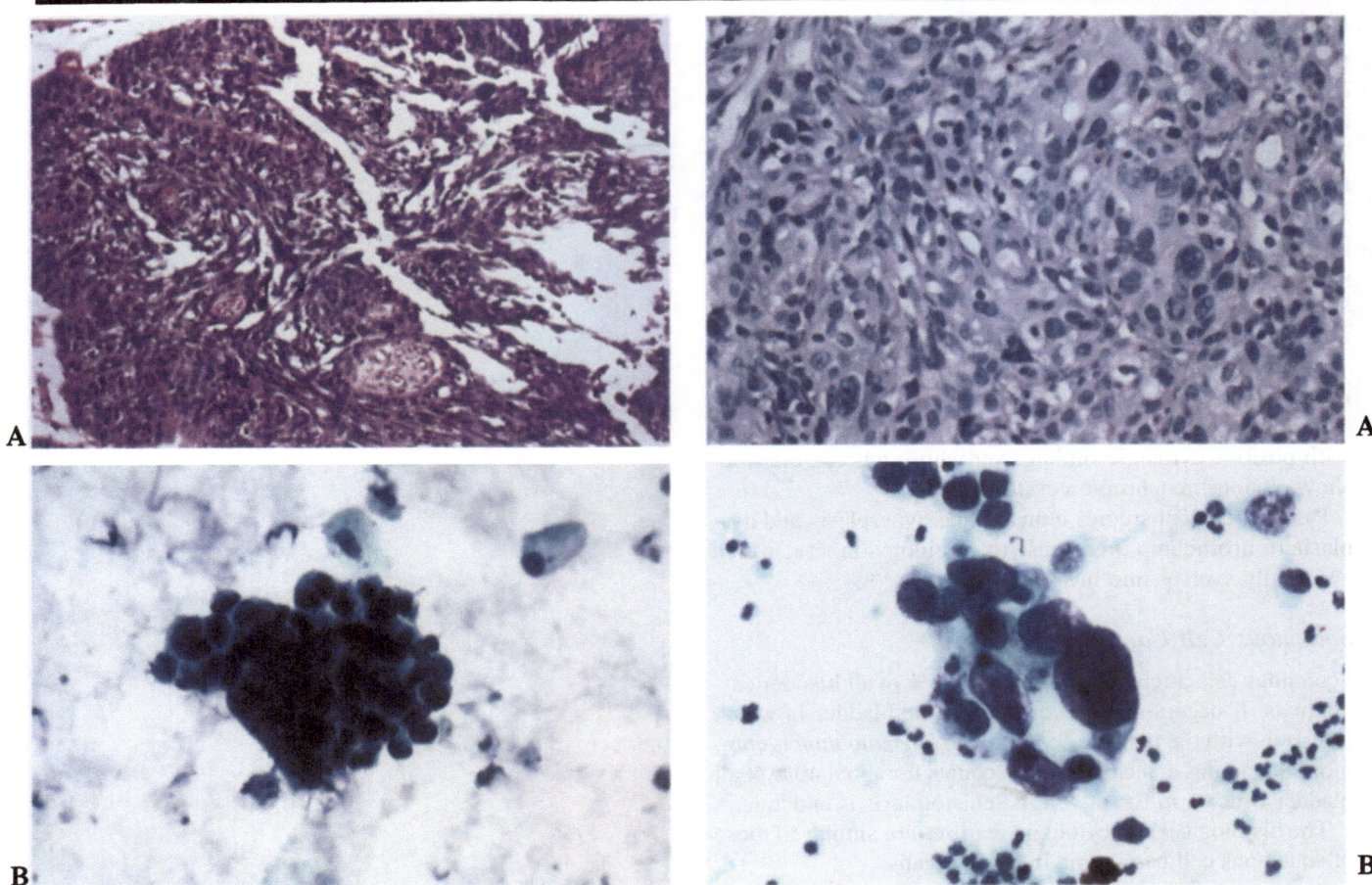

FIGURE 14.8 Papillary transitional cell carcinoma, Grade II. A: Biopsy specimen showing confluent papillary structures covered by urothelial cells exhibiting slight pleomorphism and mitotic figures. **B**: Urine containing papillary clusters of urothelial cells with pleomorphic nuclei and a high nucleocytoplasmic ratio.

FIGURE 14.9 Transitional cell carcinoma, Grade III. A: Biopsy specimen showing sheets of pleomorphic carcinoma cells. **B**: Urine cytology containing a syncytial aggregate of pleomorphic tumor cells.

Carcinoma in situ

Carcinoma in situ refers to a nonpapillary, malignant lesion confined to the mucosa. The lesions are flat and consist of anaplastic cells with total loss of cell polarity (Fig. 14.10A, B). The cytologic features are similar to those of Grade III transitional cell carcinomas (Fig. 14.10C). Carcinomas in situ are most frequently detected in patients known to have or have had bladder cancer and occasionally they are detected by urine cytology screening in populations at risk. Bladder mapping studies on cystectomy specimens for transitional cell carcinoma showed carcinoma in situ in up to 90% of the cases.[3]

Cystoscopically, carcinoma in situ is not remarkable, and may exhibit some mucosal discoloration or a velvety texture. Multiple cystoscopic biopsies are recommended in patients with positive cytologic findings yet whose mucosa does not show obvious neoplasm on cystoscopy.

Past and current studies indicate that hyperplasia and dysplasia of urothelium predispose to carcinoma in situ, which eventually evolves into invasive carcinoma.[4-6]

Squamous Cell Carcinoma

Squamous cell carcinoma accounts for 5% of all bladder carcinomas. It occurs more frequently in the bladder in which infection with the parasite *Schistosoma haematobium* is common. Squamous cell carcinoma accounts for about 40% of all bladder cancers in Egypt where Schistomiasis is endemic.

The histological and cytologic features are similar to those of squamous cell carcinoma in other organs.

Adenocarcinoma

Adenocarcinomas of the bladder account for fewer than 1% of all bladder carcinomas. They may arise from urachal remnants or periurethral or periprostatic glands. Adenocarcinomas arising from the urachal remnants occur at the dome of the bladder (Fig. 14.11A). In urine the cells occur in loose aggregates and clusters. They may show a columnar configuration with amphophilic cytoplasm. The nuclei are round to oval and hyperchromatic and have prominent nucleoli (Fig. 14.11B). Histologically, they are mucin-secreting adenocarcinomas (Fig. 14.11C). The prognosis of adenocarcinoma of the bladder is poor, and metastasis occurs early.

Clinical Course of Bladder Cancer

Hematuria is the most common clinical presentation of bladder cancer. Although most bladder cancers are histologically low grade, they have a strong tendency to recur after excision. Therefore, every patient with bladder cancer should be followed closely with urine cytology and cystoscopy. The prognosis depends on the histologic pattern and clinical stage when first diagnosed.

Death from bladder cancer is usually caused by obstructive uropathy, a consequence of local extension of the cancer to the ureters, and by bacterial infection (Fig. 14.12).

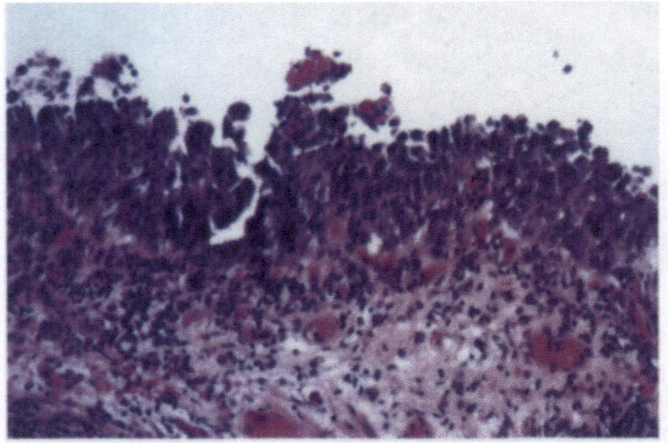
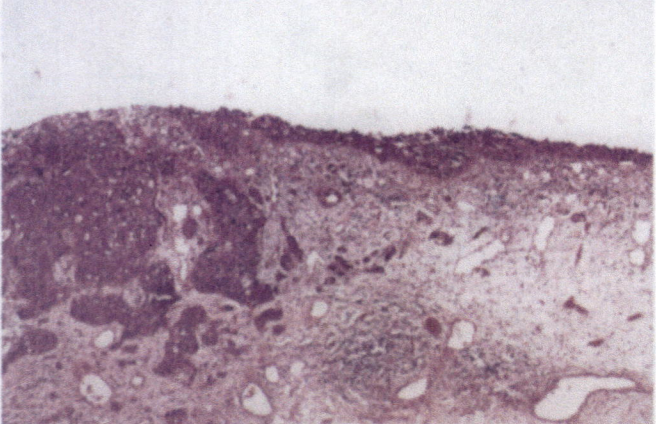
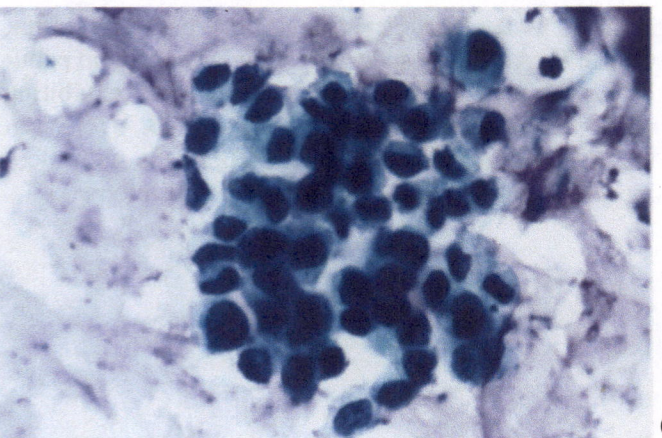

FIGURE 14.10   Carcinoma in situ of urinary bladder. A: Biopsy specimen showing anaplastic cells confined to bladder mucosa. B: Early invasive transitional cell carcinoma for comparison. C: Urine containing syncytial aggregates of anaplastic tumor cells.

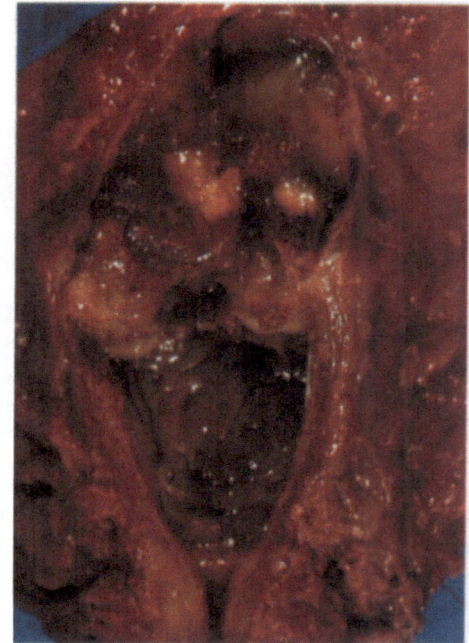

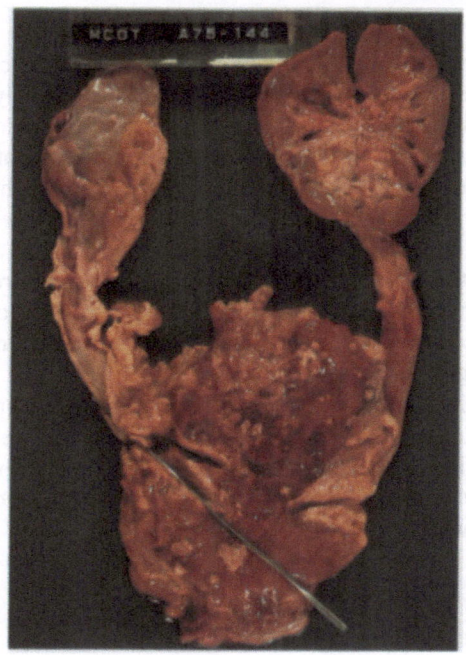

FIGURE 14.12 Obstructive uropathy due to advanced transitional cell carcinoma of urinary bladder. Obstruction of the ureteral orifices, hydroureters, hydronephrosis, and chronic pyelonephritis (necropsy).

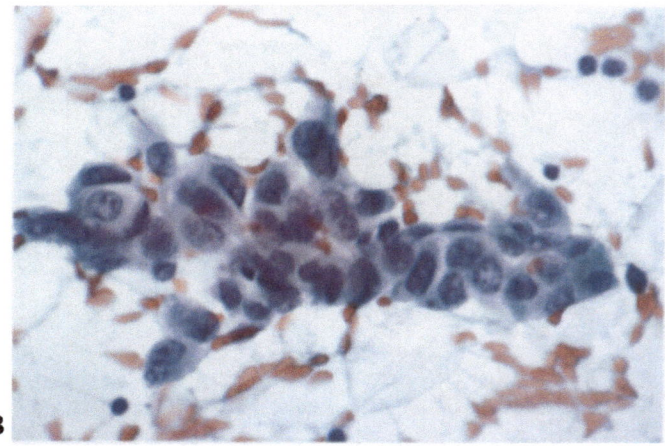

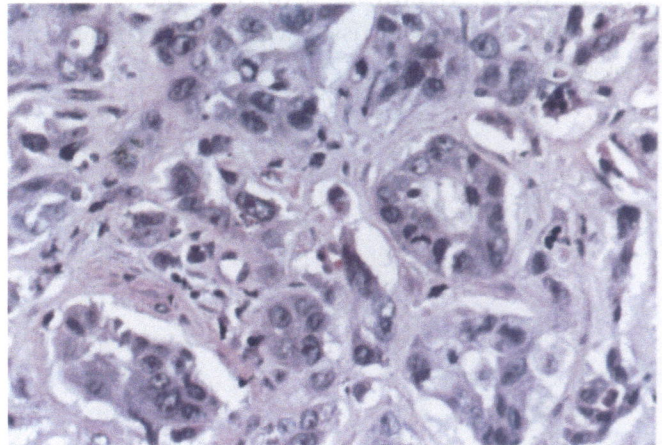

FIGURE 14.11 Adenocarcinoma of urinary bladder. A: The tumor arises in the bladder dome and grows along the urachal remnant. B: Urine showing loose aggregate of tumor cells with a columnar configuration. C: Histologic section showing neoplastic glands and clusters infiltrating the wall.

Diseases of Ureter

Inflammatory disease of the ureter may occur as one component of urinary tract infections and it is histologically similar to that in the bladder. A great variety of pathologic lesions may obstruct the ureters, causing obstructive uropathy with hydroureter, hydronephrosis, and pyelonephritis. The causes of ureteral obstruction are intrinsic ureteral disease and extrinsic lesions compressing the ureters.

The intrinsic causes are calculi, ureteral stricture due to trauma or chronic inflammation, tumors, and blood clot. The common extrinsic causes are neoplasms and inflammation of pelvic organs and retroperitoneum.

The primary malignant tumor of the ureter is transitional cell carcinoma, histologically similar to that of the bladder (Fig. 14.13). The neoplasm may be multifocal in the ureter and may occur synchronously with tumors of the bladder and renal pelvis.

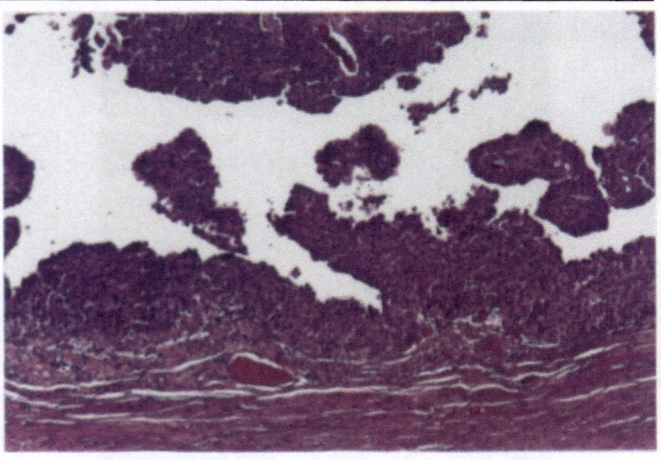

FIGURE 14.13 **Papillary transitional cell carcinoma of the ureter.** The neoplasm arising in the ureteral mucosa obstructs the ureteral lumen.

Tumors of Urethra

Caruncle

Urethral caruncle is an inflammatory polypoid lesion at the external urethral meatus in older women. They present as a red, painful, friable mass, 1 to 2 cm in diameter. Histologically, it consists of highly vascularized, young fibrous connective tissue infiltrated with leukocytes (Fig. 14.14). The overlying epithelium is either of transitional or squamous type.

Carcinoma

Carcinoma of the urethra is an uncommon lesion, usually occurring at the external urethral meatus in older women. Most of these neoplasms are squamous cell carcinomas.

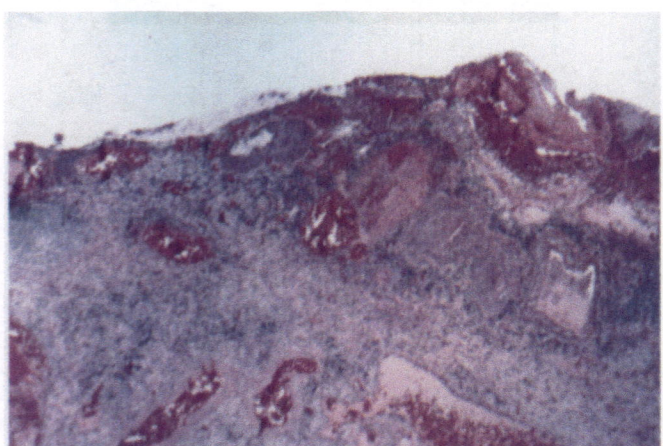

FIGURE 14.14 **Urethral caruncle.** Highly vascularized young connective tissue with leukocytic infiltration (biopsy).

References

1. Moyana TN, Kontozoglou T. Urinary bladder paragangliomas. An immunohistochemical study. *Arch Pathol Lab Med*. 1988;112:70–72.
2. Murphy WM. Current topics in the pathology of bladder cancer. *Pathol Annu*. 1983;18:1.
3. Koss LG. Mapping of the urinary bladder: Its impact on the concepts of bladder cancer. *Hum Pathol*. 1979;10:553.
4. Koss LG. Evaluation of patients with carcinoma in situ of the bladder. *Pathol Annu*. 1982;17:353.
5. Fukui I, et al. Carcinoma in situ of the urinary bladder. *Cancer*. 1987;59:164.
6. Hofstadter F, et al. Urothelial dysplasia and carcinoma in situ of the bladder. *Cancer*. 1986;57:356.

15
Prostate Gland

The prostate gland weighs approximately 20 g in the normal adult. It encircles the bladder neck and urethra, and comprises five lobes: a posterior, middle, and anterior lobe and two lateral lobes. In the course of development the five become fused into three distinct lobes—two major lateral lobes and one fused small median and posterior lobe.

Histologically, the prostate is a compound tubuloalveolar gland. The glands are lined by two layers of cells, a basal layer of cuboidal epithelium covered by a layer of columnar epithelium. The glands have distinct basement membranes and are separated by abundant fibromuscular stroma (Fig. 15.1).

Nodular Hyperplasia

Nodular hyperplasia of the prostate is an extremely common disorder in men over age 50 years in Western countries. The disorder increases in frequency with increasing age, being present in 70% of men by age 60 years. The major clinical manifestations are urinary frequency, incomplete evacuation of the bladder, and dribbling of urine secondary to compression of the urethra by large hyperplastic nodules. However, only 10% of men with this disease eventually require surgical treatment for the relief of urinary tract obstruction.

The prostate is large, soft, and nodular, particularly around the urethra, corresponding to the inner periurethral portion of the middle and lateral lobes. This is a striking contrast to prostatic carcinoma, which usually involves the posterior lobe. On rectal palpation, the prostate is found to contain multiple large and soft nodules. On cross section, the gland is nodular, soft, and bulging.

Histologically, prostate nodular hyperplasia exhibits abundant large glands with multiple intraluminal epithelial tufts covered by two distinct cuboidal and columnar cell layers. The glands are separated by abundant fibromuscular stroma (Fig. 15.2). Fine needle aspirates show benign small epithelial cells arranged in sheets with a characteristic orderly honeycomb appearance.

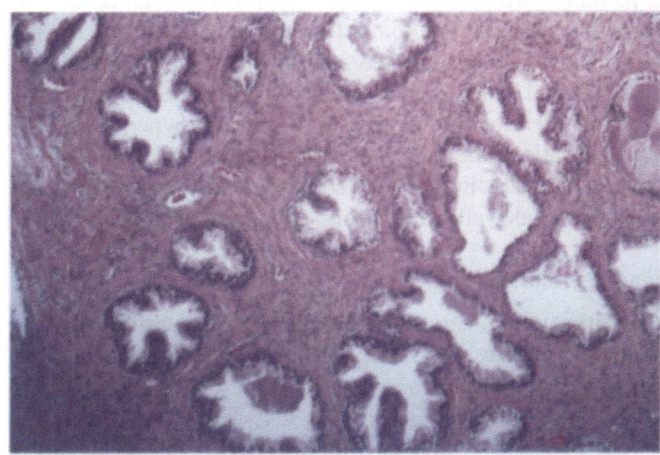

FIGURE 15.1 **Normal prostate gland.** Tubuloglandular spaces separated by abundant fibromuscular stroma.

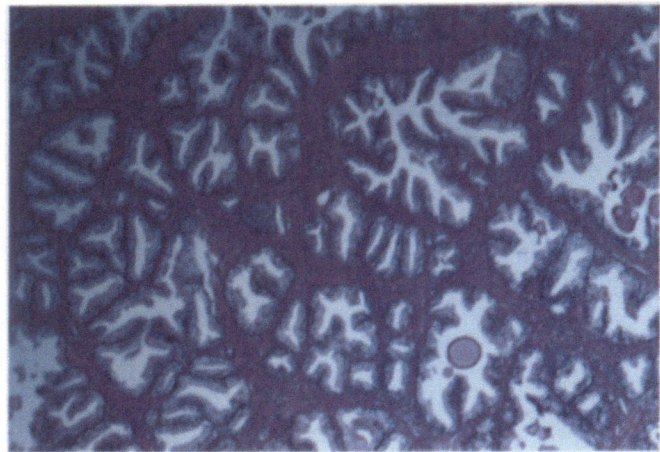

FIGURE 15.2 **Hyperplasia of prostate.** Small and large glands with outpouching and intraluminal tufting.

Adenocarcinoma of Prostate

Adenocarcinoma of the prostate is the most common form of cancer in men and the third leading cause of cancer death in men in the United States.[1] There are remarkable national and racial differences in the prevalence of this disease. Prostatic cancer is rare in Orientals, and more prevalent among blacks than whites in the United States.[2] It is a disease of men over age 50 years, with the highest incidence rate after age 70 years.

Although there are remarkable differences in incidence in terms of age, race, endocrine status, and environmental factors, little is known about causes of prostatic cancer. There is no substantive evidence of a relationship between nodular hyperplasia and the development of prostatic cancer.[3] Almost all patients with prostatic cancer first present at an advanced stage with urinary symptoms. In fewer than 10% of patients are prostatic cancers detected at early stage (stage A or B) by routine rectal palpation or in specimens obtained by transurethral resection of the prostate for nodular hyperplasia. On rectal palpation, the neoplastic nodules are firm and distinct from the surrounding uninvolved tissue. On section, they are pale gray to pale yellow, firm, and flat or retracted (Fig. 15.3).

Histology and Cytology

Most prostate cancers are adenocarcinomas with a distinct glandular pattern and scanty intervening stroma. Grading of adenocarcinomas of the prostate correlates well with clinical stage and prognosis. Failure to achieve reliability and reproducibility in histologic grading has limited the value and general acceptance of many suggested protocols.[4-6]

The grading system developed by Gleason in conjunction with the Veterans Administration Cooperative Urologic Research Group is based on the degree of glandular differentiation and the growth pattern of the carcinoma in relation to the stroma.[7] This system has shown a remarkable correlation with mortality rate and is applied in many pathology departments. Figure 15.4 illustrates five patterns and final grading. Tumor is assigned to a category according to grade on the basis of shape and arrangement of the glands. It ranges from grade 1, most well differentiated pattern, to grade 5, most poorly differentiated pattern. A tumor may consist of a single type of grade throughout the tumor or two dissimilar grades admixed. A combined grade is obtained by adding predominant grade (primary grade) and the other grade (secondary grade) when present. When tumor has the same grade throughout, its combined grade is obtained by doubling the value of this grade.

Gleason grade 1 adenocarcinoma: Uniform tubular glands in closely packed masses with smooth limiting edges (Fig. 15.5).

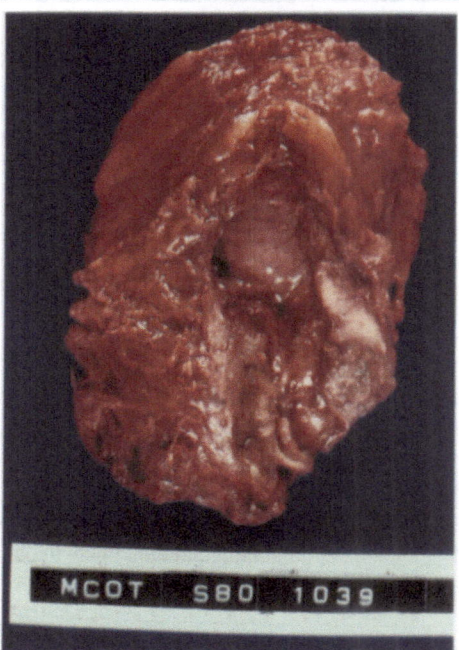

FIGURE 15.3 Adenocarcinoma of prostate. Longitudinal bisection of the prostate showing retracted granular firm tumor in the posterior lobe.

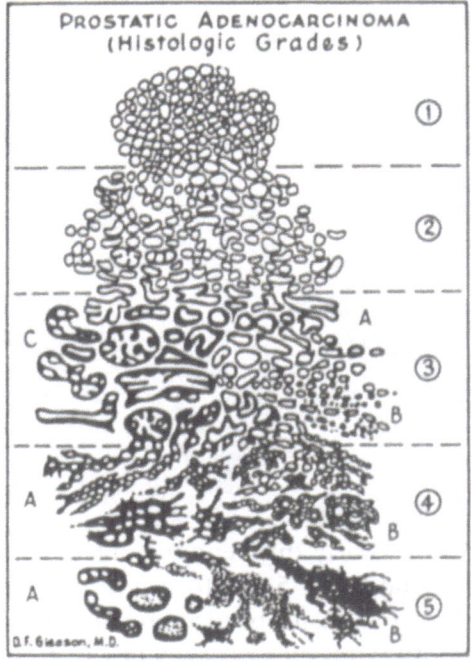

FIGURE 15.4 Gleason grading system of prostatic adenocarcinoma. (Reproduced from Gleason DF, Mellinger DT. Histologic grading and clinical staging of prostatic carcinoma. In: Tannenbaum M, ed. *Urologic Pathology: The Prostate*. Philadelphia: Lea & Febiger, 1977.)

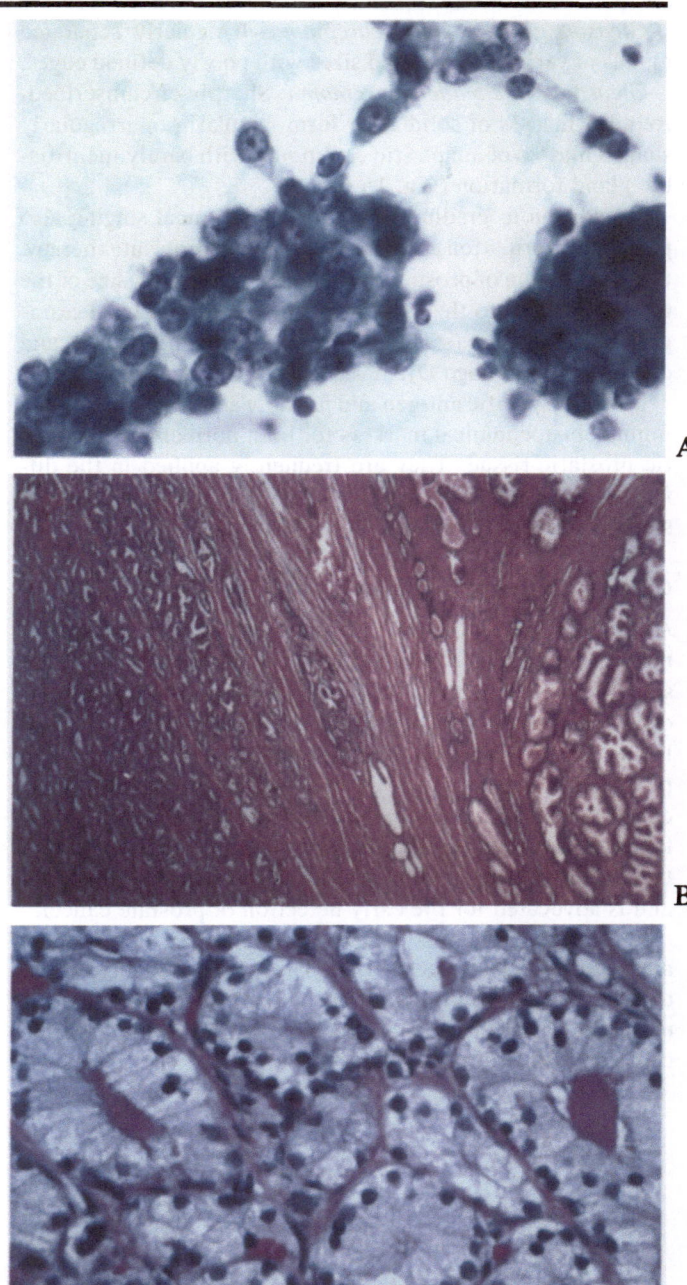

FIGURE 15.5 Well differentiated adenocarcinoma (Gleason's grade 1 + 1 = 2) of prostate. A: FNA smear showing a syncytial aggregate and a cluster of uniform cuboidal to round tumor cells. **B:** Biopsy section showing a compact mass of carcinoma with a smooth limiting edge. **C:** Uniform tubular glands lined by single layer of uniform cuboidal cells.

Gleason grade 3 adenocarcinoma: Irregularly separated glands of various shapes and sizes with poorly defined edges.

Gleason grade 5 adenocarcinoma: Sharply circumscribed, rounded masses of solid cribriform neoplasm or irregularly shaped masses of anaplastic carcinoma with barely identifiable gland formation (Fig. 15.6).

In addition to grading of the tumors, clinical staging also provides information as to prognosis and appropriate therapy. Clinical staging of prostate carcinomas is based on size of the tumor confined to the prostate (stage A and B), local extraprostatic extension (stage C), and spread to lymph nodes and distant viscera (stage D).[8]

Prostate-specific antigen and prostate acid phosphatase are immunohistochemical markers for both normal and neoplastic prostatic tissue. They are frequently applied in the differential diagnosis of metastatic carcinomas where a prostatic origin is in question (Fig. 15.7A–C).

Clinical Course

A few prostatic cancers are discovered incidentally at necropsy or in tissue removed because of prostatic hyperplasia from patients clinically not suspected of having prostatic cancer. This type of prostate cancer is designated as occult or latent cancer (stage A). About 5% to 10% of patients with prostatic cancer do not have urinary symptoms, and the cancer is discovered by the finding of a suspicious nodule on rectal examination (stage B). Transrectal ultrasound may detect twice as many stage A cancers as digital rectal examination and is advocated for the early detection of prostate cancer.[9]

More than 75% of patients with prostatic cancer present at an advanced stage (stage C or D). They come to clinical attention because of urinary symptoms or back pain caused by vertebral metastatic deposits. Osteoblastic metastasis to bone is characteristic of prostatic cancers (Fig. 15.7D).

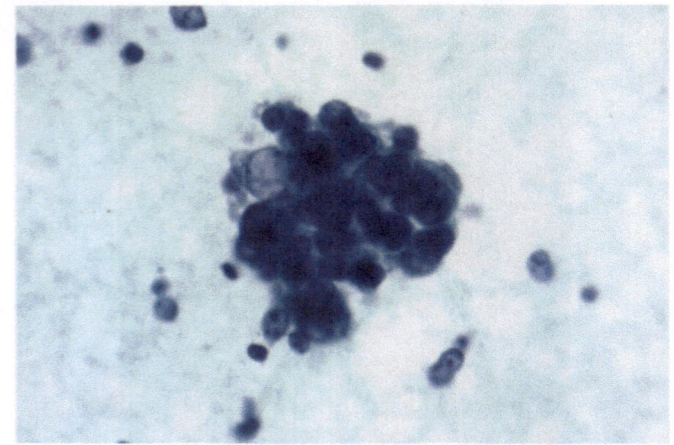

A

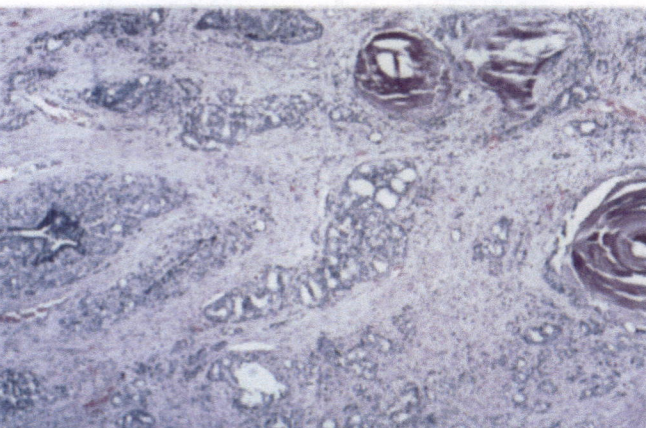

B

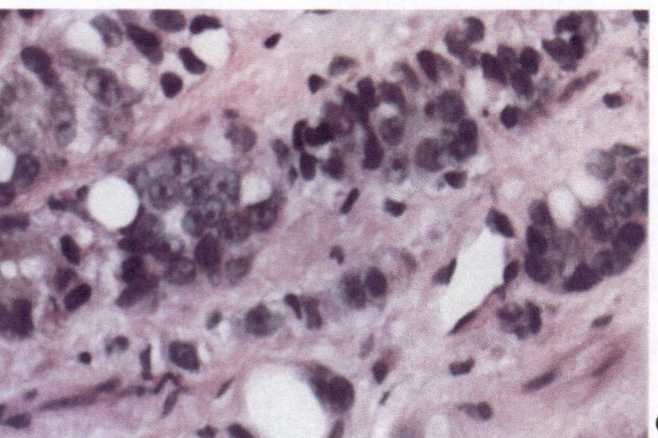

C

FIGURE 15.6 **Poorly differentiated adenocarcinoma (Gleason's grade 5 + 5 = 10) of prostate. A:** FNA smear showing a cluster of pleomorphic tumor cells. **B:** Diffuse infiltrating masses of carcinoma. **C:** Clusters and cords of pleomorphic carcinoma cells.

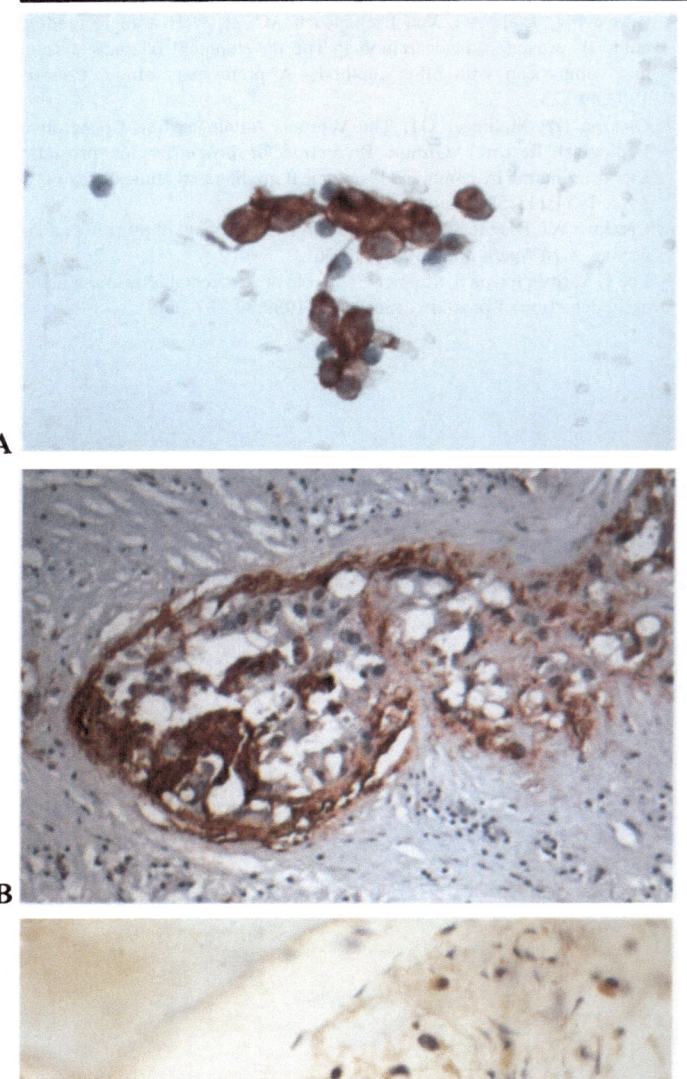

A

B

C

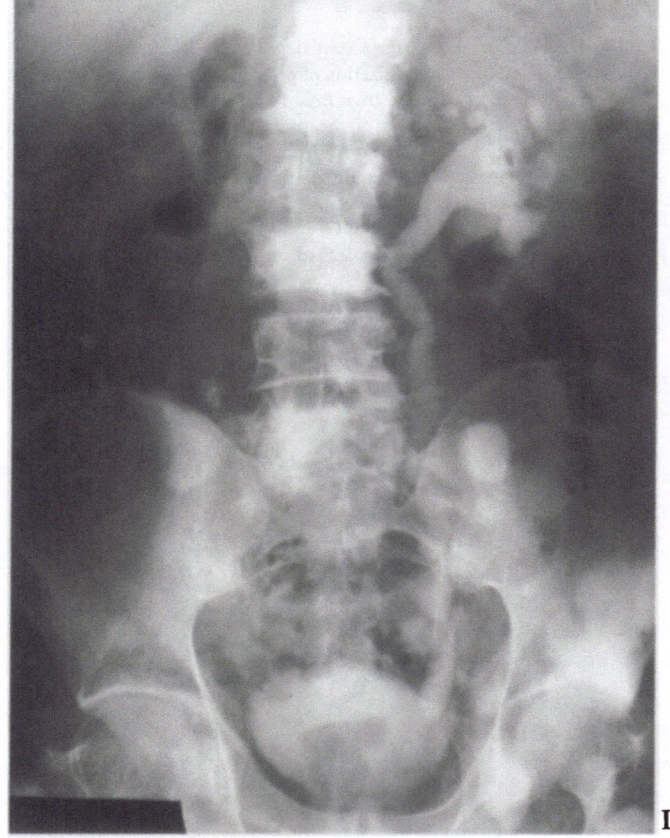

D

FIGURE 15.7 Metastatic adenocarcinoma of prostate. **A**: FNA smear obtained from a retroperitoneal mass showing a cluster of carcinoma cells giving a positive immunochemical reaction for prostatic acid phosphatase. **B**: Biopsy specimen of the carcinoma showing a positive immunocytochemical reaction for prostatic acid phosphatase. **C**: Biopsy specimen from an osteoblastic lesion in a vertebra showing adenocarcinoma giving a positive reaction for prostate specific antigen. **D**: Radiograph demonstrating metastatic prostate adenocarcinoma to a vertebra and obstructive uropathy of the left kidney and ureter.

References

1. Silverberg E, Lubera J. Cancer Statistics, 1989. *CA*. 1989;39:3.

2. Jackson MS, et al. Characterization of prostatic cancer among blacks. A continuation report. *Cancer Treat Rep*. 1977;61:167.

3. Greenwald P, et al. Cancer of the prostate among men with benign prostatic hyperplasia. *J Natl Cancer Inst*. 1974;53:335.

4. Mostofi FK. Grading of prostatic carcinoma. *Cancer Chemother Rep*. 1975;59:111.

5. Gaeta JF, Asirwatham JE, Miller G, et al. Histologic grading of primary prostatic cancer: A new approach to an old problem. *J Urol*. 1980; 123:689.

6. Brawn PN, Ayala AG, Von Eschenbach AC, et al. Histologic grading study of prostate adenocarcinoma: The development of anew system and comparison with other methods—A preliminary study. *Cancer*. 1982;49:525.

7. Gleason DF, Mellinger GT. The Veterans Administration Cooperative Urological Research Group: Prediction of prognosis for prostatic adenocarcinoma by combined histological grading and clinical staging. *J Urol*. 1974;111:58–64.

8. Catalona WJ. Diagnosis, staging and surgical treatment of prostatic carcinomas. *Arch Intern Med*. 1987;147:361.

9. Lee F, Torp-Petersen S, Siders D. The role of transrectal ultrasound in the early detection of prostate cancer. *CA*. 1989;39:337–360.

16
Testis

Tumors of Testis

About 95% of testicular tumors are of germ cell origin, and they are quite aggressive and spread widely. Testicular tumors of non-germ cell origin are generally benign, and some of them elaborate steroid hormones resulting in endocrinologic syndromes.

The World Health Organization (WHO) Pathologic Classification of Testicular Tumors differs only in minor aspects from the Mostofi classification.[1] It is based on the concept that germ cells may differentiate into seminoma (gonadal differentiation) or into totipotential tumor cells represented by embryonal carcinoma, choriocarcinoma and yolk sac tumor. Teratoma, on the other hand, results from the differentiation of embryonic carcinoma cells along the lines of all three germ cell layers, thus resulting in a variety of neoplastic tissue.[2]

Germ Cell Tumors

Although germ cell tumors are rare, they are the most common testicular tumors in the 15- to 34-year-old age group of men, and cause about 10% of all cancer deaths. Two smaller peaks of incidence are encountered in infancy and in later life. About 30% to 40% of germ cell tumors comprise a single cell type, and the rest of them have mixed patterns.

Seminoma

Seminoma is the most common type of germ cell tumor, and occurs most often in the fourth decade. Patients present with unilateral testicular enlargement. Grossly, seminomas are well circumscribed, lobular masses. On section, they are pale, gray, with a homogeneous cut surface, and they partly or totally replace the testis (Fig. 16.1A).

Histologically, the typical seminoma consists of large, polyhedral cells arranged in sheets divided into a lobular pattern by delicate fibrous septae. The cells are large and have vacuolated cytoplasm and large, round, central hyperchromatic nuclei with prominent macronucleoli. Mitotic figures are infrequent. The septae are infiltrated with lymphocytes or histiocytes (Fig. 16.1B). The anaplastic seminoma exhibits greater cytologic atypia and frequent mitotic figures.

Fine needle aspiration is rarely performed to distinguish malignant from benign testicular tumors. In aspirates, the cells occur singly and in loose aggregates. The cells are large, polyhedral, and have vacuolated cytoplasm. The nuclei are large, round, and hyperchromatic, and have prominent macronucleoli (Fig. 16.1C).

Spermatocytic Seminoma

Spermatocytic seminoma is a unique and distinctive type of neoplasm. It occurs usually in patients over the age of 65 years, and they are slowly growing tumors that rarely metastasize. Grossly, spermatocytic seminomas tend to be larger than classic seminomas and present with a pale, gray, soft, and friable cut surface.

Histologically, they consist of a mixture of cells varying in size and arranged in haphazard sheets. The nuclei are round and vary in size. Mitotic figures are infrequently seen. Ultrastructurally, the cells show clear-cut evidence of spermatocytic differentiation.[3,4]

Embryonal Carcinoma

Embryonal cell carcinomas occur mostly in the 20- to 30-year-old age group, and they are more aggressive than seminomas. Grossly, they present as a small to large, poorly demarcated mass. On section, the tumors are pale, gray, soft, and punctuated by multifocal necrosis and hemorrhage. Extension through the tunica albuginea, epididymis, or cord is common (Fig. 16.2A).

Histologically, the cells grow in glandular, alveolar, or tubular patterns and sometimes as poorly differentiated sheets. The cells have epithelial features, and are large, anaplastic, and variable in size and shape. The nuclei are large, pleomorphic, and hyperchromatic, and have prominent macronucleoli. Mitotic figures and tumor giant cells are frequent (Fig. 16.2B). Human chorionic gonadotropin (HCG) or alpha-fetoprotein (AFP) may be identified focally by immunocytochemistry.

Yolk Sac Tumor (Endodermal Sinus Tumor)

There are two distinct patterns of yolk sac tumor: 1) pure yolk sac tumor with the classical organoid appearance described by Teilum, which occurs in infants and children and has an excellent prognosis, and 2) mixed germ cell tumor with a yolk sac component, which occurs in adults and has a poor prognosis.

Grossly, the pure form of yolk sac tumor of infants is non-encapsulated and on section it presents a homogeneous, pale gray, mucinous appearance.

Histologically, the tumor consists of numerous microcystic spaces lined by flat to cuboidal epithelial cells. Endodermal sinuses, a characteristic feature of this neoplasm, consist of a mesodermal core with a central capillary and a visceral and parietal layer of cells reminiscent of a primitive glomerulus (Schiller-Duval body) (Fig. 16.3A, B). Eosinophilic, periodic acid-Schiff (PAS)-positive hyaline droplets are usually present within and outside the cells. AFP can be demonstrated in the cells by immunocytochemical staining (Fig. 16.3C).

Choriocarcinoma

Choriocarcinoma is a highly malignant tumor that occurs rarely in the testis. The tumor occurs in placental tissue and ovary and is identified more often as focal components of mixed germ cell tumors. Grossly, it may present as a small hemorrhagic mass in the testis or as an extratesticular metastatic deposit. On the other hand, it may present as a hemorrhagic, large, bulky mass in the testis.

Histologically, the tumor is similar to those of the ovary and placenta, consisting of syncytiotrophoblastic and cytotrophoblastic cells. Syncytiotrophoblastic cells are large and pleomorphic, and have abundant eosinophilic cytoplasm and pleomorphic, hyperchromatic nuclei. Immunocytochemical stains may demonstrate HCG in the cells. Cytotrophoblastic cells are polygonal with distinct cell borders and clear cytoplasm, and have uniform nuclei.

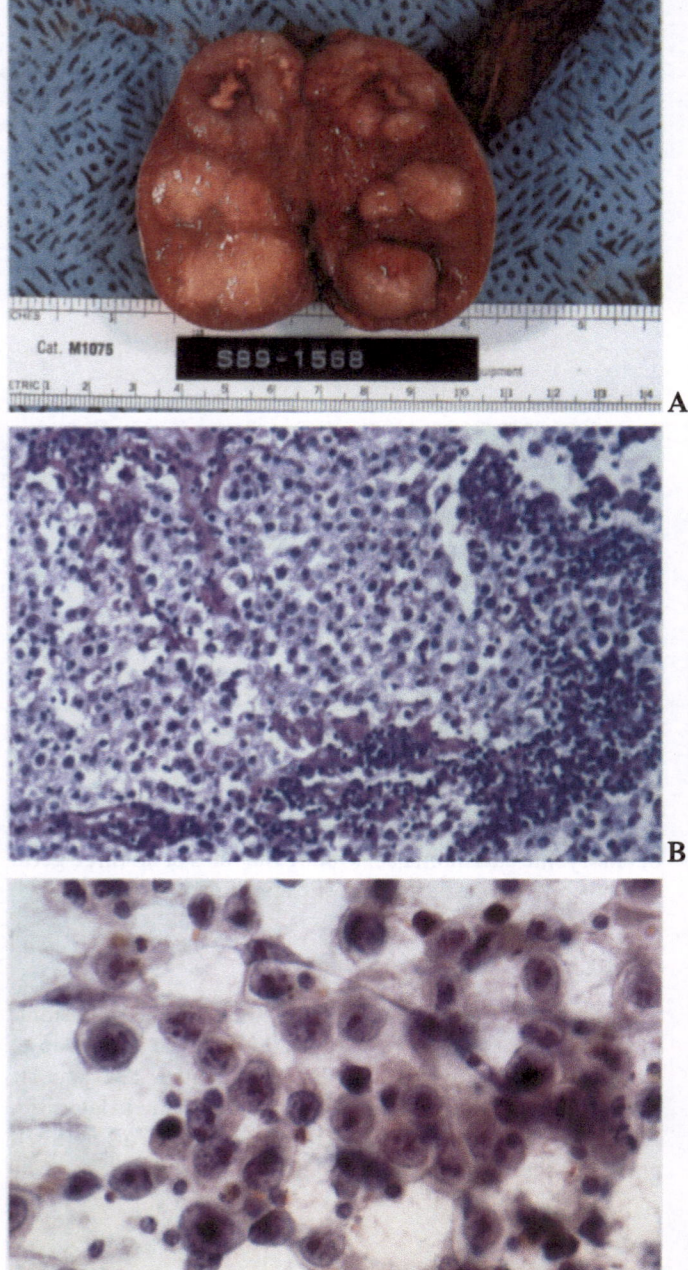

FIGURE 16.1   Seminoma of testis. A: Well defined lobular mass on cross section (gross). B: Histologic section showing large round tumor cells arranged in sheets separated by delicate fibrous septae. C: FNA smears showing loose aggregates of large round tumor cells.

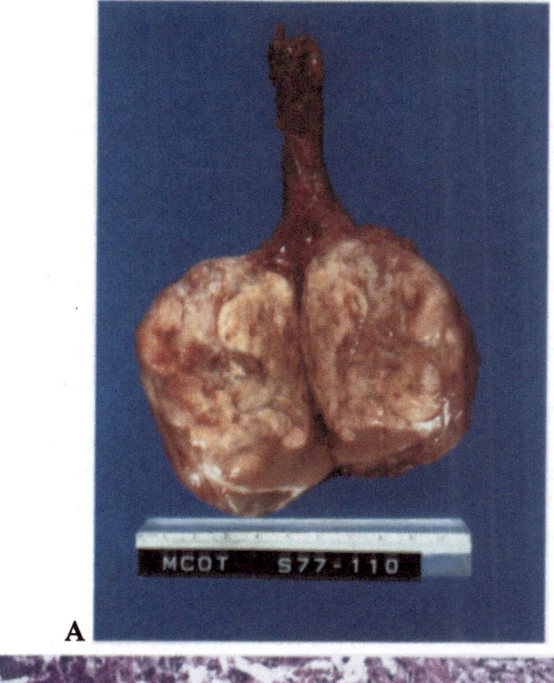

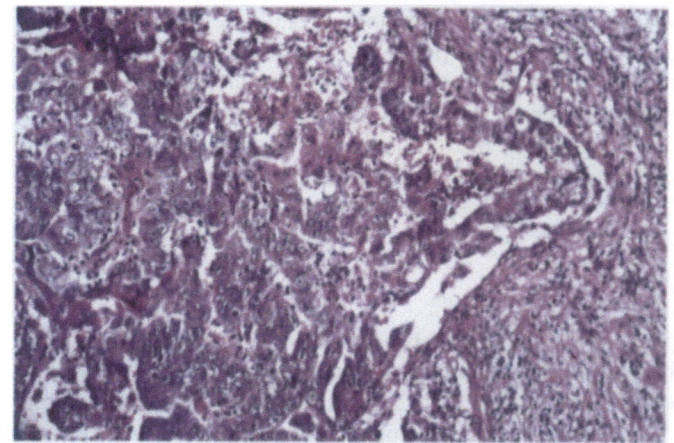

FIGURE 16.2 Embryonal cell carcinoma of testis. A: Pale gray, soft tumor mass infiltrating to the tunica albuginea (cross section of the testis). **B**: Histologic section showing large polygonal tumor cells arranged in glands, cords, and sheets.

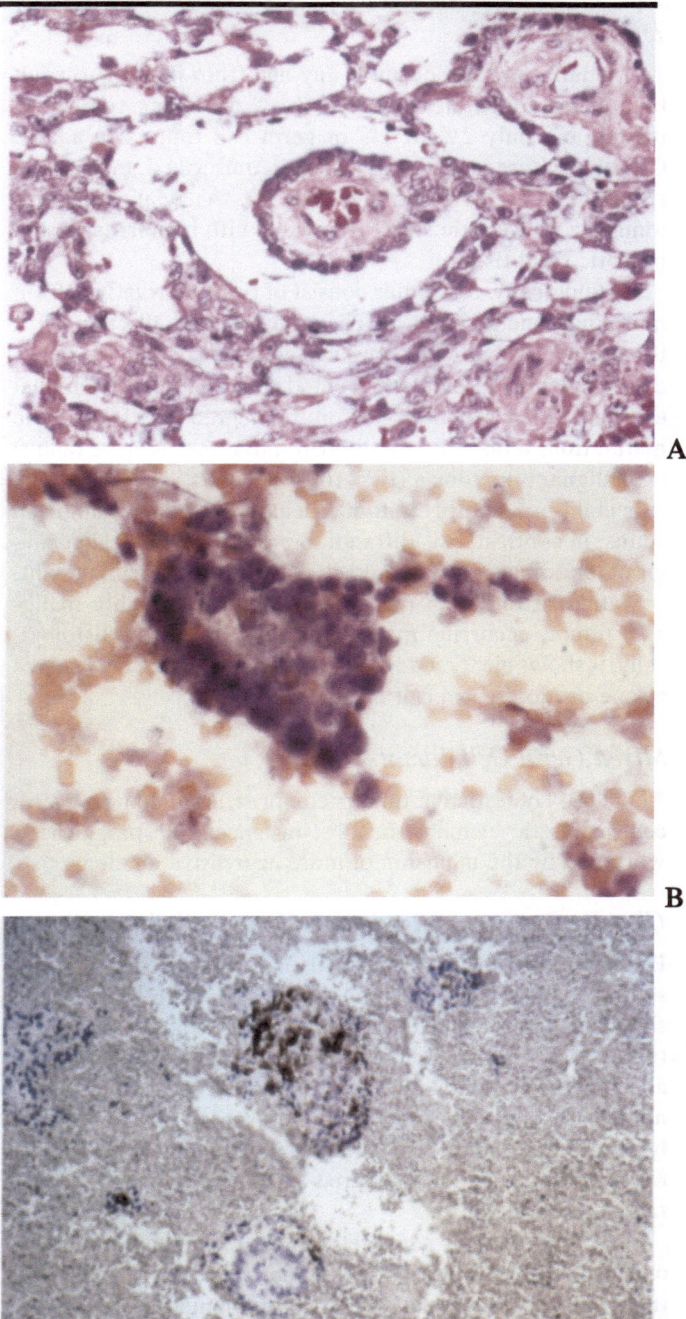

FIGURE 16.3 Yolk sac tumor of testis. A: Histologic section showing characteristic Schiller-Duval bodies. **B**: FNA smears obtained from a retroperitoneal metastatic deposit showing a cluster of neoplastic cells forming a Schiller-Duval body. **C**: A positive reaction for alpha-fetoprotein in the tumor cells (immunostain).

Teratoma

Testicular teratomas occur at any age from infancy to adult life. They constitute about 40% of testicular tumors in infants, but only 2% to 3% of germ cell tumors in adults. Grossly, mature teratoma is a well circumscribed, multicystic structure with foci of cartilage (Fig. 16.4A). Malignant teratoma is a multicystic structure mixed with hemorrhagic and necrotic solid tissue.

Histologically, teratomas consist of tissue derivatives from more than one germ layer. They may contain all or some of the following elements: neural or squamous elements (ectoderm), glandular elements (entoderm), and mesenchymal elements (mesoderm). Based on the degree of cell or tissue maturation, teratomas are divided into either mature (adult) or malignant teratomas (Fig. 16.4B).

In children, mature teratomas behave as a benign tumor. In adults, in contrast, it is difficult to predict the clinical behavior of teratomas. They should all be considered as malignant.

Malignant teratoma (teratocarcinoma) is a highly malignant tumor, occurring more commonly in adults. Histologically, it shows clear evidence of malignancy in the derivatives of one or more germ cell layers.

Mixed Germ Cell Tumors

About 60% of testicular tumors comprise more than one germ cell neoplastic element. In most instances, the prognosis is worsened by the inclusion of more aggressive elements.

Clinical Features of Testicular Germ Cell Tumors

Painless enlargement of the testis is the most common presenting feature. Unless proved otherwise, any testicular mass should be considered to be neoplastic. Testicular germ cell tumors can be separated into two broad categories: seminoma and nonseminomatous germ cell tumors (NSGCT). Seminomas are radiosensitive. They first spread to the regional lymph nodes; later they spread by hematogenous routes. Most seminomas are discovered at an early stage. The cure rate is more than 90%.

Nonseminomatous germ cell tumors encompass tumors of one histologic type other than seminoma and those with more than one histologic pattern. Nonseminomatous germ cell tumors usually present at an advanced stage clinically and are relatively radioresistant.

Tumors of Sex Cord–Gonadal Stroma

Leydig's (Interstitial) Cell Tumor

Leydig's cell tumors account for only 2% of testicular tumors and occur at any age. The most common clinical presentation is testicular swelling, occasionally with gynecomastia. Leydig's cell tumors may elaborate androgens or androgens and estrogens, and rarely corticosteroids. If the tumors occur in children, they may present with precocious puberty. Grossly, the tumors range from small nodules to a large mass. On section, they are well circumscribed, yellow-brown, and soft.

Histologically, the tumors consist of polyhedral cells arranged in solid sheets or in trabecular pattern. The cells have abundant, granular, eosinophilic cytoplasm. Rod-shaped cytoplasmic crystalloids of Reinke are frequently observed. The nuclei are small and round. Only 10% of Leydig's cell tumors show evidence of malignancy with metastasis to lymph nodes, liver, and lung.

Sertoli's Cell Tumor (Androblastoma)

Sertoli's cell tumors are derived from the sex cord and comprise Sertoli's cells. They may produce estrogens or androgens but rarely cause precocious masculinization or feminization. Grossly, the tumors appear as firm nodules. On section, they are homogeneous, pale gray to yellow.

Histologically, the tumors consist of columnar or polyhedral cells arranged in cords reminiscent of seminiferous tubules. The cells have abundant, vacuolated cytoplasm and small, round nuclei. Ten percent of these tumors are malignant.

Testicular Lymphoma

Malignant lymphomas account for 5% of all testicular tumors, but it is the most common testicular tumor in men over the age of 60 years. About 8% to 20% of children with acute lymphocytic leukemia have leukemic involvement of the testis.

In most cases, disseminated lymphoma follows detection of the testicular mass; only rarely does it remain confined to the testis.[5] In most cases the histologic type is diffuse, large cell lymphoma (Fig. 16.5).

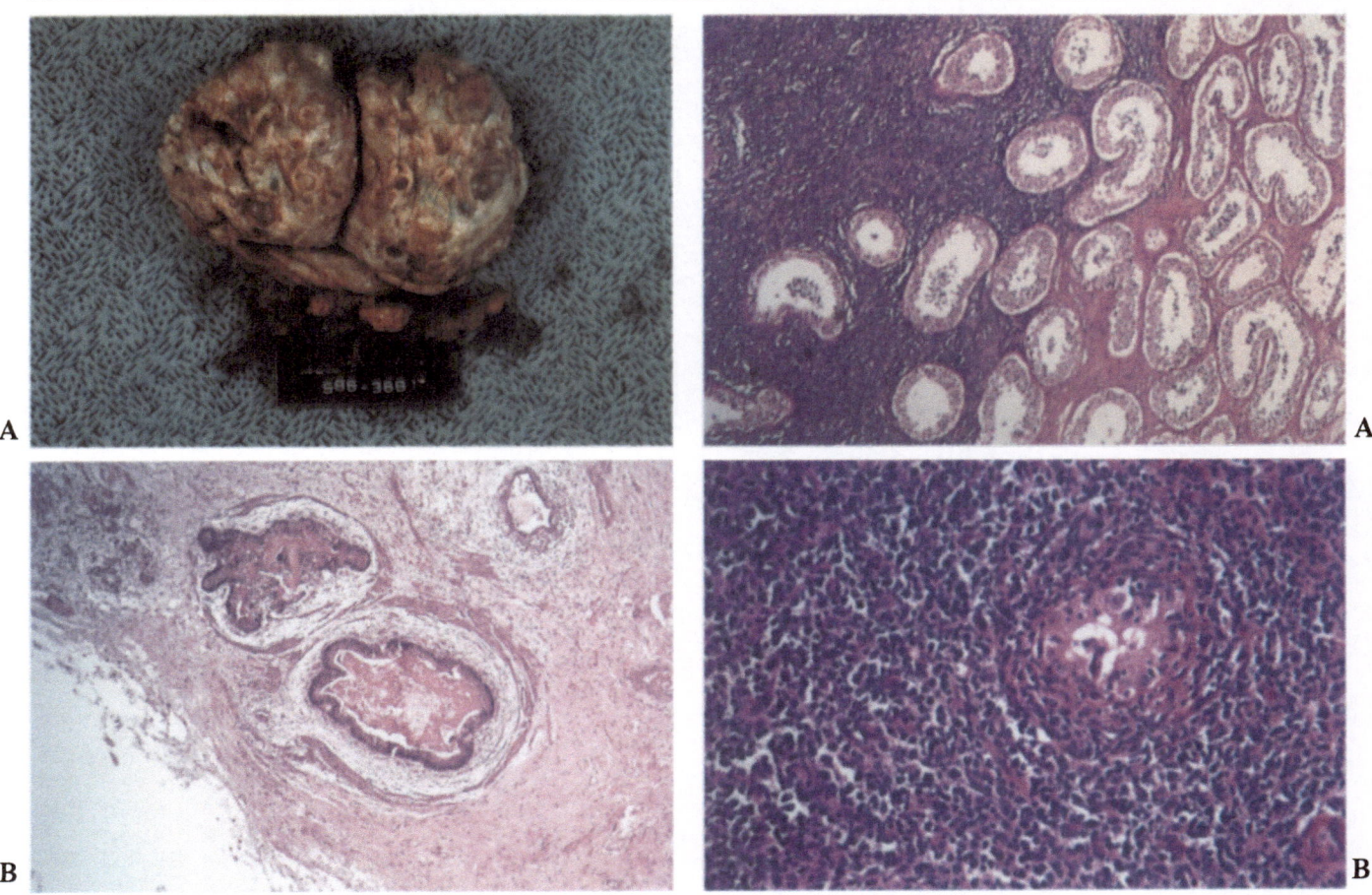

FIGURE 16.4 **Teratoma of testis. A**: Multicystic tumor mass replacing the entire testis (cross section). **B**: Histologic section showing tubuloglandular tissue, an entodermal derivative.

FIGURE 16.5 **Lymphoma of testis. A**: Neoplastic lymphoid cells infiltrate the testis diffusely. **B**: Lymphoma cells compressing the seminiferous tubules.

References

1. Mostofi FK, Sesterhenn IA. Pathology of germ cell tumors of testes. *Prog Clin Biol Res*. 1985;203:1.
2. Pierce GG, Jr, Abell MA. Embryonal carcinoma of the testis. In: Sommers SC, ed. *Pathology Annual*. New York: Appleton-Century-Crofts, 1970:27.
3. Rosai J, Khodadoust K, Silber I. Spermatocytic seminoma. II. ultrastructural study. *Cancer*. 1969;24:103–106.
4. Talerman A, Fu YS, Okagaki T. Spermatocytic seminoma. Ultrastructural and microspectrophotometric observations. *Lab Invest*. 1984;51:343–349.
5. Doll DC, Weiss RB. Malignant lymphoma of testes. *Am J Med*. 1986; 81:515.

17
Vulva and Vagina

Infectious and Inflammatory Diseases of the Lower Female Genital Tract

A number of infectious diseases involve the female genital tract, most of them being identified by culture. Some infectious diseases that may be diagnosed or at least suspected by cytology or histopathology will be reviewed.

Among the microorganisms commonly causing venereal diseases are *Gardnerella vaginalis* (*Haemophilis vaginalis*), *Trichomonas vaginalis*, Herpes simplex virus Type II, Human Papilloma Virus, *Chlamydia trachomatis*, and *Neisseria gonorrhoeae*. In women in the reproductive phase of life, the vagina maintains an acidic pH by the production of lactic acid by acidogenic bacilli, which metabolize the glycogen in intermediate squamous cells. This acidic environment helps to maintain a normal balance of microorganisms.

Instrumentation, trauma (including surgery), immunosuppression, hormonal imbalances, and metabolic disorders are some of the factors known to predispose to the development of nonvenereal bacterial and candidal vulvovaginitis.

Gardnerella Vaginitis

Gardner and Dukes pointed out that the changes of "nonspecific vaginitis" were usually related to the presence of organisms initially classified as *Haemophilis vaginalis*.

Gardnerella vaginitis is clinically characterized by malodorous vaginal discharge in the absence of trichomoniasis, candidiasis and gonorrhea. The causative organism, *Corynebacterium vaginale*, is a nonmotile gram-negative bacillus that is sexually transmitted.

In 1980, the designation *Gardnerella vaginalis* was proposed. Either in wet mounts or Papanicolaou smears, tiny grainy bacillary structures are seen stuck on the surface of squamous epithelial cells ("clue cells") (Fig. 17.1). When "clue cells" are observed in cellular samples, *G. vaginalis* is identified by culture in more than 87% of the cases.[1] Because no significant tissue change is present, biopsy is not necessary.

Trichomoniasis

Trichomoniasis is a common venereal disease of the reproductive years, with a prevalence ranging from 15% (private patients) to 90% (prostitutes). Trichomoniasis is clinically characterized by malodorous vaginal secretion, or it may be asymptomatic. The causative organism is a flagellate protozoan with an oval shape, 10 to 20 μm in length and 5 to 10 μm in width. Wet mounts are considered to be the optimal practical method for identifying the organism, which is actively motile. In Papanicolaou-stained smears, the organisms appear as small, oval, pear-shaped forms with a lightly cyanophilic cytoplasmic staining reaction. In some trichomonads, an eccentric, pale-staining, almond-shaped nucleus may be seen (Fig. 17.2). Biopsy is not necessary to make the diagnosis.

Herpes Simplex Virus Type II Infection

There are two types of Herpes simplex virus (HSV): Types I and II. On the basis of antigenic and biologic differences, recent evidence suggests that 85% to 90% of the genital herpetic infections are caused by HSV Type II, and 10% to 15% by HSV Type I.[2] Most herpetic genital infections are transmitted sexually. The virus has strong infectivity and oncogenic potential.

Symptoms develop usually within 3 to 7 days after exposure. In primary infections, the changes are widespread and may involve the vulva, perianal skin, cervix, and vagina. With the development of vesicles, there may be pain and systemic symptoms. The vesicles subsequently give rise to shallow ulcers. With recurrent infection, the lesions are less conspicuous. Cytologic samples from women with genital herpes simplex are characterized in their early stage by smooth, "glassy"-appearing chromatin and later by enlarged squamous cells containing large multiple or multilobulated nuclei that contain eosinophilic inclusions (Fig. 17.3). The cytologic identification of herpetic viral infections in pregnant patients is important because of possible damage to the infant. Biopsy is not commonly used to establish the diagnosis.

The histopathologic features of herpes simplex are acantholysis and acute inflammation. Cells containing intranuclear viral inclusions are observed at the margin of the ulcer.

Gonorrhea

The diagnosis of gonorrhea is based primarily on clinical observations supplemented by culture. Identification of *Neisseria gonorrhoeae* by cytologic technique is not recommended.

Chlamydia Trachomatis Infections (C. Trachomatis)

Chlamydial infection, the most common sexually transmitted disease in the United States and Europe, is the leading cause of infertility and ectopic pregnancy.[3] About 4.6 million cases of chlamydial infections occur annually, with the infections being found in 1 in 13 women younger than age 25 years. *Chlamydia trachomatis* has properties shared by viruses and bacteria. Like viruses, they grow only intracellularly. Unlike viruses, they contain both DNA and RNA, divide by binary fission, and have cell walls similar to those observed in gram-negative bacteria.[4-6]

Chlamydia trachomatis may cause acute mucopurulent cervicitis and acute pelvic inflammatory disease. Since as many as 70% of women infected with the organism are asymptomatic, routine screening of women categorized as at risk for chlamydial infection is recommended. Chlamydial organisms preferentially infect glandular epithelial cells; consequently vaginal infection is rare.[4-6] The cytologic identification of *C. trachomatis* is not reliable. Smears obtained from the cervix show aggregates of finely granular, uniform, eosinophilic, or cyanophilic bodies in the cytoplasm of columnar or squamous metaplastic cells. Sometimes the inclusion bodies (elementary bodies) are identified in the vacuolated cytoplasm (Fig. 17.4). *Chlamydia trachomatis* cervicitis is diagnosed most accurately by culture or immunofluorescence technique, using monoclonal antibodies to *C. trachomatis*.

Non-Neoplastic Epithelial Disorders of the Vulva

The diagnosis of most vulvar lesions should be confirmed by biopsy. Cytology is usually unrewarding for vulvar lesions. The following lesions will be considered because they are relatively frequent and clinically they may simulate malignancy.

Squamous Hyperplasia

Squamous hyperplasia is usually found in women between 30 and 60 years of age as a nonspecific response of vulval skin to a wide variety of irritants. It accounts for about one half of all vulval epithelial changes. Grossly, the lesions may be white, red, or bright pink. The surface may be wrinkled and raised or scaly and eczematoid. In the absence of epithelial atypia, such a benign squamous epithelial hyperplasia has no relationship to carcinoma (Fig. 17.5).

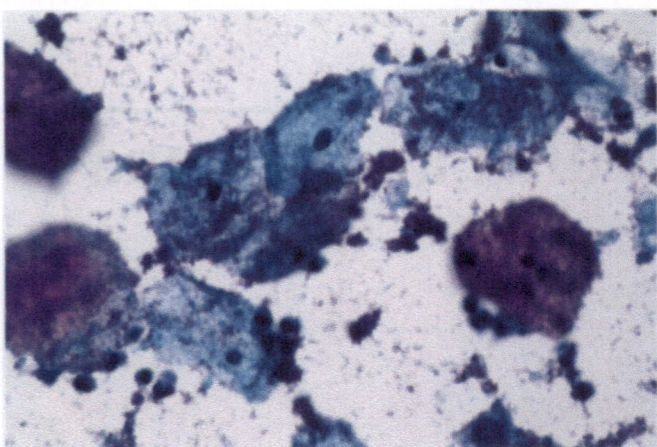

FIGURE 17.1 *Gardnerella vaginalis* ("clue cells") (Papanicolaou smear). Grainy structures, stuck on the surface of squamous epithelial cells.

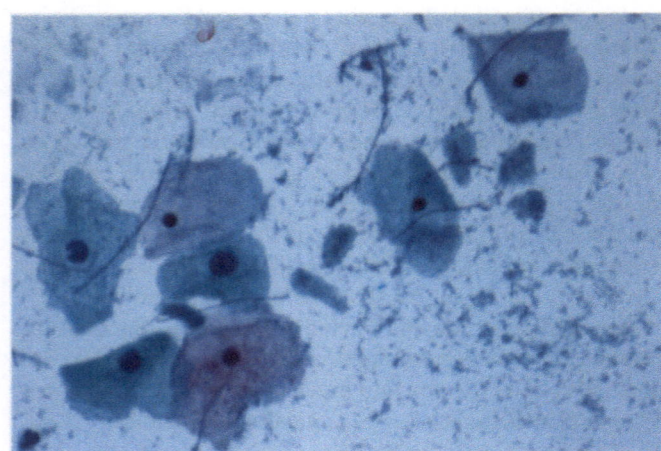

FIGURE 17.2 *Trichomonas vaginalis* (Papanicolaou smear). Small oval to pear-shaped organisms.

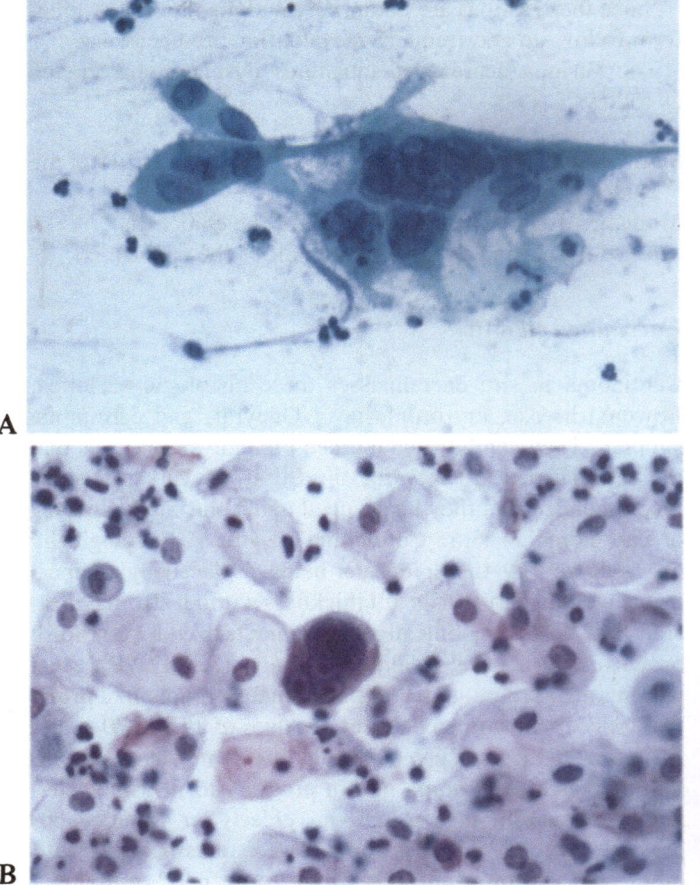

A

B

FIGURE 17.3 Herpes genitalis (Papanicolaou smear). A: Multinucleate herpes giant cells with multiple "ground glass" nuclei (early phase). **B**: Multinucleate herpes giant cells with intranuclear eosinophilic inclusions.

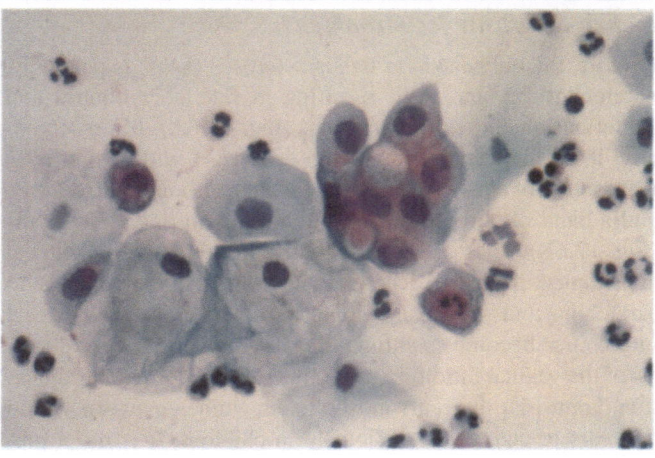

FIGURE 17.4 *Chlamydia trachomatis* (Papanicolaou smear). Intracytoplasmic eosinophilic bodies and granular bodies in the vacuoles.

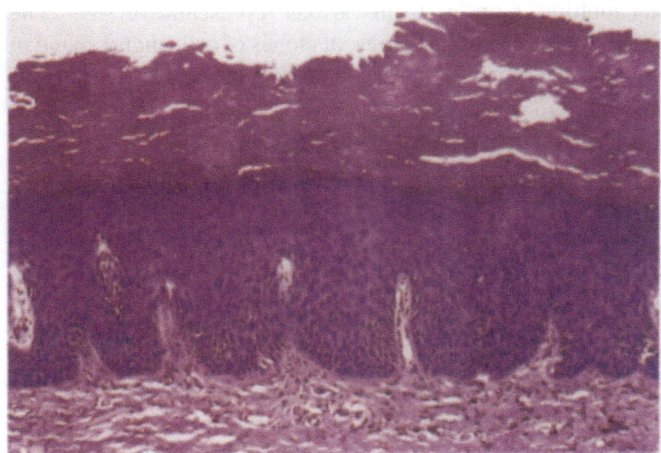

FIGURE 17.5 Squamous epithelial hyperplasia of vulva. Epidermal thickening caused by hyperplasia of benign squamous cells and hyperkeratosis. (Courtesy of A.S.C.P., F. Vellios, MD)

Lichen Sclerosus (et Atrophicus)

Grossly, the vulval skin in lichen sclerosus (LSA) is pale gray, parchmentlike, and thin, resulting in flat labia minora and agglutination of the preputial folds (Fig. 17.6A). Microscopically, it is characterized by a thin epidermis with loss of rete ridges, loss of elastic fibers with collagenization in the dermis, and a band of chronic inflammatory cells in the deep dermis (Fig. 17.6B). Lack of pigment contributes to the white clinical appearance. Pruritus accompanying these changes leads to scratching and subsequent irritation and soreness. If sexual intercourse becomes painful and is no longer practiced, stenosis of the vaginal introitus can result from lack of regular dilatation (kraurosis). It occurs most often in women between 45 and 55 years of age, and occasionally in children. It is not a premalignant lesion, and usually responds to topical treatment.

Mixed Vulvar Squamous Hyperplasia and LSA

Both conditions, epidermal hyperplasia and LSA, may affect different areas of the same vulva at the same time, necessitating multiple biopsies from various representative sites. The different area seems to represent clones of cells that respond in different ways to the same general but unidentified stimulus.

Vulvar Intraepithelial Neoplasia

Classification of Vulvar Intraepithelial Neoplasia (VIN)

VIN I   Slight dysplasia
VIN II   Moderate dysplasia
VIN III Severe dysplasia or carcinoma in situ
Paget's disease

(Developed by the International Society for the Study of Vulvar Disease, 1986.)[7]

Since these lesions are potentially malignant, careful long-term follow-up and frequent reevaluation are necessary.

The various degrees of squamous dysplasia are graded as follows:

Slight dysplasia (atypical change in the lower one third of the epidermis)
Moderate dysplasia (up to one half of the epidermis)
Marked dysplasia (more than one half of the epidermis).

Carcinoma in situ

Carcinoma in situ encompasses three histologic varieties: Bowen's disease, erythroplasia of Queyrat, and carcinoma simplex. They exhibit such marked biologic similarities that the International Society for the Study of Vulvar Disease recommended that they be grouped under the single heading of carcinoma in situ. Carcinoma in situ is histologically characterized by the epidermis being replaced by atypical primitive cells through its full thickness without stromal invasion (Fig. 17.7A). Clinically, it is characterized by a reddish brown or whitish (leukoplakic) raised area (Fig. 17.7B). Most patients are asymptomatic, although many complain of pruritus. It occurs in women between the ages of 25 and 70 years. Increasing numbers of cases are being found in young women. Some cases of carcinoma in situ progress to invasive squamous cell carcinoma, usually in elderly or immunosuppressed women.[8,9] There is a high degree of association with other sexually transmitted diseases (especially condyloma acuminatum and herpes simplex). Twenty five to 30% of patients have preexisting or concomitant carcinoma in situ of the cervix. For this reason, cytology and colposcopically directed biopsy of the cervix should be performed in all cases.

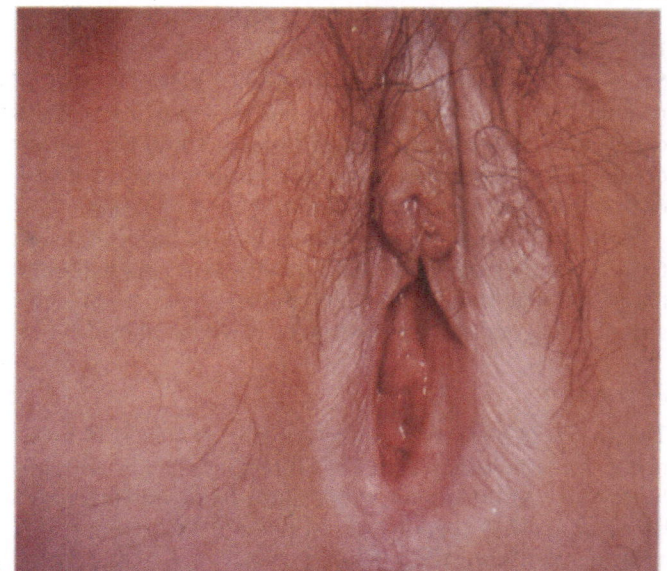

A

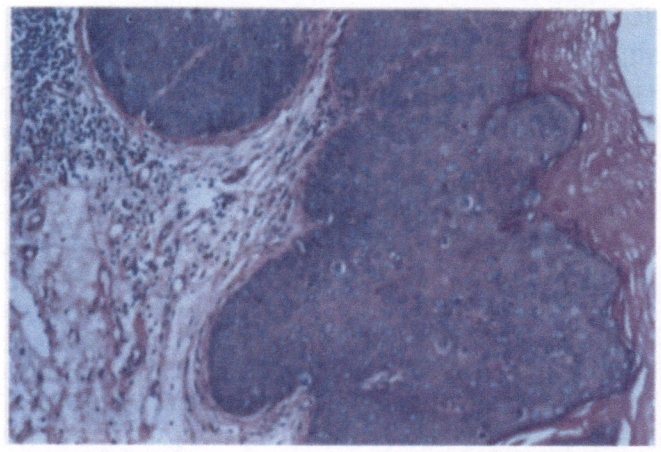

A

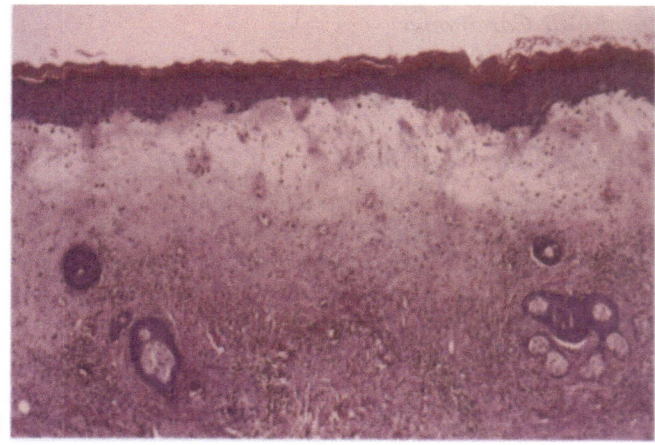

B

FIGURE 17.6   Lichen sclerosus. A: Thin vulval skin and flat labia minora (gross). **B**: Thin epidermis, subepithelial collagenization replacing elastic fibers, and a band of chronic inflammatory cells in the deep dermis. (Courtesy of A.S.C.P., F. Vellios, M.D.)

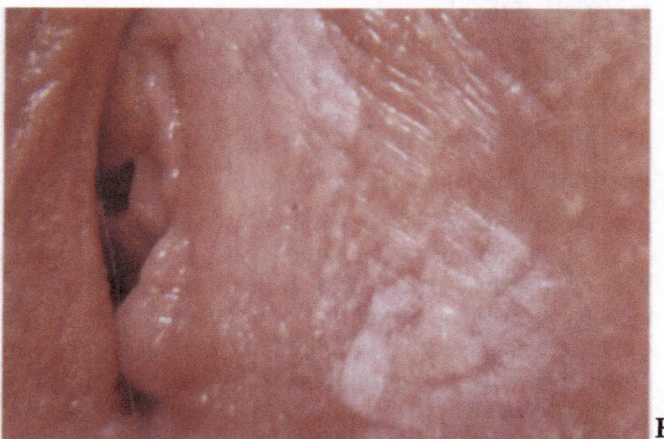

B

FIGURE 17.7   Carcinoma in situ of vulval skin. A: The full thickness of the epidermis is replaced by atypical squamous cells and is covered by a thick layer of keratin. **B**: Carcinoma in situ (gross). Raised leukoplakic surface.(Courtesy of A.S.C.P., F. Vellios, M.D.)

Paget's Disease of Vulva

Clinically, Paget's disease of vulva is characterized by a red, crusted, sharply demarcated lesion, usually of the labium majora or perineum or both. Microscopically, Paget's cells, singly or in clusters, infiltrate the epidermis. The underlying adnexal epithelium may also share the same change. Paget's cells are large round cells with perinuclear halos or optically clear cytoplasm and small atypical nuclei (Fig. 17.8). The cells contain mucopolysaccharide, which can be demonstrated by the periodic acid-schiff (PAS) or mucicaramine stain. Paget's cells appear to be of apocrine or eccrine duct cell origin.

In contrast to Paget's disease of the nipple, which is almost always accompanied by an underlying ductal carcinoma of the breast, vulvar lesions are most frequently confined to the epidermis of the skin.

To prevent local recurrence, wide excision, including the underlying fibromuscular layer, is recommended.

Malignant Neoplasms of the Vulva

Invasive Squamous Cell Carcinoma

Invasive squamous cell carcinoma of the vulva accounts for 3% to 4% of all female genital malignancies and more than 90% of all vulvar cancers. It is primarily a cancer of post-menopausal women. Fewer than 6% of patients are premenopausal. They present with pruritus and endophytic or exophytic lesions of long duration, which occur on any part of the vulva (Fig. 17.9A). Histologically, the lesion consists of large, pleomorphic cells arranged in sheets and cords infiltrating the underlying dermis (Fig. 17.9B). These carcinomas tend to metastasize at an early stage to regional lymph nodes. Clinical staging of squamous carcinoma of the vulva is shown in Table 17.1.

Table 17.1. Clinical staging of squamous carcinoma of the vulva.

Stage	Description
I	Carcinoma confined to the vulva, 2 cm or less in diameter, without suspicious groin nodes
II	Carcinoma confined to the vulva, exceeding 2 cm in diameter, without suspicious groin nodes
III	Extension beyond the vulva, without suspicious groin nodes, or lesions of any size with suspicious groin nodes
IV	Grossly positive groin nodes, regardless of extent of primary, or evidence of metastasis elsewhere.

The corrected 5-year survival of all patients treated with radical surgery is 70%, for Stage I and II patients, 90%, and for Stage III and IV patients, less than 20%. Eleven percent of patients with early invasive carcinoma (less than 5 mm depth of penetration) had lymph node metastasis. Thirty five percent of well differentiated carcinomas had positive nodes, whereas 62% of poorly differentiated tumors showed metastasis.

Verrucous carcinoma is a special type of highly differentiated squamous carcinoma that presents as a large fungating tumor. It resembles condyloma accuminatum but is locally invasive. It rarely metastasizes and can be cured by wide excision.

Melanoma

Two to 9% of most series of vulvar cancers consist of melanoma. Its pathologic features and biologic behavior are similar to those of other sites of the skin. Its highly aggressive behavior and low overall survival rate (30%) account for its clinical importance.

Basal Cell Carcinoma

The pathologic features and biologic behavior of basal cell carcinoma are similar to those of other sites of skin.

Bartholin Gland Carcinoma

Bartholin gland carcinoma is a rare neoplasm. It carries a poor prognosis because of the rich lymphatic supply of the area, the deep occult site of involvement, and the tendency to dismiss enlargement of the area being benign. One half of the carcinomas are adenocarcinomas, one third are of squamous type, and the remainder are of interdeterminate type.

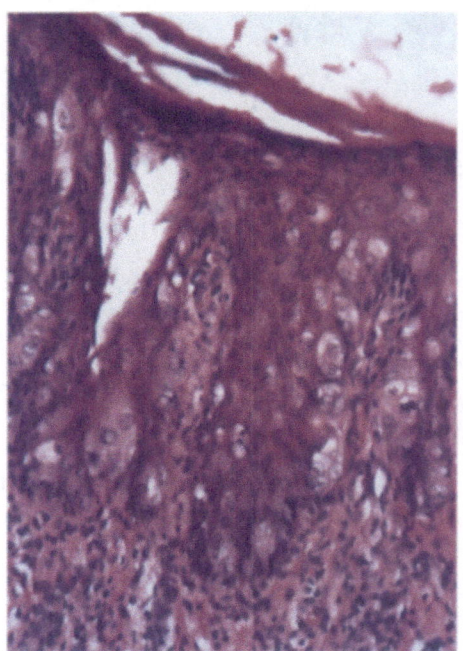

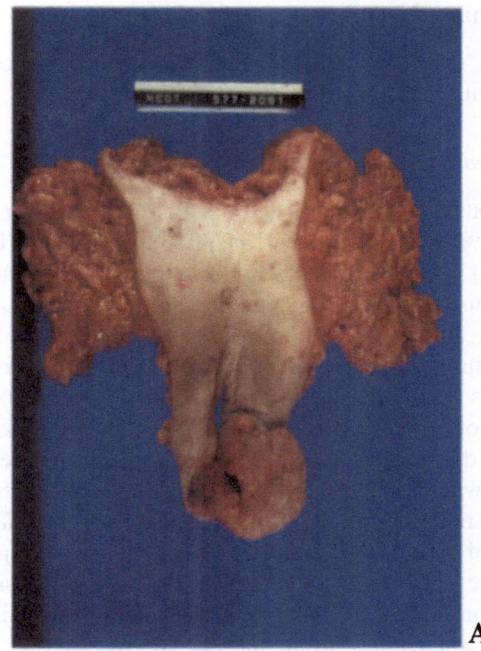

FIGURE 17.8 **Paget's disease of vulva.** Paget's cells infiltrating the lower layer of the epidermis singly and in clusters.

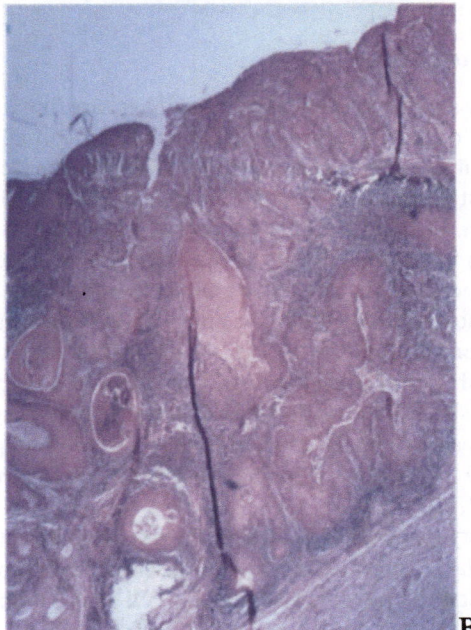

FIGURE 17.9 **Squamous cell carcinoma of vulva.** **A:** Fungating tumor in the left labium majus (gross). **B:** The neoplasm infiltrates the underlying dermis as sheets and cords of atypical squamous cells.

Malignant Neoplasms of the Vagina

Primary malignant neoplasms of the vagina are uncommon, representing 1% of all gynecologic cancers.

Squamous Cell Carcinoma

Squamous cell carcinomas of the vagina occur in older women, with 70% of the cases occurring after age 50 years. The most common site is the upper portion of the posterior wall. They present usually as an exophytic growth extending into the submucosa, and later into the paracolpos, parametria, bladder, and rectum. Histologically, squamous cell carcinoma of the vagina is similar to that of other organs (Fig. 17.10). Twenty percent of the cases have pelvic lymph node metastasis at the time of diagnosis. Inguinal node metastasis increases in frequency when the tumor involves the lower vagina. The 5-year survival rate for early lesions (Stage I) is 80% to 90% and for advanced (Stage III and IV) lesions only 20%. The poor survival rate is attributed to the inability to excise the lesion completely or to provide adequate radiotherapy without incurring considerable damage to the bladder and rectum.

Adenocarcinoma

Primary adenocarcinoma of the vagina is rare, but it is unique because of the increased frequency of clear cell adenocarcinomas in young women whose mothers had been treated with diethylstilbesterol (DES) during pregnancy for threatened abortion. Official Registry for these tumors shows that they occur in fewer than 0.14% of the women who were exposed to DES during the pregnancy of their mothers. The carcinoma most often occurs in the anterior wall of the vagina and can extend to the cervix (Fig. 17.11A). Histologically, it is identical to clear cell adenocarcinoma of the ovary, consisting of solid sheets and tubulocystic structures comprising of cells with clear cytoplasm (Fig. 17.11B). The tumors may be detected cytologically in their early stage of development (Fig. 17.11C).

Surgery and radiation therapy have successfully eradicated DES-related tumors in up to 80% of cases, in contrast to the poor survival rates for squamous cell carcinoma and for adenocarcinoma not related to DES.

Probably the precursor of DES related adenocarcinoma is vaginal adenosis, a condition in which glandular epithelium of mullerian type replaces part of the vaginal squamous epithelium. Vaginal adenosis presents clinically as red, granular areas. Adenosis has been reported in 35% to 90% of the offspring of estrogen-treated mothers.

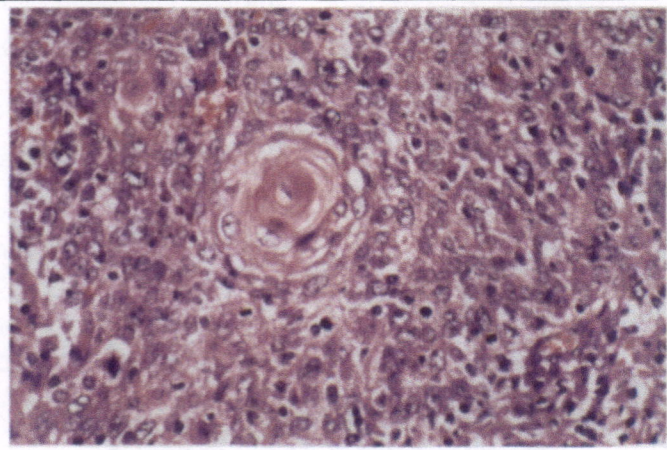

FIGURE 17.10   Invasive squamous cell carcinoma of vagina. Sheets of neoplastic squamous cells and keratin pearls.

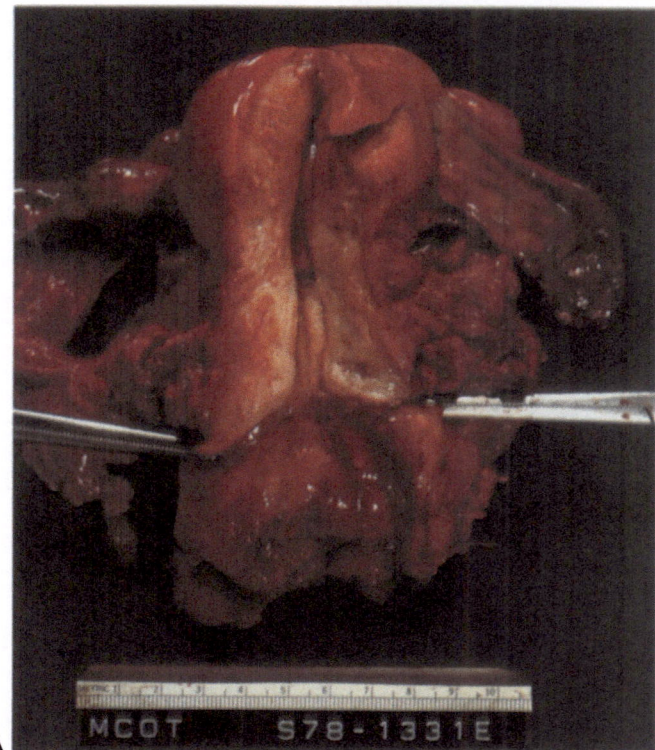

A

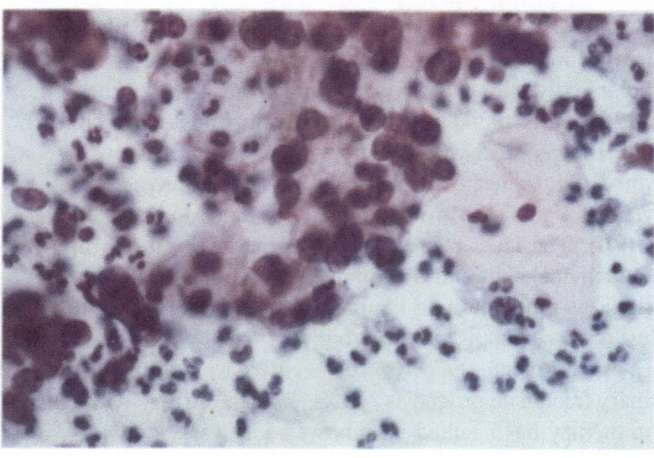

C

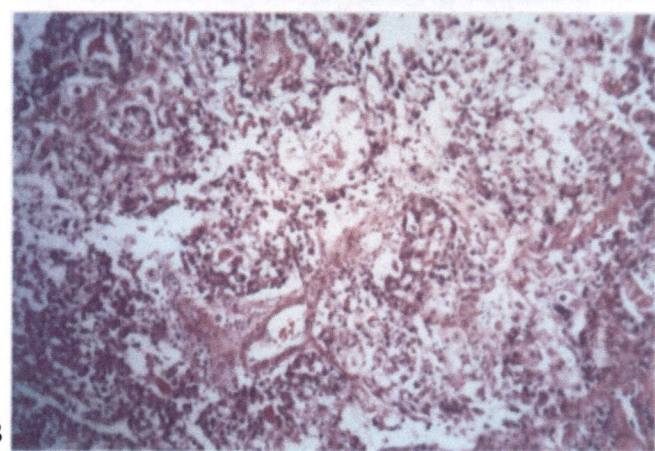

B

FIGURE 17.11 **Adenocarcinoma of vagina. A**: The tumor arises in the anterior wall, replaces the upper vagina, and extends to the cervix. **B**: Solid sheets and tubulocystic structures of clear cell adenocarcinoma. The patient, who was 29 years old, had a history of intrauterine exposure to DES (biopsy). **C**: The cells occur in sheets and have abundant clear cytoplasm and large round nuclei (Papanicolaou smear).

Sarcoma Botryoides (Embryonal Rhabdomyosarcoma)

Sarcoma botryoides is a rare neoplasm, which presents as multilobular polypoid mass protruding from the vagina (Fig. 17.12A). It is found most frequently in infants and children under the age of 5 years. Histologically, the neoplasm is seen immediately beneath the intact mucosa as a layer (cambium layer) of spindle or round cells and rhabdomyoblasts (Fig. 17.12B). The layer next to this comprises elongated primitive mesenchymal cells and rhabdomyoblasts (Fig. 17.12C). Metastasis takes place through lymphatic and hematogenous routes. Most of these neoplasms tend to invade locally and cause death by penetration into the peritoneal cavity or by obstruction of the urinary tract. The prognosis is poor. Radical surgery with radiation therapy has resulted in improved survival.

Malignant Melanomas

The vagina is not a common site for malignant melanoma. Melanomas usually develop in the lower third of the vagina and are often pigmented. The prognosis is poor.

Metastatic Carcinoma of the Vagina

Carcinomas metastatic to the vagina are more common than primary cancers of the vagina. Endometrial and cervical carcinomas are the most common sources of metastasis. Metastatic deposits are usually seen in the upper third and anterior wall. They may be small and can resemble granulation tissue. Such lesions may be diagnosed by a cytologic scraping or by biopsy.

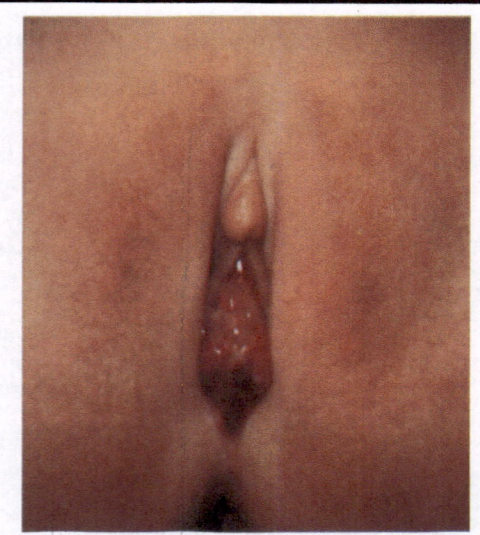

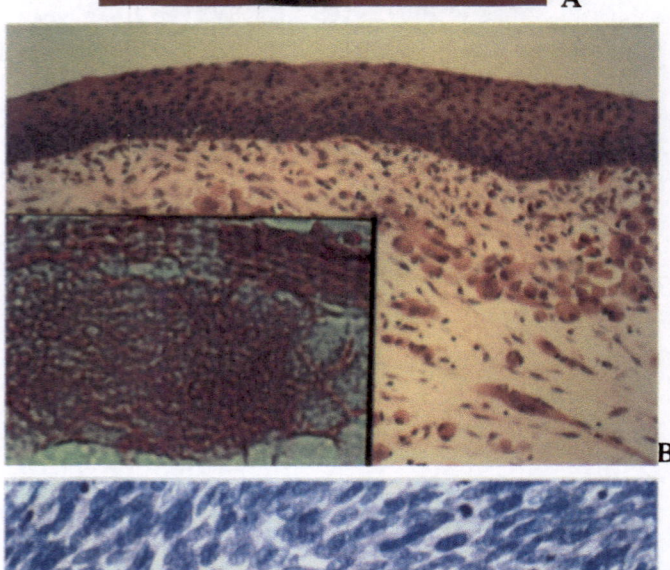

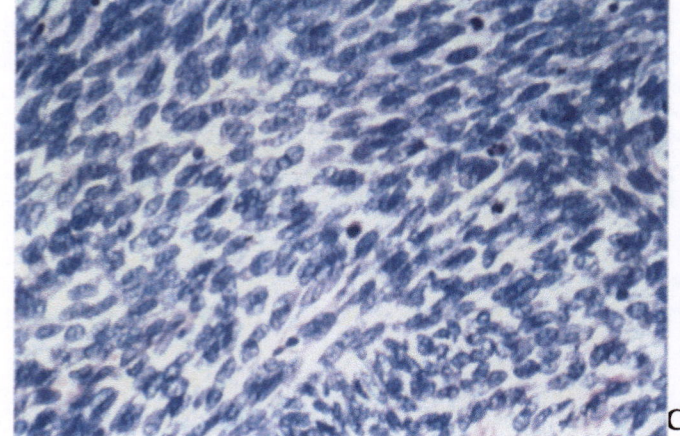

FIGURE 17.12 Sarcoma botryoides of vagina. A: Multilobular polypoid mass protruding from the vagina of a 3-year-old girl (gross). B: Beneath the intact mucosa is the cambium layer comprising spindle cells and rhabdomyoblasts. Cross striations of the neoplastic rhabdomyoblast (*inset*). C: In the deep layer are primitive mesenchymal cells and rhabdomyoblasts.

References

1. Lewis JF, O'Brien M. Diagnosis of *Haemophilus vaginalis* by Papanicolaou smears. *Tech Bull Req Med Tech*. 1969;39:34.
2. Reeves WC, Corey L, Adams HG, et al. Risk of recurrence after first episodes of genital herpes. Relation to HSV type and antibody response. *N Eng J Med*. 1981;305:315.
3. CDC Report, 1988.
4. Schachter J. Chlamydial infections (first of three parts). *N Engl J Med*. 1978;298:428.
5. Schachter J. Chlamydial infections (second of three parts). *N Engl J Med*. 1978;298:490.
6. Schachter J. Chlamydial infections (third of three parts). *N Engl J Med*. 1978;298:540.
7. Report of the ISSUD Terminology Committee. Proc VIII World Congress, Stockholm, Sweden. *J Reprod Med*. 1986;31:973.
8. Crum CP, Liskow A, Petras P, Keng WC, Frick HC. Vulvar intraepithelial neoplasia (severe dysplasia and carcinoma in situ). *Cancer*. 1984; 54:1429.
9. Friedrich EG, Wilkinson EJ, Fu YS. Carcinoma in situ of the vulva: A continuing challenge. *Am J Obstet Gynecol*. 1980;130:830.

18
The Uterine Cervix

Histology

The ectocervix and vagina are lined by stratified squamous epithelium, which can be divided into several different layers during the reproductive phase of life. From the deepest layer, they are: 1) the basal layer (stratum cylindricum), 2) the parabasal zone (deep spinous layer), 3) the intermediate zone (superficial spinous layer), and 4) the superficial layer (stratum corneum) (Fig. 18.1). The upper two layers, the intermediate and superficial layers, change in thickness under the influence of ovarian hormones. Because of its sensitivity to estrogen and progesterone, a scraping of the lateral wall of the vagina provides a specimen suitable for evaluating the hormonal state. Hormonal evaluation of a smear is based on the proportion of the various types of squamous cells.

The squamocolumnar junction of the cervix is the border between ectocervical stratified squamous epithelium and endocervical columnar epithelium (Fig. 18.2).

In most women during the reproductive phase of life, the columnar epithelium of the endocervix tends to move down on to the ectocervix to form an ectropion with its new squamocolumnar junction below the external os. Ectropion is a normal finding and is most extensive in younger women. The columnar epithelium of ectropion gradually becomes replaced by squamous epithelium, causing the squamocolumnar junction to move toward the external os. In older and postmenopausal women the squamocolumnar junction is almost always above the external os. The newly formed squamous epithelium replacing the ectropion up to the original squamocolumnar junction is referred to as the transformation zone.

Scraping and sampling of the squamocolumnar junction of the transformation zone is important because almost all cervical squamous neoplasms begin at this junction and the extent and limits of cervical intraepithelial neoplasia coincide with the distribution of the transformation zone. Localization of the transformation zone can be enhanced during colposcopy by the application of 3% acetic acid.

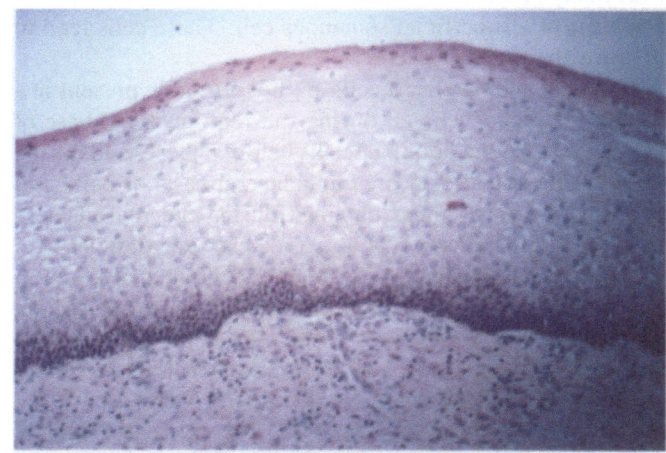

FIGURE 18.1 **Normal ectocervical mucosa.** Stratified squamous epithelium comprising the basal layer, parabasal zone, intermediate zone, and superficial layer.

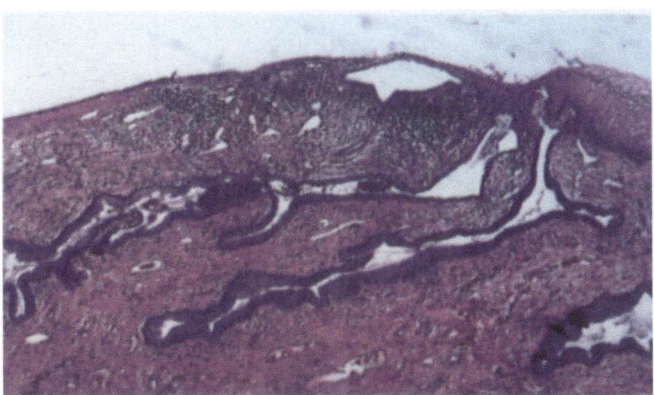

FIGURE 18.2 **Squamocolumnar junction and cervical glands of a normal cervix.** Stratified squamous epithelium (*right*) covering the distal portion of the ectocervical os, and a single layer of columnar epithelium covering the proximal portion and cervical canal.

Normal Cells of the Uterine Cervix

As in histologic preparations, there are four types of squamous cells seen in cervical smears. The most common types are superficial squamous and intermediate squamous cells. Superficial squamous cells are polygonal and are the largest squamous cells seen in routine cellular specimens, with a mean diameter of 40 to 50 μm. They occur singly isolated or in loose aggregates or sheets. The cytoplasm is translucent and eosinophilic in staining. The nucleus is central, round, small, and pyknotic.

Intermediate squamous cells are polygonal and smaller than superficial squamous cells. The cytoplasm is denser and is cyanophilic. The nucleus is central, round, and vesicular, with finely granular chromatin, two to three times the size of a nucleus of a superficial squamous cell. These cells tend to occur in sheets (Fig. 18.3).

The basal and parabasal cells are not normally present in a cervical smear of women during the reproductive phase of life, but may be the dominant cells before puberty and during and after menopause. A predominance of basal or parabasal cells in a cervical smear obtained during the reproductive phase of life is indicative of a marked estrogen deficiency.

Endocervical columnar cells occur singly, in strips, and in sheets. They vary in appearance, depending on the perspective from which they are viewed. When viewed on end, the cells appear small and polygonal and form sheets that have a honeycomb arrangement. When viewed from the lateral aspect, the cells have a columnar configuration. The cytoplasm may be diffusely vacuolated and variable in its staining reaction.

Benign Proliferative Reactions

Keratosis and Parakeratosis

Keratosis and parakeratosis occur as a protective reaction to unusual external stimuli. An example of this reaction is frequently seen in uterine prolapse when thickening of the ectocervical squamous epithelium takes place with keratin production. Clinically, the uterine cervix may show white patches (leukoplakia), and smears obtained from such areas contain numerous anucleated squames (Fig. 18.4).

The surface layers of the squamous epithelium showing parakeratosis of cervix consist of compact densely eosinophilic miniature squames, visible in smears as sheets or as isolated cells (Fig. 18.5). Occasionally, hyperkeratosis or parakeratosis may be a part of the surface change overlying atypical epithelium.

Squamous Metaplasia and Reserve Cell Hyperplasia

The term metaplasia refers to the change in form of mature cells with the substitution of one cell type for another. Squamous metaplasia is extremely common in the uterine cervix, most often taking place in the columnar epithelium of the transformation zone (Fig. 18.6A).

Cytologically, squamous metaplastic cells occur in loose aggregates and singly. Squamous metaplastic cells are round, oval, or polygonal. Their mean cell area is less than half that of mature (intermediate and superficial) squamous epithelial cells. The cytoplasm of squamous metaplastic cells is abundant with dense cyanophilic staining and has a distinct and smooth border. The nuclei are centrally located with a round or oval configuration, and are slightly larger than those of intermediate cells. The chromatin pattern is finely granular and evenly dispersed (Fig. 18.6B).

(*Discussion continued on p. 244*)

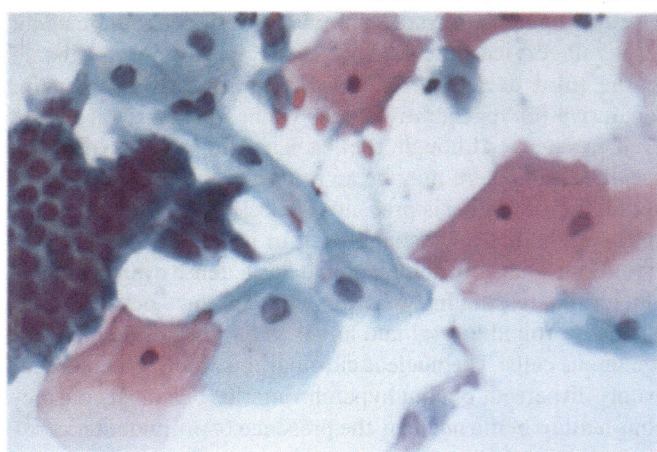

FIGURE 18.3   Normal cells in a cervical smear. Three superficial squamous cells (two, *right upper*, and one, *lower left*), intermediate squamous cells in the center, and sheets of endocervical columnar cells (*left*). (Papanicolaou stain)

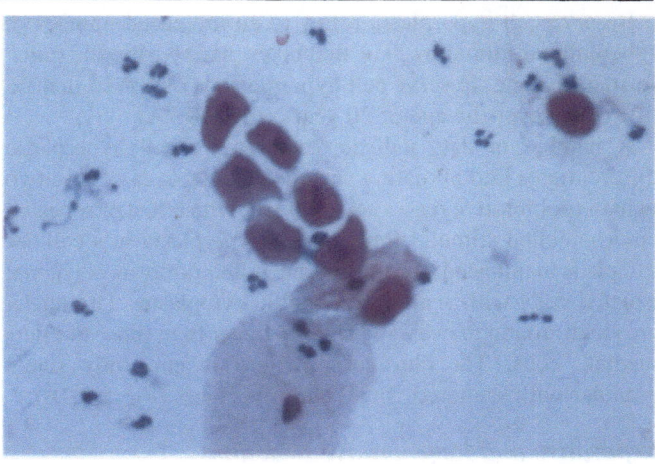

FIGURE 18.5   Parakeratosis. Eosinophilic miniature squames, a manifestation of parakeratosis (Papanicolaou stain).

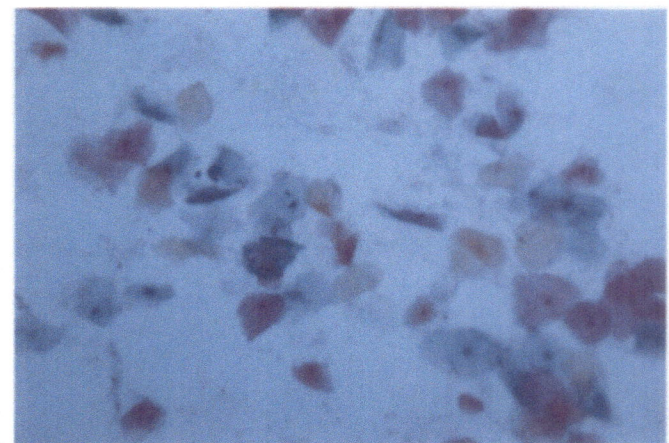

A

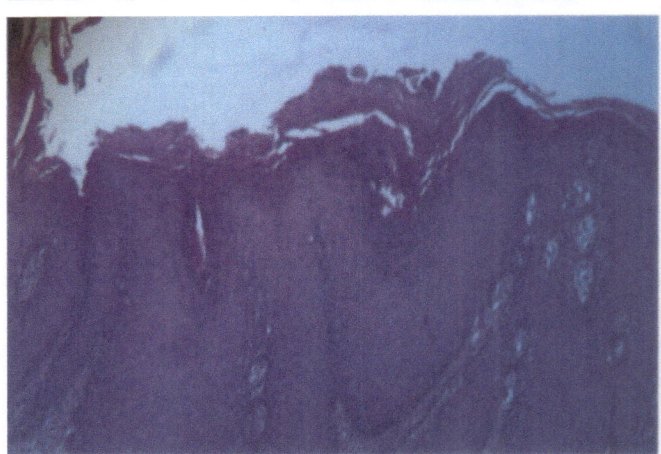

B

FIGURE 18.4   Hyperkeratosis. A: Anucleate squames, a manifestation of keratosis (Papanicolaou stain). **B**: Thick keratin layer on the surface.

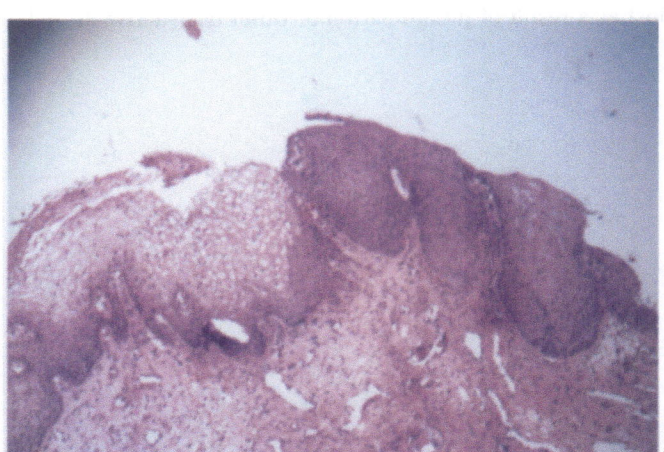

A

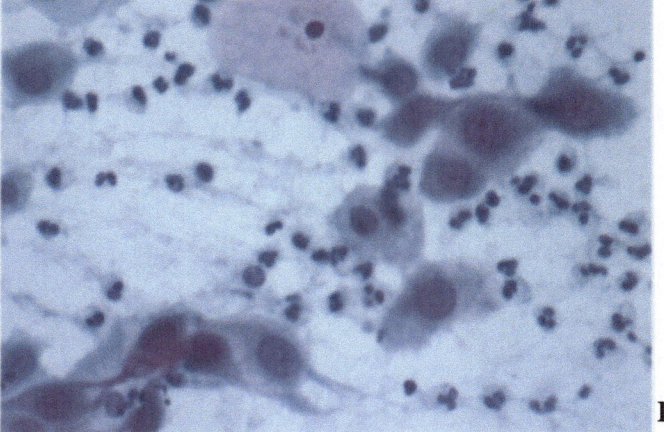

B

FIGURE 18.6   Squamous metaplasia. A: The cervical epithelium is replaced by sheets of metaplastic cells (*right*) in contrast to normal nonmetaplastic stratified squamous epithelium (*left*). **B**: Squamous metaplastic cells. Round, oval, or polygonal cells in loose aggregates and singly (Papanicolaou stain).

Reserve cell hyperplasia refers to an increased number of subcolumnar immature cells that takes place within the transformation zone. Reserve cell hyperplasia is observed in 40% of women over the age of 20 years (Fig. 18.7A).

A number of data indicate that reserve cell hyperplasia differentiates into immature squamous metaplasia. These two benign proliferative reactions result from the effect of repeated environmental stimuli.[2] Reserve cell hyperplasia in a cellular sample is manifested as compact sheets and rarely as polygonal isolated cells with scanty cyanophilic cytoplasm. The nuclei are small, round to oval, and slightly larger than those of intermediate cells. The chromatin pattern is uniformly finely granular with scattered, small chromocenters (Fig. 18.7B).

Reparative and Regenerative Reactions

The term "repair" in the context of cervical cytology originated with Reagan and Patten. Bibbo et al. documented the morphologic and biologic significance of "reparative cells" in the uterine cervix. Repair or regeneration of epithelium implies that new immature cells appear to replace epithelium lost as a result of inflammation or other destructive stimuli.

The cytologic manifestation of this condition is seen in about 1% of all cervical smears, with the highest prevalence being in the third decade. In cellular samples from the cervix, reparative (or regenerative) cells occur in sheets; rarely are they isolated. Although the background of the smear is usually clean, there may be an acute inflammatory exudate, but no tumor diathesis present. The cells are variable in size and are columnar, polygonal, oval, or irregular in shape. The cytoplasm is usually abundant and has a dense cyanophilic or indeterminate staining reaction with distinct borders. The nuclei are round to oval and larger than those of metaplastic squamous cells. The nuclear chromatin is finely granular and evenly dispersed, but not hyperchromatic. The most conspicuous feature of the nuclei is the presence of prominent macronucleoli (Fig. 18.8).

The practical importance of correctly recognizing the cellular changes of repair is to distinguish it from adenocarcinoma and nonkeratinizing squamous cell carcinoma of the cervix (Figs. 18.9 and 18.10). The biologic significance of reparative process is that in 10% to 15% of cases it may coexist with cervical intraepithelial neoplasia.

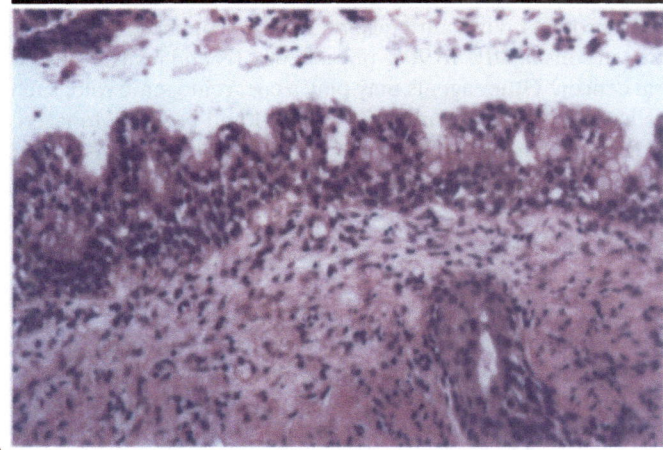

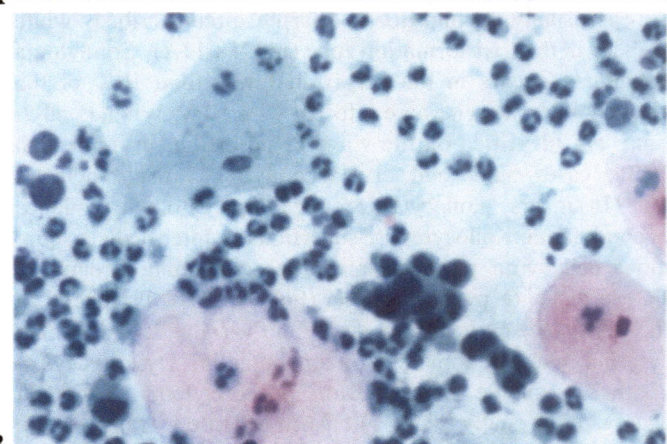

FIGURE 18.7 Reserve cell hyperplasia. A: Multiple layers of small cells between the columnar cells and basement membrane. **B:** Compact sheets of small polygonal cells with scanty cyanophilic cytoplasm (Papanicolaou stain).

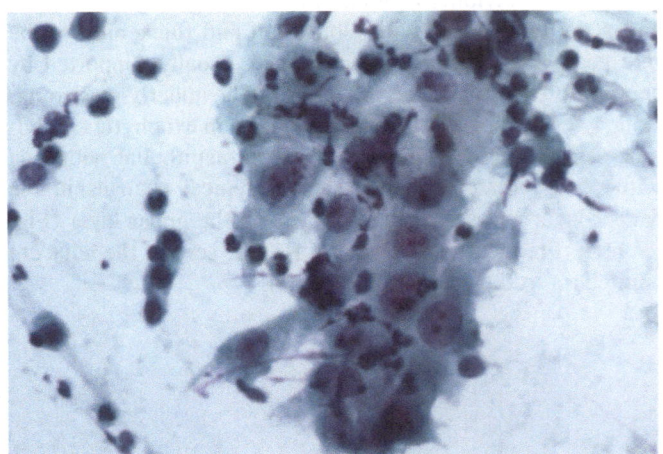

FIGURE 18.8 Reparative cells of uterine cervix. Sheets of polygonal and elongated cells with cyanophilic cytoplasm and round nuclei with prominent macronucleoli (Papanicolaou stain).

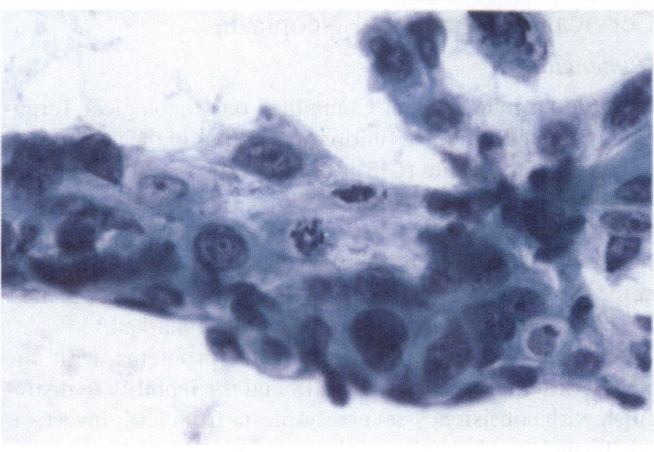

FIGURE 18.9 Adenocarcinoma of uterine cervix. In contrast to the cells of the reparative process, the cells of adenocarcinomas show nuclear atypia (Papanicolaou stain).

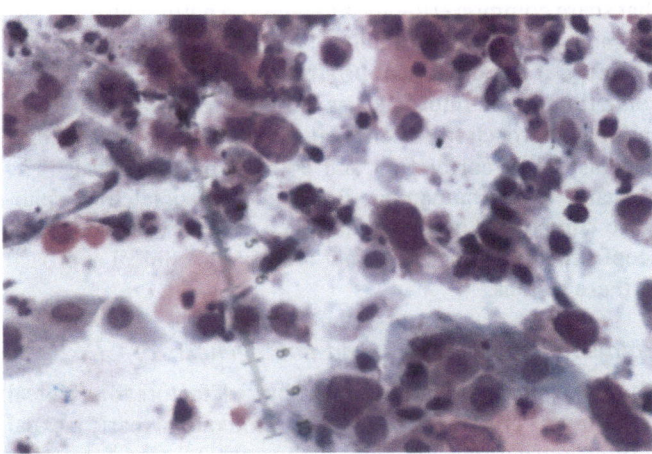

FIGURE 18.10 Squamous cell carcinoma of uterine cervix. Cells showing pleomorphism, nuclear atypia, and scanty cytoplasm (Papanicolaou stain).

Cervical Intraepithelial Neoplasia

Nomenclature

In 1961 the International Committee on Histological Terminology created several definitions for lesions of the uterine cervix. Carcinoma in situ (CIS) was defined as atypical primitive cells involving the whole thickness of epithelium of the surface and/or the glands in the absence of invasion. Dysplasia of the cervix was defined as all other disturbances of differentiation in the squamous epithelial lining of the surface and/or glands. Dysplasia may be characterized as slight to marked.[3]

Because of management associated problems with the classification of dysplasia and CIS and the inability to distinguish with consistency severe dysplasia from CIS, investigators turned to a definition of the precursors of cervical cancer based on the biologic behavior of these lesions. A number of studies demonstrated that the cellular changes of dysplasia and CIS were quantitatively similar and remained constant throughout the histologic spectrum. Based on these studies, Richart introduced the term "cervical intraepithelial neoplasia" (CIN),[4] which defines a spectrum of histologic changes that share common etiology, biology, and natural history. The diagnostic term "CIN" implies a malignant precursor lesion, that may, if left untreated, progress to invasive carcinoma at some time in the future.[4-6] Use of the CIN system provides a rational approach to patient management based on cytologic and histologic correlation and colposcopic findings.[7,8] The presence of any human papilloma virus-associated morphologic component may be mentioned as a part of the microscopic diagnosis but should not modify the clinical approach to these lesions.

Epidemiology, Etiology, and Pathogenesis of CIN

The following are the most important risk factors for cervical carcinoma: 1) early age at first intercourse: early sexual activity during development of the cervical transformation zone appears to play a pivotal role in susceptibility to carcinogens, 2) multiple sexual partners: there is a stronger potential of exposure to carcinogens, for example, human papilloma virus (HPN), herpes simplex virus, 3) high-risk male sexual partners, that is, promiscuous male cohorts who have a former wife with cervical cancer or who have a history of penile condyloma acuminatum. In addition to epidemiologic risk factors, there is strong convincing evidence that HPV plays an important role in cervical carcinogenesis. Human papilloma virus infection frequently coexists with CIN; HPV-viral proteins, viral antigens, and DNA sequences are identified in cells of 80% to 90% of cases of CIN and invasive cervical cancer.[9] Other agents may play a cocarcinogenic role, such as herpes simplex virus (HSV) type II and possibly tobacco. The association of HSV type II infection with cervical cancer is not as persuasive as the association with HPV.

Cytology and Pathology of CIN

Cervical Condyloma

Cervical condyloma is intimately associated with cervical carcinogenesis. Ninety percent of cervical condylomas occur as clinically invisible flat condylomas. On colposcopic examination, after application of 3% acetic acid, flat condylomas appear usually as multifocal, sharply circumscribed, white plaques in the transformation zone (Fig. 18.11A). Condyloma acuminata occurs in the cervix in fewer than 10% of the women whose cervices are infected with HPV. When condylomas are identified on the vulva or perineum, in more than 70% of cases vaginal and cervical condylomas are also detectable.[10] In smears, "koilocytes" are the salient cytologic evidence of condyloma. Koilocytes are superficial or intermediate squamous cells with perinuclear cavities containing irregularly shaped dense or pyknotic nuclei (Fig. 18.11B). Peripheral to the cavity, the cytoplasm is dense and variable in its staining reaction, the phenomenon of amphophilia. Dyskaryocytes, another cytologic manifestation of condyloma, occur in aggregates or singly. Their cytoplasm is densely orangeophilic and their nuclei are pyknotic and hyperchromatic. Occasionally, cells derived from atypical condyloma have large, irregular, hyperchromatic nuclei and eosinophilic or orangeophilic cytoplasm (Fig. 18.11C).

Histologically, flat condylomas show abundant koilocytes in the upper layer and slight acanthosis with well preserved maturation (Fig. 18.11D). Surface parakeratosis and keratosis are usually slight.

Typical condyloma acuminatum is a papillary, exophytic, and acanthotic lesion with elongation and thickening of the rete pegs. The papillary structures are usually supported by central fibrovascular cores arising from the underlying stroma. Koilocytes are not observed as frequently in exophytic condyloma as in flat condyloma. Cervical intraepithelial neoplasia with condylomatous change shows atypical changes in the deeper layer and scattered koilocytes in the upper layer (Fig. 18.11E). Frequently, condylomas may be seen at the adjacent epithelium to the atypical epithelium.

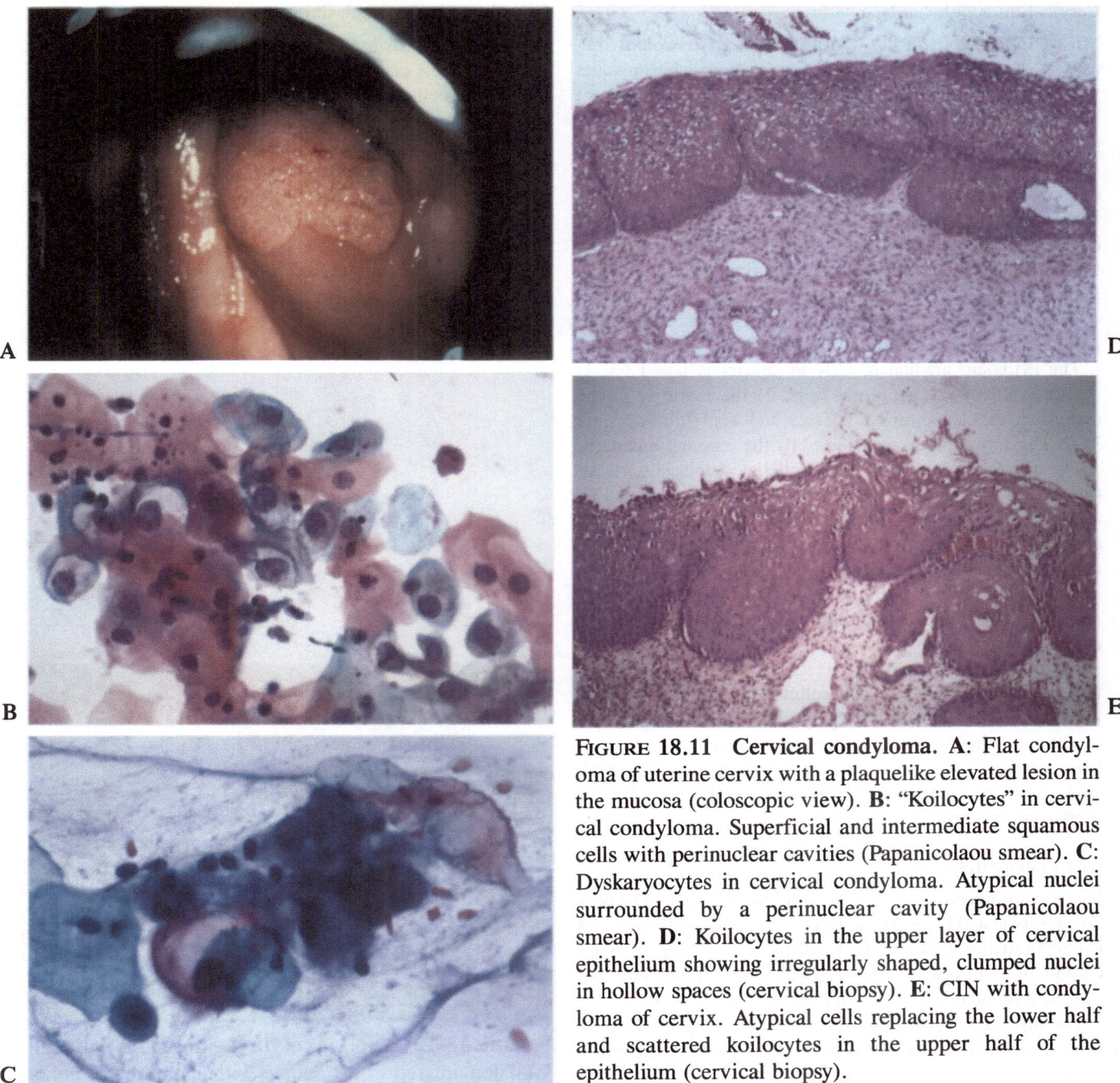

FIGURE 18.11   Cervical condyloma. A: Flat condyloma of uterine cervix with a plaquelike elevated lesion in the mucosa (coloscopic view). B: "Koilocytes" in cervical condyloma. Superficial and intermediate squamous cells with perinuclear cavities (Papanicolaou smear). C: Dyskaryocytes in cervical condyloma. Atypical nuclei surrounded by a perinuclear cavity (Papanicolaou smear). D: Koilocytes in the upper layer of cervical epithelium showing irregularly shaped, clumped nuclei in hollow spaces (cervical biopsy). E: CIN with condyloma of cervix. Atypical cells replacing the lower half and scattered koilocytes in the upper half of the epithelium (cervical biopsy).

Cervical Intraepithelial Neoplasia

Most CIN develops in the transformation zone. Colposcopically, CIN appears as fairly well demarcated, white plaques with a mosaic or punctate pattern (Fig. 18.12). Since most CIN occurs in the transformation zone and a small proportion of cases originate in the endocervical epithelium in the proximal cervix, cellular samples from the ectocervix and the endocervix are desirable for cytologic screening. Cervical intraepithelial neoplasia can be graded I to III to reflect the degree of epithelial abnormality, provided that no prognostic significance is attached to this classification. The implication of the CIN concept is that all patients with such abnormalities, whatever their grade, must be referred for colposcopic examination for further evaluation.[11]

The cytologic grading of CIN in smears is based on: 1) the total number of abnormal cells, 2) the maturity of the cytoplasm as characterized by size and configuration, and 3) nuclear morphology as reflected by the chromatin pattern.

The histologic grading of intraepithelial neoplasia is classically based on the proportion of the epithelium occupied by atypical primitive cells, reflecting a progressive loss of epithelial maturation: CIN grade 1: atypical cells occupying the lower third of the epithelium; CIN grade 2: atypical cells occupying the lower two thirds of the epithelium; CIN grade 3: atypical cells occupying two thirds to the full thickness of the epithelium.

Patten proposed the following classification of dysplasia on the correlation of histologic and cellular material: 1) keratinizing dysplasia, 2) nonkeratinizing dysplasia, and 3) metaplastic dysplasia. Although biologic differences between the morphologic subclasses of dysplasia might become apparent through analysis of their cytologic behavior, it has little clinical or therapeutic relevance.

CIN I (slight dysplasia)

In smears most cells occur singly, with some in sheets. The cells are polygonal and large. The nuclei are large, round to oval, and hyperchromatic with uniformly distributed, finely granular chromatin. The cytoplasm is predominantly cyanophilic, but may be eosinophilic or indeterminate (Fig. 18.13A, B).

The histologic feature of CIN I is atypical squamous cells occupying the lowest one third of the epithelium. The component cells are most often nonkeratinizing dysplastic cells; occasionally they are keratinizing or metaplastic dysplastic cells (Fig. 18.13C).

CIN II (moderate dysplasia)

The abnormal cells in CIN II tend to be more numerous than in CIN I. Most cells occur as isolated cells and some are in sheets. The cells may vary in size and are round to oval, polygonal, or pleomorphic in configuration. Round to oval cells have predominantly cyanophilic cytoplasm, smooth cytoplasmic borders, and a relatively high nucleocytoplasmic ratio. The nuclei are round to oval and moderately hyperchromatic with an evenly distributed finely granular chromatin pattern (Fig. 18.14A). The histologic feature is atypical cells occupying the lowest and middle two thirds of the epithelium with scattered abnormal mitotic figures (Fig. 18.14B).

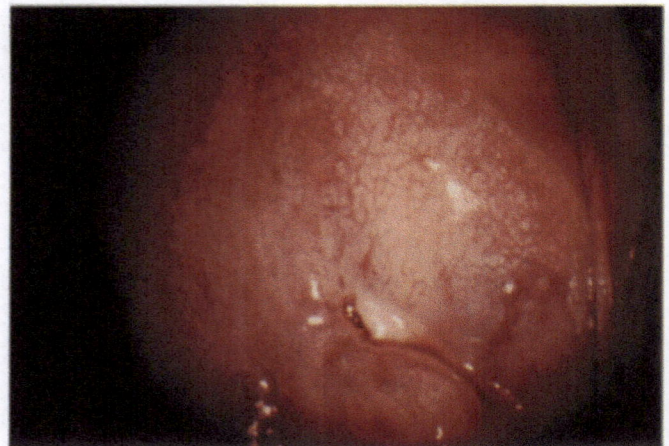

FIGURE 18.12   CIN of cervix (colposcopic feature). Well demarcated white plaques with a mosaic and punctate pattern. (Courtesy of E.H. Vogel, M.D., Toledo, Ohio)

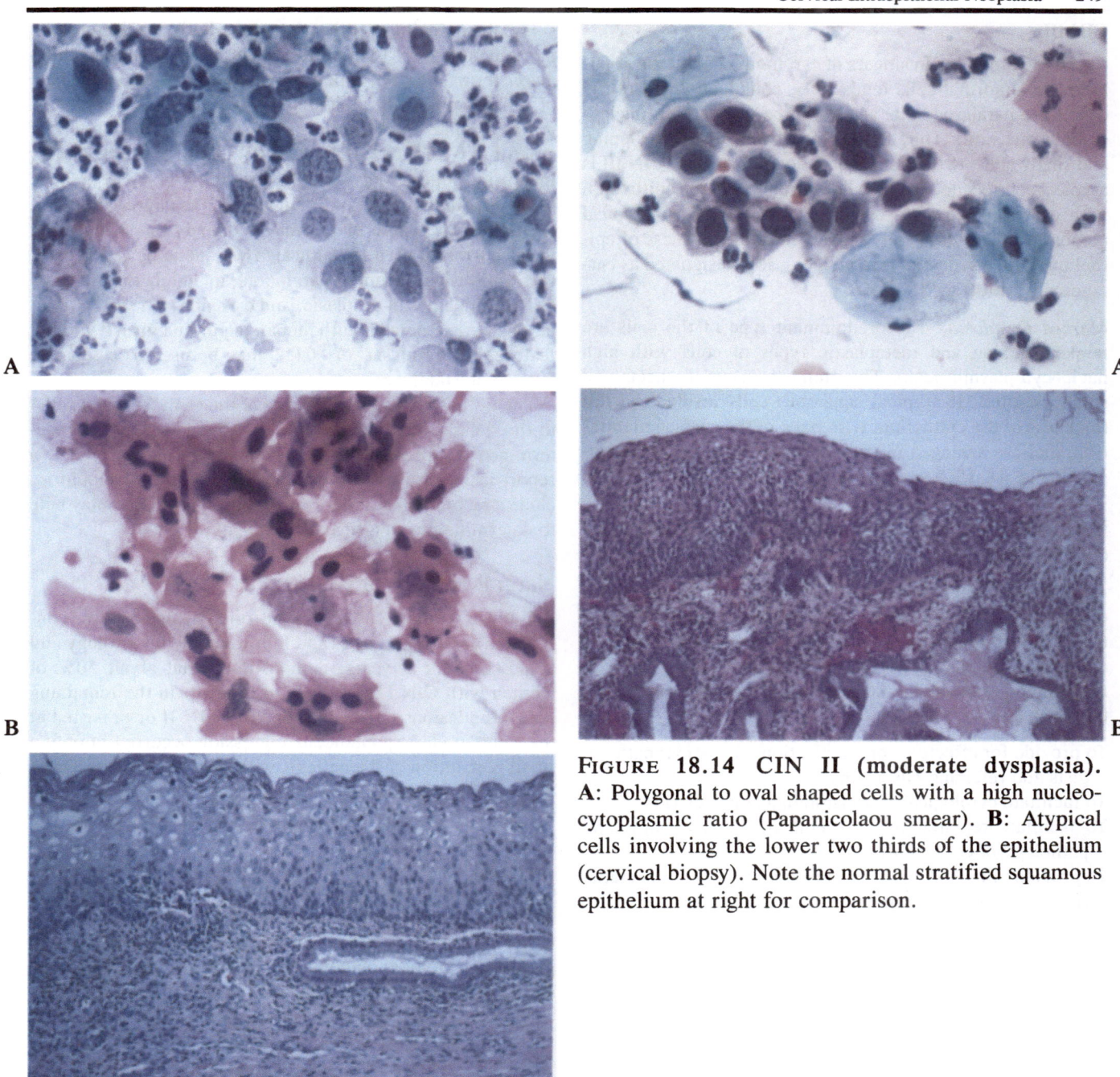

FIGURE 18.14 CIN II (moderate dysplasia). A: Polygonal to oval shaped cells with a high nucleo-cytoplasmic ratio (Papanicolaou smear). B: Atypical cells involving the lower two thirds of the epithelium (cervical biopsy). Note the normal stratified squamous epithelium at right for comparison.

FIGURE 18.13 CIN I (slight dysplasia). A, B: Large polygonal and pleomorphic cells occurring in sheets and singly (Papanicolaou smear). C: Atypical squamous cells involving the lower one third of the epithelium (cervical biopsy).

CIN III

Carcinoma In Situ. In smears of carcinoma in situ the population of abnormal cells tends to be abundant. Most of the dysplastic parabasal cells are of a type with a high nucleocytoplasmic ratio. They tend to occur in syncytial grouping and singly (Fig. 18.15A). The histologic feature of CIN III is atypical cells occupying the whole thickness of the epithelium with or without a trace of surface maturation. If atypical parabasal dyskaryotic cells replace the full thickness of epithelium with a syncytial arrangement, it is designated as carcinoma in situ (Fig. 18.15B).

Marked Dysplasia. The predominant type of the cells are nonkeratinizing and metaplastic types of cells with high nucleocytoplasmic ratio. They tend to occur in sheets and singly isolated. If atypical squamous cells involve the full thickness of the epithelium with trace of the surface maturation, and are arranged in sheets, marked dysplasia is designated (Fig. 18.15C).

Bethesda System for Reporting Cervical/Vaginal Cytological Diagnosis

As a result of ambiguous terminology and controversial subclassification, the Division of Cancer Prevention and Control of the National Cancer Institute convened a workshop of expert consultants to review existing terminology and to recommend effective methods of reporting.[12] The aim of system is as follows:

To provide for effective communication among cytopathologists and referring physicians

To facilitate cytological-histopathological correlation

To facilitate research into the epidemiology, biology, and pathology of cervical disease

To provide reliable data for national and international statistical analysis and comparison.

Finally, to facilitate utilization of the Bethesda System, the participants agreed to minimize the introduction of new diagnostic terms. Years of experience have demonstrated the lack of reproducibility in assigning cervical lesions to the categories of mild, moderate, or severe dysplasia, carcinoma in situ (or to CIN I, CIN II, or CIN III). As a result, the participants introduced only two terms: "Low-grade squamous intraepithelial lesion" and "High-grade squamous intraepithelial lesion." These two terms encompass the spectrum of terms currently used to delineate the squamous cell precursors of invasive squamous carcinoma, including the grades of CIN, the degrees of dysplasia, and carcinoma in situ. "Cellular changes associated with human papilloma virus," without features of "dysplasia" or "CIN" may be used as a separate diagnostic statement.

The Bethesda System limits use of the term "atypical cells" to those cases in which the cytological findings are of undetermined significance. To assist the referring physician, a report in which cells are described as "atypical" should include a recommendation for further evaluation that may help to determine the significance of the atypical cells.

Natural History of CIN

A study of women with CIN, confirmed by two or three consecutive abnormal smears and followed only by cytology and colposcopy for 9 years, demonstrated that about 50% of women with CIN I progressed to CIN III. In the remaining cases, the lesions either developed to CIN II or persisted at the same grade.[7] Spontaneous regression occurred in only a small population of the patients with mild dysplasia (CIN I). The median transit time to CIN III was 6 months to 3 years for CIN I, 2 years for CIN II, and 4 years for all the CIN I–II lesions taken together.[7,13,14]

Carcinoma in situ, CIN III, rarely regressed spontaneously, but persisted unchanged during the period of surveillance in some cases, and in less than one half of the reported cases of CIN III progressed to invasive cancer.[15] It is impossible to predict the biologic outcome of CIN III. As yet, there is no accurate means for separating the CIN that will ultimately become invasive carcinoma from that which will not.

Fu and Reagan investigated the biologic potential of CIN on the basis of DNA ploidy analysis and HPV DNA typing and demonstrated a subset of aneuploid lesions that have high malignant potential.[16]

Analysis of HPV type in CIN by in situ hybridization revealed that CIN I is associated more often with HPV Types 6 and 11 with a low malignant potential, and CIN II–III is usually associated with HPV types 16, 18, and 31 with a high malignant potential.[16]

Management of CIN

Cervical cytology has achieved a high detection rate and a high degree of diagnostic predictability for cervical cancer. When cytology and colposcopy are combined to evaluate women with abnormal smears, their diagnostic accuracy approaches 100%.

In the investigation of CIN the colposcope is an essential instrument, which achieves excellent reproducible results. However, colposcopy alone is not a practical screening method for cervical pathology. It is time consuming and expensive and requires a skilled, experienced clinician for successful use.

Colposcopic examination of the cervix is limited to the portio and distal part of the endocervical canal and is inadequate for the evaluation of endocervical lesions.

Treatment of CIN is basically cryosurgery or laser therapy under colposcopic guidance if the entire lesion is visible and limited to the cervix. Diagnostic cervical conization can be avoided in more than 95% of patients.

Indications for diagnostic cervical conization are as follows: 1) normal colposcopy in a patient with persistent abnormal cytology or positive endocervical curettage, 2) abnormal cytology and a squamocolumnar junction that is not visualized, 3) the limits of lesion are not visualized, 4) biopsy reveals microinvasive carcinoma or colposcopy is suspicious for invasive carcinoma, 5) adenocarcinoma in situ on biopsy or endocervical curettage, and 6) a lack of correlation between cytologic, colposcopic, and histologic findings.

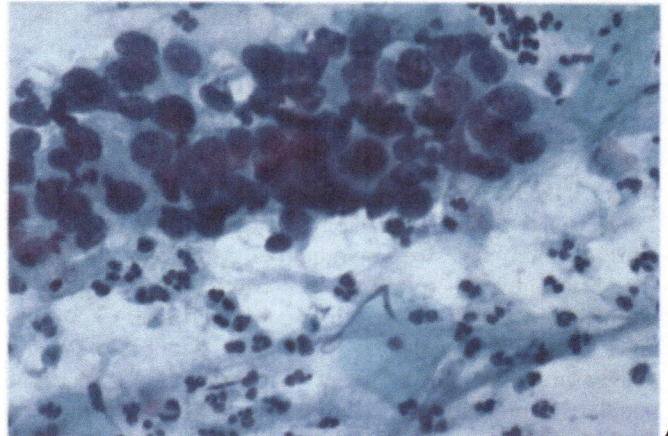

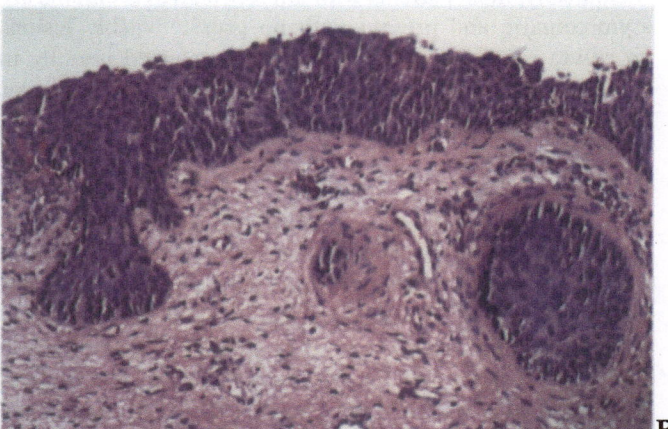

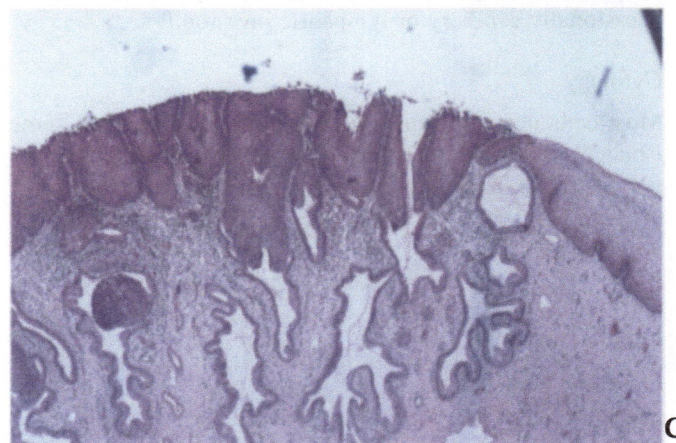

FIGURE 18.15   CIN III. **A**: The cells occur in syncytial aggregates and singly. They have cyanophilic cytoplasm with indistinct cell borders and large, round to oval hyperchromatic nuclei (Papanicolaou smear). **B** (carcinoma in situ): Atypical cells involve the full thickness of the epithelium of the surface and/or glands (cervical biopsy). **C**: CIN III (marked dysplasia). Atypical cells replace more than two thirds of the epithelium. A trace of surface maturation may be present (cervical biopsy).

Invasive Squamous Cell Carcinoma

Microinvasive Squamous Cell Carcinoma

Although it is not usually possible to predict if CIN will progress to invasive carcinoma, there is evidence that CIN I lesions are more prone to regress spontaneously and that CIN II and CIN III are more likely to persist or progress.[7,13,14] There is a distinct progression from CIN III (carcinoma in situ) to frankly invasive squamous cell carcinoma of the cervix. Microinvasive squamous cell carcinoma is arbitrarily defined as squamous cell carcinoma with stromal penetration up to 5 mm or less in depth. The depth of penetration should be measured from the basement membrane of the base of the neoplastic epithelium by a calibrated ocular micrometer.

Clinically, most patients with microinvasive carcinoma are asymptomatic and present with no grossly visible lesions on pelvic examination. Most cases are detected initially in cytology and are confirmed by punch biopsy, conization, or hysterectomy.

Histology

Microinvasive squamous cell carcinoma consists of sharply penetrating tonguelike foci of well differentiated squamous cells at the base of CIN into the underlying stroma. The cells are of a distinctive squamous nature, with abundant eosinophilic cytoplasm and prominent macronucleoli. The stroma reacts to invasion by lymphoplasmacytic infiltration and fibroblastic proliferation (Fig. 18.16A, B). The penetrating neoplastic down growths may be multiple and confluent, and occasionally capillary or lymphatic invasion is seen.

Cytology

Most cells occur in syncytia, and some in sheets and some isolated. Most cells are round to oval; less frequently they are polyhedral or irregular in contour with a small amount of cytoplasm. The nuclei are round to oval and similar in size to those of carcinoma in situ. The nuclear chromatin is coarsely granular and irregular in distribution (Fig. 18.16C).

According to the review of Fu and Berek on microinvasive carcinoma of the cervix, there is a strong correlation between the frequency of lymph node metastasis and the depth of penetration. Carcinomas with invasion 0.1 to 3.0 mm in depth had lymph node metastasis in only 1% to 3% of 375 cases, and with 3.1 mm to 5.0 mm in depth had lymph node metastasis in 6% to 8% of 132 cases.[17] The suggested therapeutic modality is simple total hysterectomy for microinvasive carcinomas to a depth of 0.1 to 3.0 mm, and total hysterectomy with or without lymphadenectomy for those with invasion 3.1 to 5.0 mm in depth.

Invasive Squamous Cell Carcinoma

The incidence of invasive cervical squamous cell carcinoma has been markedly reduced where cervical cancer detection programs have been established. In contrast, cervical cancer is still among the leading cause of cancer deaths among women where no detection program exists.[1,18] Mass cytologic screening for cervical cancer will contribute to the reduction of the morbidity and mortality of cervical cancer by detection of the cancer in its early and curable stage.

It is a human tragedy that cervical cancer is still one of the leading causes of cancer deaths among women in many countries where mass cytology screening programs have not been established.

Since the introduction of cytologic screening to the general female population in Western countries three or more decades ago, there has been a dramatic reduction in the morbidity and mortality of invasive cervical carcinoma. This change is the most rewarding application of mass screening by cytology.[1] In contrast, the incidence rate of CIN (dysplasia and carcinoma in situ) has been steadily increasing (Fig. 18.17).

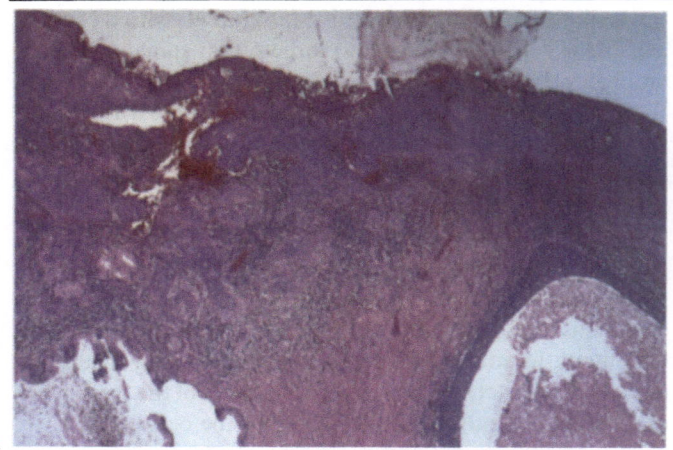

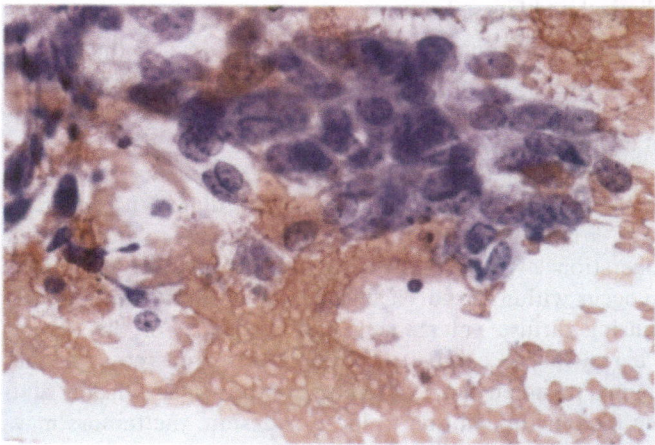

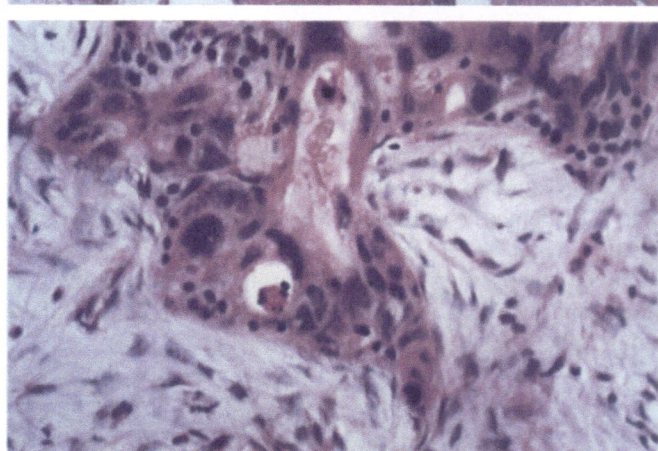

FIGURE 18.16 Microinvasive squamous cell carcinoma of the cervix. A: Microinvasive squamous cell carcinoma of the cervix. Neoplastic down growths penetrate the stroma and are accompanied by an inflammatory reaction (cervical biopsy). B: Microinvasive squamous cell carcinoma of the cervix. A tonguelike down growth penetrates the stroma (cervical biopsy). C: Syncytial aggregates of atypical cells with scanty cytoplasm, nuclear clearing, and irregularly distributed chromatin (Papanicolaou smear).

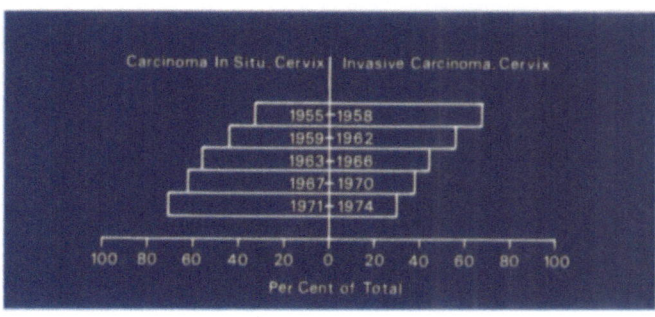

◄

FIGURE 18.17 Changing trends in the ratio of CIN and invasive cervical cancer. (From K. Kim et al.: Cancer 42:2439, 1978, with permission)

Clinical and Gross Features

Almost all patients with invasive carcinoma of the cervix complain of painless vaginal bleeding. Weakness, weight loss, edema of lower limbs, and hematuria are symptoms and signs of advanced disease.

In the early stage, cervical cancer presents as poorly defined "eroded" lesion with contact bleeding. With progression, a nodular, polypoid, or verrucous lesion with central ulceration develops (Fig. 18.18). The endophytic lesions tend to occur within the cervical canal and infiltrate into stroma, causing diffuse enlargement and hardening of the cervix ("barrel-shaped cervix"). Locally, the tumors spread to the vagina, parametrium, and the base of the urinary bladder and the rectum. In addition to local extension, the tumors may spread to the internal and external iliac lymph nodes.

Diagnosis is based on cytology, colposcopy, and biopsy. Rectovaginal examination, intravenous pyelography (IVP), cystoscopy, proctosigmoidoscopy, and a skeletal survey are required to assess the clinical stage of the tumor.

Cytology and Histology

The histologic subclassification of invasive squamous cell carcinoma of the uterine cervix has been controversial for decades. Broders' grading system was based on the degree of differentiation of the carcinoma and does not correlate with the response to radiotherapy.[19,20] Martzloff classified cervical squamous cell carcinomas into three types: spinal cell, transitional cell, and spindle cell.[21] Subsequently, Wentz and Reagan modified Martzloff's concept of classification.[22] Based on the cells derived from squamous cell carcinoma of the cervix, their classification consisted of (large cell) nonkeratinizing, keratinizing, and small cell carcinoma.

The cells may occur singly or in syncytial aggregates in a granular proteinaceous background (tumor diathesis). Compared with superficial squamous cells, the cells of invasive squamous cell carcinoma are small, similar in size to those of carcinoma in situ and microinvasive carcinoma. There are distinct differences in the cytologic features of the three types of invasive squamous cell carcinoma of the cervix.

Nonkeratinizing Squamous Cell Carcinoma

The cells in nonkeratinizing squamous cell carcinoma are relatively large and vary slightly in size. The smears usually show a distinct granular proteinaceous background. The nuclei are round to oval and have coarsely granular and irregularly dispersed chromatin. Macronucleoli may be conspicuous (Fig. 18.19A).

Histologically, (large cell) nonkeratinizing squamous cell carcinomas. Cells grow in sheets and nests of neoplastic squamous cells. Keratin pearls are absent (Fig. 18.19B).

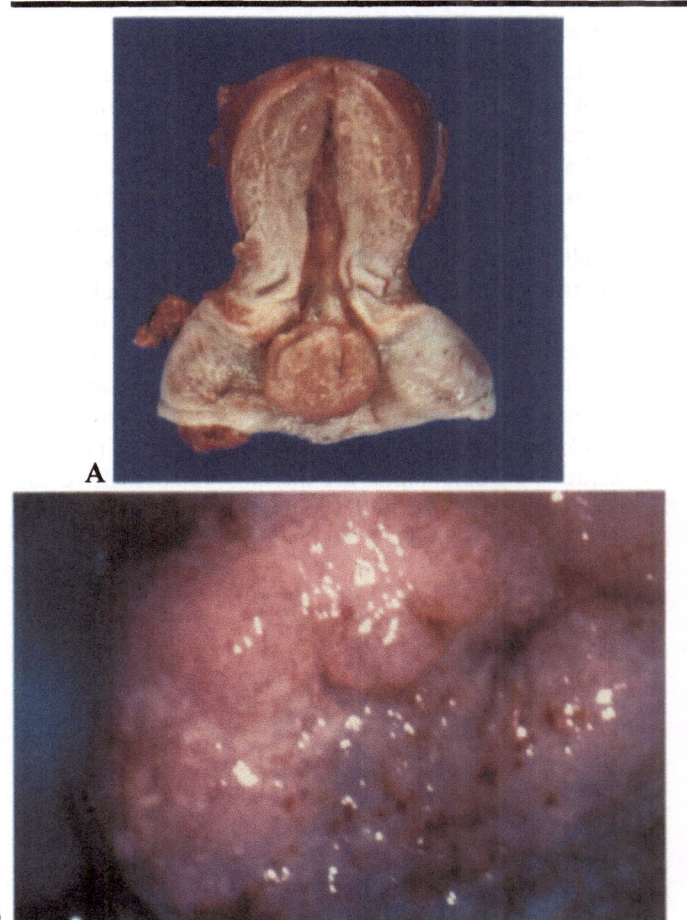

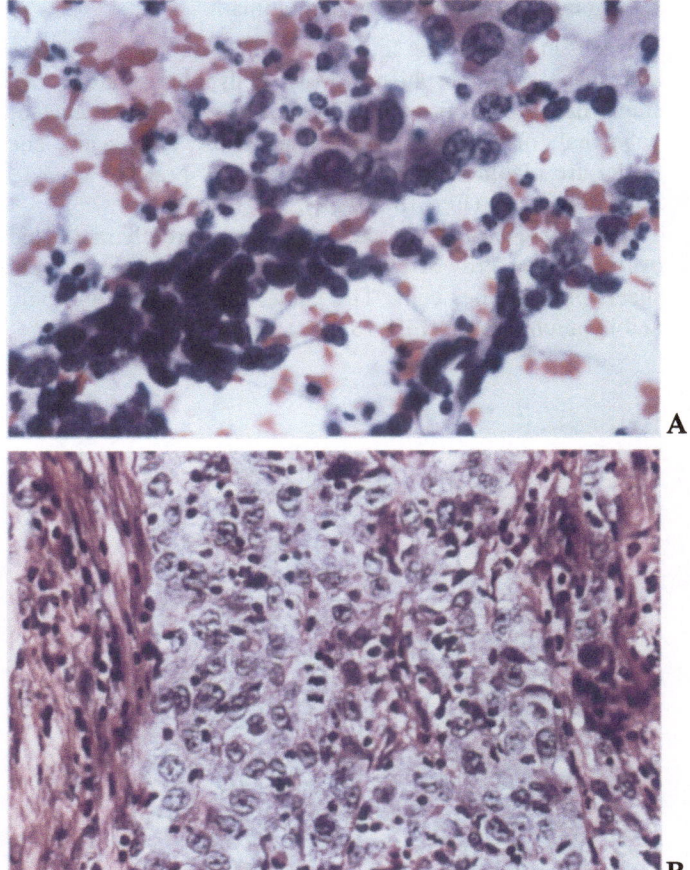

FIGURE 18.18   Invasive squamous cell carcinoma of the cervix. A: Exophytic fungating squamous cell carcinoma. **B**: Invasive squamous cell carcinoma (colposcopic view). Coarsely nodular surface with an irregular vascular pattern and hemorrhagic spots. (Courtesy of E.H. Vogel, M.D., Toledo, Ohio)

FIGURE 18.19   Nonkeratinizing squamous cell carcinoma of the cervix. A: The cells occur in syncytial group and have scanty cyanophilic cytoplasm and large, round to oval nuclei with irregularly dispersed clumped chromatin and prominent macronucleoli (Papanicolaou smear). **B**: Sheets and nests of neoplastic cells infiltrating fibrous stroma (cervical biopsy).

Keratinizing Squamous Cell Carcinoma

The cells in keratinizing squamous cell carcinoma vary in size and shape (pleomorphism). Most cells are isolated. The smear background is usually clean. The cells are elongated, polygonal, or caudate, with orangeophilic cytoplasm. The nuclei are pleomorphic and have coarsely granular or pyknotic chromatin (Fig. 18.20A,B).

Keratinizing squamous cell carcinomas are characterized by infiltrative growth patterns forming keratin pearls and sheets of squamous cells. The nuclei are large pleomorphic and hyperchromatic (Fig. 18.20C).

Small Cell Carcinoma

The cells in small cell carcinoma are relatively small and round or oval and have scanty cyanophilic cytoplasm. There is a prominent tumor diathesis in the background. The nuclei are oval and have coarsely granular chromatin. Macronucleoli are not frequently observed (Fig. 18.21A). Small cell carcinomas grow in a diffusely infiltrative manner, simulating small cell carcinomas of other organs. The cells have scanty cytoplasm and round to oval, hyperchromatic nuclei with coarsely granular chromatin and inconspicuous nucleoli. Squamous differentiation is not present (Fig. 18.21B).

Using the criteria of Wentz and Reagan, most squamous carcinomas are of nonkeratinizing type (59%), followed by those of keratinizing type (28%) and small cell type (13%).[23] Nonkeratinizing carcinomas are the most radiosensitive and have the best prognosis, followed by keratinizing carcinoma and small cell carcinoma.

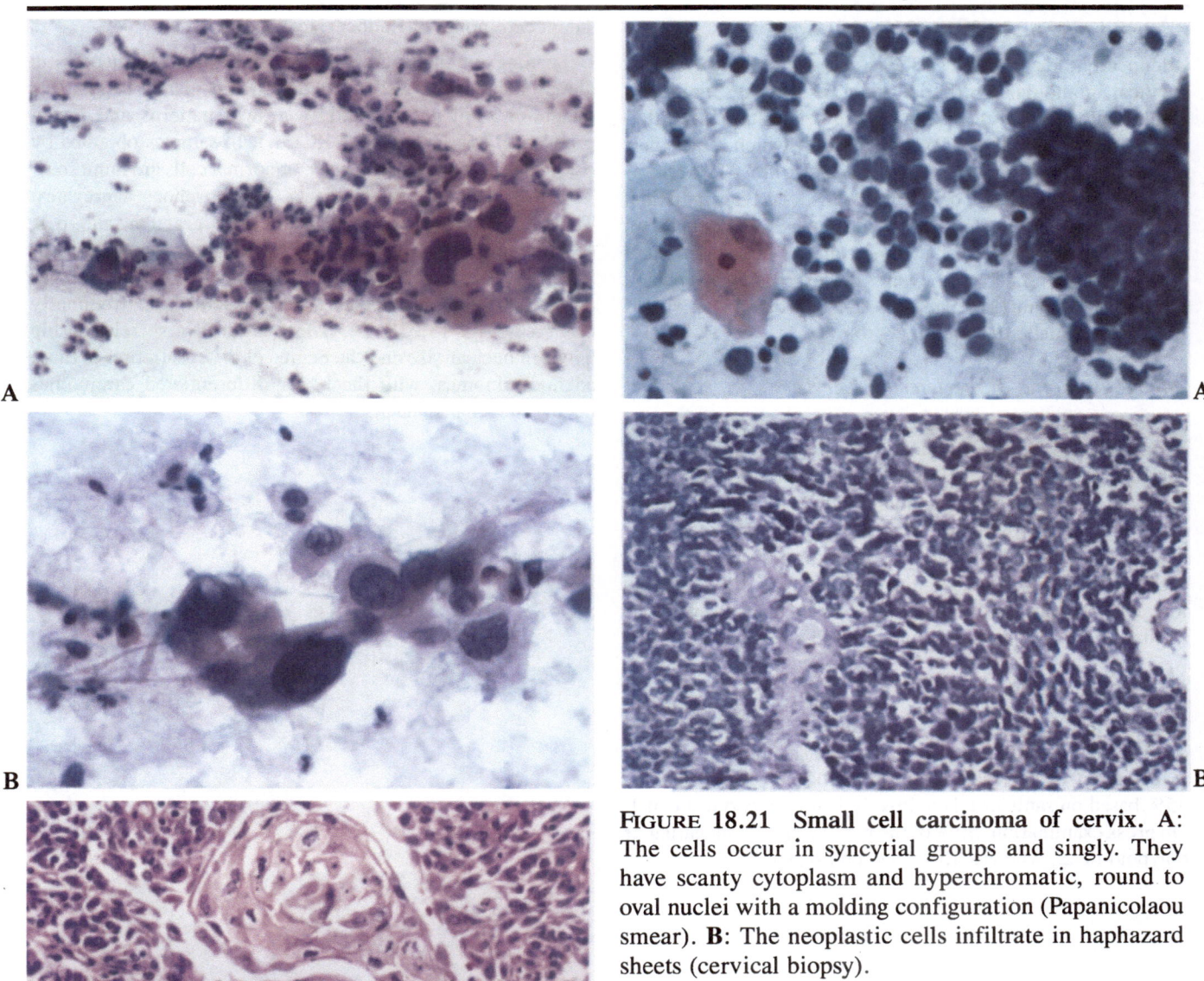

FIGURE 18.21 Small cell carcinoma of cervix. A: The cells occur in syncytial groups and singly. They have scanty cytoplasm and hyperchromatic, round to oval nuclei with a molding configuration (Papanicolaou smear). B: The neoplastic cells infiltrate in haphazard sheets (cervical biopsy).

FIGURE 18.20 Keratinizing squamous cell carcinoma of cervix. A, B: The cells occur in syncytial groups and singly. They are pleomorphic and have abundant eosinophilic cytoplasm and hyperchromatic pyknotic-appearing nuclei. Macronucleoli are not conspicuous (Papanicolaou smear). C: The neoplastic cells infiltrate in sheets, with prominent keratin pearls (cervical biopsy).

Adenocarcinoma In Situ *of Uterine Cervix*

Adenocarcinoma in situ (ACIS) is characterized by retained cervical glandular epithelial cells exhibiting malignant change but without evidence of invasion. The atypical epithelium is confined to the preexisting glands, which retain their normal branching pattern. Cells derived from ACIS occur as strips of columnar cells, or rosettes and sheets with indistinct cell borders. The nuclei are round to oval and larger than those of normal endocervical gland cells. The chromatin pattern is finely granular and evenly dispersed. Macronucleoli are usually absent (Fig. 18.22). Adenocarcinoma in situ is rare and is usually detected by cytology.

Adenocarcinoma of the Uterine Cervix

Six to 16% of all cervical carcinomas show glandular differentiation. The relative frequency of adenocarcinoma among cervical cancers has increased in recent years, with the increase found mainly in women younger than 35 years of age.[24] A study from Toledo, Ohio showed that cervical carcinomas with glandular differentiation composed 14% of 983 cases of all cervical cancers during a 20-year period.[1] Stage for stage the prognosis of endocervical adenocarcinoma is similar to that of cervical squamous cell carcinoma.

Clinical and Pathologic Features

Vaginal bleeding is the most common presenting symptom in cervical adenocarcinoma. The diagnostic accuracy of cytology in detection of cervical adenocarcinoma can reach 90% to 95% based on samples taken directly from the cervical canal. On gross examination, 50% of the patients have a fungating or polypoid mass, whereas 15% have no gross lesion.

Adenocarcinoma of Endocervical Type

Depending on the degree of differentiation, the neoplastic glands range from well formed crowded glands to abortive glands or solid nests. Papillary growth patterns and mucin production may occur (Fig. 18.23A). In samples obtained by cervical aspiration or cytobrush, abnormal cells are numerous. The cells occur in strips, sheets, or amorphous aggregates. They are columnar or polygonal, with granular and pale eosinophilic cytoplasm. The nuclei are large, round, oval, or irregular in shape. The chromatin is finely to coarsely granular and sometimes clumped. Macronucleoli are frequently observed (Fig. 18.23B–D). There is an inverse relationship between nuclear size and the degree of differentiation of these adenocarcinomas, with the better differentiated carcinomas having the smaller nuclei.

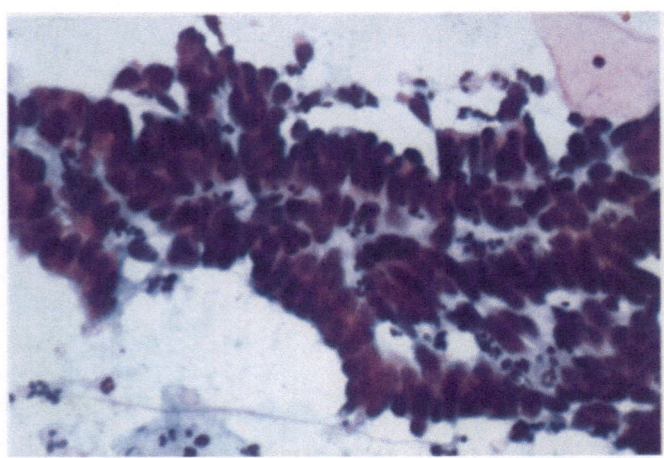

A

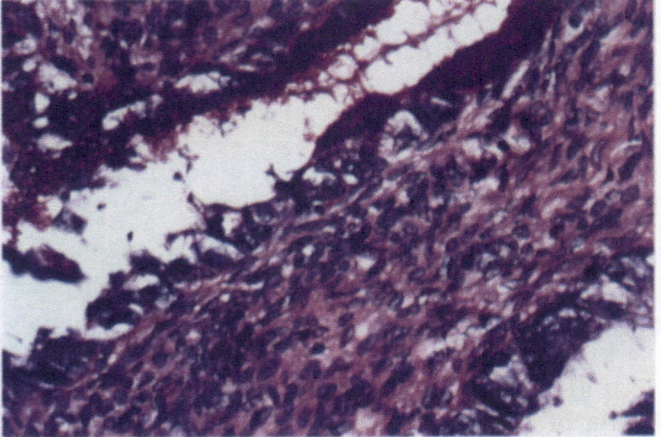

B

FIGURE 18.22 **Adenocarcinoma in situ of cervix. A:** The cells occur in strips and have a columnar configuration with round to oval, hyperchromatic nuclei. Macronucleoli are not conspicuous (Papanicolaou smear). **B:** The epithelium of the cervical glands is replaced by neoplastic cells. No stromal invasion is present (biopsy, PAS stain).

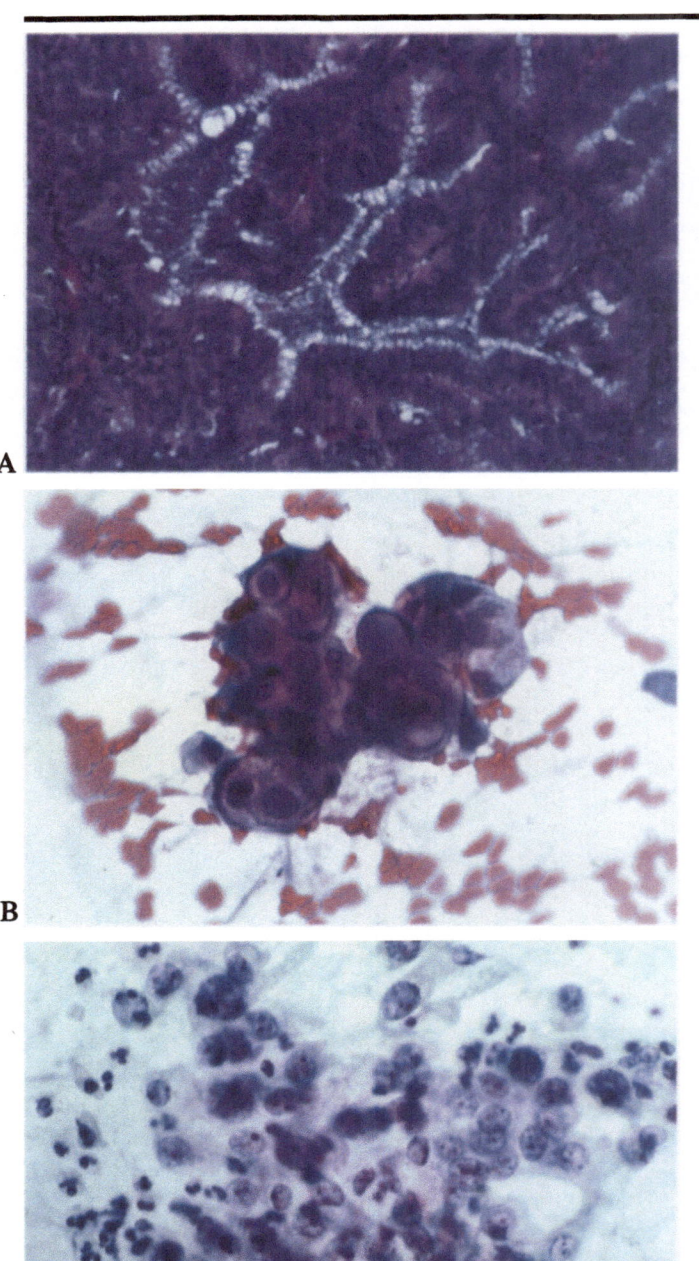

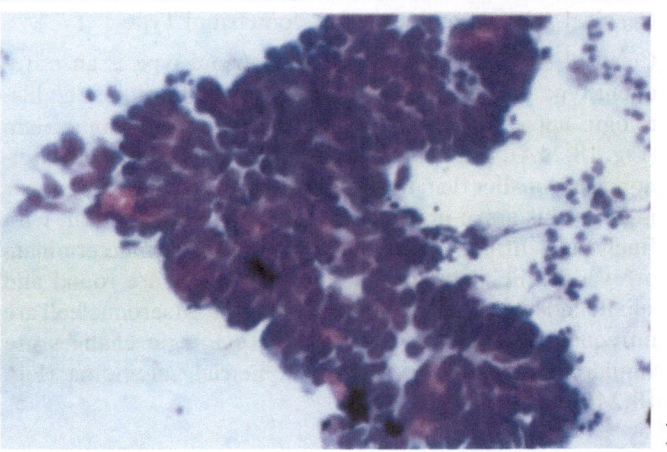

FIGURE 18.23 **Cervical adenocarcinoma of endocervical type.** A: The neoplasm consists of glands, nests, or papillary structure, separated by fibrous stroma (biopsy). **B, C, D**: Cervical adenocarcinoma of endocervical type (Papanicolaou smear). The cells occur in clusters (**B**), loose aggregates (**C**), or strips (**D**).

Cervical Adenocarcinoma of Endometrioid Type

Cervical adenocarcinoma of endometrioid type is an infrequent type of cervical adenocarcinoma that mimics the histologic appearance of its counterpart in the endometrium (Fig. 18.24A). The cells derived from this type of adenocarcinoma are smaller than those of endocervical type. They occur in loose clusters or in sheets. The cells are round to oval, with finely and diffusely vacuolated cytoplasm of indeterminate or cyanophilic staining reaction. The nuclei are round and small, and have finely granular chromatin. Macronucleoli are infrequently observed. Overall, the cytologic changes are similar to those observed in endometrial carcinoma (Fig. 18.24B, C).

Clear Cell Adenocarcinoma

Clear cell adenocarcinoma may arise in the vagina, cervix, endometrium, or ovary. The tumors are solid, cystic, or papillary. Papillary or cystic tumors may show "hobnail" carcinoma cells in the lining epithelium. The cytoplasm is optically clear because of glycogen loss in the processing of tissue (Fig. 18.25A). The cells occur singly, in clusters, or in sheets. The cytoplasm is poorly defined, finely and diffusely vacuolated. The nuclei are enlarged, round, or oval and hyperchromatic. The nuclear chromatin is finely to coarsely granular without clumping. Macronucleoli are prominent in most cells (Fig. 18.25B). The neoplasms involving the vagina and uterine cervix occur in young women, with a mean age at detection of 17 years. Most patients have a history of intrauterine exposure to diethylstilbestrol.[25] Mesonephric adenocarcinoma resembles or is identical to clear cell carcinoma.

Adenoacanthoma

Adenocanthoma consists of malignant glandular elements and benign squamous elements (Fig. 18.26). In cell samples, the cells are those of endocervical adenocarcinoma and benign squamous cells.

Adenosquamous Carcinoma

Adenosquamous carcinoma comprises neoplastic glandular and neoplastic squamous elements, and is divided into mature cell type, signet cell type, and glassy cell type (Fig. 18.27). The cells derived from these tumors are those of squamous cell carcinoma and endocervical adenocarcinoma. This neoplasm is highly aggressive; compared with other types of cervical adenocarcinoma this has a bad prognosis.

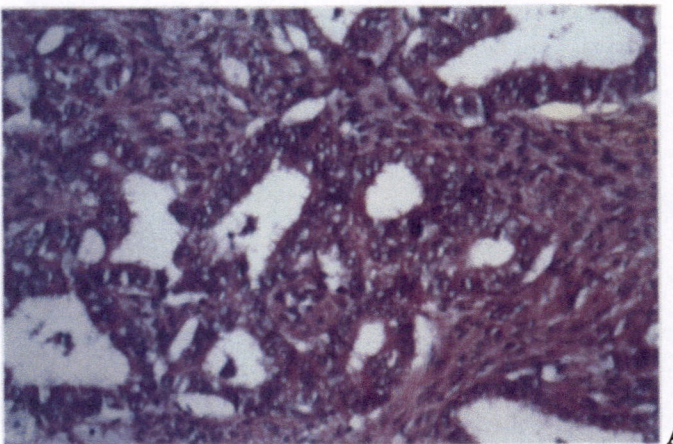

A

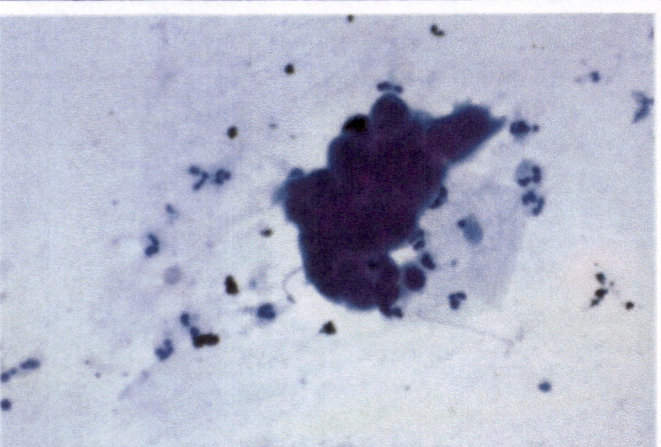

B

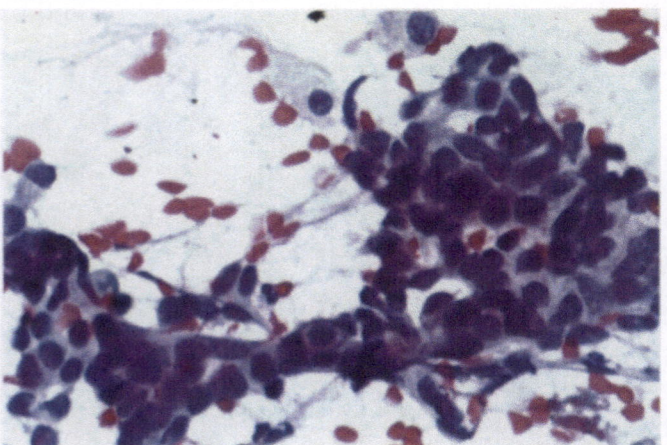

C

FIGURE 18.24 Cervical adenocarcinoma of endometrioid type. A: The neoplasm consists of compactly arranged glands and mimics the histologic appearance of endometrial adenocarcinoma (biopsy). B, C: The cells occur in clusters or sheets and have discernible cyanophilic cytoplasm and round to oval hyperchromatic nuclei (Papanicolaou smear).

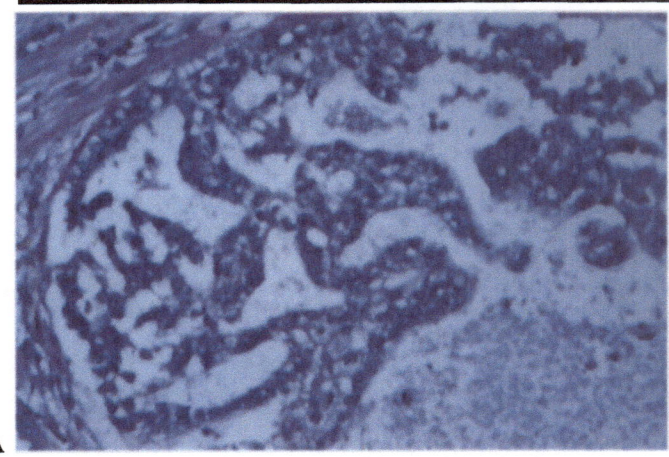

A

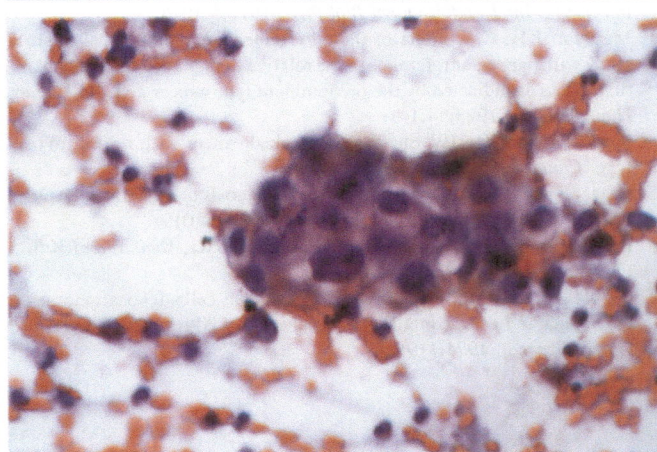

B

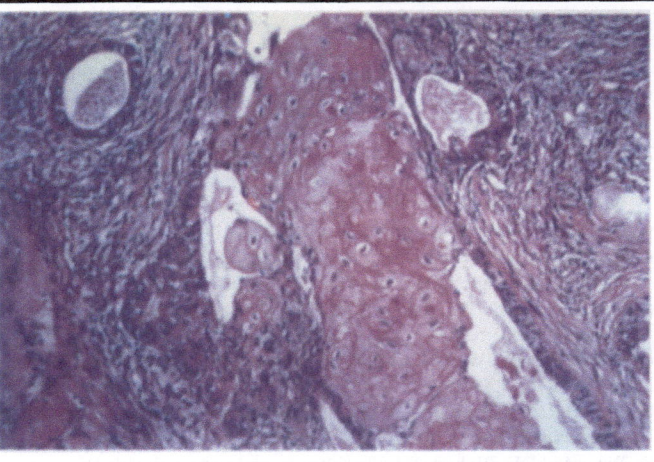

FIGURE 18.26 Adenoacanthoma of cervix (biopsy). Glandular neoplastic element and benign squamous element (*center*).

FIGURE 18.25 Clear cell adenocarcinoma of cervix. A: Cystic and papillary structures lined by optically clear cells (biopsy). **B**: Clear cell adenocarcinoma. The cells occur in clusters and have abundant clear cytoplasm (Papanicolaou smear).

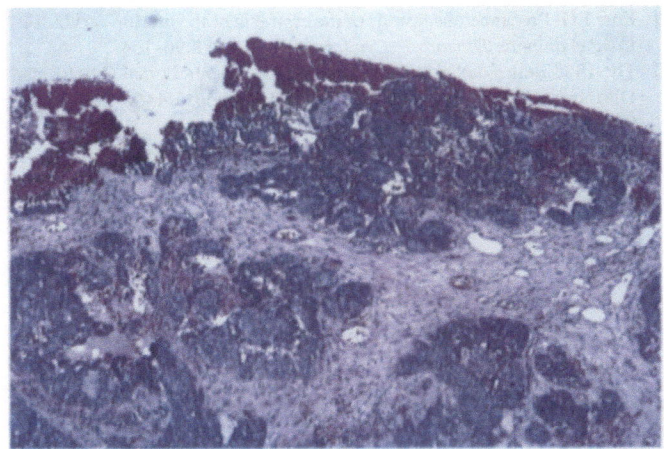

FIGURE 18.27 Adenosquamous carcinoma of cervix (biopsy). Both glandular and squamous neoplastic elements are present.

References

1. Kim K, et al. The changing trends of uterine cancer and cytology: A study of morbidity and mortality trends over a twenty year period. *Cancer*. 1978;42:2439.

2. Patten SF. *Benign Proliferative Reactions of the Uterine Cervix*. In: *Compendium on Diagnostic Cytology*. 6th ed. 1988.

3. Weid GL. *Proceedings of the First International Congress on Exfoliative Cytology*. 1st ed. Philadelphia: JB Lippincott, 1961.

4. Richart RM. *Cervical Intraepithelial Neoplasia. Pathology Annual*. Norwalk, Conn: Appleton-Century-Crofts, pp 301–328.

5. Fu YS, Reagan JW, Richart RM. Definitions of precursors. *Gynecol Oncol*. 1981;12:5220.

6. Fu YS, Reagan JW, Richart RM. Precursors of cervical cancer. *Cancer Surv*. 1983;2:359.

7. Richart RM, Barron BA. A follow-up study of patients with cervical dysplasia. *Am J Obstet Gynecol*. 1969;105:386.

8. Townsend DE, Richart RM. Cryotherapy and carbon dioxide laser management of cervical intraepithelial neoplasia. A controlled comparison. *Obstet Gynecol*. 1983;61:75.

9. Meisels A, et al. Human papilloma virus (HPV), venereal infections and gynecologic cancer. *Path Annu*. 1983;18(2):277.

10. Roy M, Meisels A, Fortier M, et al. Vaginal condylomata: A human papilloma virus infection. *Clin Obstet Gynecol*. 1981;24:261.

11. Koss LG. Precancerous lesions of the epithelia of the uterine cervix. In: *Compendium on Diagnostic Cytology*. 6th ed. 1988;96–104.

12. The 1988 Bethesda System for Reporting Cervical/Vaginal Cytological Diagnosis. National Cancer Institute Workshop. *JAMA*. 1988;262:931–934.

13. Barron BA, Cahill MC, Richart RM. A statistical model of the natural history of cervical carcinoma. II. Estimates of the transition time from dysplasia to carcinoma in situ. *J Natl Cancer Inst*. 1978;45:1025.

14. Barron BA, Cahill MC, Richart RM. A statistical model of the natural history of cervical carcinoma in situ. *Gynecol Oncol*. 1978;6:196.

15. Old JW, Wielenga G, von Haam E. Squamous carcinoma in situ of the uterine cervix. I. Classification and histogenesis. *Cancer*. 1965;18:1596.

16. Fu YS, Reagan JW. Pathology of the uterine cervix, vagina and vulva. In: *Major Problems in Pathology, Vol. 21*. Philadelphia: WB Saunders Co; 1989;248–251.

17. Fu YS, Berek JS. Minimal cervical cancer: Definition and histology. In: *Minimal Neoplasia—Diagnosis and Therapy. Recent Results in Cancer Research, Vol. 106*. Berlin: Springer-Verlag; 1988;47–56.

18. Silverberg E, Dubera JA. Cancer statistics. *CA*. 1989;39:3–20.

19. Broders AC. Carcinoma: Grading and practical application. *Arch Pathol*. 1926;2:376–381.

20. Reagan JW, Fu YS. Histologic types and prognosis of cancers of the uterine cervix. *Int J Radiat Oncol Biol Phys*. 1979;5:1015.

21. Martzloff KH. Carcinoma of the cervix uteri. A pathological clinical study with particular reference to the relative malignancy of the neoplastic process as indicated by the predominant type cancer cell. *Bull Johns Hopkins Hosp*. 1923;34:141.

22. Wentz WB, Reagan JW. Survival in cervical cancer with respect to cell type. *Cancer*. 1959;12:384.

23. Reagan JW, Fu YS. Histologic types and prognosis of cancers of the uterine cervix. *Int J Radiat Oncol Biol Phys*. 1979;5:1019.

24. Fu YS, Reagan JW. *Pathology of the Uterine Cervix, Vagina, and Vulva*. Philadelphia: WS Saunders Co; 1989;289–326.

25. Herbst AL, Robboy SL, Scully RE, et al. Clear cell adenocarcinoma of the vagina and cervix in girls: An analysis of 170 registry cases. *Am J Obstet Gynecol*. 1974;119:713.

19
The Uterine Corpus

Anatomy and Histology of the Uterine Corpus

During the reproductive years, the size and weight of a normal uterus vary according to parity. Nulliparous uteri weigh 40 to 100 g and measure about 8 cm in length, 5 cm in width at the fundus, and 2.5 cm in anteroposterior thickness. Multiparous uteri weigh up to 250 g and measure 12 cm × 5–7 cm × 3.5 cm.

The endometrial mucosa (endometrium) lines the uterine cavity above the internal os and measures a few millimeters in thickness. During the reproductive years the endometrium undergoes cyclic morphologic change, more prominent in the zona functionalis (inner two thirds) and minimal in the zona basalis (deeper one third) (Fig. 19.1). In postmenopausal life, the endometrium is thin, with sparse glands, and is devoid of cyclic change.

During a 28-day cycle, proliferation of the endometrium occurs from day 5 to day 14. This is referred to as the proliferative or follicular phase. Early in the proliferative phase the glands are sparse and tubular; later they become more tortuous and closely spaced. The epithelial cells lining the glands are simple cuboidal or columnar in the early proliferative phase and become enlarged in the later phase. Mitotic figures frequently are observed. The stroma is compact and comprises spindle-shaped or stellate cells with mitotic figures (Fig. 19.2). In terms of evaluating histopathologic changes of the endometrium, proliferative endometrium is generally regarded as the normal prototype.

After ovulation, the endometrium becomes thick with closely arranged tortuous glands with dilated lumens. This is the secretory or luteal phase. Distinctive histologic change of the secretory phase begins to occur on day 17, postovulatory day (POD) 3, when the endometrium shows S-shaped glands with conspicuous subnuclear vacuolization and nuclear palisading. The stroma is relatively edematous (Fig. 19.3). These changes are the first morphologic evidence of ovulation. As the cycle advances, the glands are dilated and tortuous and the stroma becomes more edematous. At day 23 (POD 9), the stroma contains prominent spiral arteries with periarterial deciduoid change (Fig. 19.4). Subsequently, the glands become more tortuous and the stroma shows diffuse deciduoid change.

Acute Endometritis

The cervix acts as a barrier to the entry of microorganisms into the endometrial cavity. This barrier is less effective during menstruation, abortion, delivery, instrumentation, and the wearing of an intrauterine contraceptive device (IUD).

Common causative agents of acute endometritis are *Streptococcus*, *Staphylococcus*, *Neisseria gonorrhoeae*, and *Clostridium welchi*.

The histologic diagnosis of acute endometritis is based on finding aggregates of neutrophil leukocytes in the stroma and gland lumens (Fig. 19.5).

Chronic Endometritis

Patients with chronic endometritis may present with menometrorrhagia, mucopurulent cervical discharge or uterine tenderness, but some are asymptomatic. Chronic endometritis has been observed in 3% to 10% of women undergoing an endometrial biopsy for irregular bleeding.[1,2] It has been associated with abortion in 41% of cases, with salpingitis in 25%, with an IUD in 14%, and with a recent pregnancy in 12%.[3]

The histologic diagnosis is made by identifying plasma cells in the stroma, and enlarged spindle-shaped stromal cells arranged in a pinwheel pattern around the glands (Fig. 19.6).

An important diagnostic clue for the pathologist is difficulty in dating the endometrium because of a wide variation in the maturation of the glands or a discordance between the glands and stroma. The diagnosis of chronic endometritis in an asymptomatic patient should be followed by an endocervical culture for gonococci and Chlamydia.

Dysfunctional Uterine Bleeding

The term "dysfunctional uterine bleeding" is used for uterine bleeding without an underlying organic pathologic condition. The bleeding results from derangements in the magnitude or duration of the effect of estrogen and progesterone on the endometrium. Abnormalities along the hypothalamic-pituitary-ovarian axis may result in derangement of follicular maturation, ovulation, or corpus luteum development, with subsequent abnormal hormone secretion.

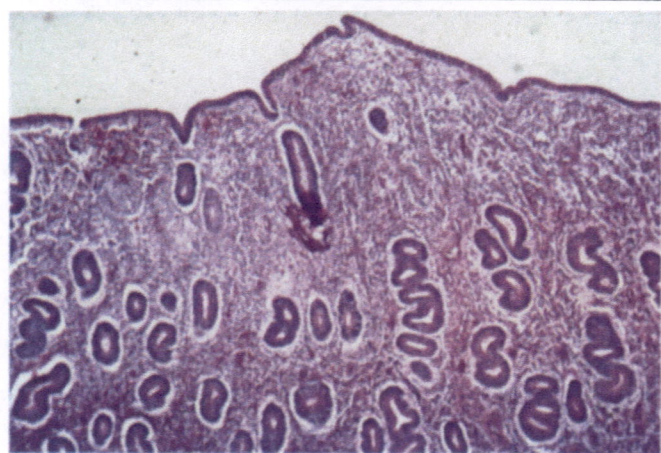

FIGURE 19.1   Endometrial mucosa of proliferative phase. Tubuloglandular structures separated by abundant compact stroma.

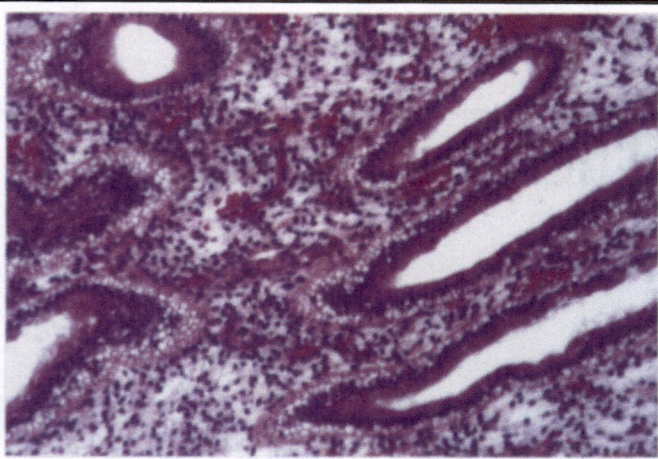

FIGURE 19.3   Endometrium of early secretory phase (day 17). Dilated glands lined by a single layer of columnar cells with subnuclear secretory vacuoles.

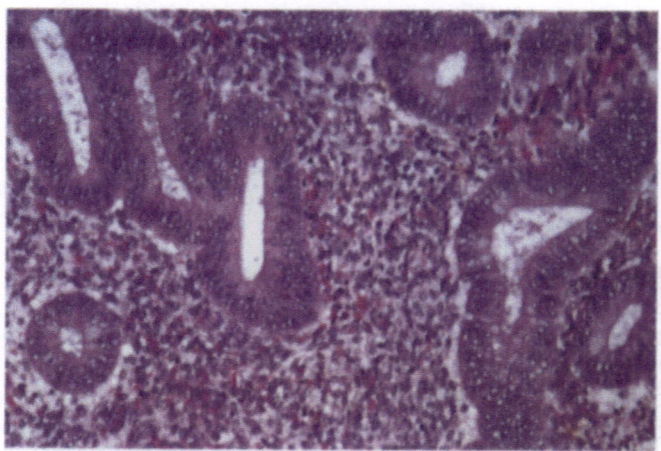

FIGURE 19.2   Endometrial glands and stroma of proliferative phase. The glands are lined by pseudo-stratified columnar cells, and the stromal cells are abundant and compact.

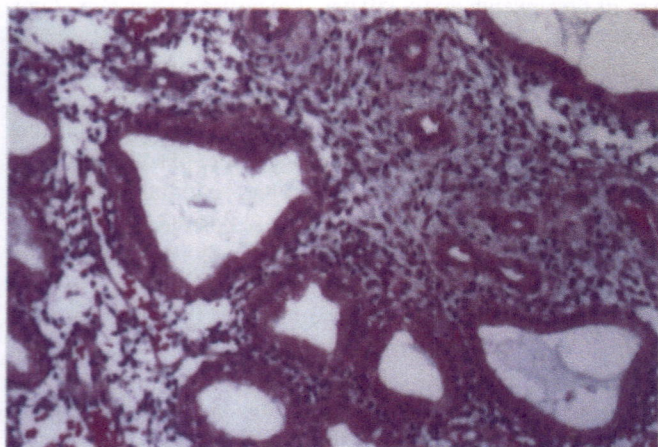

FIGURE 19.4   Endometrium of secretory phase (day 23). Dilated glands lined by a single layer of columnar cells. The stroma has prominent spiral arteries with periarterial deciduoid change.

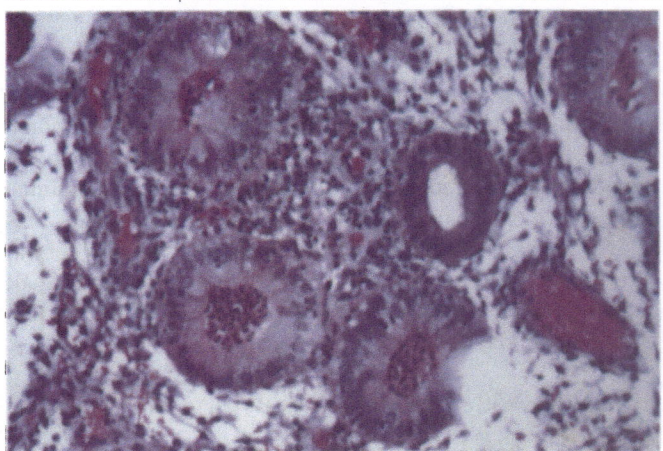

FIGURE 19.5 Acute endometritis. Aggregates of polymorphonuclear leukocytes in the stroma and glands.

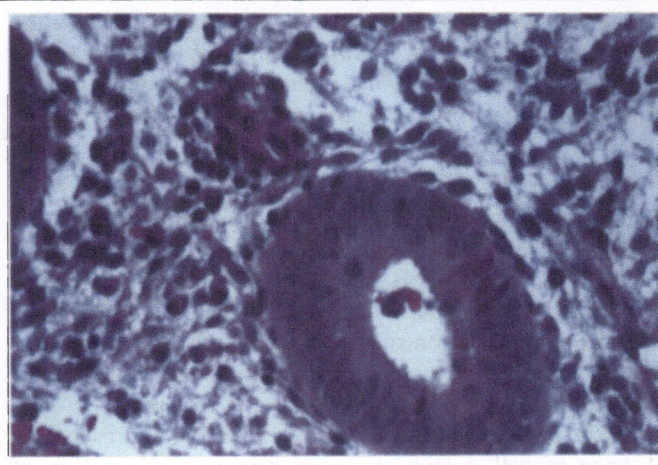

FIGURE 19.6 Chronic endometritis. Scattered plasma cells in the stroma.

Estrogen withdrawal as a result of anovulatory cycles is the most common cause of dysfunctional uterine bleeding, but luteal phase defect and failure of the corpus luteum to regress at the appropriate time (irregular shedding) are other causes.

Endometrial Hyperplasia

Endometrial hyperplasia produces endometrial bleeding and has the potential to evolve into endometrial carcinoma. Endometrial hyperplasia occurs most often in perimenopausal or postmenopausal women. It is caused by relative or absolute hyperestrogenism, such as is seen with polycystic ovaries, anovulatory cycles, estrogen-producing ovarian tumors, and prolonged use of exogenous estrogen.

On the basis of glandular architecture and the presence or absence of cell atypia, the conventional classification of endometrial hyperplasia is cystic hyperplasia, adenomatous hyperplasia, and atypical hyperplasia. Recently, the International Society of Gynecologic Pathologists proposed a classification based on the presence or absence of cytologic atypia and the natural history of the disease. It is known that fewer than 2% of hyperplasias without cytologic atypia progress to carcinoma regardless of architectural pattern, whereas 23% of hyperplasias with cytologic atypia (atypical hyperplasia) progress to carcinoma.[4]

Hyperplasia Without Atypia

The endometrial glands are active and increased in number in hyperplasia without atypia. They are cystically dilated with occasional outpouching and are separated by abundant stroma (simple hyperplasia) (Fig. 19.7). If the glands are crowded with prominent infolding and outpouching and lined by stratified epithelial cells with frequent mitotic figures, it is designated as complex hyperplasia (adenomatous hyperplasia) (Fig. 19.8). The epithelial cells may be slightly enlarged, but their nuclei are bland and similar to those of the normal proliferative glands.

Hyperplasia With Atypia (Atypical Hyperplasia)

Atypical hyperplasia is similar in architecture to that of hyperplasia without atypia. However, the epithelial cells are atypical, with loss of polarity. The cells show an increased nucleocytoplasmic ratio. The nuclei are enlarged, round, and hyperchromatic, with coarse chromatin, and have prominent nucleoli (Fig. 19.9).

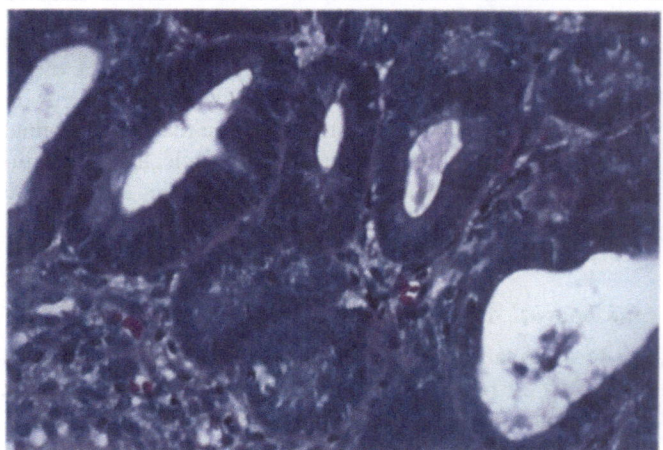

FIGURE 19.7 Simple hyperplasia of endometrium (cystic hyperplasia). Tubular and cystically dilated glands and abundant intervening stroma. The epithelial cells are active, but there is no nuclear atypia.

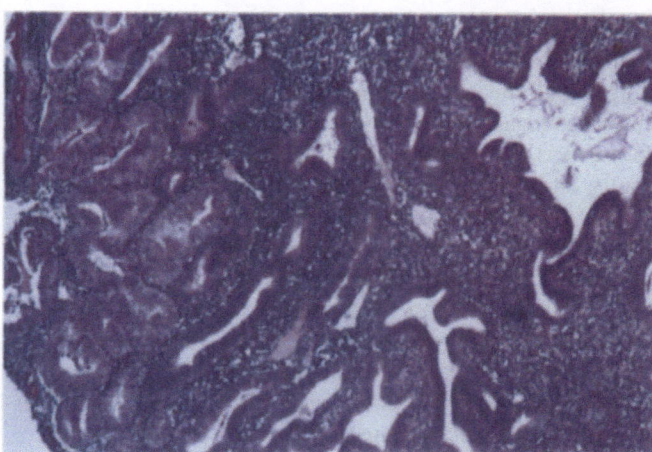

FIGURE 19.9 Hyperplasia with atypia (atypical hyperplasia) of endometrium. Atypical change of the glandular epithelial cells with large hyperchromatic nuclei. The glands are small and tightly arranged (*left*).

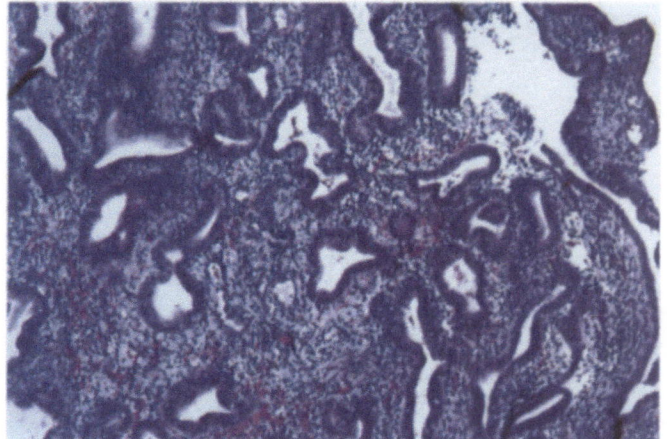

FIGURE 19.8 Complex hyperplasia of endometrium without atypia (adenomatous hyperplasia). Endometrial glands with infolding and outpouchings.

Cytology of Endometrial Hyperplasia

Compared with adenocarcinoma of the endometrium, the cells of endometrial hyperplasia retain in various degrees the mutual adhesiveness of their normal counterpart. Since in endometrial hyperplasia the number of cells is likely to be scanty and the cytologic changes subtle, the cytologic features of this condition have not been well documented. Samples obtained directly from the endometrium and cervical canal are recommended for evaluation of the endometrium. Cells originating from endometrial hyperplasia occur in sheets and are rarely isolated. Their size varies and depends on the degree of atypia. The nuclei are slightly enlarged and round. Nuclear chromatin is finely granular and evenly distributed. Macronucleoli are rarely observed (Fig. 19.10).

Management of Endometrial Hyperplasia

In long-term follow-up, 11% to 23% of women with atypical hyperplasia develop well differentiated endometrial carcinoma. Hysterectomy is reserved for the perimenopausal and postmenopausal women with a high grade of atypical hyperplasia. Young women with low grade atypical hyperplasia may be treated conservatively, either by ovarian suppression with progestins or by induction of ovulation, but close follow-up and periodic endometrial biopsies are necessary.[4]

Endometrial Polyp

Endometrial polyps are usually sessile polypoid masses, measuring up to 3.0 cm in diameter. They usually occur in menopausal or perimenopausal women and may cause vaginal bleeding due to mucosal ulceration. Histologically, they comprise normal or hyperplastic endometrium covered by endometrial mucosa and have a central fibrovascular core (Fig. 19.11). Malignant change in an endometrial polyp is rare.

Endometrial Adenocarcinoma in situ

The term adenocarcinoma in situ of the endometrium was introduced by Hertig et al., and the histopathologic criteria for its diagnosis were modified by Buehl et al.[5] Adenocarcinoma in situ is characterized by a small lesion involving no more than five or six glands, with cytologic atypia, but in which there is no evidence of invasion. The cells are large, with loss of polarity, and have abundant amphophilic or eosinophilic cytoplasm. The nuclei are enlarged, round, and hyperchromatic, with clumping of chromatin and irregular outlines. Macronucleoli are prominent (Fig. 19.12).

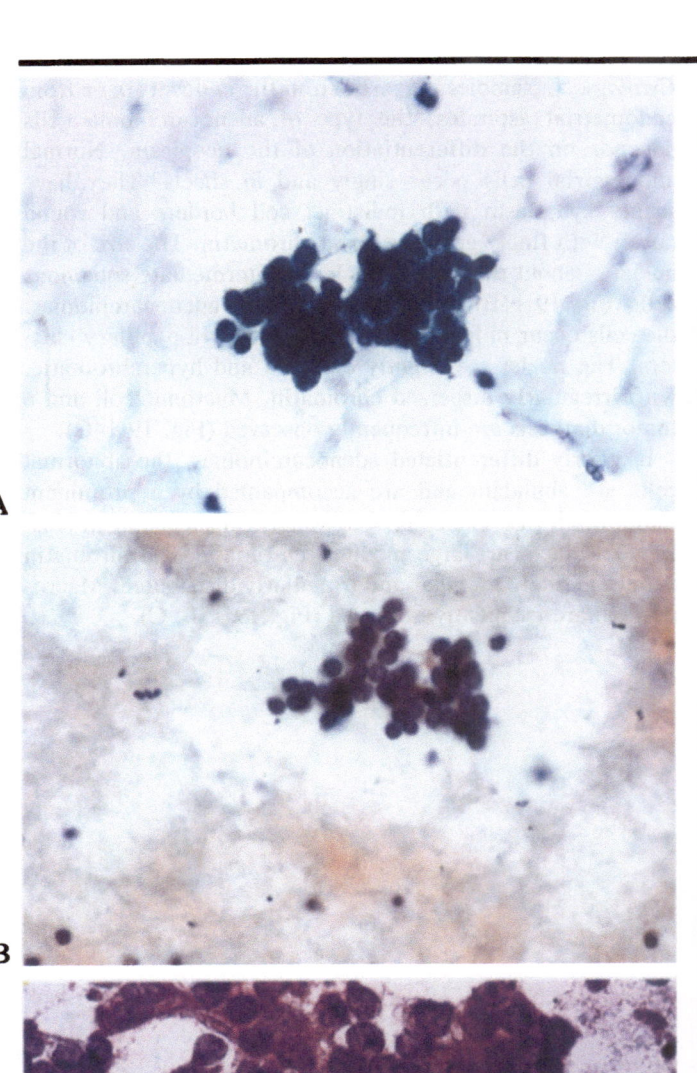

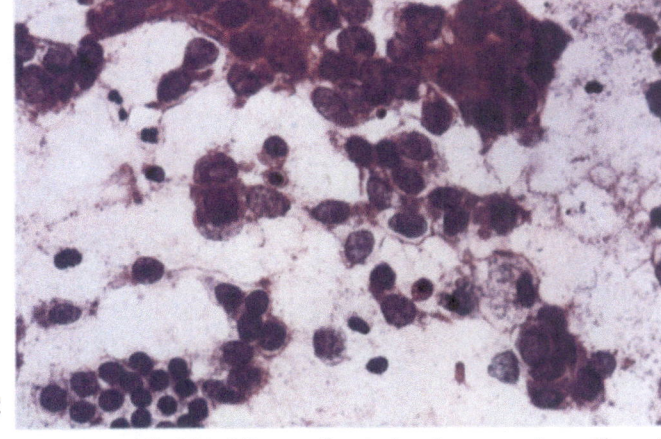

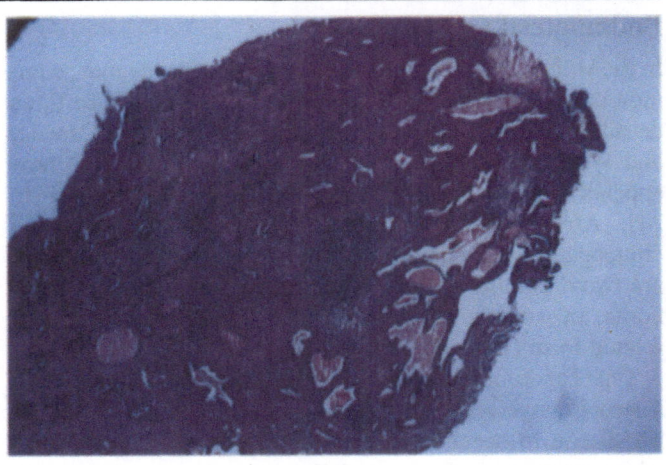

FIGURE 19.11 Endometrial polyp. Polypoid mass covered by endometrial mucosa on three sides and comprising hyperplastic endometrial glands.

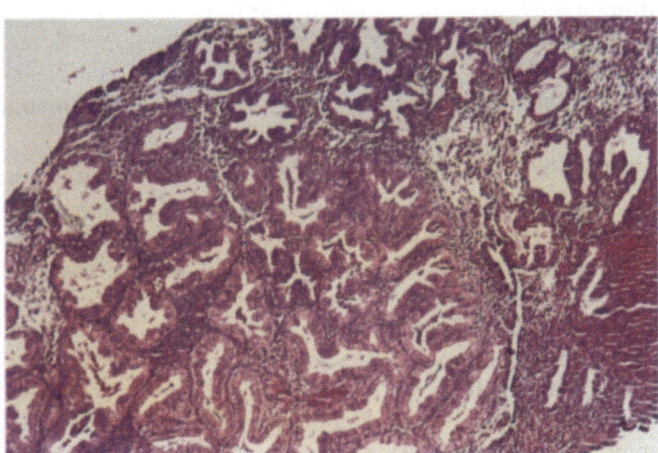

FIGURE 19.12 Adenocarcinoma in situ of endometrium. Well circumscribed compact neoplastic glands (*lower left*) in a background of adenomatous hyperplasia (*right*).

FIGURE 19.10 Normal and abnormal cells of endometrium. A: Endometrial hyperplasia showing cell aggregates with loss of cell polarity and nuclear enlargement (endometrial aspirate). **B**: Normal endometrial epithelial cells (endometrial aspirate). Sheets of normal endometrial cells. **C**: Normal endometrial cells (*left lower*) and cells of endometrial adenocarcinoma (*top*) (endometrial aspirate).

Endometrial Carcinoma

In the United States, endometrial carcinoma is the most common cancer of the female genital tract. Over the past three decades its incidence has risen in the United States, Canada, and Western Europe, although in the United States it now appears to be leveling off.[6] The incidence is much lower in Asia, Africa, and South America.[7] Several epidemiologic and clinicopathologic studies support the hypothesis that there are two dissimilar pathogenetic forms of endometrial carcinoma, an estrogen-related form (Type I) and a non–estrogen-related form (Type II).[8-10]

Type I endometrial carcinomas are more common and have a strong association with unopposed estrogen stimulation. They tend to occur in premenopausal and perimenopausal white women, to be well differentiated, to coexist with endometrial hyperplasia, and to have a better prognosis.

In contrast, Type II endometrial carcinomas are less common and not associated with estrogenic stimulation, and tend to occur in older postmenopausal black women, to be poorly differentiated, to occur without hyperplasia, and to be clinically aggressive.

Adenosquamous carcinoma, serous carcinoma and clear cell carcinoma belong to the type II endometrial carcinoma.

Clinical and Pathologic Features

The first clinical presentation of endometrial carcinoma is irregular vaginal bleeding, reflecting erosion and ulceration of the neoplastic mucosa. The endometrial lesion is shaggy, granular, and soft, and diffuse or circumscribed (Fig. 19.13). By direct extension the adenocarcinoma may involve the myometrium, peritoneum, uterine tubes, ovaries, cervix, and vagina. The lymphatic system of the uterus may facilitate the spread of uterine adenocarcinoma to pelvic and paraaortic lymph nodes, uterine cervix, vagina, external genitalia, and other pelvic organs.

Histopathology and Cytology

Adenocarcinoma

Seventy percent of malignant endometrial neoplasms are adenocarcinomas. In these lesions, the glands are increased in number, vary in size and shape, and are arranged back to back with scanty stroma. Well differentiated adenocarcinomas (Grade I) tend to reproduce in varying degrees the normal glandular pattern (Fig. 19.14A). Poorly differentiated adenocarcinoma (Grade III) has an inconspicuous glandular or a more discernible papillary pattern (Fig. 19.15A). Moderately differentiated adenocarcinoma (Grade II) has an irregular but definite glandular pattern combined with medullary sheets and poorly formed glands.

Cytology. In samples prepared from the endocervix or from endometrial aspirates, the type of adenocarcinoma cells depends on the differentiation of the neoplasm. Normal endometrial cells occur singly and in sheets. They have scanty cytoplasm with indistinct cell borders and round nuclei with finely granular bland chromatin. The size of the nuclei is about that of the nuclei of intermediate squamous cells (Fig. 19.14B). In well differentiated adenocarcinomas, the cells occur in loose aggregates or in tight papillary clusters. The nuclei are slightly enlarged and hyperchromatic, with irregularly dispersed chromatin. Macronucleoli and a tumor diathesis are infrequently observed (Fig. 19.14C).

In poorly differentiated adenocarcinomas, the abnormal cells are abundant and are accompanied by a prominent tumor diathesis. The cells occur singly, in sheets, or in clusters. The nuclei are large and hyperchromatic. The chromatin pattern is finely granular and irregularly distributed. Macronucleoli are frequently observed (Fig. 19.15B, C).

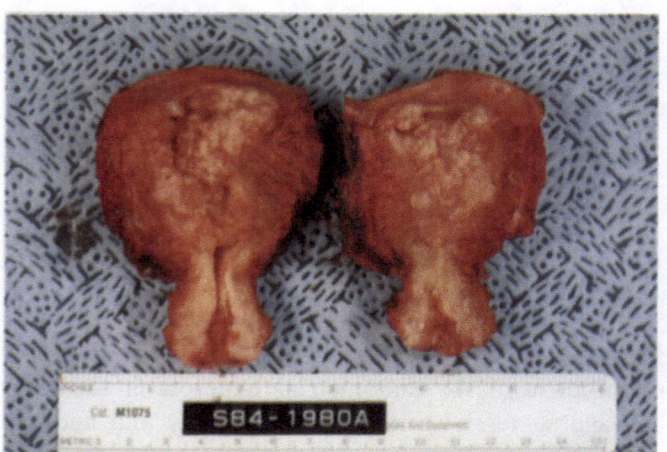

FIGURE 19.13 **Adenocarcinoma of endometrium.** Neoplasm replaces the uterine cavity (bisected uterus).

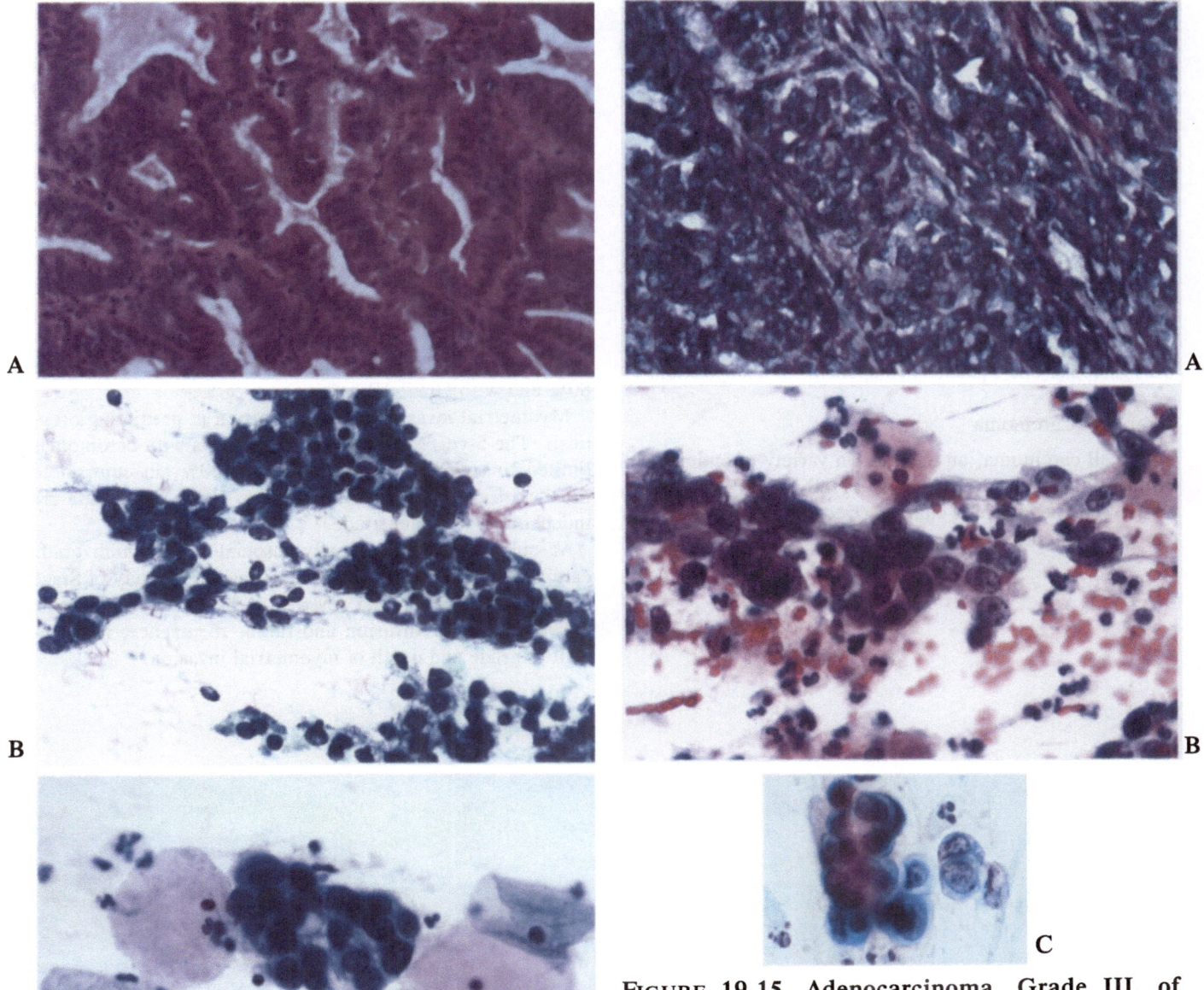

FIGURE 19.14 Adenocarcinoma, Grade I. A: Well formed glands arranged back to back with scanty intervening stroma (endometrial curettage). B: Normal endometrial cells in sheets with scanty cyanophilic cytoplasm and uniform round nuclei (endometrial aspiration smear). C: Three-dimensional clusters of cells of adenocarcinoma, Grade I, of endometrium. Compare their nuclear size to that of nuclei of intermediate squamous cells.

FIGURE 19.15 Adenocarcinoma, Grade III, of endometrium. A: Sheets of neoplastic cells with inconspicuous glands (biopsy). B: The cells occur in loose aggregates and have large nuclei and prominent macronucleoli (endocervical aspirate). C: Papillary cluster of cells from a papillary adenocarcinoma, Grade III (endocervical aspirate).

Adenoacanthoma

Adenoacanthoma consists of adenocarcinoma with a benign metaplastic squamous epithelial component. The glandular element is usually well differentiated (Fig. 19.16). Ten to 15% of all endometrial carcinomas are of this type.

Adenosquamous Carcinoma

Adenosquamous carcinomas, accounting for 10% to 15% of all endometrial carcinomas, have a poor 5-year survival. The neoplasm is characterized by malignant glandular and squamous elements. The glandular element tends to be poorly differentiated, and in 80% of cases the squamous component is nonkeratinizing (Fig. 19.17). The cells occur singly and in aggregates, with glandular and squamous components in juxtaposition.

Clear Cell Carcinoma

Clear cell carcinoma, an uncommon variety of endometrial carcinoma, comprises only 1% of all endometrial carcinomas. The neoplasm is characterized by sheets, tubules, or papillary structures.

The cells are large with optically clear cytoplasm. Their nuclei are large, round, and hyperchromatic, and have prominent macronucleoli. Cells that have discharged their glycogen and lost most of their cytoplasm are characterized by a naked or near naked nucleus, and are referred to as "hobnail" cells (Fig. 19.18A). In cellular samples, the cells occur singly, in sheets, or in clusters. Their cytoplasm is poorly defined and diffusely vacuolated. The nuclei are enlarged, round, or oval, with clumped chromatin and prominent nucleoli (Fig. 19.18B).

Pathologic Risk Factors of Endometrial Carcinomas

Histologic grading is closely correlated with survival. The 5-year survival rate for patients with Grade I carcinomas is 80% and with Grade III carcinomas, 50%.[11]

Myometrial invasion is also important in predicting prognosis. The 5-year survival rate for patients with carcinomas limited to superficial myometrium is 80%, in contrast to those with deep myometrial invasion, 60%. These data are independent of tumor grade.[11]

Vascular invasion is usually associated with high grade carcinomas and deep myometrial invasion. A study of Stage I endometrial carcinoma revealed a significant correlation between vascular invasion and tumor recurrence, independent of grade and depth of myometrial invasion.[12]

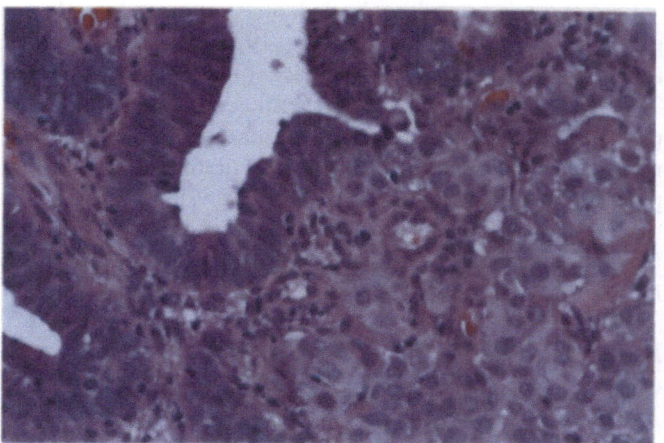

FIGURE 19.16 **Adenoacanthoma of endometrium.** Well formed neoplastic glands mixed with a benign squamous neoplastic element.

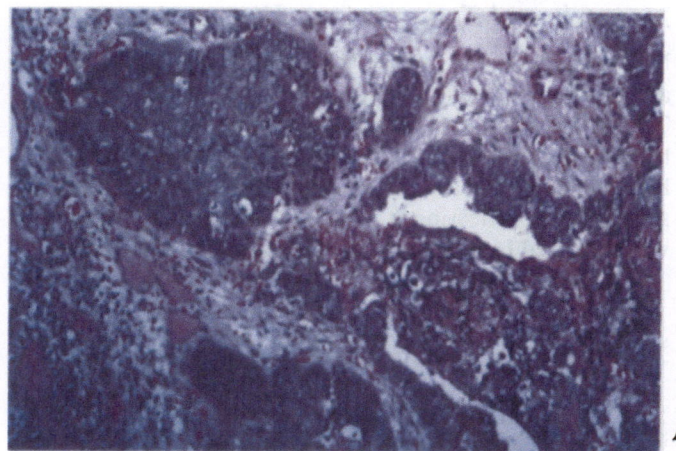

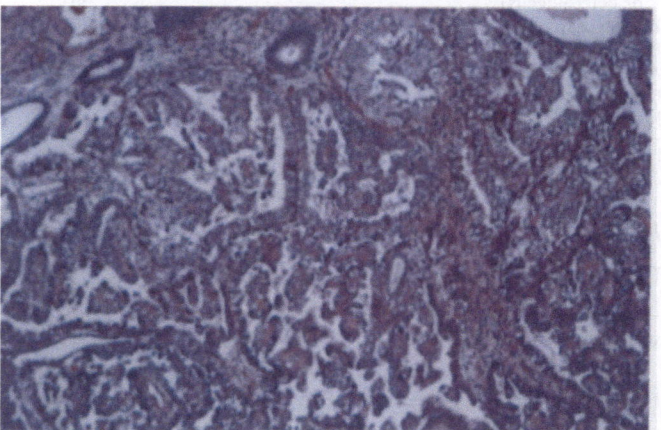

FIGURE 19.18 **Clear cell adenocarcinoma of endometrium. A**: Sheets and papillary and cystic structures of clear cells. **B**: Clear cell clusters of the same case (endocervical aspirate).

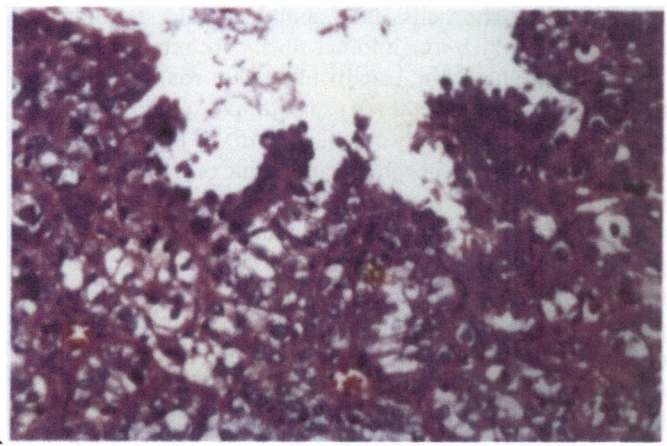

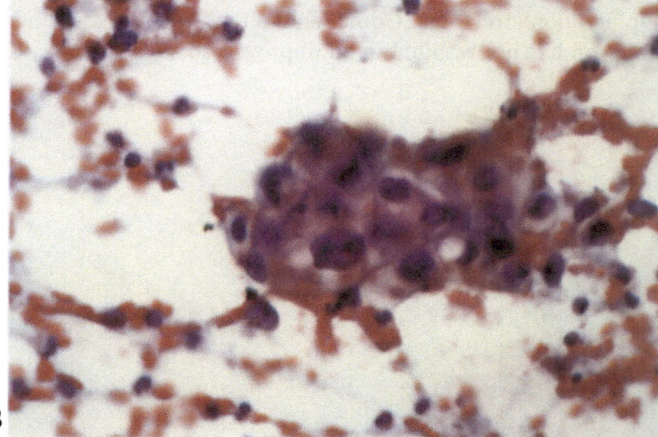

FIGURE 19.17 **A**: Adenosquamous cell carcinoma of endometrium consisting of malignant glandular and squamous elements. **B**: Serous endometrial carcinoma resembling ovarian popillary serous adeno-carcinoma (for comparison with adenosquamous cell carcinoma).

Mesenchymal Tumors of the Uterus

Mesenchymal tumors of the uterus, other than leiomyomas, are uncommon, constituting only 3% of uterine cancers.[13] They arise from the mesodermal premordium that is to become the uterus, and may express their multipotentiality by a mixture of epithelial and mesodermal components. A simplified classification of mesenchymal tumors of the uterus was proposed by Zaloudek and Norris[14] (Table 19.1).

Table 19.1. Classification and relative frequency of uterine sarcoma.

Type	Percent of uterine sarcomas
Mixed müllerian tumor (carcinosarcoma homologous or heterologous)	30
Leiomyosarcoma	27
Endometrial stromal sarcoma	26
Adenosarcoma	8
Unclassified sarcoma	6
Miscellaneous sarcomas	3

From Zaloudek C, Norris HJ. In: Kurman (ed): *Blaustein's Pathology of the Female Genital Tract*. 3rd ed. New York: Springer-Verlag.

Leiomyoma

Leiomyoma, a benign tumor of smooth muscle cells, is the most common uterine neoplasm, occurring in 20% to 30% of women more than 30 years of age.

The clinical presentation depends on their size and location. Most patients with uterine leiomyomas are asymptomatic; usually the neoplasms are detected at a routine pelvic examination. The most common symptoms are pelvic pain, a sensation of pressure in the pelvis, and excessive uterine bleeding. Leiomyomas may involve intramural, subserosal, or submucosal sites. The neoplasms are well circumscribed but not encapsulated. On section they are bulging and resilient (Fig. 19.19A). Large leiomyomas may show various degenerative changes: hemorrhage, necrosis, cyst formation, and hyalinization.

Leiomyomas comprise whorled, anastomosing fascicles of elongated smooth muscle cells (Fig. 19.19B). The neoplasms are well demarcated from the adjacent normal myometrium. The cells tend to run in parallel with each other. They have pale eosinophilic cytoplasm and bland elongated nuclei. No mitotic activity is present. Sarcomas seldom, if ever, arise in preexisting leiomyomas.

Several subtypes of leiomyomas must be distinguished from leiomyosarcoma. They are cellular leiomyoma, atypical leiomyoma, and epithelioid leiomyoma.

Leiomyosarcoma

Vaginal bleeding, lower abdominal pain, and a pelvic mass are the usual symptoms and signs of leiomyosarcoma. A rapid increase in the size of a uterine tumor in a postmenopausal woman should arouse suspicion of sarcoma.

Leiomyosarcomas are large, usually more than 10 cm in diameter, soft, fleshy, and pale gray. Multifocal necrosis and hemorrhage frequently are observed (Fig. 19.20A). Histologically, leiomyosarcomas consist of interlacing bundles of spindle cells. The cells have abundant pale, eosinophilic cytoplasm in which longitudinal fibrils are often identified. The nuclei are fusiform, usually blunted or rounded end, and hyperchromatic. Nucleoli are usually inconspicuous. Mitotic figures are seen, usually not less than 10 per high power fields. Cellular pleomorphism and giant cells with multiple nuclei are common (Fig. 19.20B, C).

Neoplasms with fewer than nine mitotic figures per 10 high power fields and moderate to marked cellular atypia are regarded as leiomyosarcoma, but the behavior of the neoplasms with a comparable degree of mitotic activity and minimal cell atypia is uncertain. The latter are designated as smooth muscle tumors of uncertain malignant potential. The overall survival rate of patients with leiomyosarcoma is 20%. Leiomyosarcomas are treated by hysterectomy and bilateral salpingo-oophorectomy. Combined therapy with surgery and radiation has not resulted in an improved survival.[15]

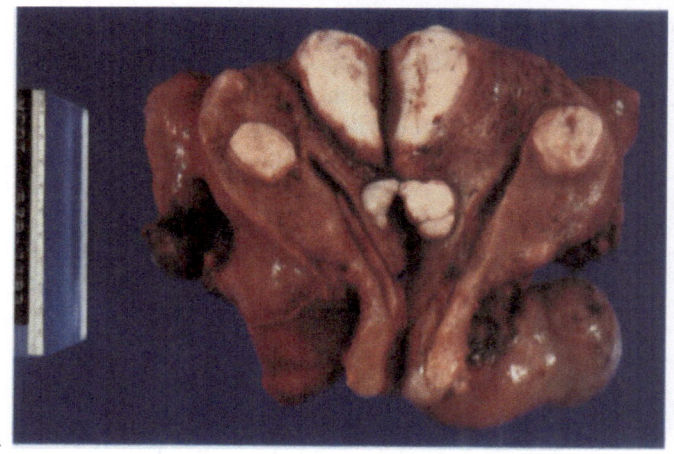

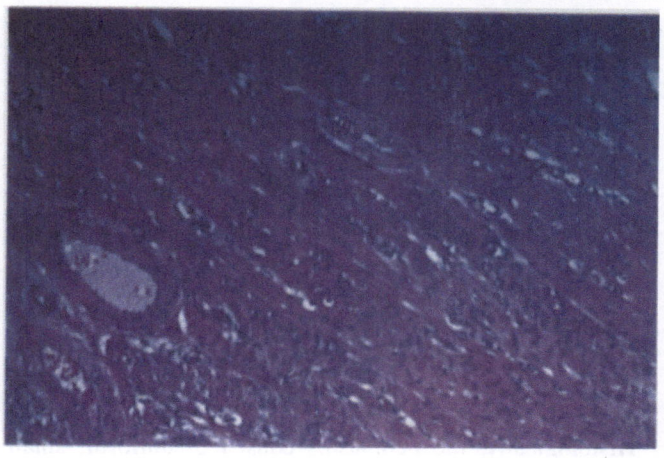

FIGURE 19.19 Leiomyomas of uterus. A: Bisected uterus showing multiple, soft, bulging tumors. **B**: Histo-logic section of the same case. Interlacing bundles of benign smooth muscle cells.

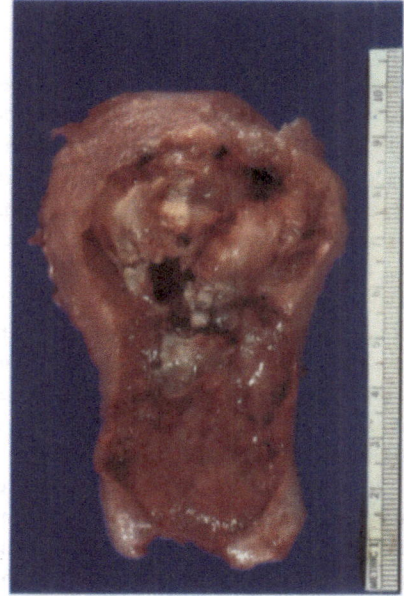

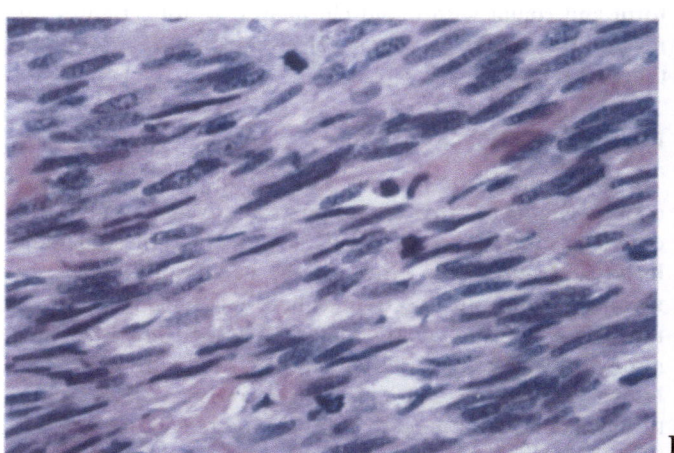

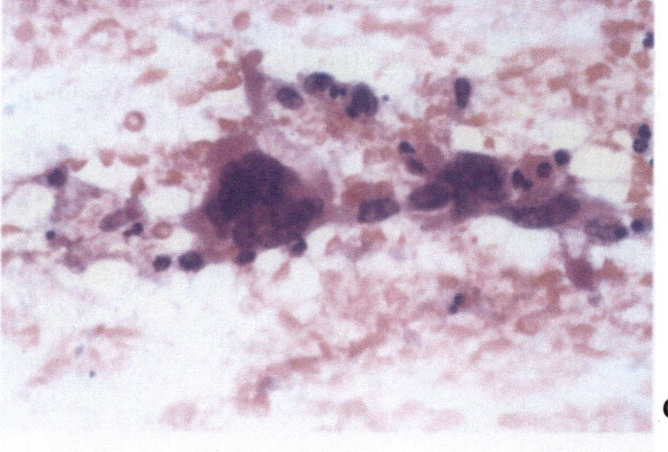

FIGURE 19.20 Leiomyosarcoma of uterus. A: Soft, fleshy mass involving the uterine cavity and cervix. **B**: Histologic section of the same case. Parallel running bundles of elongated neoplastic cells with multiple mitotic figures. **C**: Cervical smear from the same case. Loose aggregates of cells with abundant eosinophilic cytoplasm and large fusiform nuclei with rounded ends.

Endometrial Stromal Tumors

Based on the morphologic and biologic features, endometrial stromal tumors are divided into two distinct types: endometrial stromal nodule and endometrial stromal sarcoma.

Endometrial Stromal Nodule

Endometrial stroma nodule is a rare type of neoplasm, occurring usually in women of reproductive age. Vaginal bleeding, menorrhagia, and pelvic discomfort are the common clinical presentations. The neoplasms are well circumscribed and may involve submucosal, intramural, or subserosal sites. The nodules measure up to 5 cm in diameter. On section, they are bulging, pale yellow, and fleshy.

Histologically, the neoplasms consist of uniform, small cells arranged in compact sheets, tubules, or in a cordlike pattern. The neoplasm is expansile and has a "pushing" rather than an infiltrative border. The cells are rather uniform and round to polygonal with scanty neoplasm. The nuclei are uniform and round with bland chromatin. Mitotic figures are rarely observed (Fig. 19.21). Hysterectomy is appropriate therapy. Recurrence is rare.

Endometrial Stromal Sarcoma

The mean age of the patients with endometrial stromal sarcoma is similar to that of endometrial stromal nodule. The common clinical presentations are vaginal bleeding and lower abdominal pain. Grossly, the neoplasm involves the myometrium or endometrium as poorly defined pale gray to tan, fleshy, soft, polypoid nodules. Histologically, low grade stromal sarcomas infiltrate the myometrium with prominent lymphatic invasion. The cells are relatively uniform, similar to those of stromal nodules. Mitotic figures are usually less than nine per 10 high power fields. High grade stromal sarcomas consist of atypical stromal cells haphazardly infiltrating the myometrium. Mitotic figures are usually more than 10 per 10 high power fields (Fig. 19.22). Hysterectomy with bilateral salpingo-oophorectomy is appropriate treatment. Postoperative radiation therapy is recommended.

Mixed Mesodermal Tumors

Mixed mesodermal tumors consist of stromal and epithelial neoplastic elements. Depending on their cytologic components, there are several distinct types.

Adenofibroma

Adenofibromas are polypoid lesions comprising benign glandular epithelium and benign fibrous stroma. They are covered by a single layer of cuboidal to columnar cells. Hysterectomy is the preferred treatment.

Adenosarcoma

Adenosarcoma consists of malignant fibrous stromal elements and benign glandular epithelium. By definition, the sarcomatous element should have more than four mitotic figures per 10 high power fields. Adenosarcoma is not as aggressive as malignant mixed müllerian tumor. Common sites of metastasis are the vagina or elsewhere in the pelvis.

Mixed Müllerian Tumor (Carcinosarcoma)

Mixed müllerian tumor is the most common type of uterine sarcomas and occurs in postmenopausal women.[16-18] The common clinical presentations are vaginal bleeding and abdominal discomfort and mass. Norris and Taylor found 17 postradiation sarcomas in a review of 136 malignant mesenchymal tumors of the uterus.[19] Curettage is an effective means of establishing the diagnosis.

The neoplasms are polypoid and fill the endometrial cavity. Sometimes the polypoid mass protrudes from the external os. On section, the neoplasms are fleshy, soft, and tan, with areas of necrosis and hemorrhage. Histologically, mixed müllerian tumors consist of malignant epithelial and malignant stromal elements. The malignant epithelial component typically is adenocarcinoma, rarely squamous carcinoma. The common homologous stromal components are fibrosarcoma, endometrial stromal sarcoma, and leiomyosarcoma (Fig. 19.23). The common heterologous components are rhabdomyosarcoma and chondrosarcoma.

Treatment and Prognosis of Uterine Sarcomas

Compared with that of endometrial carcinomas, the overall survival from uterine sarcomas is poor. The most significant prognostic factors are the clinical stage and depth of myometrial invasion. Total abdominal hysterectomy and bilateral salpingo-oophorectomy are recommended for Stage I and II. An extensive surgical procedure is not recommended for Stage III and IV. Most oncologists recommend postoperative radiation therapy.

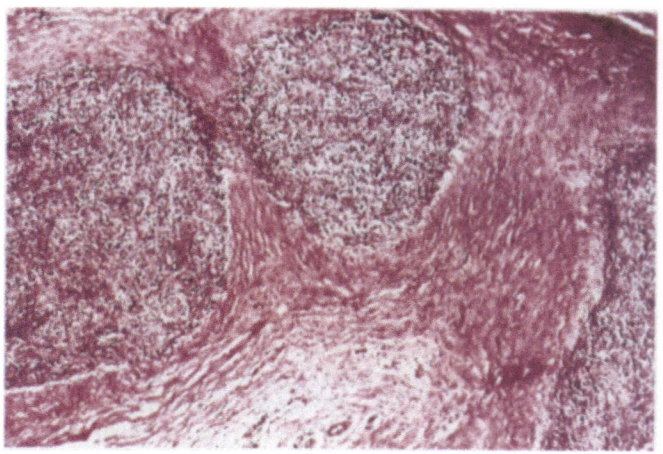

FIGURE 19.21 Endometrial stromal nodule. Expanding nodules with "pushing" margins.

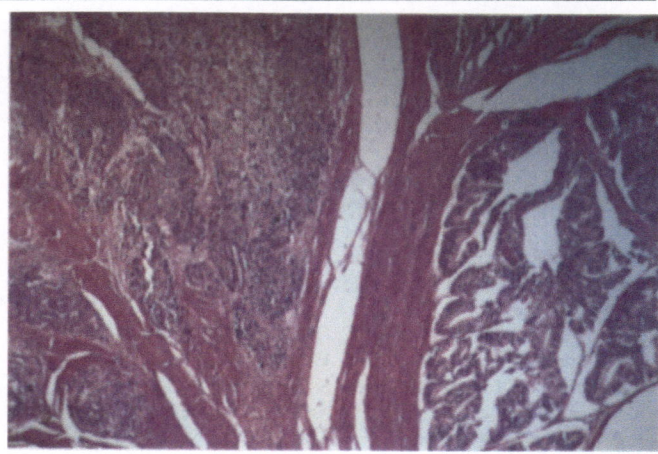

FIGURE 19.23 Carcinosarcoma of uterine corpus. The neoplasm comprises malignant epithelial elements (adenocarcinoma, *right*) and malignant stromal elements (stromal sarcoma, *left*).

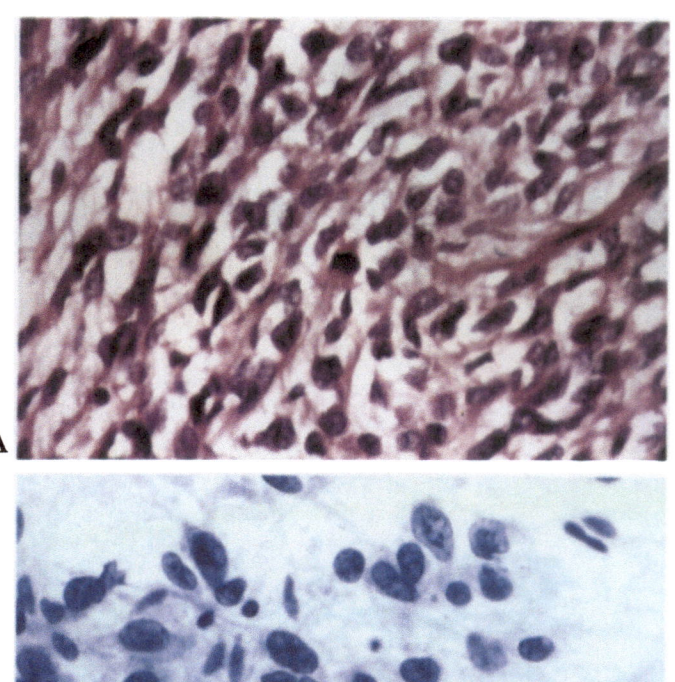

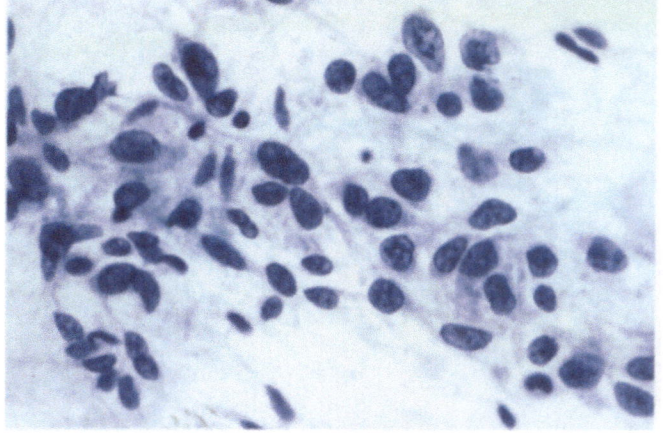

FIGURE 19.22 Endometrial stromal sarcoma. A: Round to spindle-shaped tumor cell infiltration. B: Cervical smear from the same case showing loose aggregates of round to spindle-shaped cells.

References

1. Greenwood SM, Moran JJ. Chronic endometritis: Morphologic and clinical observations. *Obstet Gynecol*. 1981;58:176.

2. Rotterdam H. Chronic endometritis: A clinicopathologic study. *Pathol Annu*. 1978;13:209.

3. Cadena D, Cavanzo FJ, Leone CL, Taylor HB. Chronic endometritis: A comparative clinicopathologic study. *Obstet Gynecol*. 1973; 1:733.

4. Kurman RJ, Kaminski PF, Norris HJ. The behavior of endometrial hyperplasia. A long-term study of "untreated" hyperplasia in 170 patients. *Cancer*. 1985;56:403.

5. Buehl IA, Vellios F, Carter JE, Huber CP. Carcinoma in situ of the endometrium. *Am J Clin Pathol*. 1964;42:594.

6. Silverberg E, Lubera JA. Cancer Statistics. *CA*. 1989;39:3.

7. Doll R, Muir C, Waterhouse J. *Cancer Incidence in Five Continents. International Union Against Cancer*, vol. 2. Berlin: Springer-Verlag; 1970.

8. Bokhman JV. Two pathogenetic types of endometrial cancer. *Gynecol Oncol*. 1983;15:10.

9. Smith M, McCarthey AJ. Occult, high-risk endometrial cancer. *Gynecol Oncol*. 1985;22:154.

10. Robboy SJ, Bradley R. Changing trends and prognostic features in endometrial cancer associated with exogenous estrogen therapy. *Obstet Gyneol*. 1979;54:269.

11. Jones HW. Treatment of adenocarcinoma of endometrium. *Obstet Gynecol Surv*. 1975;30:147.

12. Hanson MB, Van Nagell JR, Powell DE, et al. The prognostic significance of lymph-vascular space invasion in Stage I endometrial cancer. *Cancer*. 1985;55:1753.

13. Christopherson WM, Williamson EO, Gray LA. Leiomyosarcoma of the uterus. *Cancer*. 1972;29:1512.

14. Zaloudek C, Norris HJ. In: Kurman, ed. *Blaustein's Pathology of the Female Genital Tract*. 3rd ed. New York: Springer-Verlag.

15. Vongtama V, Karlen JR, Piver SM, et al. Treatment, results and prognostic factors in stage I and II sarcomas of the corpus uteri. *Am J Roentgenol*. 1976;126:139.

16. Marchese MJ, Liskow AS, Cram CP, et al. Uterine sarcomas: A clinicopathologic study, 1965–1981. *Gynecol Oncol*. 1984;18:299.

17. Salazar OM, Bonfiglio TA, Patten SF, et al. Uterine sarcomas. Natural histology, treatment and prognosis. *Cancer*. 1978;42:1152.

18. Wheelock JB, Krebs H-B, Schneider V, et al. Uterine sarcoma: Analysis of prognostic variables in 71 cases. *Am J Obstet Gynecol*. 1985;151:1016.

19. Norris HJ, Taylor HB. Postirradiation sarcomas of the uterus. *Obstet Gynecol*. 1965;26:684.

20
Ovary and Fallopian Tube

Ovary

Although the incidence of ovarian cancer is lower than that of cervical and endometrial cancers, its mortality rate is higher than that of cancers of the cervix and endometrium combined, indicating its lethal biologic behavior. The diagnostic yield by cervical cytology of ovarian and fallopian tube neoplasms is poor. Since most adnexal masses need to be resected or debulked for diagnosis or treatment, percutaneous fine needle aspiration (FNA) is not the primary diagnostic approach except for advanced neoplasms beyond exploration.

Non-neoplastic cysts of the ovary are common but generally harmless.

Primary inflammation of the ovaries is rare and may be involved in pelvic inflammatory disease. The ovary is frequently secondarily affected in endometriosis. In this chapter, discussion is limited to neoplasms of the ovary, and polycystic ovaries in terms of their clinicopathologic significance.

Polycystic Ovaries

Polycystic ovaries are enlarged up to twice their normal size. The outer cortex is pale gray and smooth (Fig. 20.1A). On section, the cortex is studded with cysts 0.5 to 1.5 cm in diameter. Histologically, there is a thick cortical fibrosis beneath which are multiple cysts lined by granuloma cells (Fig. 20.1B). Corpora lutea are usually not identified.

Polycystic ovarian disease occurs usually in young women after menarche and is clinically characterized by oligomenorrhea, hirsutism, infertility, and sometimes obesity. These manifestations, considered to be secondary to excessive production of estrogen and androgens by the multiple cystic follicles, are referred to as the Stein-Leventhal syndrome. The principal biochemical abnormalities are excessive production of androgens, a high level of luteinizing hormone (LH), and a low level of follicle-stimulating hormone (FSH). It is believed that the ovarian and hormonal changes are probably the result of unbalanced or asynchronous release of FSH and LH by the pituitary, which is in turn related to some disruption of hypothalamic control of pituitary secretion.[1] Wedge resection of the ovaries may correct the condition.

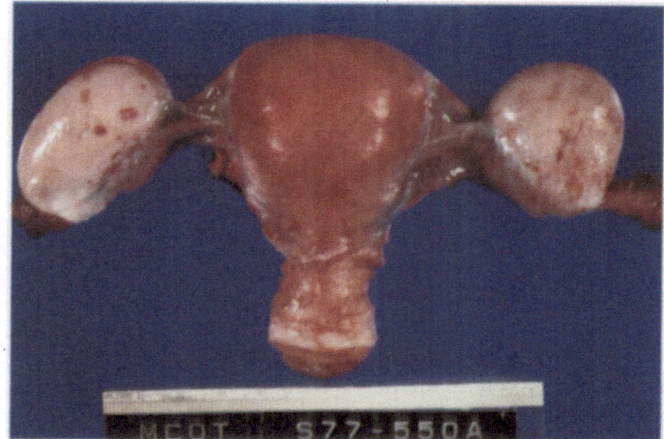
A

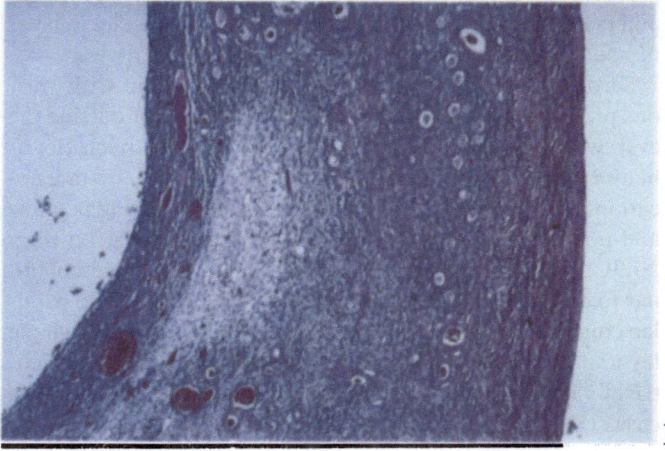
B

FIGURE 20.1 Polycystic ovaries. A: The ovaries are 2 to 3 times their normal size. The cortex of the ovaries is pale gray and smooth. B: Histologic section of the ovarian cortex showing fibrosis beneath which are multiple cysts.

Tumors of the Ovary

Ovarian cancer ranks as the fourth leading cause of cancer deaths in women, after cancers of the lung, breast, and large intestine.[2] Ovarian cancers are locally aggressive neoplasms that do not produce symptoms and signs until advanced. Thus, they are often discovered at the stage beyond complete resection.

Based on their histogenesis and morphologic features, ovarian neoplasms are classified into three major groups: tumors of the multipotential surface (coelomic) epithelium, tumors of germ cell origin, and tumors of sex-cord stromal origin.

Tumors of Surface Epithelial Origin

Seventy percent of all ovarian neoplasms compose this group of neoplasms. The group comprises several types of neoplasm with different cell types. On the basis of the degree of cytologic atypia, histologic features, and biologic behavior, each type of neoplasm is divided into benign, borderline (intermediate), and malignant (carcinoma).[3] Fifteen to 30% of the surface epithelial tumors are bilateral.

Serous Tumors

Serous tumors are the most common of the ovarian tumors, encountered usually between the ages of 30 and 40 years. Two thirds are malignant. Grossly, the tumors are cystic with various proportions of solid neoplasm, and measure from just a few up to 40 cm in diameter. Benign, serous cystadenomas are typically thin-walled cysts with a smooth lining (Fig. 20.2A). Microscopically, they consist of tiny cysts, alveoli, and occasional papillations lined or covered by a single layer of columnar cells with bland nuclei (Fig. 20.2B).

Serous cystadenocarcinomas are usually cystic with various proportions of solid neoplasm either inside or outside the cyst wall. The solid portion may be focally necrotic or hemorrhagic (Fig. 20.3A, B). Microscopically, cystadenocarcinomas consist of microcystic structures bearing papillae and poorly formed glands exhibiting stromal invasion (Fig. 20.3C). The neoplastic glands are lined by stratified columnar to cuboidal cells with hyperchromatic nuclei. The papillae consist of delicate fibrovascular cores covered by a single layer of atypical columnar cells. Psammoma bodies (concentrically laminated calcospherites) are identified in 40% of the cases (Fig. 20.3D, E).

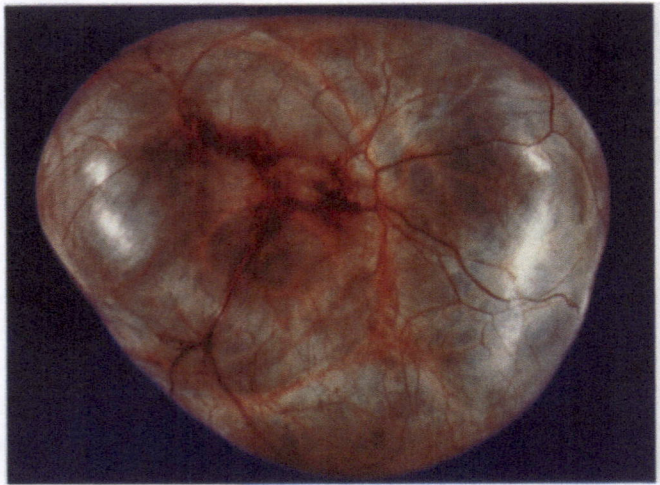

A

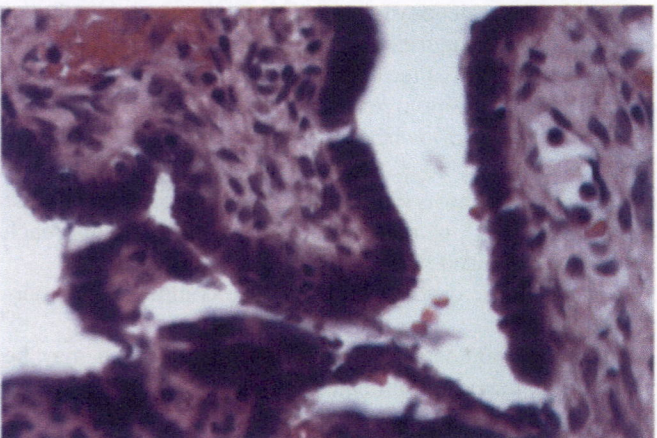

B

FIGURE 20.2   Serous cystadenoma of ovary. A: Cystic structure with a smooth surface, prominent vessels, and a watery cystic content. B: Histologic section of the same case showing a single layer of uniform serous epithelial cells lining the inner wall.

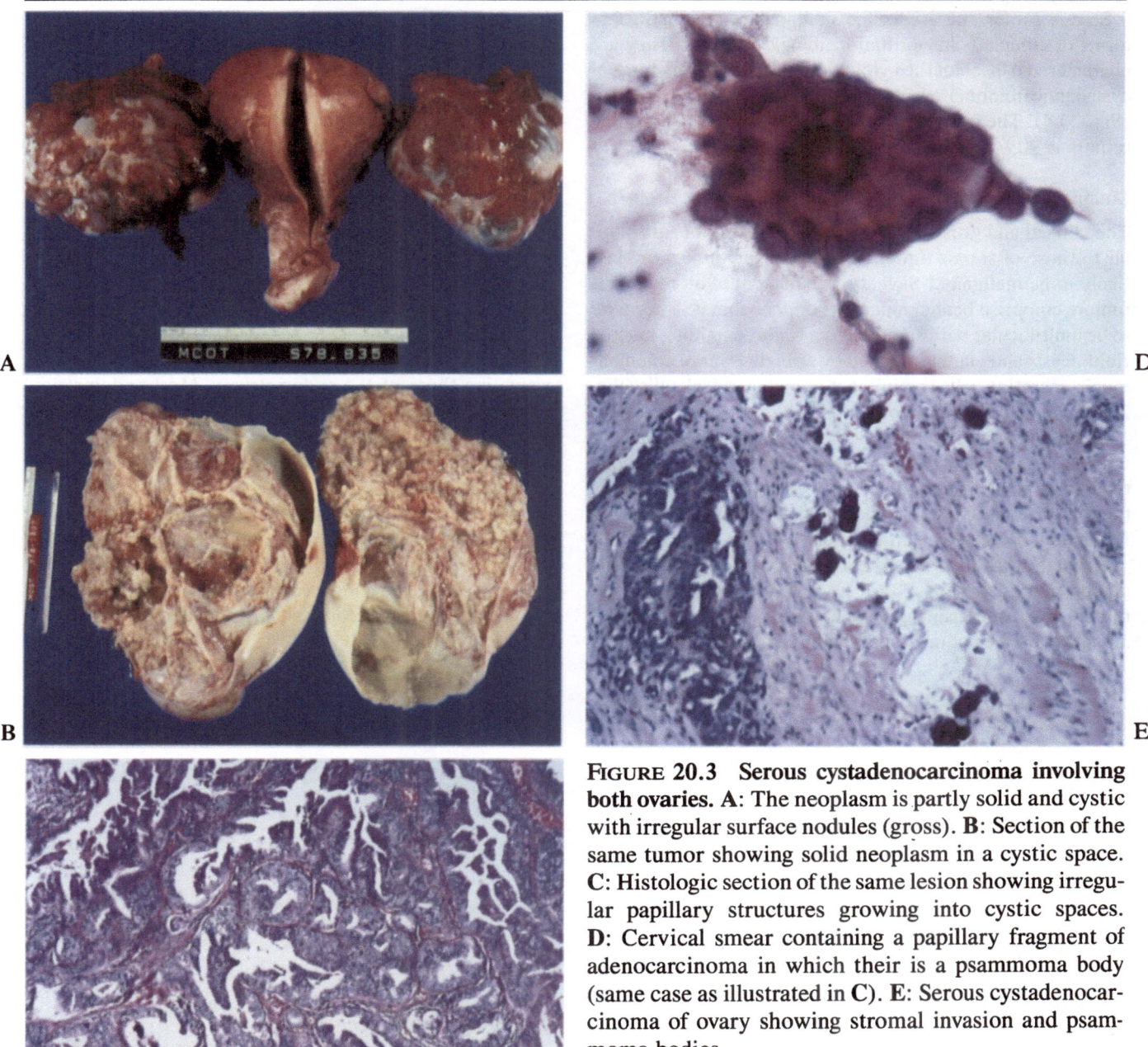

FIGURE 20.3   Serous cystadenocarcinoma involving both ovaries. A: The neoplasm is partly solid and cystic with irregular surface nodules (gross). **B**: Section of the same tumor showing solid neoplasm in a cystic space. **C**: Histologic section of the same lesion showing irregular papillary structures growing into cystic spaces. **D**: Cervical smear containing a papillary fragment of adenocarcinoma in which their is a psammoma body (same case as illustrated in **C**). **E**: Serous cystadenocarcinoma of ovary showing stromal invasion and psammoma bodies.

Serous tumors of borderline malignancy are distinct in terms of clinical behavior and histologic features. They are characterized by all of the cytologic and histologic features of cystadenocarcinoma except that they lack stromal invasion (Fig. 20.4). The overall 5-year survival for serous borderline tumors is 90% to 95%.[3]

Mucinous Tumors

The clinical and gross features of mucinous tumors are similar to those of serous tumors, but mucinous tumors are less likely to be malignant. Seventy-five percent of all mucinous tumors comprise benign mucinous cystadenomas. They tend to be multilocular with smooth, thin walls containing mucoid fluid. Cysts and glands are lined by a single layer of columnar mucin-secreting cells reminiscent of endocervical cells (Fig. 20.5). Papillae are rarely observed.

Fifteen percent of all mucinous tumors are mucinous cystadenocarcinomas. Grossly, they are multicystic, with distinct solid areas and papillary projections. Microscopically, the tumors consist of cysts and glands lined by pseudostratified mucin-secreting columnar cells.

Stromal invasion as a cordlike pattern or as poorly formed glands is present (Fig. 20.6). Ten percent of all mucinous tumors are of borderline malignancy and are characterized by all of the features of mucinous carcinoma except for the lack of stromal invasion. The overall 5-year survival rate for borderline tumors is more than 90%.

Pseudomyxoma Peritonei. Rupture or metastasis of mucinous tumors may result in massive mucinous ascites with multiple tumor implants and neoplastic adhesions between the abdominal viscera, a condition referred to as pseudomyxoma peritonei. This condition may also result from rupture of a mucocele of the appendix or appendiceal adenocarcinoma.

Endometrioid Tumors

Endometrioid tumors are characterized by neoplastic glands resembling those of the endometrium. Most endometrioid tumors are malignant; benign and borderline forms are rare. Fifteen to 30% of cases have a coexisting endometrial carcinoma. The relationship between the ovarian and endometrial carcinomas is unclear.

The gross features of these neoplasms are similar to those of other common epithelial tumors except for frequently observed chocolate-colored fluid in endometrioid tumors. Microscopically, the tumors consist of tubular glands lined by columnar cells reminiscent of endometrial adenocarcinoma (Fig. 20.7).

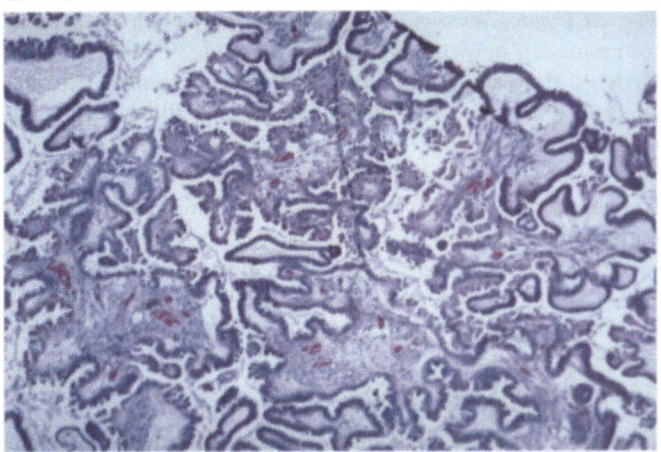

FIGURE 20.4 **Ovarian serous cystadenoma of borderline malignant potential.** Irregular papillary and cystic structures reminiscent of cystadenocarcinoma. No stromal invasion was identified.

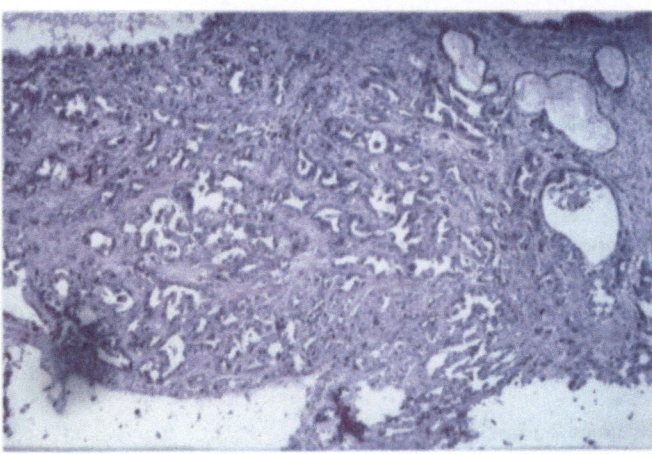

FIGURE 20.6 **Mucinous cystadenocarcinoma of ovary.** Irregular glandular and cystic structures are lined by pseudostratified mucin-secreting columnar cells with atypical nuclei.

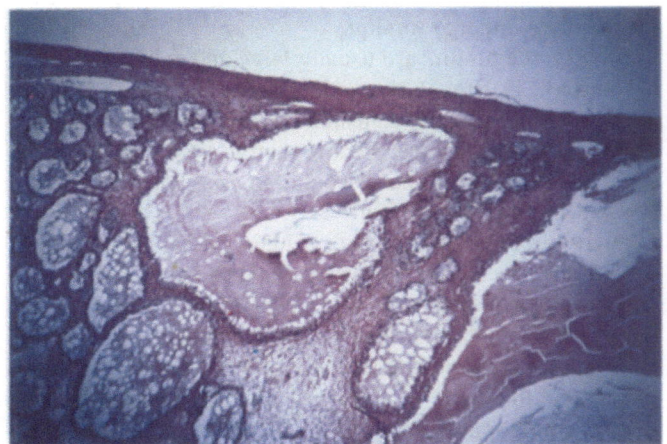

FIGURE 20.5 **Mucinous cystadenoma of ovary.** Well formed glands and cysts are lined by a single layer of uniform mucin-secreting columnar cells.

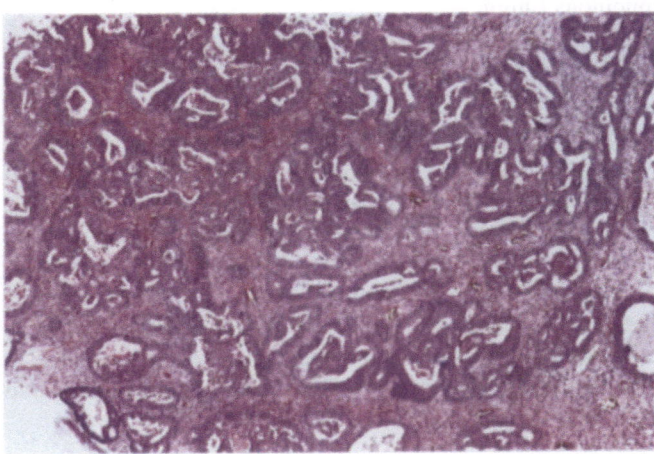

FIGURE 20.7 **Endometrioid carcinoma of ovary.** Tubular glands are arranged compactly, reminiscent of endometrial adenocarcinoma.

Clear Cell Adenocarcinoma

Clear cell adenocarcinomas are rare neoplasms that resemble clear cell renal adenocarcinoma and consist of tubules or papillary projections into cystic space lined by columnar to polygonal cells with optically clear cytoplasm. A characteristic cytologic feature of the cells is the presence of "hobnail" cells, cells with large, prominent nuclei, protruding toward the apex of the cell (Fig. 20.8). On the basis of their frequent coexistence with endometrioid carcinomas and similar ultrastructural features similar to those of other common epithelial neoplasms, these neoplasms are considered to be of müllerian origin.

Brenner Tumor

Brenner tumor is an uncommon, benign, solid ovarian neoplasm detected incidentally in hysterectomy or pelvic surgery for other reasons. Microscopically, the tumor consists of nests of transitional type epithelium resembling that of the urinary bladder embedded in dense fibrous stroma (Fig. 20.9). Sometimes this tumor appears as a focal area within a mucinous tumor.

Germ Cell Tumors

About 15% to 20% of all ovarian tumors are of germ cell origin, and more than 90% of germ cell tumors are benign cystic teratomas. The remaining 5% to 10% of germ cell tumors are immature and malignant teratomas, dysgerminomas, embryonal carcinomas, entodermal sinus tumors, and choriocarcinomas. More than one half of germ cell tumors occur in the first two decades of life, and the younger the patient, the greater the likelihood of malignancy. Germ cell tumors arise most often in the ovary and testis, and rarely arise in the retroperitoneum, mediastinum, pineal gland, and sacroccygeal area.

Teratoma

Teratoma is defined as a neoplasm containing elements representative of more than one germ layer. They arise most often in the ovary, where 99% of them are benign, whereas testicular teratomas are relatively rare and 99% are malignant.

Benign Cystic Teratoma. About 80% of benign cystic teratomas occur in women between 20 and 30 years of age. Grossly, they are cystic with a smooth, glistening external surface. On sectioning, the cystic space is filled with sebaceous secretion, hair ball, bone, cartilage, or teeth (Fig. 20.10A). Microscopically, the cystic wall is lined by mature squamous epithelium with underlying skin appendages, an ectodermal element (Fig. 20.10B). Occasionally, nests of bronchial or gastrointestinal epithelium, an entodermal element, are identified. Malignant transformation is present in less than 1% of the tumors, usually taking the form of squamous cell carcinoma. Torsion is the most frequent complication, occurring in about 10% to 15% of cases.

Immature Teratoma. Immature teratomas comprise immature or embryonal structures derived from the three germ layers, which may be focal or diffuse, in a background of mature tissue. Fewer than 1% of ovarian teratomas are immature teratomas, which occur most commonly in the first two decades of life. The tumor is usually asymptomatic until it reaches a considerable size, when it manifests itself as a pelvic mass causing pressure symptoms and a feeling of heaviness. It may undergo torsion.

Grossly, the tumors are usually large and solid. The external surface is irregularly nodular. The neoplasm may be perforated, resulting in adhesion to adjacent organs. On sectioning, the tumors are predominantly solid, trabeculated, and lobulated. Cystic spaces containing serous, mucinous, or greasy fluid may be present.

Microscopically, the tumors contain immature or embryonic tissues focally or in a multifocal fashion. Ectodermal elements are neuroblastic tissue and squamous or sweat gland structures. Entodermal elements are bronchial or gastrointestinal type epithelium with a tubular pattern. Mesodermal elements are muscular or bony tissue and undifferentiated embryonic mesenchyme.

Immature teratoma is a malignant neoplasm that spreads locally and to regional lymph nodes and distant organs. The overall 5-year survival is about 20%. There is a good correlation between the histologic appearance of the tumor and prognosis. Histologic grading is of prognostic value, and is based on the relative amounts of immature and mature tissue, and the degree of differentiation and mitotic activity within the immature components. These neoplasms are graded as Grade 0 through Grade 3.[4,5]

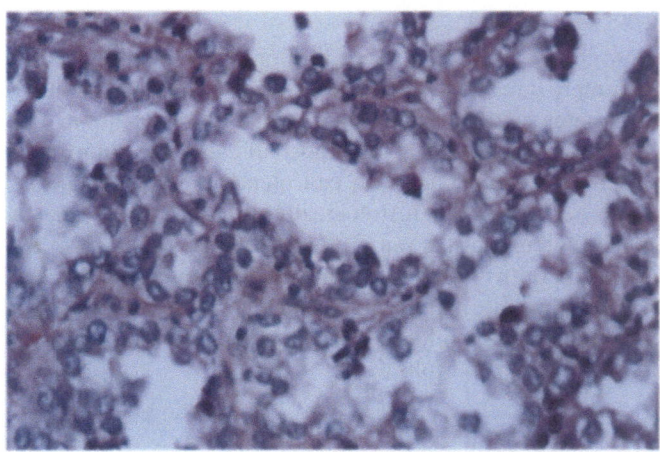

FIGURE 20.8 Clear cell adenocarcinoma of ovary. Cystic and papillary structures and solid sheets of clear cells.

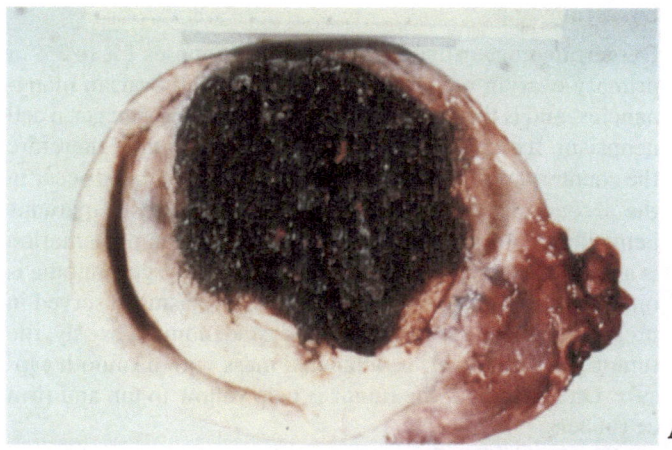

A

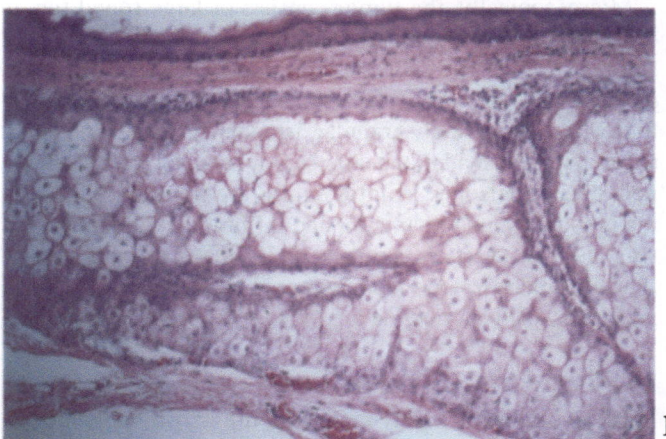

B

FIGURE 20.10 Benign cystic teratoma of ovary. A: Cystic tumor with a smooth external surface. It contains greasy material, a ball of hair, and bone. **B:** Histologic section of the same tumor showing a cyst wall lined by squamous epithelium and sebaceous glands.

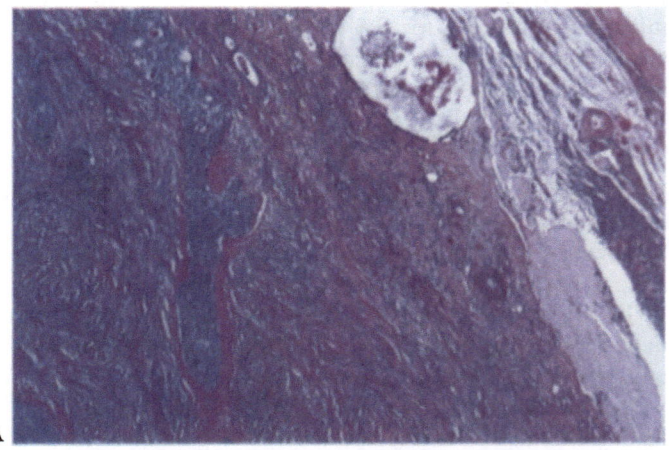

A

B

FIGURE 20.9 Brenner's tumor of ovary. A: Epithelial cell nests embedded in dense stroma. **B:** Epithelial element in Brenner's tumor resembles urothelial epithelium.

Dysgerminoma

Dysgerminoma, an uncommon tumor, composes 1% to 2% of primary ovarian neoplasms, 3% to 5% of all ovarian malignancies, and is the most common malignant ovarian germ cell neoplasm. It comprises primordial germ cells and is therefore the counterpart of seminoma of the testis. Most cases occur in the second and third decades of life, with 80% of patients being under 30 years of age. The most common presentation is abdominal enlargement and pelvic mass. Dysgerminoma is one of the two most common ovarian neoplasms observed in pregnancy, the other being serous cystadenoma. Grossly, the tumor is a solid, oval, or lobulated mass with a smooth capsule. On sectioning, the tumor is pale yellow to tan and firm or rubbery.

Microscopically, the tumor consists of large round tumor cells arranged in sheets and islands surrounded by delicate fibrous stroma. The cells are large and round with abundant pale, granular, or clear cytoplasm. The nuclei are large, round to oval, and have finely granular, irregularly distributed chromatin with a vesicular appearance. Most nuclei have a prominent macronucleolus. Mitotic figures are frequent. The stroma is usually small in amount and infiltrated by lymphocytes (Fig. 20.11). Dysgerminomas tend to spread to regional and then to paraaortic nodes before metastasizing elsewhere. They are radiosensitive, yielding a 65% to 95% 5-year survival.

Endodermal Sinus (Yolk Sac) Tumor

Yolk sac tumor is a highly malignant tumor, probably arising from undifferentiated and multipotential elements by selective differentiation toward yolk sac or vitelline structures. The tumors occur most often in the second decade of life, but may occur from infancy to middle age. The common clinical presentation is abdominal enlargement and pain. Occasionally, torsion of the tumor may present as an acute abdominal emergency.

Yolk sac tumors are usually unilateral and encapsulated, round, or lobulated. On sectioning, they are pale yellow and solid with frequently necrotic and hemorrhagic foci. Multifocal cysts containing gelatinous fluid are common.

Microscopically, the tumors resemble the yolk sac, comprising a loose meshwork of cysts and channels lined by flattened, vacuolated cells. The cells may contain cytoplasmic droplets, rich in alpha-fetoprotein (AFP), alpha-antitrypsin, or both, demonstrable by immunocytochemistry.

Papillary structures in cystic spaces covered by a single layer of epithelium and supported by fibrovascular core (Schiller-Duval body) are frequently observed (Fig. 20.12). Since most yolk sac tumors produce alpha-fetoprotein, monitoring of serum level of AFP is highly recommended. This tumor is radioresistant and chemotherapy imparts no significant benefit.

Choriocarcinoma

Non-gestational choriocarcinoma of the ovary is an extremely rare and highly malignant germ cell tumor that differentiates toward trophoblastic structures. It occurs in children and young women. In almost all cases, the tumor contains other neoplastic germ cell elements. Non-gestational choriocarcinomas are histologically similar to those of gestational type except for the presence of these other germ cell elements. Both types produce human chorionic gonadotropic (HCG) hormone, and the hormonal level is closely correlated with viable tumor volume. It is an excellent tumor marker for monitoring clinical follow-up.

Sex-Cord Stromal Tumors

Sex-cord stromal tumors consist of sex cord and stromal derivatives capable of differentiating in an ovarian direction (granulosa cells, theca cells), in a testicular direction (Sertoli's cells, Leydig's cells), in a stromal direction to remain fibromatous, or in a bigonadal direction (Sertoli's and/or Leydig's cells and granulosa cells and/or theca cells).[6] These tumors compose 5% to 10% of all ovarian tumors but only about 2% of all ovarian cancers. Some produce steroid hormones, usually estrogenic but sometimes androgenic.

Granulosa Cell Tumor

Most granulosa cell tumors arise in postmenopausal women and may induce hyperestrogenism, resulting in endometrial hyperplasia and adenocarcinoma. Occasionally, the tumors arise in prepubertal girls to induce precocious puberty.

Grossly, these neoplasms form an encapsulated, solid mass. On sectioning, they are pale gray to pale yellow with multifocal hemorrhagic necrosis or cysts.

Their microscopic features are quite variable. The predominant pattern is of sheets and islands of granulosa cells in which there are microfollicular spaces containing the debris of disintegrated tumor cells in amorphous material (Call-Exner body) (Fig. 20.13). Other frequently seen microscopic patterns are macrofollicular, trabecular, gyriform, "water-silk," and diffuse forms. The cells have scanty cytoplasm and pale, oval to angular grooved nuclei. Most granulosa cell tumors are Stage I. These tumors are treated by bilateral salpingo-oophorectomy and hysterectomy in postmenopausal women, and by a conservative approach for preservation of fertility in younger women. The 10 year survival is almost 100% for small Stage I tumors and 25% to 50% for advanced large tumors.[7]

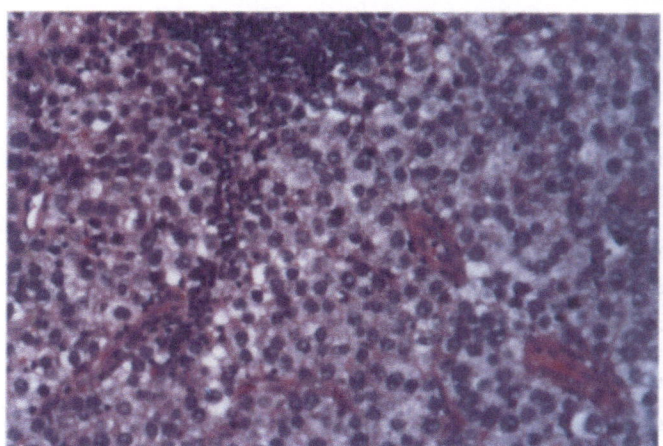

FIGURE 20.11   **Dysgerminoma of ovary.** Large round tumor cells arranged in sheets and islands separated by fibrous stroma infiltrated by lymphoid cells.

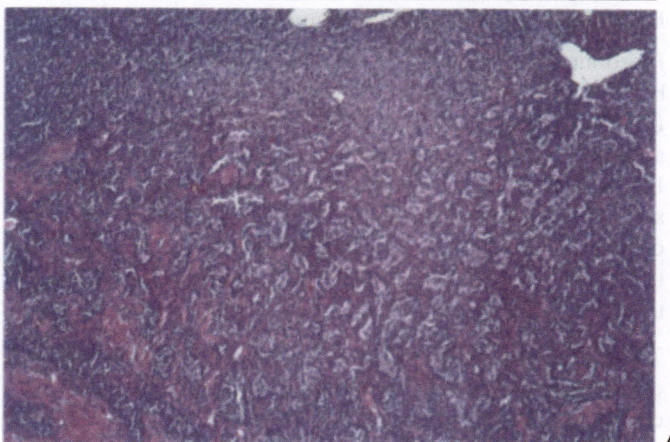

A

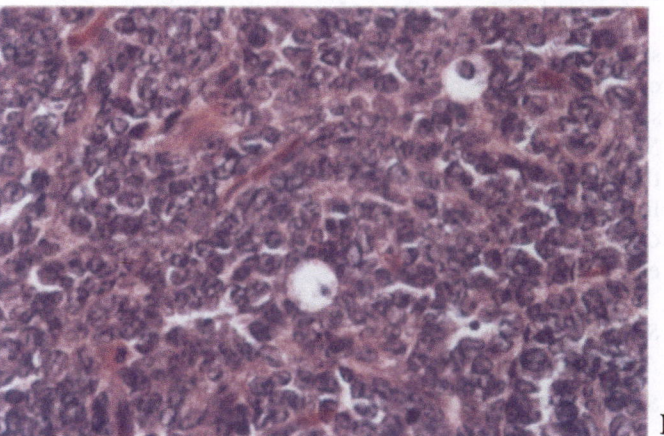

B

FIGURE 20.13   **Granulosa cell tumor of ovary.** **A**: Sheets, microfollicles, and anastomotic cords of round to cuboidal cells. **B**: High magnification of the same tumor showing a Call-Exner body.

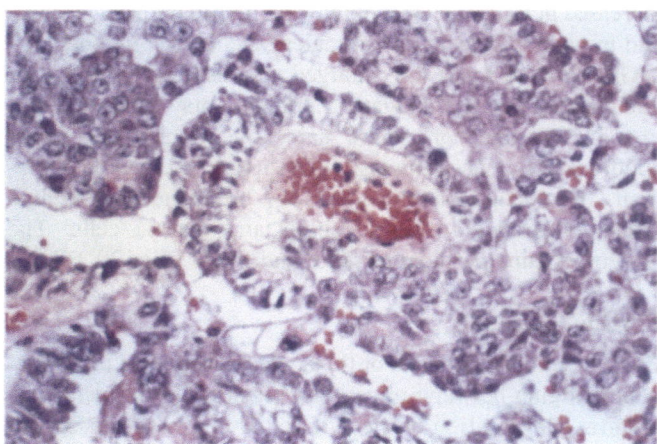

FIGURE 20.12   **Yolk sac tumor (endodermal sinus tumor) of ovary.** Papillary structure in cystic spaces covered by a single layer of epithelium and supported by a fibrovascular core (Schiller-Duval body).

Fibroma-Thecoma-Luteoma Tumors

Fibroma-thecoma-luteoma tumors range from typical fibroblastic lesions (fibroma) to neoplasms comprising plump fibroblasts with abundant intracytoplasmic lipid (thecoma) and neoplasms comprising typical lutein cells (luteoma). Fibroma is usually a small, gray, solid, encapsulated mass seldom exceeding 10 cm in diameter. They occur in women over 40 years of age and are hormonally inert. Large tumors tend to be associated with ascites and hydrothorax, the condition of "Meigs' syndrome."

Thecomas. Thecomas occur in postmenopausal women and elaborate estrogen, resulting in endometrial hyperplasia or carcinoma with uterine bleeding in 20% to 30% of cases. Grossly, they are a pale yellow, rubbery, solid mass (Fig. 20.14A).

Microscopically, the tumors consist of plump spindle-shaped or oval cells with granular or vacuolated cytoplasm containing abundant lipid (Fig. 20.14B). Biochemical analysis revealed this lipid at least in part to comprise estrogen. Most thecomas contain luteinized cells focally (luteinized thecoma). In contrast, luteoma consists predominantly of lutein cells. In almost all cases of luteomas, there is evidence of hyperthecosis elsewhere in the ovary. Luteomas may be estrogenic or androgenic.

Sertoli-Leydig Cell Tumors (Androblastoma, Arrhenoblastoma)

Sertoli-Leydig cell tumors are considered to arise from primitive mesenchymal elements in the ovary that differentiate in a masculine direction. Most elaborate a variety of androgens causing masculinization, although some are nonfunctional or may even be estrogenic. These tumors account for less than 0.5% of all ovarian tumors, with most occurring in young women. Grossly, they are lobulated, pale yellow, solid tumors.

Microscopically, they are quite variable. Rarely these tumors comprise Sertoli's cells only with closely packed tubules lined by cuboidal to columnar epithelial cells (Fig. 20.15). Cytologic atypia or mitotic activity is rarely observed.

Most of these tumors consist of a mixture of Sertoli's cells and Leydig's cells with various amounts of Leydig's cells occurring in sheets, aggregates, or clusters. Leydig's cells are large, polygonal cells with granular, eosinophilic cytoplasm that sometimes contain pointed crystals of Reinke. The nuclei are small, round, and hyperchromatic.

Gynandroblastoma

Gynandroblastoma is extremely rare and consists of male directed cells, Sertoli-Leydig cells, and female-directed cells, granulosa-theca cells.

Fallopian Tubes

The most common pathologic process involving the fallopian tubes is inflammation, almost always as part of pelvic inflammatory disease (PID). Ectopic tubal pregnancy is less common, but is a catastrophic lesion. Much less frequent are tubal endometriosis and primary neoplasms of the tubes.

Salpingitis

Salpingitis may be divided into three major types: acute, chronic, and granulomatous.

Acute Salpingitis

Acute salpingitis is a purulent inflammatory process secondary to bacterial infection spreading from the uterine cavity to the tube. The common causative organisms are *N. gonorrhoeae*, *Chlamydia trachomatis*, anaerobic bacteria, and *E. coli*.

N. gonorrhoeae spreads via the epithelial surface and thus causes mucosal changes. Other bacteria tend to spread into the tube by vascular or lymphatic channels. Acute salpingitis is increased in frequency in women with multiple sexual partners and in women carrying an intrauterine contraceptive device.

Grossly, the tubes are enlarged, reddish, and edematous and contain purulent exudate. Salpingitis may produce fever, lower abdominal or pelvic pain, and sometimes upper abdominal pain when the organism spreads to the upper abdomen. Microscopically, the tubes show broadened and blunted plicae infiltrated with neutrophils and plasma cells. The lumen contains purulent exudate and fibrin (Fig. 20.16).

Chronic Salpingitis

Healing and organization of the acute process lead to permanent bridging between plications, resulting in follicular salpingitis. Obliteration of the fimbriated end with subsequent dilatation of the tube results in a thin-walled distended structure containing serous fluid known as hydrosalpinx.

Tuberculous Salpingitis

The frequency of tuberculous salpingitis in women studied for infertility ranges from 1% in the United States to more than 10% in countries where tuberculosis is common.[8] The organism is blood-borne from the lung or extrapulmonary sources. Pelvic pain and sterility are the most common complaints. Grossly, the tubes are enlarged and adherent to the ovaries, and the fimbriae and tubal ostium may be obliterated, resulting in accumulation of exudate within the tube, which becomes progressively distended. Microscopic features are caseating granulomas in the mucosa and elsewhere in the wall. Because of repeated seeding of the endometrium with *M. tuberculosis* from the infected tubes, mycobacterial culture and the histologic findings on curettage of the endometrium can establish the diagnosis.

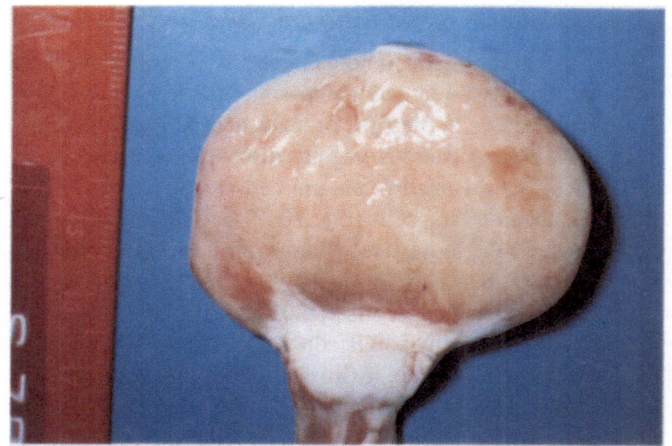

A

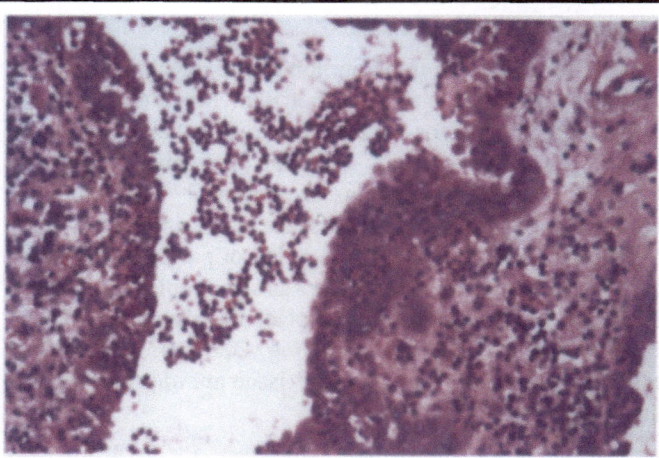

FIGURE 20.16 Acute salpingitis (acute PID). Numerous polymorphonuclear leukocytes in the tubal mucosa and lumen.

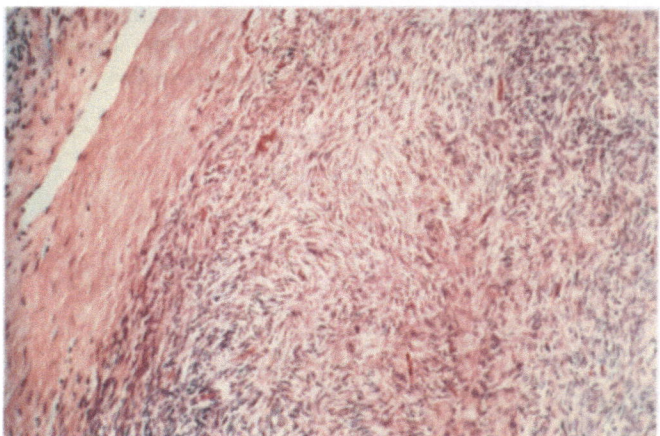

B

FIGURE 20.14 Thecoma of ovary. A: Pale yellow solid mass. B: Histologic section of the same thecoma showing interlacing bundles of plump spindle-shaped cells.

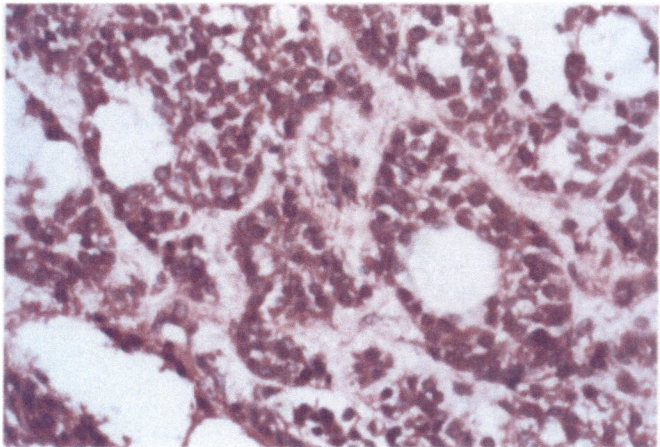

FIGURE 20.15 Androblastoma (Sertoli-Leydig cell tumor) of ovary. Sheets and tubules of cuboidal to round cells.

Ectopic Pregnancy

Ectopic pregnancy is implantation of the developing blasto-cyst at a site other than endometrium. More than 95% of ectopic pregnancies occur in the fallopian tube. Rupture of the ectopic tubal pregnancy is a grave emergency. Currently, 1% to 2% of all conceptions are ectopic.[9,10] A history of previous pelvic inflammatory disease is the single most common antecedent factor in 35% to 45% of patients.[11] Grossly, the affected tubal segment appears as an irregular sausagelike dilatation filled with blood and placental tissue. In 75% of cases an embryo may be found (Fig. 20.17A). Microscopically, chorionic villi and decidual tissue are identified in the tubal wall (Fig. 20.17B).

Neoplasms of the Fallopian Tube

Several types of benign neoplasms occur in the fallopian tubes: epithelial polyps, leiomyoma, adenomatoid tumor, benign teratoma, and paratubal cyst.

Adenocarcinoma of the Fallopian Tube

Adenocarcinoma of the fallopian tube is probably the least common primary malignant neoplasm of the female genitalia. The tumor occurs in the fifth or sixth decade of life and presents with serosanguinous vaginal discharge or bleeding, or pelvic pain. Occasionally, cervical cell samples may demonstrate adenocarcinoma cells (Fig. 20.18A). Under the impression that the patient has an endometrial lesion, the clinician and pathologist may be frustrated to find that endometrial curettings do not demonstrate a lesion. When advanced, the lesion may be felt as a doughy pelvic adnexal mass. Grossly, the tube is enlarged, reminiscent of hydrosalpinx or tubovarian abscess. On opening the lumen is found to be filled by a polypoid or solid mass with shaggy mucosal surface. Histologically, the neoplasm consists of glandular or papillary structures infiltrating the tubal wall and lumen (Fig. 20.18B). The neoplasm is highly aggressive, exhibiting transperitoneal spread.

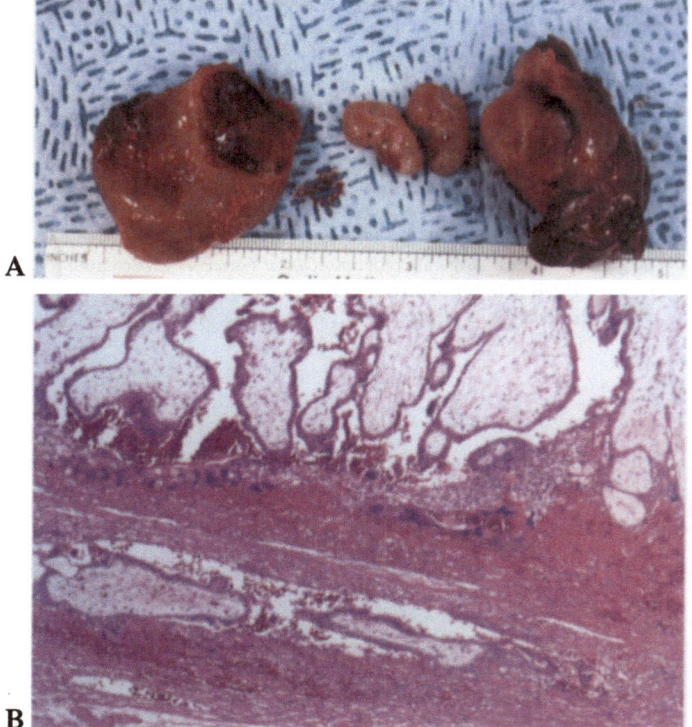

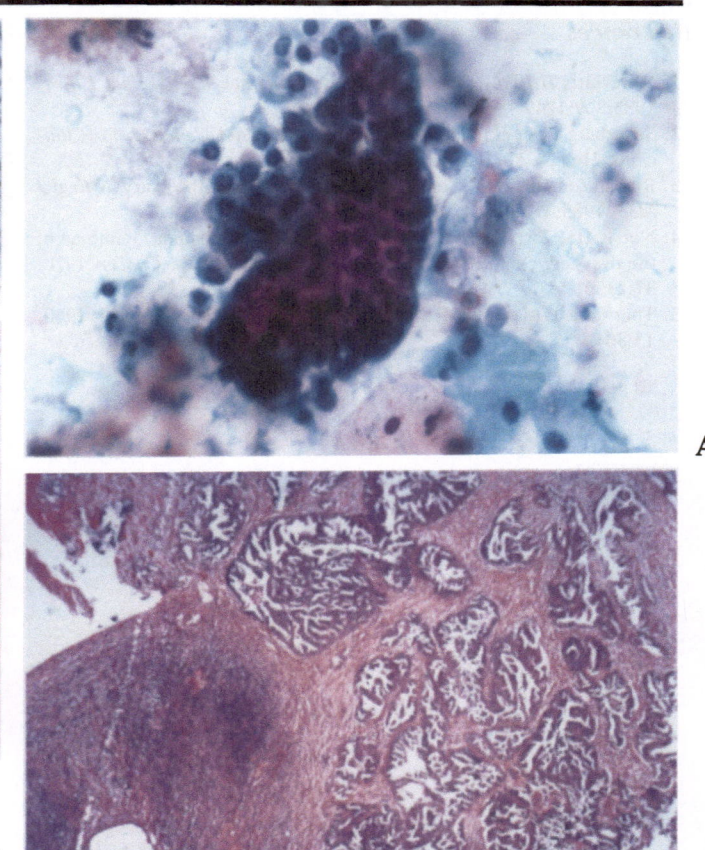

FIGURE 20.17   Ectopic tubal pregnancy (twin). A: Twin fetuses (*center*) and blood clot in a dilated tube. B: Histologic section of the tube showing chorionic villi in the tubal wall.

FIGURE 20.18   Adenocarcinoma of a fallopian tube. A: Cervical aspirate containing adenocarcinoma cells exfoliated from a fallopian tube. B: Histologic section of fallopian tubes of the same case showing glandular and papillary structures infiltrating the wall.

References

1. Vaitukaitis JL. Polycystic ovary syndrome—what is it? *N Engl J Med.* 1983;309:1249.

2. Silverberg E, et al. Cancer Statistics, 1990. *Ca-A Cancer J. for Clinicians.* Holheb A, et al. (ed.) 1990;40:9-26.

3. Richardson GS, et al. Common epithelial cancer of the ovary. *N Engl J Med.* 1985;312:415–474.

4. Norris HS, Zirkin HS, Benson NL. Immature (malignant) teratoma of the ovary. A clinical and pathologic study of 58 cases. *Cancer.* 1976; 37:2359.

5. Thurlbeck WM, Scully RE. Solid teratoma of the ovary. *Cancer.* 1960; 13:804.

6. Young RH, Scully RE. Ovarian sex cord-stromal tumours: Recent advances and current status. *Clin Obstet Gynecol.* 1984;11:93.

7. Bjorkholm E, Silfvergward C. Prognostic factors in granulosa-cell tumors. *Gynecol Oncol.* 1981;11:261.

8. Schaefer G. Tuberculosis of the female genital tract. *Clin Obstet Gynecol.* 1970;13:965.

9. Rubin GL, Peterson HB, Dorfman SF, Layde PM, Maze JM, Ory HW, Cates WJ. Ectopic pregnancy in the United States, 1970 through 1978. *JAMA.* 1983;249:1725.

10. Weinstein L, Morris MG, Dotters D, Christian CD. Ectopic pregnancy—A new surgical epidemic. *Obstet Gynecol.* 1983;61:698.

11. Brenner PF, Roy S, Mishell DR, Jr. Ectopic pregnancy. A study of 300 consecutive surgically treated cases. *JAMA.* 1980;243:673.

21
Breast

The traditional methods of diagnosing breast disease have been open biopsy or core-needle biopsy of palpable lumps. Over the last decade, with the development of mammography, fine needle aspiration (FNA) biopsy has become increasingly popular for establishing the diagnosis of breast lesions. Aspiration can be performed in the office, and its complications are virtually negligible. Its diagnostic sensitivity is greater than 90% and positive predictive value is nearly 100%. Advantages of FNA of breast are cost effectiveness, the rapid psychological relief of patients, and its ability to expedite treatment.

Anatomy and Histology

Each breast consists of 15 to 20 lobes, and each lobe drains through a lactiferous duct into the nipple. The lactiferous duct extends to periphery with multiple branchings leading to the terminal ducts. After the menarche, the terminal ducts proliferate, giving rise to numerous ductules or acini. Each terminal duct and its ductules or acini compose the terminal duct lobular units (Fig. 21.1). Smaller peripheral ducts and ductules are lined by ductal epithelium and subepithelial flat myoepithelial cells. These ductules (acini) are enclosed in a loose, delicate, myxomatous stroma (intralobular connective tissue), and the individual lobules are enclosed within a dense, collagenous, fibrous interlobular stroma.

Inflammatory Breast Diseases

Acute Mastitis and Breast Abscess

Acute inflammatory breast disease occurs most often during the early weeks of nursing and rarely in women with dermatologic problems in the nipple. Staphylococcus is the most common causative agent and tends to produce a localized infection with abscess formation. Surgical drainage and antibiotic therapy are usually required. Streptococcus is a less common agent and tends to cause a diffuse spreading infection (Fig. 21.2).

Mammary Duct Ectasia (Plasma Cell Mastitis)

Mammary duct ectasia is characterized by dilatation of ducts with inspissated secretion and chronic periductal inflammation. The disease occurs most often in multiparous women and is considered to result from obstruction of ducts by secre-

tion (Fig. 21.3). This lesion is of clinical significance because it can be mistaken for a carcinoma clinically and mammographically.

Fat Necrosis

Fat necrosis is characterized by an isolated, sharply localized palpable lump in the breast. Most patients give a history of trauma. Histologically, the lesion consists of a central focus of necrotic fat surrounded by lipid-filled macrophages and neutrophils (Fig. 21.4). Later when the lesion becomes organized by fibroblastic tissue, it can be mistaken for carcinoma.

Fibrocystic Disease

Fibrocystic disease (fibrocystic change) refers to non-neoplastic, miscellaneous lesions encompassing cyst formation, fibrosclerosis, and various types of epithelial hyperplasia including sclerosing adenosis. It is the most common breast disorder and accounts for more than one half of all surgical operations on the female breast. Hormonal imbalance is considered to be basic to the development of this disorder. Its major clinical significance is that it forms palpable lumps, frequently indistinguishable clinically from cancer.

Cysts and Fibrosis (Simple Fibrocystic Change)

The dominant clinical presentation of cysts and fibrosis is poorly defined nodularity, either as a solitary lesion or multiple lesions (Fig. 21.5). Grossly, they are characterized by cystic dilation of ducts with increased fibrous stroma. After aspiration the cysts usually collapse. If the aspirated fluid of the cyst is bloody and a residual mass remains, the cyst may rapidly recur. Cytologic examination of the cyst fluid is recommended. One to 2% incidence of carcinoma from cystic fluid of 1700 cases of mammary fibrocystic disease of the breast has been reported.[1,2]

Histologically, fibrocystic change consists of small and large cysts surrounded by dense collagenous fibrous connective tissue. The cysts may be lined by a single layer of cuboidal epithelium or may have no discernible epithelial lining (Fig. 21.6A). Some cysts are lined by tall eosinophilic columnar cells with intraluminal piling up of the cells (apocrine metaplasia) (Fig. 21.6B).

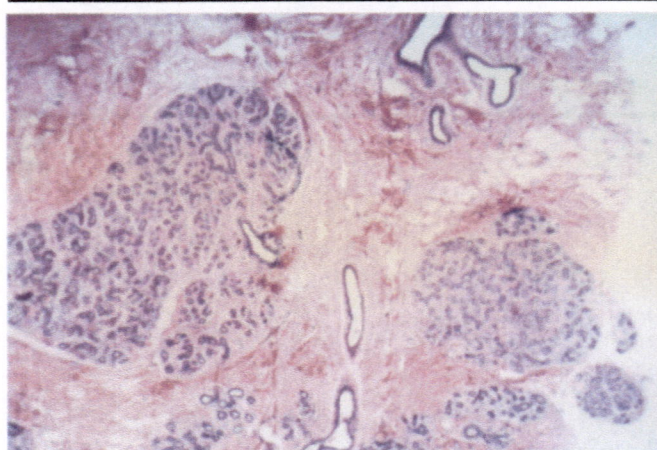

FIGURE 21.1   **Normal breast.** Lobules and interlobular ducts enclosed within stroma.

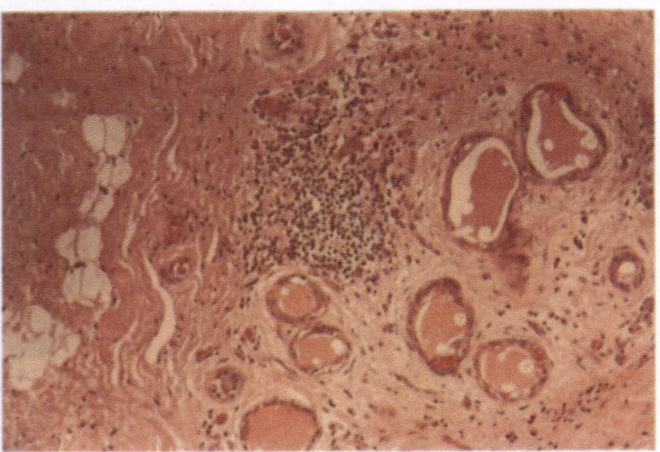

FIGURE 21.3   **Mammary duct ectasia.** Dilated ducts with inspissated secretion in the lumina and periductal mononuclear cell infiltration.

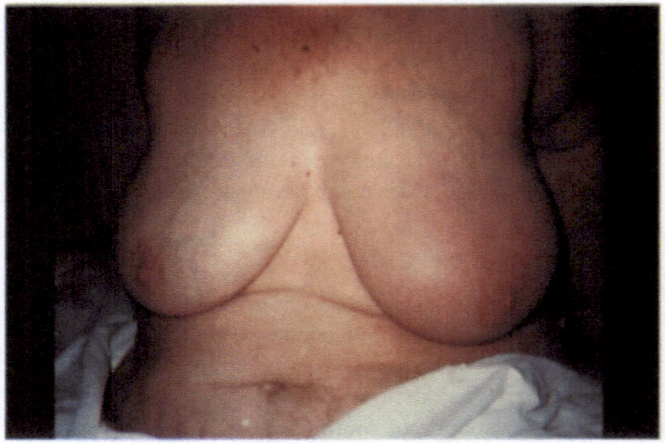

FIGURE 21.2   **Acute mastitis.** Diffuse swollen breast with reddish discoloration.

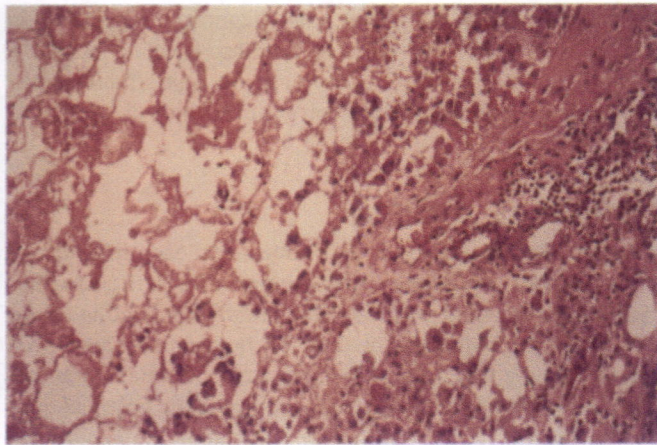

FIGURE 21.4   **Fat necrosis of breast.** Necrotic fat cells surrounded by lipid-laden macrophages.

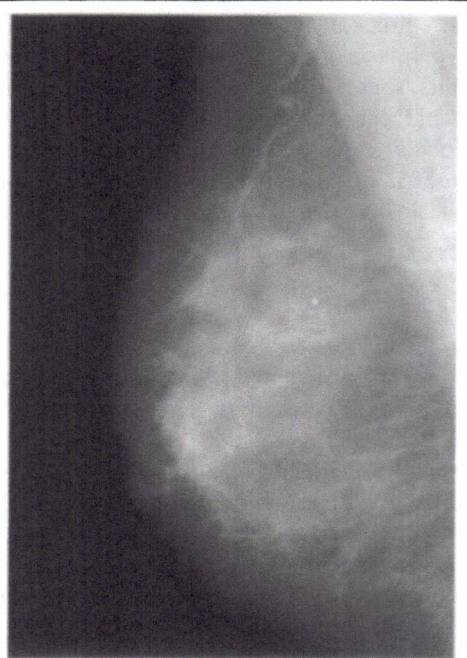

◄

FIGURE 21.5   Fibrocystic disease of breast (mammogram). Confluent radio dense lesion in the center.

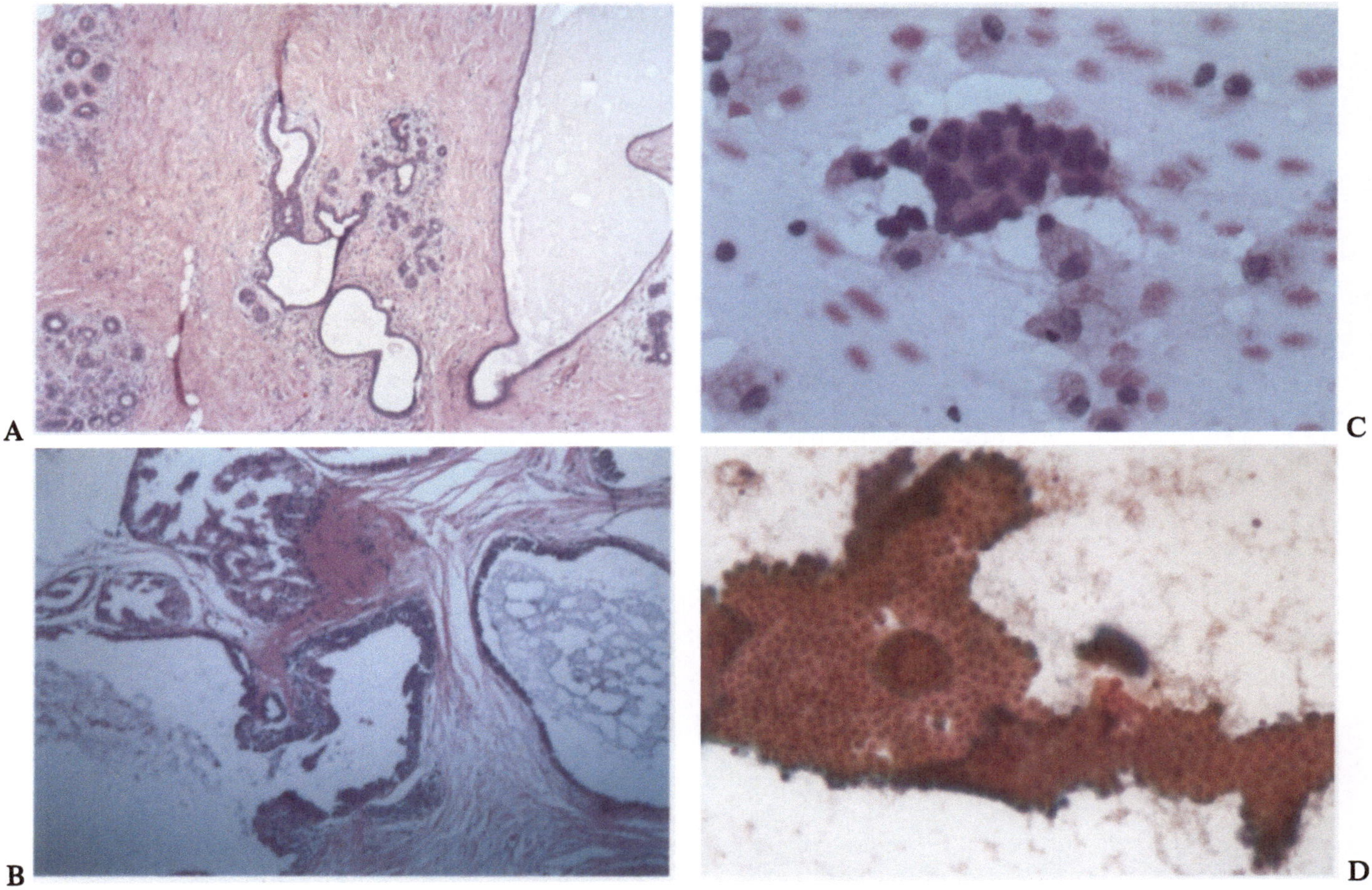

A

B

C

D

FIGURE 21.6   Fibrocystic disease of breast. A: Small and large cysts lined by single layer of cuboidal epithelium. B: Fibrocystic disease with apocrine cystic change. Multiple cysts with papillary projections covered by eosinophilic columnar cells. C: Aspirate showing sheet of ductal lining cells and singly isolated foam cells. D: Aspirate showing sheets ("honeycomb") of apocrine metaplastic cells.

Aspirated cells occur mainly singly, and are large, foam cells with small, round, bland nuclei. Occasionally, aspirated cells occur in sheet of active ductal lining cells (Fig. 21.6C). Cells of apocrine metaplastic cysts occur in sheets and singly and have abundant eosinophilic cytoplasm and small, round, bland nuclei (Fig. 21.6D).

Epithelial Hyperplasia

Epithelial hyperplasia is the most important histologic variant of fibrocystic breast disease in terms of its possible relationship to carcinoma. Grossly, it is unremarkable. Histologically, it usually involves the terminal duct lobular unit and is characterized by proliferation of duct-lining epithelium beyond the usual double layers (Fig. 21.7A).

Proliferated epithelium may fill the duct lumina to result in multiple irregular intraductal spaces. If the lumina are totally or almost totally filled by proliferated epithelium the condition is designated ductal papillomatosis (Fig. 21.7B).

In fine needle aspirates, the cells occur most often as monolayer sheets and occasionally as cell balls. They are relatively uniform in shape and size and have a columnar configuration, with homogeneous basophilic cytoplasm and round to oval, bland nuclei (Fig. 21.7C).

Atypical epithelial hyperplasia is characterized by exaggerated hyperplasia of the terminal ducts and ductules (acini) and exhibits some features of lobular carcinoma in situ or intraductal carcinoma (Fig. 21.8). The cells resemble those of lobular carcinoma in situ but do not fill or distend more than 50% of the terminal ductal units. Atypical lobular hyperplasia is associated with an increased risk of invasive carcinoma.[3,4]

Sclerosing Adenosis

Sclerosing adenosis is a less common histologic variant and is characterized by intralobular fibrosis and proliferation of ductules. Grossly, it is a poorly circumscribed, homogeneous, firm, resilient mass.

Histologically, sclerosing adenosis consists of proliferation of terminal ductal epithelial and myoepithelial cells within fibrous stroma. A lobular arrangement may be maintained or the areas of proliferation may be confluent (Fig. 21.9). Occasionally, fibrous growth may totally compress the ductules to create solid cords or strands of cells embedded in dense stroma, a picture reminiscent of carcinoma.

Fine needle aspirates contain small, uniform cells arranged in groups.

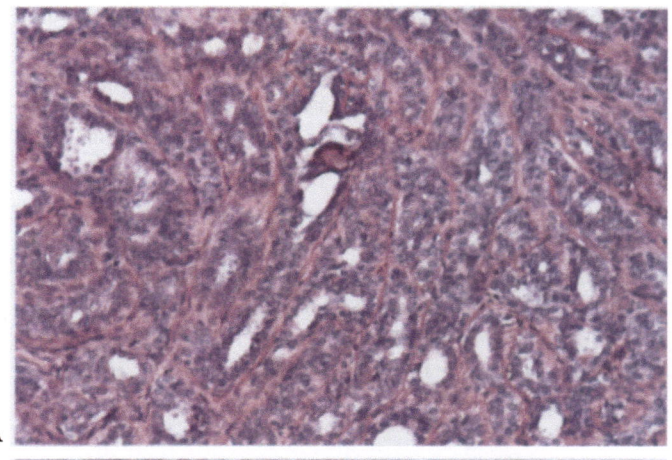

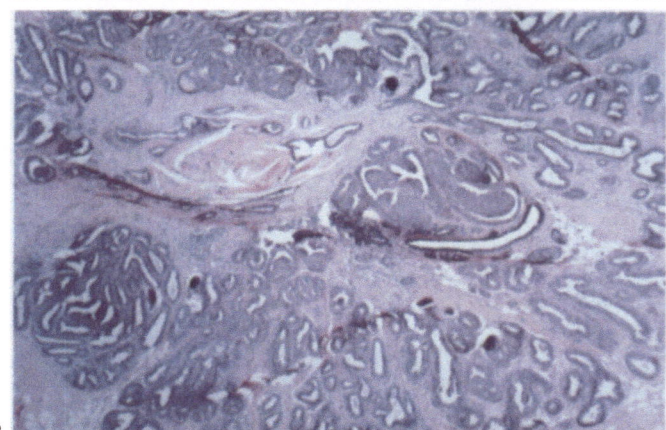

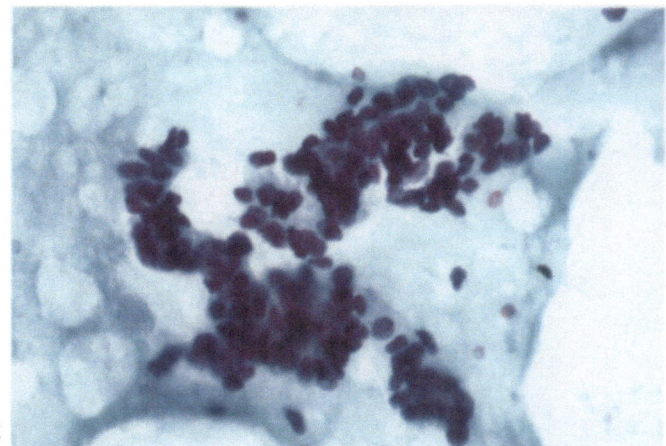

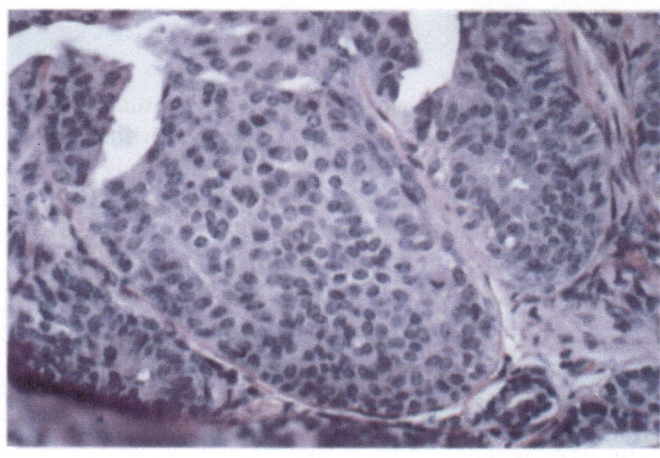

FIGURE 21.8 Atypical epithelial hyperplasia of breast. Atypical epithelial cells filling the terminal ducts and lobular acini.

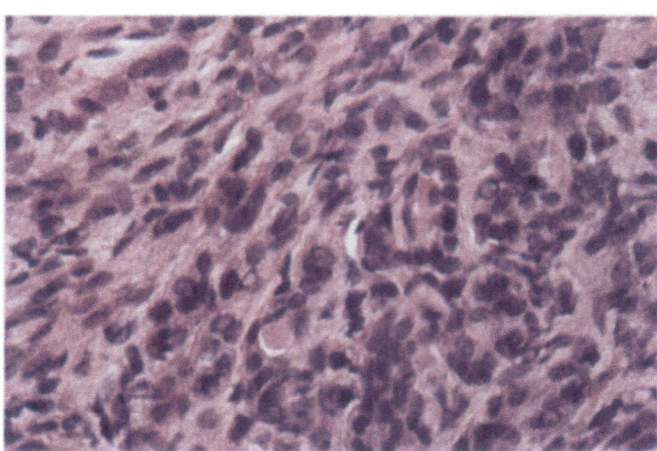

FIGURE 21.9 Sclerosing adenosis of breast. Confluent epithelial and elongated myoepithelial cell proliferation.

FIGURE 21.7 Epithelial hyperplasia (lobular hyperplasia) of breast. A: Proliferation of lobular acini and terminal ducts. B: Ductal papillomatosis of breast. Ductal epithelial cell proliferation filling the lumina. C: Aspirate showing sheets of uniform columnar cells.

Benign Tumors

Fibroadenoma

Fibroadenoma is the most common benign tumor of the female breast and occurs usually in women before age 30 years. It characteristically presents as a sharply circumscribed and freely movable spherical nodule (Fig. 21.10A). Grossly, fibroadenomas range from a few centimeters to several centimeters in diameter. On section, they are well circumscribed, homogeneous, pale gray, firm, and rubbery (Fig. 21.10B).

Histopathology. Fibroadenomas consist of glandular structures separated by cellular fibroblastic stroma. The glandular structures are lined by single or multiple layers of benign epithelial cells (pericanalicular fibroadenoma) (Fig. 21.10C).

In other areas, more active stromal growth results in glandular compression with cleftlike spaces or epithelial strands (intracanalicular fibroadenoma) (Fig. 21.10D). These histologic variants may coexist in the same tumor and are of no clinical significance. Fibroadenomas may require surgical excision to verify their benign nature.

Cytology. Fine needle aspirates contain fronds and sheets of cells as well as isolated cells. The fronds are large cell groups in cohesive clusters (Fig. 21.10E). Singly isolated cells are columnar in shape with vesicular nuclei and micronucleoli. The background of the smear contains bare spindle-shaped nuclei, believed to be myoepithelial cells (Fig. 21.10F).

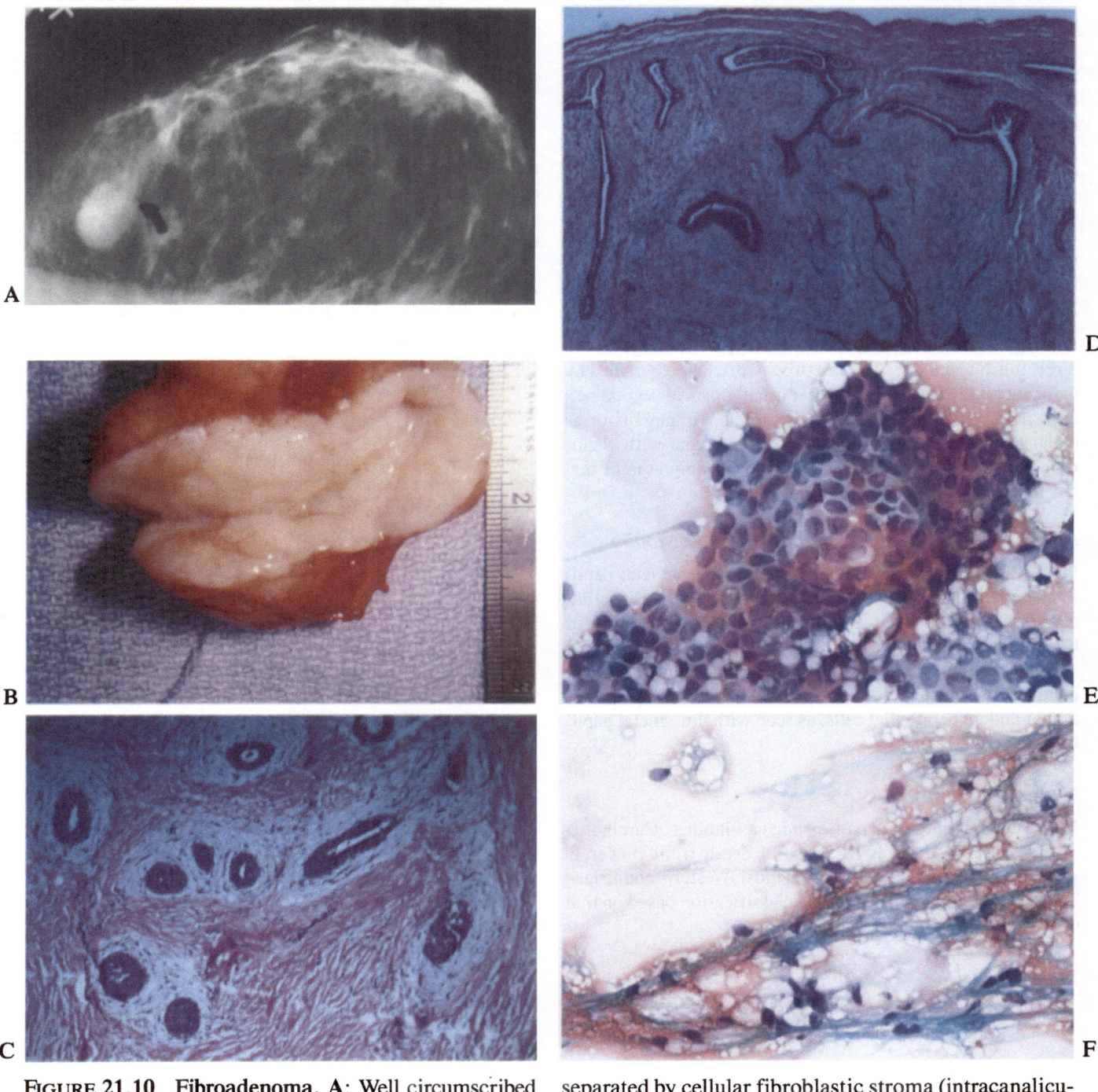

FIGURE 21.10   Fibroadenoma. A: Well circumscribed lesion with a smooth contour (mammogram). B: Encapsulated lobular mass showing pale gray rubbery consistency on cut section. C: Histologic section showing encapsulation and compressed glandular structures separated by cellular fibroblastic stroma (intracanalicular fibroadenoma). D: Hyperplastic tubular mammary ducts separated by active fibroblastic stroma. E, F: Aspirates showing sheets of benign ductal epithelial cells and fibroblastic cells.

Intraductal Papilloma

This is a papillary neoplastic growth involving the major lactiferous ducts, which occurs in the fourth or fifth decade of life. They present clinically as a result of a serous or bloody nipple discharge (Fig. 21.11A). These tumors are rarely palpable because they are usually less than 1 cm in diameter. Grossly, they consist of a friable, villous growth within a large dilated duct.

Histopathology. The lesion consists of confluent papillae supported by fibrovascular stalks. The papillae are covered by two cell layers, benign epithelial and myoepithelial cells (Fig. 21.11B).

Cytology. Smears are prepared from nipple discharge by the direct touch technique. The last drop of discharge obtained by manual compression of the breast usually provides good cellular material. The cells occur in papillary fragments or as balls. The cells are rather uniform and columnar with bland, round nuclei (Fig. 21.11C). Papilloma is a benign tumor that has no tendency to develop into carcinoma.[5]

Nipple Adenoma (Florid Papillomatosis of Nipple)

Nipple adenoma is a histologic variant of intraductal papilloma and occurs in the fourth or fifth decade of life. Its clinical presentation is enlargement of the nipple with serous or bloody discharge.

Histologically, the lesion consists of confluent branching papillations. The papillae are covered by two cell layers, columnar and myoepithelial cells, as seen with intraductal papilloma (Fig. 21.12).

Malignant Tumors

More than 90% of breast cancers are carcinomas. Carcinoma of the breast is the leading cause of death from cancer in women in the United States and most Western countries.[6] Table 21.1 presents the histologic classification based on that of the World Health Organization.

Noninvasive (In Situ) Carcinoma

Intraductal Carcinoma

More than 90% of breast carcinomas are of ductal epithelial origin. Intraductal carcinoma is defined as a carcinoma confined to the duct lumina. Grossly, the tumors are poorly defined and relatively firm. On section, some intraductal carcinomas show cordlike ducts filled with cheesy necrotic tissue that can be readily expelled upon slight pressure.

Histopathology. Ducts are dilated by carcinoma that fills the lumina. Some intraductal carcinomas have prominent central necrosis (intraductal comedocarcinoma) (Fig. 21.13A), some show a cribriform pattern (Fig. 21.13B), and others show a prominent papillary pattern (intraductal papillary carcinoma).

Cytology. Aspirated cells are relatively small and uniform and are similar to those aspirated from invasive carcinomas. A follow-up study of intraductal carcinomas over a period of 15 years showed that invasive carcinomas developed in 28% of women treated with excisional biopsy alone.[8]

Table 21.1. Histologic classification of breast tumors.

Noninvasive (noninfiltrating)
Intraductal carcinoma
Intraductal papillary carcinoma
Lobular carcinoma in situ
Invasive
Invasive ductal carcinoma—not otherwise specified (NOS)
Invasive lobular carcinoma
Medullary carcinoma
Colloid carcinoma (mucinous carcinoma)
Paget's disease
Tubular carcinoma
Adenoid cystic carcinoma
Invasive comedocarcinoma
Apocrine carcinoma
Invasive papillary carcinoma

Adopted from the World Health Organization.[7]

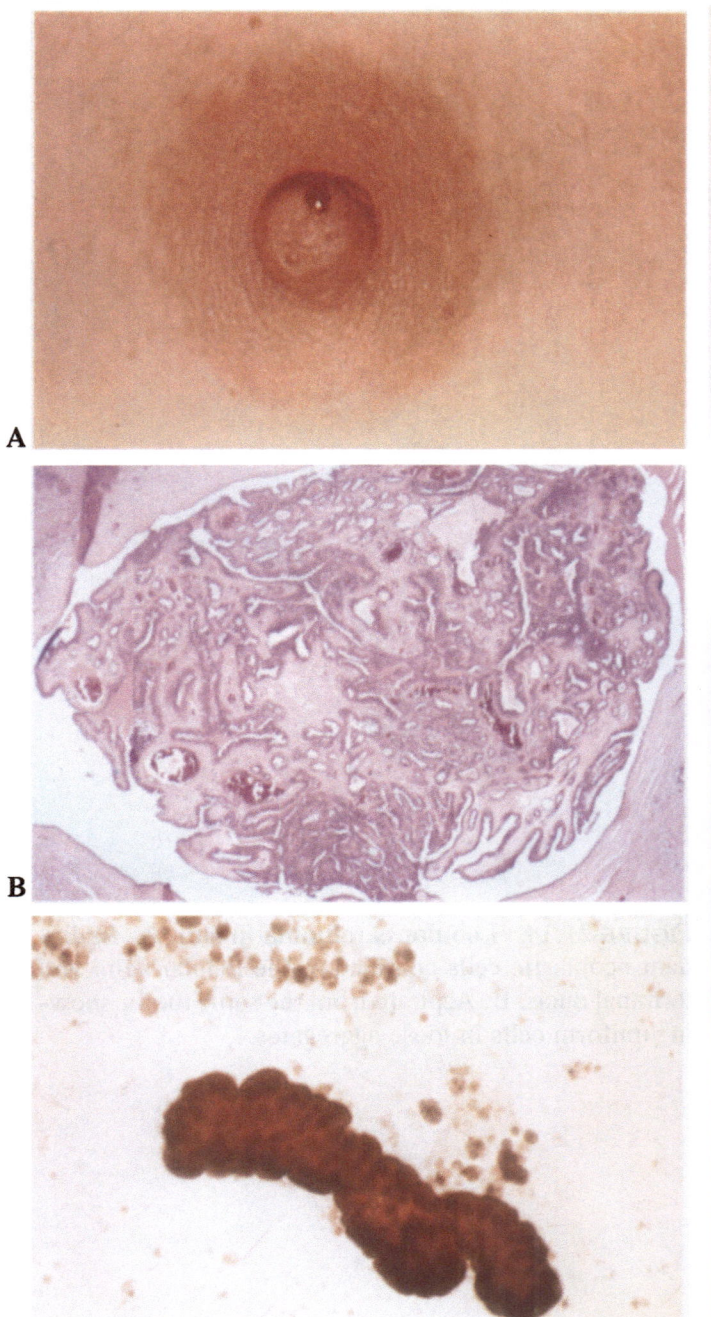

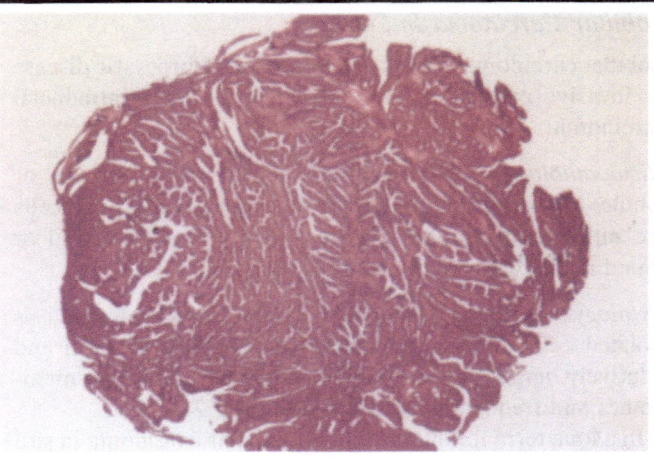

FIGURE 21.12   Nipple adenoma. Confluent papillary structures covered by columnar and myoepithelial cells.

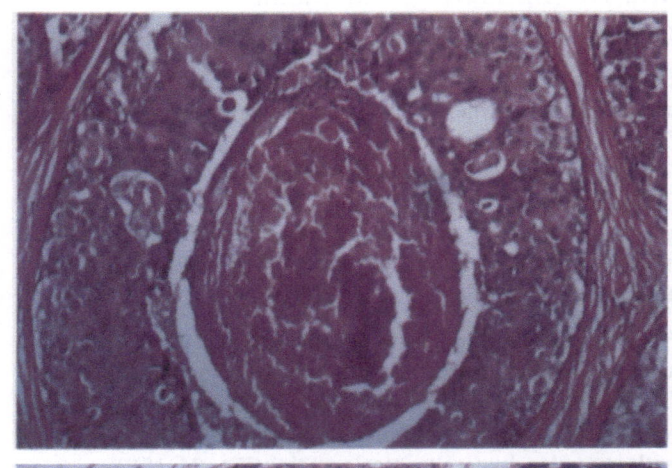

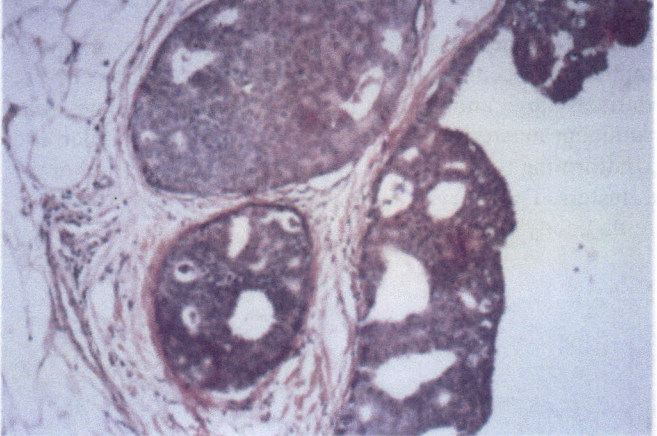

FIGURE 21.11 Intraductal papilloma of breast. A: Bloody nipple discharge in a patient with intraductal papilloma. **B**: Histologic section from the same lesion showing confluent papillary structures in the major lactiferous duct. **C**: Direct touch smear of the nipple discharge showing a dense papillary cluster.

FIGURE 21.13   Intraductal carcinoma. A: Intraductal proliferation of partly necrotic malignant epithelial cells (comedo type). **B**: Intraductal malignant cells arranged in a cribriform pattern.

Lobular Carcinoma In Situ

Lobular carcinoma in situ can be seen near fibrocystic disease or invasive carcinoma, or it may coexist with intraductal carcinoma.

Histopathology. The neoplasm involves terminal ducts or lobules as a proliferation of loosely cohesive cells. The cells are rather uniform and slightly enlarged and have oval or round nuclei with small nucleoli (Fig. 21.14A).

Cytology. Aspirated cells occur in loose aggregates and as isolated cells. They have scanty ill-defined cytoplasm and relatively large nuclei with irregular thick nuclear membranes and frequently micronucleoli (Fig. 21.14B).

In a long term follow-up study of lobular carcinoma in situ treated by lumpectomy alone, the frequency of carcinoma subsequently developing in the same or contralateral breast was 30%.[9]

Invasive (Infiltrating) Carcinoma

Invasive Duct Carcinoma

Invasive duct carcinoma is the most common type of breast cancer. Grossly, the tumors are poorly circumscribed and firm in consistency. Mammography reveals a radiodense lesion, with irregular margins resulting from infiltration (Fig. 21.15A). On section, the tumor is pale gray, chalky, granular, and firm, and retracted below the cut surface. The margin is irregular as a result of neoplastic infiltration of the adjacent tissue.

Histopathology. The lesion consists of atypical duct cells arranged in cords, nests, and glands embedded in dense fibrous stroma. The cells vary from small uniform cells with round, hyperchromatic nuclei to large, pleomorphic cells with irregular, hyperchromatic nuclei (Fig. 21.15B).

Cytology. In the scirrhous type, cells in an aspirate are few in number and occur singly or in small clusters. The cells are relatively large and have large, hyperchromatic nuclei with prominent macronucleoli (Fig. 21.15C). In the cellular and glandforming type, cells in aspirates are abundant and occur in clusters. They vary in size and shape and have features that are distinctly malignant.

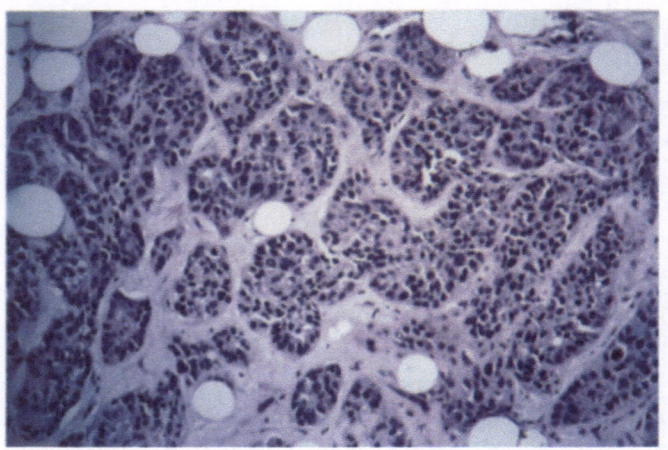

A

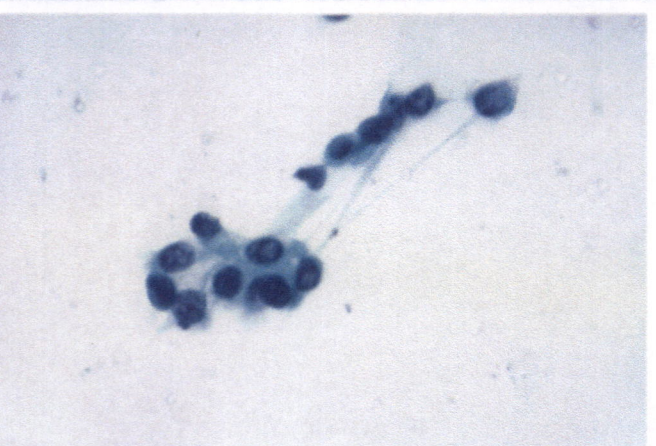

B

FIGURE 21.14 Lobular carcinoma in situ. **A**: Malignant neoplastic cells confined to the lobular acini and terminal ducts. **B**: Aspirate from the same tumor showing uniform cells in loose aggregates.

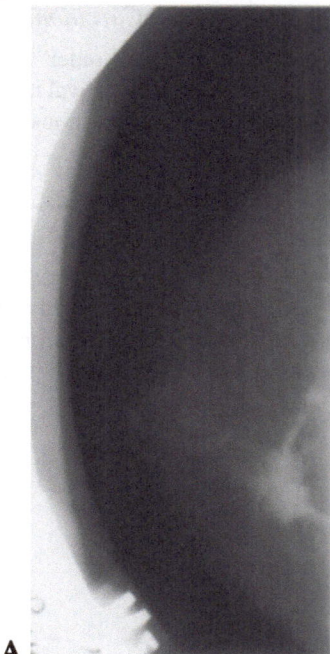

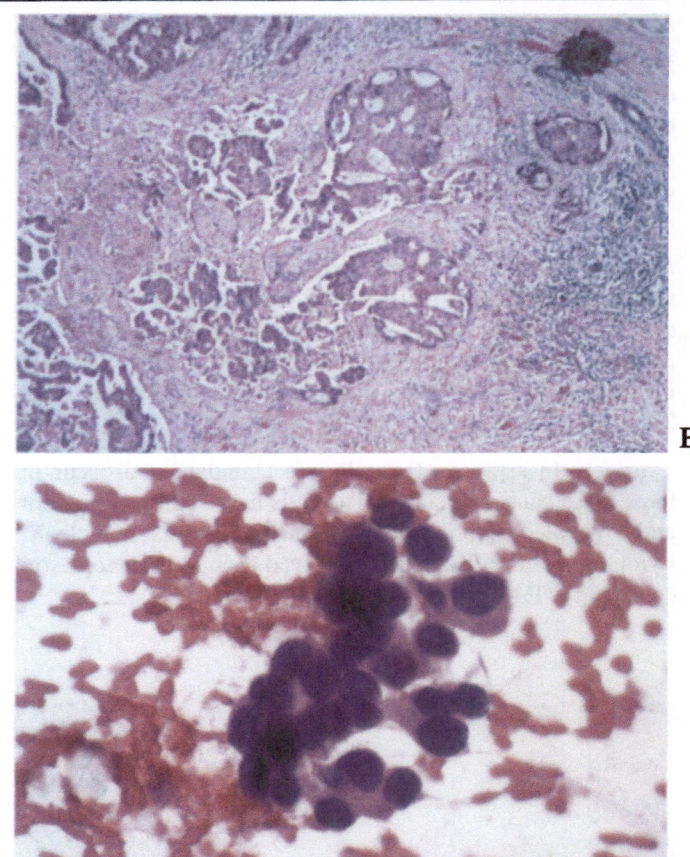

FIGURE 21.15   **Invasive duct carcinoma of breast. A**: Mammogram showing a radiodense lesion with an irregular peripheral margin. **B**: Biopsy specimen of the same lesion showing neoplastic glands and nests of malignant cells in dense fibrous stroma. **C**: Aspirate from the tumor showing loose clusters of neoplastic cells.

Medullary Carcinoma

Pure medullary carcinoma is a relatively rare variant of breast carcinoma. Grossly, the tumors tend to be large and fleshy. On section they are well circumscribed, soft, and yielding on palpation. Multifocal necrosis and hemorrhage are frequently observed. Mammography shows a large radiodense mass with smooth margins (Fig. 21.16A).

Histopathology. The tumor consists of loosely cohesive sheets of large cells, with scanty intervening stroma. The cells are large and have little cytoplasm and large, pleomorphic nuclei with prominent macronucleoli. Lymphocytic infiltration of the fibrous stroma is usually present (Fig. 21.16B).

Cytology. In aspirates the cells are abundant and occur in loose aggregates and singly. The cells have scanty cytoplasm and large, pleomorphic nuclei with prominent macronucleoli. Lymphocytes are frequently observed around the neoplastic cells (Fig. 21.16C).

Colloid Carcinoma (Mucinous Carcinoma)

Colloid carcinoma tends to occur in older women and is a slowly growing tumor with a better survival rate. Grossly, the tumor is a large, bluish, soft, and gelatinous mass.

Histopathology. The tumor consists of cell clusters and glandular structures in an abundant, amorphous, mucinous background (Fig. 21.17).

Cytology. In aspirates the cells occur in tight clusters in a mucinous background. The cells have scanty cytoplasm and small, round, hyperchromatic nuclei. Macronucleoli may be observed. Mucicarmine stain may be of help in the differential diagnosis.

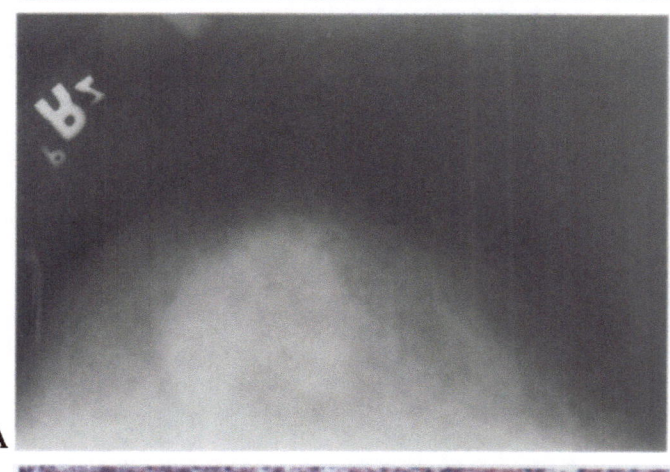

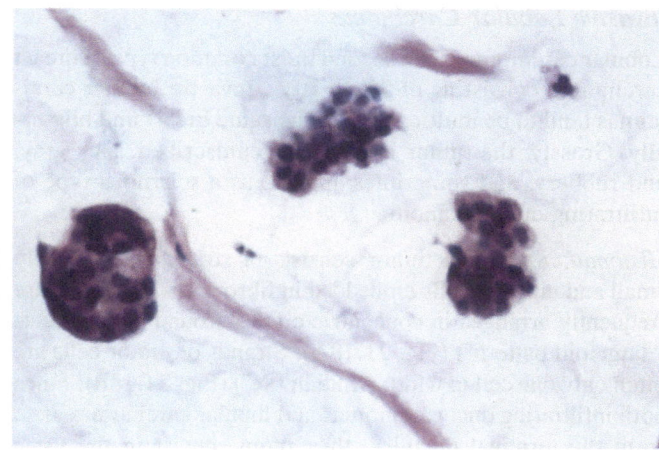

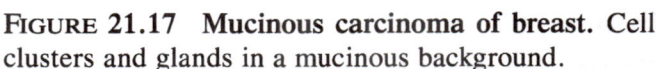

FIGURE 21.17 **Mucinous carcinoma of breast.** Cell clusters and glands in a mucinous background.

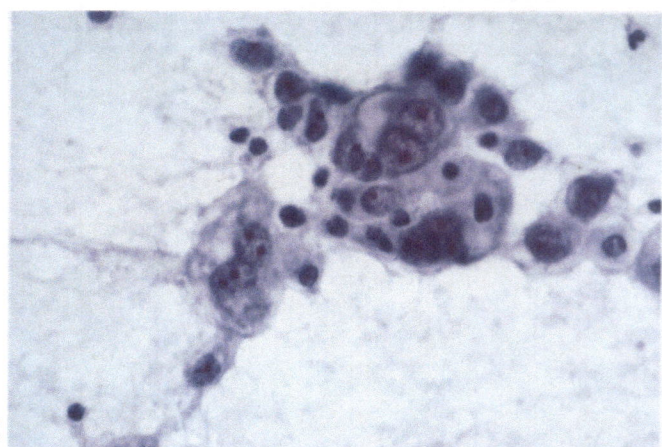

FIGURE 21.16 **Medullary carcinoma. A:** Mammogram showing a large, well defined, radiodense mass. **B:** Biopsy specimen of the mass showing loosely cohesive sheets of large pleomorphic cells and scanty intervening stroma with lymphocytic infiltration. **C:** Aspirate of the tumor showing loosely cohesive pleomorphic cells and isolated lymphocytes.

Invasive Lobular Carcinoma

Lobular carcinoma is the second most common type of breast carcinoma, consisting of 5% to 10%. Invasive lobular carcinomas tend to be multicentric in the same breast and bilaterally. Grossly, the tumor is poorly circumscribed, pale gray, and rubbery, and sometimes appears as a scirrhous type of infiltrating duct carcinoma.

Histopathology. The tumor consists of strands of relatively small and uniform cells embedded in fibrous stroma. They are frequently arranged in concentric circles around benign ducts ("targetoid pattern") (Fig. 21.18A). Strands of tumor cells are often only one cell in width ("Indian file") (Fig. 21.18B). Since both infiltrating duct carcinomas and lobular carcinomas arise from the terminal ductules, they often coexist in the same lesion.

Cytology. In aspirates the cells occur in loose aggregates and singly. The cells are relatively small and uniform, and have a moderate amount of granular or vacuolated cytoplasm and small, round, hyperchromatic nuclei with prominent small nucleoli (Fig. 21.18C).

Paget's Disease

Clinically, Paget's disease presents as an eczematoid change of the skin of the nipple, with inflammation, ulceration, and oozing (Fig. 21.19A). Paget's disease of the breast is a form of ductal carcinoma of major mammary ducts that spreads to involve the skin of the nipple and areola.

Histopathology. The neoplasm consists of large cells in the basal portion of the epidermis of the nipple. The cells may be in clusters or isolated and tend to permeate the malpighian layer (Fig. 21.19B). They have a large amount of clear cytoplasm that stains positively with alcian blue. In nearly all instances it is accompanied by an underlying breast carcinoma of ductal type with or without stromal invasion.

Inflammatory Carcinoma

The term inflammatory carcinoma was originally used because the clinical picture of this carcinoma is reminiscent of acute mastitis (Fig. 21.20A). The skin change of inflammatory carcinoma of the breast can occur with or without a dominant mass in the breast.

Histopathology. Widespread, poorly differentiated carcinoma infiltrates dermal lymphatic vessels (Fig. 21.20B). This carcinoma is aggressive and the prognosis is poor. Appropriate treatment of this neoplasm is a highly controversial matter.

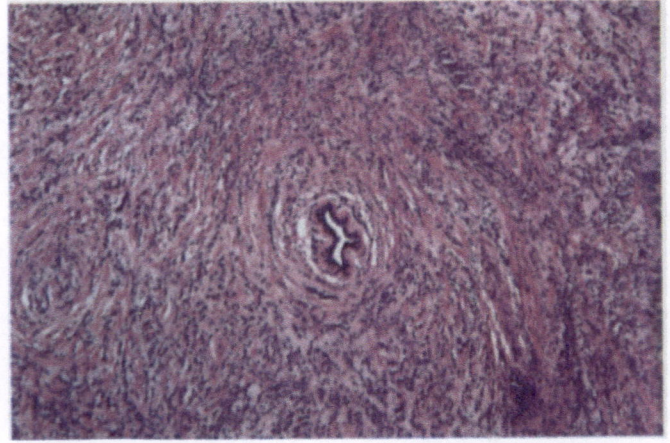

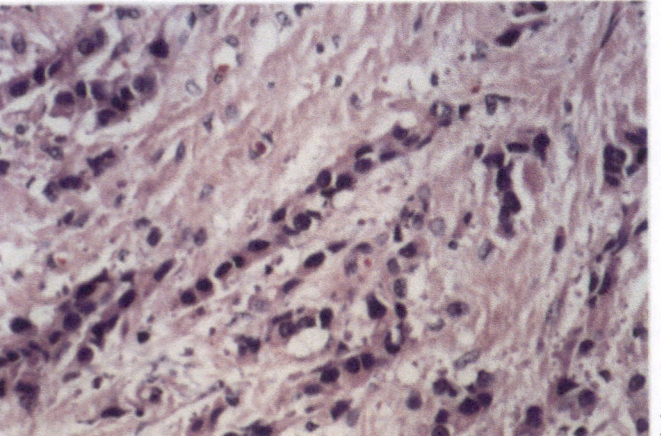

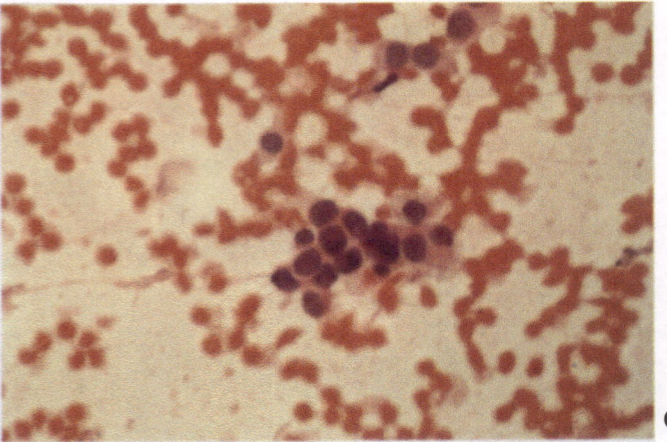

FIGURE 21.18   Invasive lobular carcinoma of breast. A: Tumor cells are arranged in a concentric configuration around the non-neoplastic ducts ("targetoid" pattern). **B:** Single or double strands of carcinoma cells. **C:** Aspirate showing loose aggregates of small uniform carcinoma cells.

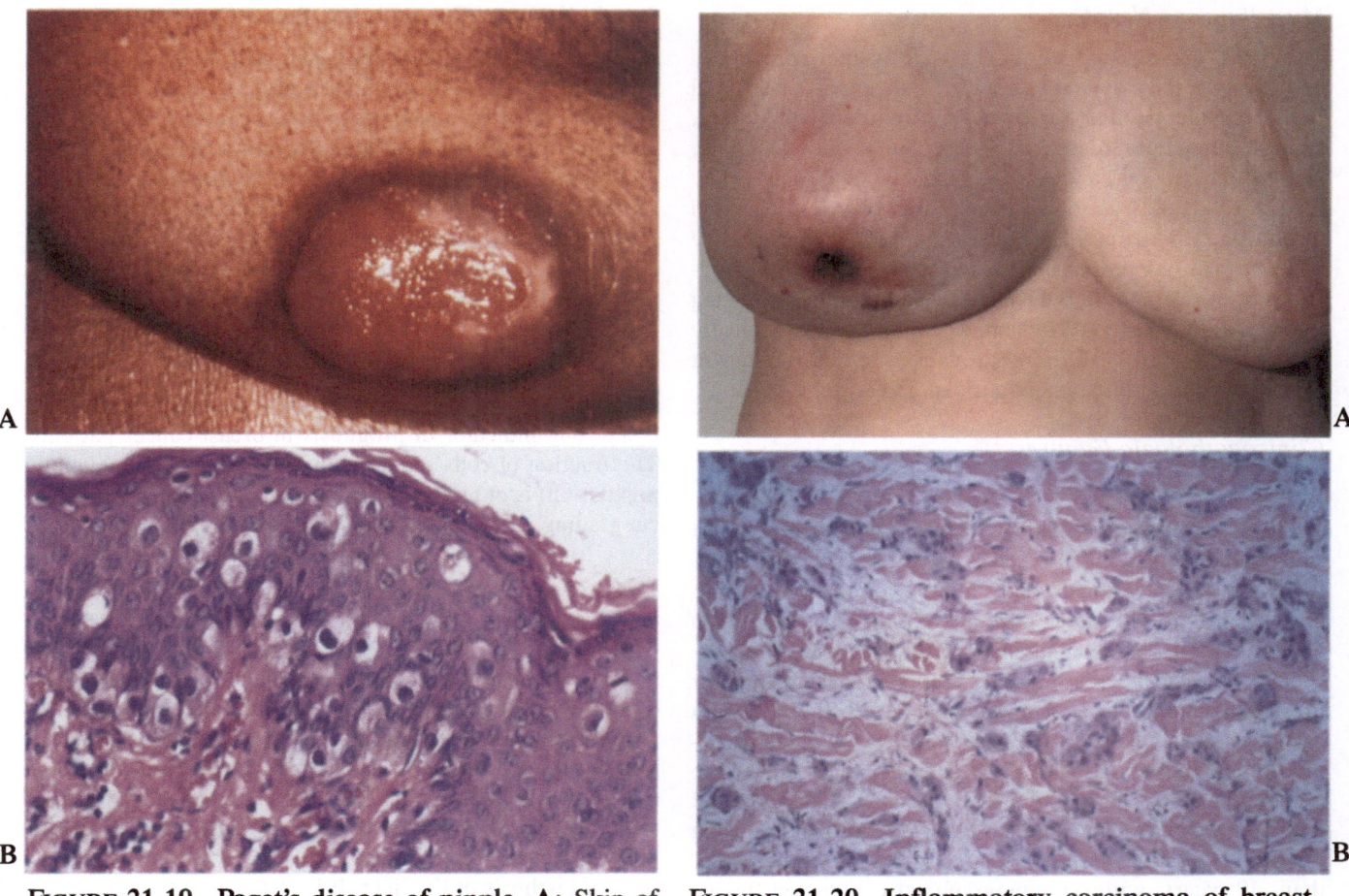

FIGURE 21.19   Paget's disease of nipple. A: Skin of nipple with oozing and eczematoid change. **B**: Histologic section of the nipple showing large clear neoplastic cells in clusters and singly in the basal portion of the epidermis.

FIGURE 21.20   Inflammatory carcinoma of breast. A: Reddish discoloration of skin, reminiscent of acute mastitis. **B**: Histologic section of the same lesion showing clusters of neoplastic cells infiltrating dermal lymphatic spaces.

Miscellaneous Neoplasms

The breast can develop any of the well recognized primary neoplasms of the skin and its adnexa. Cancers of the stromal tissue include stromal sarcomas, cystosarcoma phyllodes, fibrosarcoma, liposarcoma, angiosarcoma, chondrosarcoma, and carcinosarcoma, and, rarely, primary lymphomas. They tend to produce large, bulky masses that may result in skin ulceration. Most sarcomas of the breast are highly aggressive and have a strong propensity to metastasize by the hematogenous route. Cystosarcoma phyllodes is defined as being malignant if the stromal element is cellular and cytologically atypical (Fig. 21.21). Carcinosarcoma comprises malignant epithelial cells and malignant stromal cells (Fig. 21.22).

Clinicopathologic Features

Clinical Course

The most common and major clinical presentation of breast cancer is a definite lump noticed by the patient and physician. At the time of detection of such a lump, two thirds of the neoplasms have already metastasized to axillary or other lymph nodes. The current recommended program for early detection of breast cancer is monthly self-examination, regular medical examination by a physician, and mammography at age 40 years and every 1 to 2 years thereafter. Women recognized as having a high risk of developing breast cancer are recommended to have and more frequent check-ups and mammography at an earlier age. A recent massive screening program has shown an increase in survival for women older than 40 years with mammographically detected breast cancers.[10]

Prognostic Factors

Most breast cancers spread early by lymphatics and blood vessels. The presence or absence of lymph nodal metastasis is the most important prognostic feature in predicting survival and in determining the type of treatment. Other important factors that affect prognosis are tumor size, extent of local extension of the tumor, histologic type, and nuclear grade of the tumor cells.

Steroid Hormone Receptors and Breast Cancer

Since steroid hormones (estrogen and progesterone) are thought to be a promoter in breast carcinogenesis, the amount of steroid hormone receptors in breast cancer cells may give an indication of the potential of the tumor to respond to hormonal manipulation. Seventy percent of tumors with steroid receptors respond to hormonal manipulation, whereas only 5% of those without receptors respond. Overall, breast cancers with a high level of steroid receptors have a better prognosis than those with an intermediate level or no receptors.[11]

Prognostic Significance of DNA Pattern in Breast Cancer

Current study demonstrates that tumor nuclear DNA content is a strong indicator of prognosis in breast cancer patients. The fraction of cells scattered outside the model (aneuploid population) is of utmost importance for adequate cytochemical grading of malignancy in breast cancers.[12]

Diseases of Male Breast

Gynecomastia

Gynecomastia is defined as enlargement of the male breast due to hypertrophy and hyperplasia of ductal epithelial and stromal components. It is caused by an excess of estrogen. It may develop at the time of puberty or in the very aged without any underlying pathologic basis. Gynecomastia is chiefly of importance as an indicator of hyperestrinism, suggesting the possible existence of a functional testicular tumor or the presence of cirrhosis of the liver. It is also one of the manifestations of Klinefelter's syndrome. Histologically, the lesion consists of ductal epithelial hyperplasia in dense hypertrophic hyaline collagenous connective tissue (Fig. 21.23).

Carcinoma of Male Breast

Carcinoma of male breast occurs in older men and is rare. Since the male breast has only a scanty amount of breast substance, local extension to the skin and underlying chest wall occurs early. Histologically, these carcinomas are similar to those of the female breast.

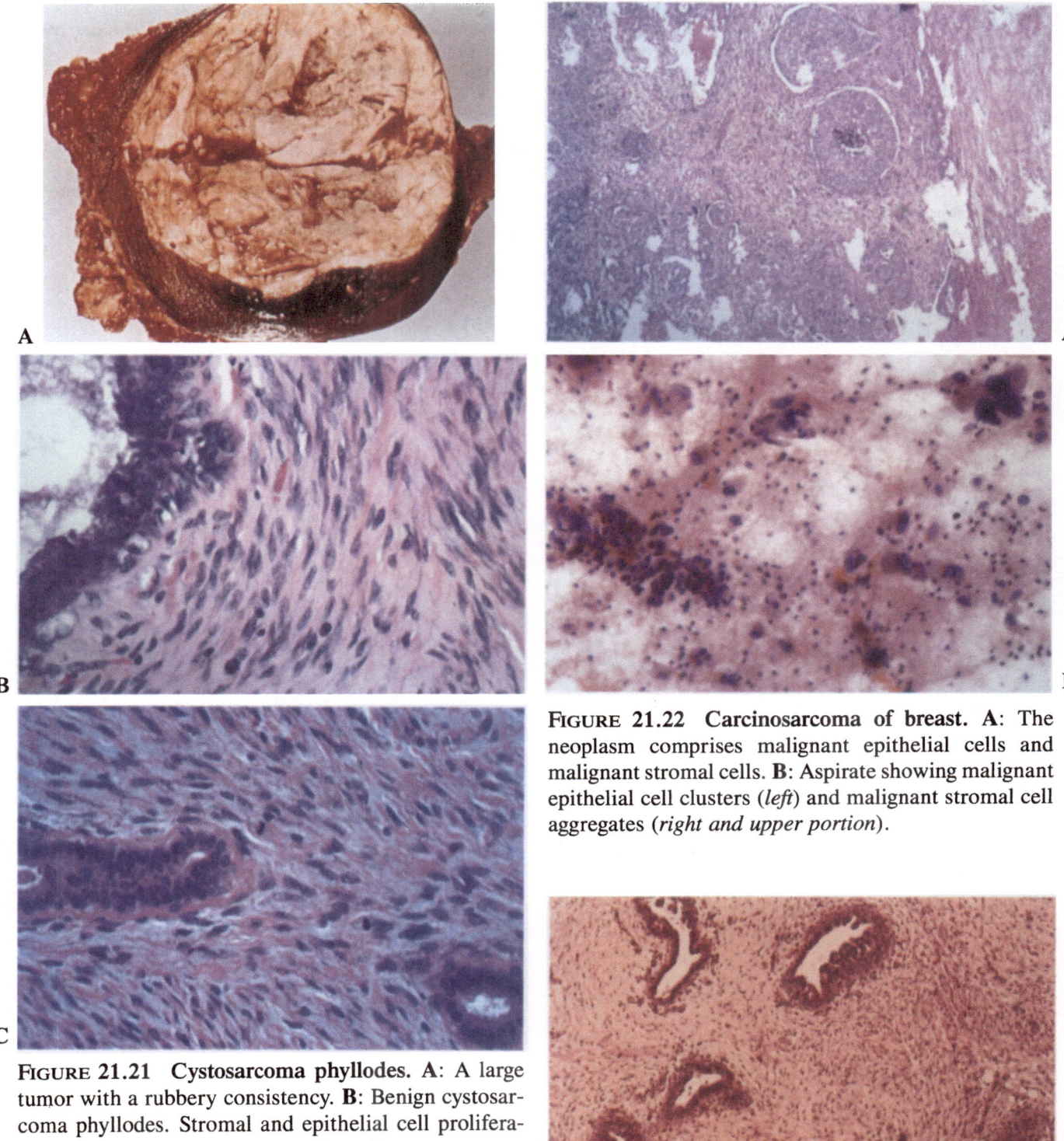

FIGURE 21.22 Carcinosarcoma of breast. A: The neoplasm comprises malignant epithelial cells and malignant stromal cells. **B**: Aspirate showing malignant epithelial cell clusters (*left*) and malignant stromal cell aggregates (*right and upper portion*).

FIGURE 21.21 Cystosarcoma phyllodes. A: A large tumor with a rubbery consistency. **B**: Benign cystosarcoma phyllodes. Stromal and epithelial cell proliferation without cytologic atypia. **C**: Malignant cystosarcoma phyllodes. A more cellular stroma containing cells with nuclear atypia and mitotic figures. The epithelial proliferation is non-neoplastic.

FIGURE 21.23 Gynecomastia. Mammary ductal hyperplasia in a dense stromal background.

References

1. Bell DA, Hajdu SI, Urban JA, et al. Role of aspiration cytology in the diagnosis and management of mammary lesions in office practice. *Cancer.* 1985;51:1182–1189.

2. Strawbridge HTG, Bassett AA, Foldes I. Role of cytology in management of lesions of the breast. *Surg Gynecol Obstet.* 1981;152:1–7.

3. Page DL, et al. Ductal involvement by cells of atypical lobular hyperplasia in the breast. *Hum Pathol.* 1988;19:201.

4. Dupont WD, Page DL. Relative risk of breast cancer varies with time since diagnosis of atypical hyperplasia. *Hum Pathol.* 1989;20:723–725.

5. Rosen PP. Arthur Purdy Stout and papilloma of the breast. Comments on the occasion of his 100th birthday. *Am J Surg Pathol.* 1986;10(Suppl1):100–107.

6. Silverberg E, Lubera JA. Cancer statistics. *CA.* 1989;39:3–20.

7. The World Health Organization Histologic Typing of Breast Tumors (2nd ed.). *Am J Clin Pathol.* 1982;78:806.

8. Page D, et al. Intraductal carcinoma of the breast: Follow up after biopsy only. *Cancer.* 1982;49:751.

9. Rosen PP. Lobar carcinoma in situ of the breast. *Am J Surg Pathol.* 1978;2:225.

10. Seidman H, et al. Survival experience in the breast cancer detection demonstration project. *Cancer.* 1987;37:258.

11. Mirecki DM, Jordan VC. Steroid hormone receptors and human breast cancer. *Lab Med.* 1985;16:287.

12. Fallenius AG, et al. Prognostic significance of DNA measurements in 409 consecutive breast cancer patients. *Cancer.* 1988;62:331.

22

The Central Nervous System

Since almost all space-occupying intracranial lesions are operated on for diagnosis, the least traumatic and most cost effective diagnostic procedure is highly desirable.

After the introduction of computed tomography (CT) in the 1970s and, subsequently, of magnetic resonance imaging (MRI), space-occupying lesions of the central nervous system can now be localized precisely and a morphologic diagnosis can be obtained by needle biopsy, which can be performed under local anesthesia.

The indications and advantages of fine needle aspiration (FNA) of space-occupying brain lesions are as follows[1]:

1. it permits differentiation between neoplastic and non-neoplastic lesions, and between primary and metastatic neoplasms
2. it is easy to gain access to deeply seated lesions or lesions close to vital structures
3. it enables fluid to be obtained from cystic lesions for culture and cell study
4. it is relatively nontraumatic.

Anatomy and Histology

The human brain is encased in the skull. The inner layer of the skull is lined by a rigid fibrous layer of meninges, the dura. Beneath the dura is the thin layer of meninges, the arachnoid, and beneath the arachnoid is the subarachnoid space filled with cerebrospinal fluid (CSF). The brain is divided into the cerebrum, cerebellum, and brain stem.

The tentorium cerebelli, a dural infolding, separates the cerebrum and cerebellum. The midline structures are the basal ganglia, thalamus, hypothalamus, and epithalamus. The cerebral cortex is the outer portion of the brain, consisting of multilayers of small and large neurons, astrocytes, and oligodendrocytes in the background of neuropil. The white matter is the inner layer of the brain, consisting of myelinated fibers, oligodendrocytes, and astrocytes (Fig. 22.1).

Cerebellar cortex consists of the outermost molecular layer, beneath which are the Purkinje cell and granular cell layers, which are next to the underlying white matter (Fig. 22.2).

Neurons

Neurons are relatively large and variable in size and shape, and have large vesicular nuclei with prominent, round nucleoli. Cytoplasm is abundant and contains Nissl substance (free ribosomal rosettes).

Neuroglial Cells

Neuroglial cells form a supporting matrix in which the neurons are embedded. They consist of astrocytes, oligodendrocytes, and ependymal cells.

Astrocytes

With silver impregnation preparations astrocytes are seen as star-shaped cells of two types: protoplasmic and fibrous astrocytes. With routine stains such as hematoxylin and eosin, only the nuclei of astrocytes are visible and they look similar. Astrocytic nuclei are fairly large and round with finely granular chromatin. The cytoplasm of individual astrocytes can be perceived only in reactive gliosis or glial neoplasia.

Oligodendrocytes

Oligodendrocytes have scanty cytoplasmic processes and in routine preparations appear as small, round, lymphocyte-sized nuclei. They are found throughout the brain, and their function is the production and maintenance of the myelin of the central nervous system (CNS). The cytoplasm of oligodendroglial cells may swell to cause the cell to resemble fried egg. Such swelling is probably due to fixation artifact.

Ependymal Cells

Ependymal cells form a single layer of cuboidal to columnar cells lining the cerebral ventricles and the central canal of the spinal cord.

Choroid plexus cells resemble ependymal cells and when exfoliated occur in loose aggregates and singly. In aspirates, they may occur in papillary clusters.

Microglial cells are probably part of the mononuclear-phagocyte system, occurring in sections in loose aggregates and singly. Their presence in aggregates usually signifies a response to tissue damage.

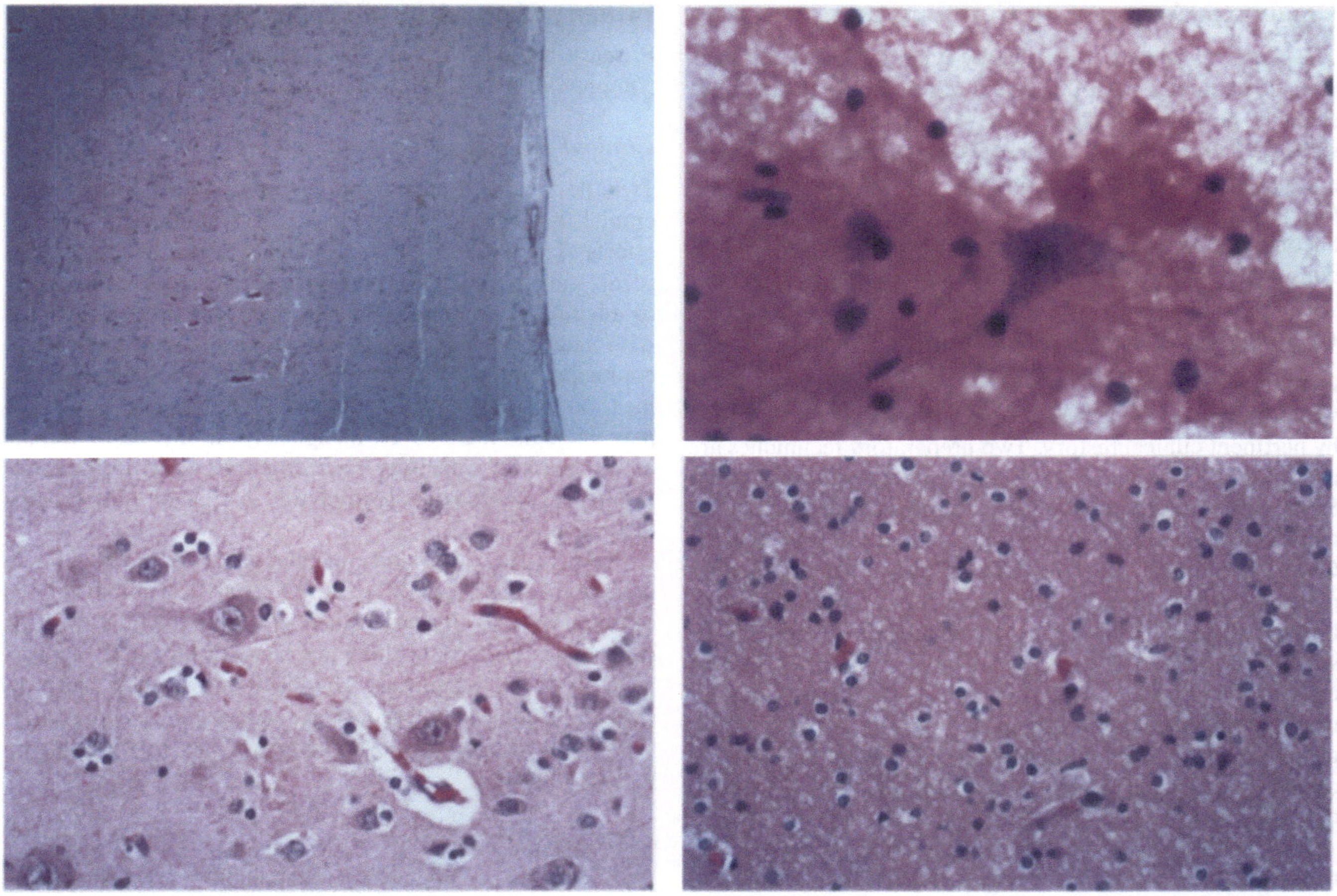

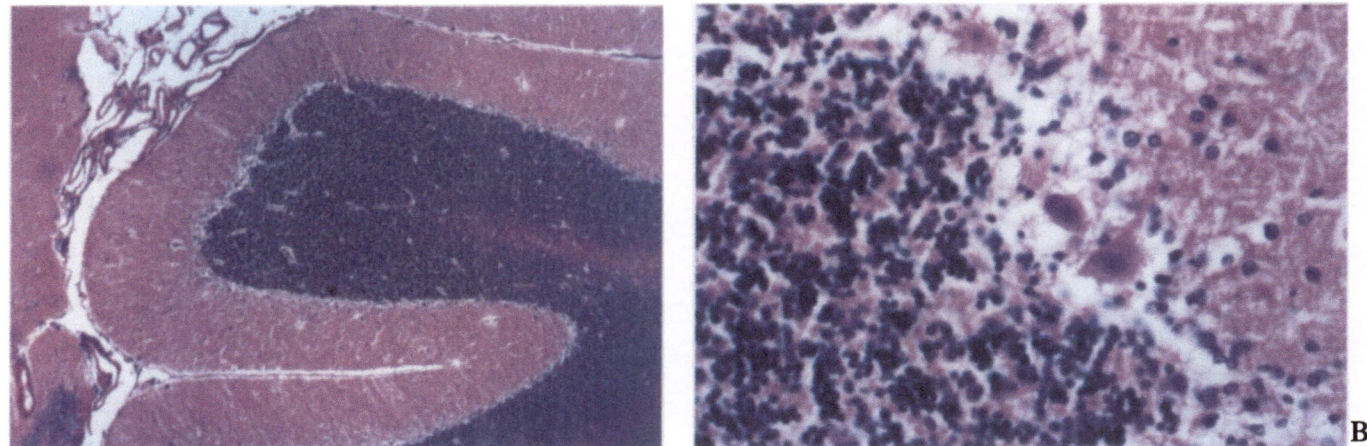

FIGURE 22.1   **Normal histology and cytology of brain.**
A: Cerebral cortex (outer layer) with overlying meninges.
B: Higher magnification showing large neurons, astrocytes (medium sized), and oligodendrocytes (small, round) with perinuclear halos. **C**: Aspiration smear showing neurons, astrocytes, and oligodendrocytes. **D**: Cerebral white matter showing oligodendrocytes and astrocytes in a background of eosinophilic granular neuropil.

FIGURE 22.2   **Normal cerebellar cortex. A**: Outer molecular layer and inner granular layer. **B**: Purkinje cell layer between the two cell layers.

Diagnostic Approach to CNS Lesions

The diagnosis of the CNS lesions by cytology of CSF has been well documented over the last three decades. Readers are strongly recommended to read two classic articles on the subject.[2,3] Open biopsy has been the traditional diagnostic approach to brain lesions.[4] However, with the introduction of CT, the cytologic diagnosis of CNS lesions by FNA has become widely used. For further information on this subject, consult the monograph on aspiration biopsy by Koss et al.[1]

Cytology of Cerebrospinal Fluid

Cytologic evaluation of CSF requires at least 3 ml of fluid, which should be processed as soon as possible, accompanied by pertinent clinical history. Two preparatory techniques are used for CSF: membrane filters and cytocentrifugation. Since both processes have advantages and disadvantages, choice of which process to use is up to the laboratory. Normal CSF may contain a few lymphocytes, monocytes, or ependymal cells. Abnormal smears can be categorized as inflammatory or neoplastic. Inflammatory conditions feature all or some of the following cells: lymphocytes, monocytes, plasma cells, or neutrophils. They are scattered singly. A monomorphic single cell population of cells scattered singly is suggestive of lymphoma or leukemia (Fig. 22.3). In contrast, cells of primary and metastatic neoplasms of the CNS tend to occur in clusters as well as singly (Fig. 22.4).

The specificity and sensitivity of CSF cytology of CNS neoplasms are extremely variable and can be summarized as follows: 66% of all patients with CNS leukemia can be expected to have a positive CSF, 50% of all patients with carcinoma metastatic to the CNS can be expected to have a positive CSF, and one third of all patients with primary tumors of the CNS can be expected to have a positive CSF.[2]

Primary Neoplasms of CNS

Primary neoplasms of the brain may occur at any age and compose 70% of all intracranial neoplasms.

Clinical Pathologic Features

Two dominant clinical manifestations characterize intracranial neoplasms: their local effects and their general effects. The local effects can be delineated by CT and MRI scans, such as a mass lesion of different density, midline shift, or edema. The general clinical effects are those associated with increased intracranial pressure: headache, vomiting, confusion, and mental slowness. Because of their anatomic location histologically benign brain neoplasms often display biologic features of malignancy. Many brain tumors have a marked propensity for infiltrative growth, with neoplastic cells extending beyond the margin of grossly visible neoplasm.

Classification of primary neoplasms of the CNS is based on a modified version of the WHO Classification of Tumors of the Nervous System. Since a major diagnostic difficulty arises because of the wide range of histologic appearance of these neoplasms, ancillary information such as clinical findings, anatomic site, radiologic imaging characteristics, and immunocytochemistry may provide important assistance.

Astrocytic Neoplasms

Astrocytic neoplasms account for about 80% of primary brain tumors of adults. They are histologically divided into three grades of increasing anaplasia and clinical aggressiveness: astrocytoma, anaplastic astrocytoma, and glioblastoma multiforme. They typically occur in middle age to the seventh decade and tend to become more anaplastic with time.

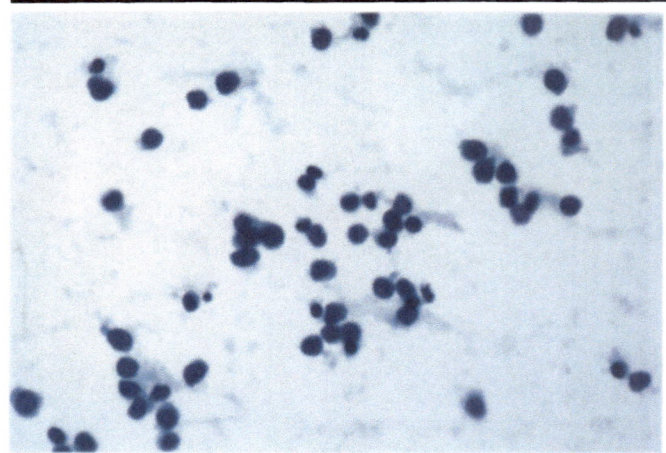

FIGURE 22.3   Acute leukemia. Monomorphic lymphoid cells occurring singly (CSF). (Nuclepore filter preparation.)

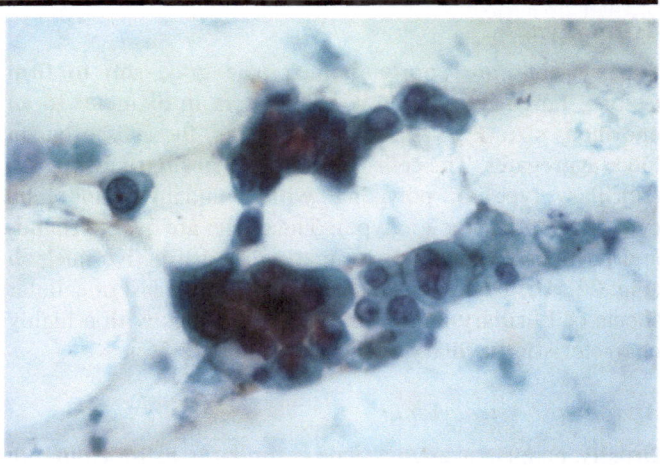

FIGURE 22.4   Metastatic adenocarcinoma of brain. Clusters of tumor cells (CSF). (Cytocentrifuge preparation.)

Astrocytoma

Astrocytomas are poorly defined pale gray, soft to firm lesions, ranging from a few centimeters in diameter to an enormous size (Fig. 22.5A). In aspirates, the cells occur in loose aggregates. The cells are oval with fibrillary cytoplasm (fibrillary type) or polygonal with abundant eosinophilic cytoplasm (gemistocytic type). The nuclei are oval to round, and have finely stippled chromatin and distinctive nucleoli (Fig. 22.5B). Histologically, astrocytomas consist of cellular sheets of fibrillary or gemistocytic astrocytes with a highly characteristic fibrillary background (Fig. 22.5C).

Anaplastic Astrocytoma

Grossly, anaplastic astrocytoma is similar to astrocytoma. In aspiration smears, the cells are abundant and show features of anaplasia: pleomorphism and nuclear atypia (Fig. 22.6A). Histologically, they consist of highly cellular sheets with pleomorphic and anaplastic cells. Vascular endothelial proliferation and mitotic figures are prominent (Fig. 22.6B).

Glioblastoma Multiforme

Grossly, the typical glioblastoma multiforme varies in color, texture, and consistency. Multifocal necrosis, hemorrhage, and cysts are common. The term "multiforme" designates its variegated appearance. In aspiration smears, the cells occur in loose aggregates and often show nuclear molding. The cells are highly pleomorphic and have pleomorphic hyperchromatic nuclei (Fig. 22.7A). Histologically, necrosis, cellular anaplasia, and striking endothelial cell proliferation imparting a "glomeruloid" appearance distinguish this neoplasm from anaplastic astrocytoma (Fig. 22.7B, C).

Clinical Course

Almost all astrocytomas in adults occur in the cerebral hemispheres. Most patients show rapid clinical deterioration.

Pilocytic Astrocytoma

Pilocytic astrocytomas are distinct from other astrocytomas in terms of their clinicopathological features. They usually occur in the cerebellum, optic nerve, and floor and wall of the third ventricle in children and young adults. Grossly, the tumors are usually cystic and well circumscribed. Histologically, the tumors consist of bipolar cells with long, thin, hairlike processes (pilocytic astrocytes). There may be endothelial proliferation, but cell anaplasia is rarely observed. The tumors grow slowly and act like hamartomas, with long-term survival.

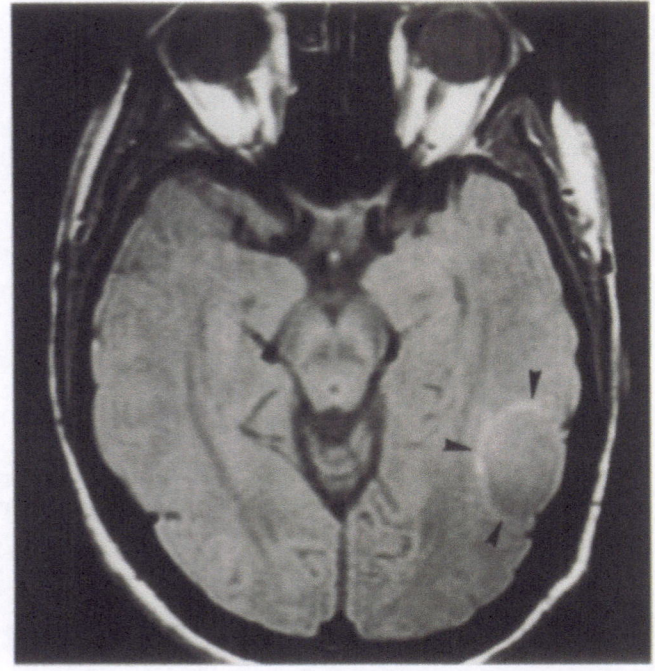

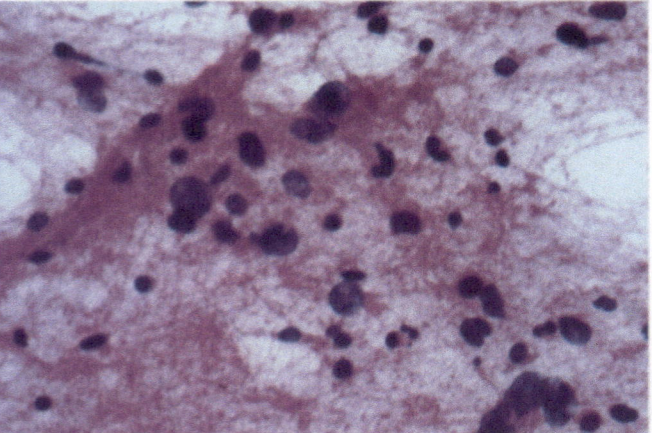

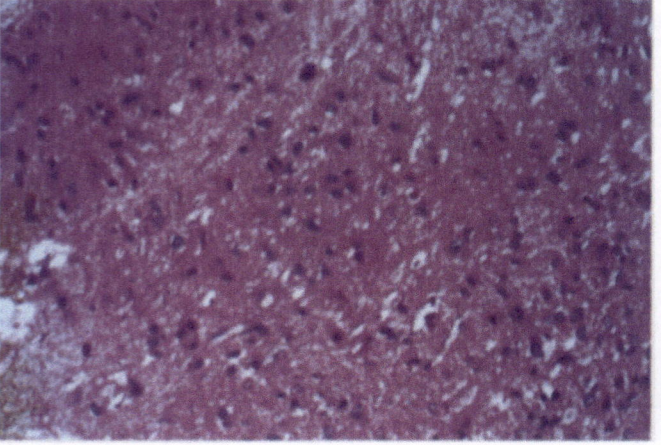

FIGURE 22.5 **Astrocytoma (low grade). A**: Solid space-occupying neoplasm in the left temporal lobe (MRI scan). **B**: Aspiration smear showing loose aggregates of neoplastic cells. **C**: Biopsy section showing relatively cellular sheets of fibrillary astrocytes.

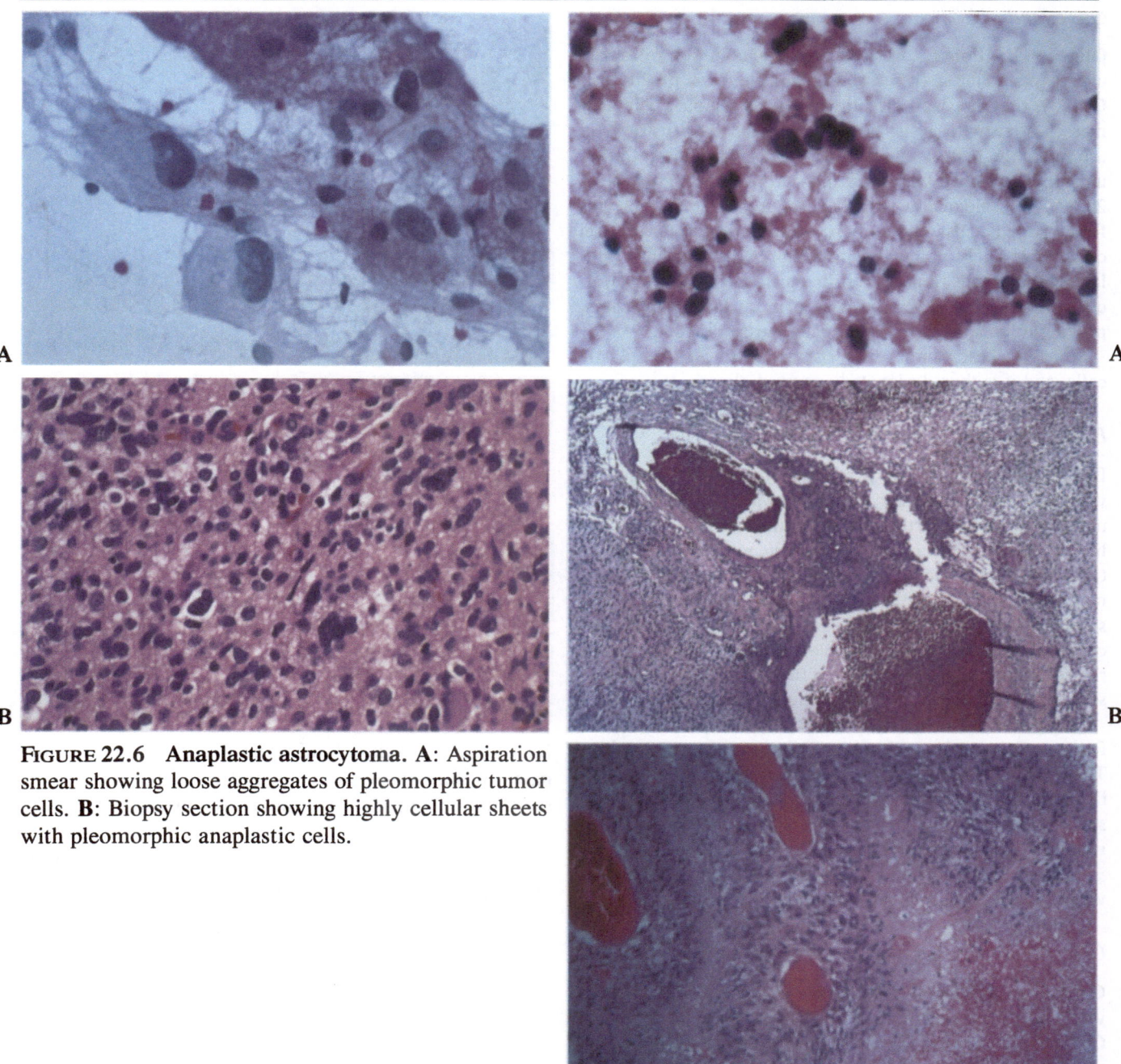

FIGURE 22.6 **Anaplastic astrocytoma. A**: Aspiration smear showing loose aggregates of pleomorphic tumor cells. **B**: Biopsy section showing highly cellular sheets with pleomorphic anaplastic cells.

FIGURE 22.7 **Glioblastoma multiforme. A**: Aspiration smear showing clusters and aggregates of highly pleomorphic and anaplastic cells in a necrotic background. **B**: Biopsy section showing necrosis, pseudopalisading of tumor cells, and prominent vascular proliferation. **C**: Prominent pseudopalisading of pleomorphic tumor cells.

Oligodendroglioma

Oligodendrogliomas are relatively uncommon gliomas, usually occurring in the cerebral hemispheres in middle age. Grossly, they are well circumscribed, gelatinous, pale gray masses often with cysts, hemorrhage, and calcification. In aspirates, the cells occur in loose aggregates and are rather uniform and round, with indistinct cytoplasmic borders (Fig. 22.8A). Histologically, oligodendrogliomas consist of uniform, round cells with clear cytoplasm and round nuclei containing finely granular chromatin. Anastomosing capillaries separate the tumor cells into clusters (Fig. 22.8B). Calcification of the neoplasms is seen in up to 90% of cases, proving to be a useful radiologic diagnostic feature.

Some of these tumors may contain astrocytic neoplastic cells, and it is then designated as mixed glioma.

Ependymoma

Ependymomas are derived from ependymal cells lining the ventricles and the central canal of the spinal cord. They occur most often in the fourth ventricle in the first two decades of life. In middle life, the spinal cord is the more common location, with ependymomas constituting a large fraction of primary intraspinal neoplasms.[5] Grossly, ependymomas are solid, filling the ventricular space, and are sharply demarcated from adjacent brain. Complete excision of the tumors of the ventricle is difficult because of their proximity to the vital structures, including nuclei of the medulla oblongata.

In aspirates or CSF, the cells occur in sheets and are uniform, round to polygonal, with distinct cytoplasmic borders. The nuclei are round to oval and have finely granular chromatin (Fig. 22.9A). Histologically, the tumor cells align themselves around tubular spaces (ependymal canals) and blood vessels (ependymal pseudorosettes) (Fig. 22.9B).

Hydrocephalus secondary to obstruction of the fourth ventricle is a frequent clinical feature.

Choroid Plexus Papilloma

Choroid plexus papillomas occur most often in the lateral ventricles in children and in the fourth ventricle in adults. Grossly, the tumors fill the ventricles with a lobular and papillary growth.

In CSF, the cells occur in papillary clusters of round or cuboidal cells reminiscent of normal choroid plexus. Histologically, the tumors consist of papillary structures covered by pseudostratified columnar cells and supported by a fibrovascular core (Fig. 22.10A). Choroid plexus carcinomas are rare, and their cytologic features are similar to those of adenocarcinomas and anaplastic ependymoma (Fig. 22.10B,C). Differential diagnosis should be based on cytomorphologic features and clinical and radiologic features.[6] Clinically, choroid plexus papillomas or carcinomas present with hydrocephalus due to obstruction of the ventricular system or to overproduction of CSF.

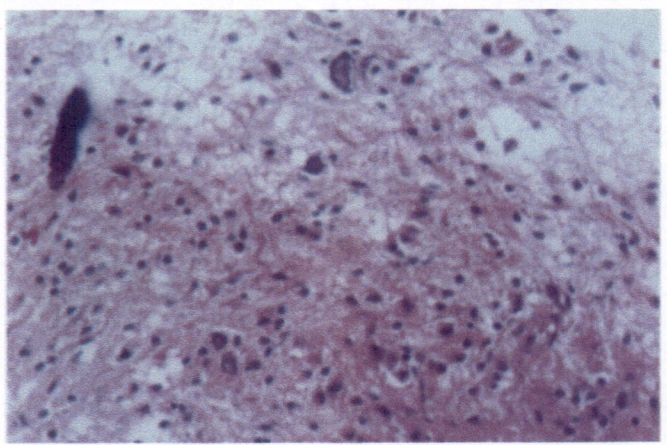

A

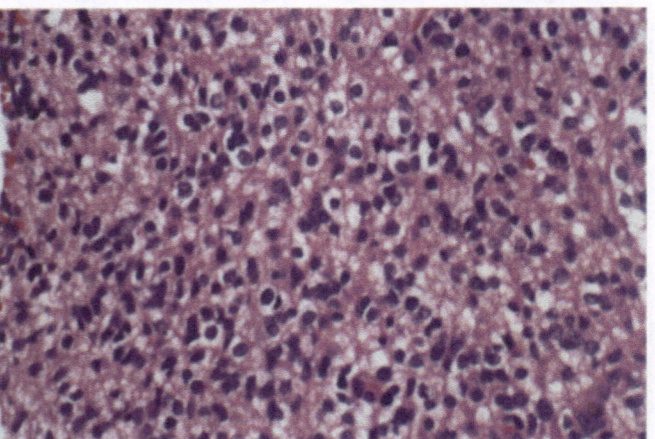

B

FIGURE 22.8 **Oligodendroglioma. A**: Loose aggregates of uniform round cells and calcospherite bodies (cell block from FNA sediment). (Courtesy of Dr. William Murphy, Memphis, Tenn.) **B**: Biopsy section showing sheets of relatively uniform tumor cells with clear cytoplasm and round nuclei.

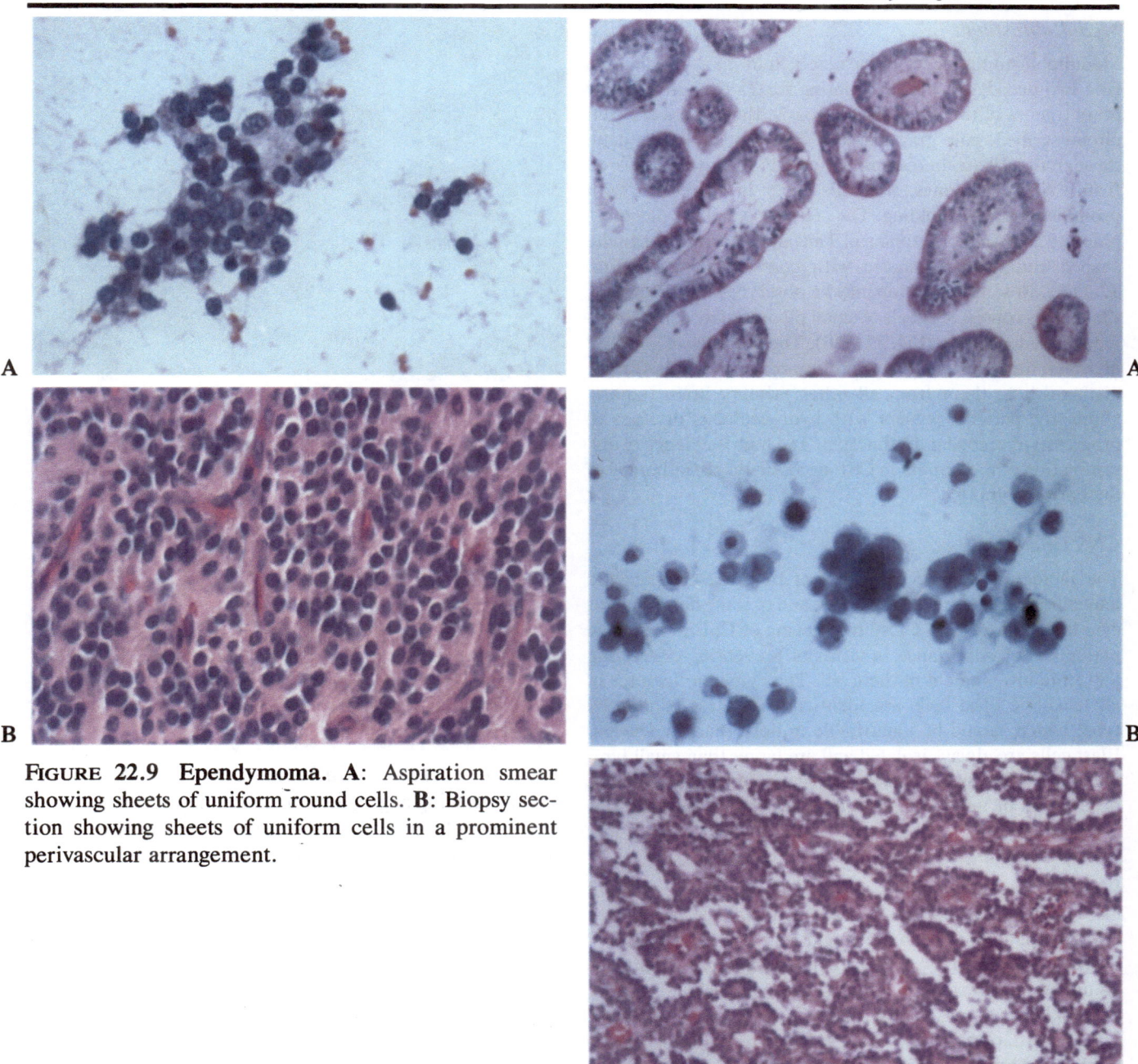

FIGURE 22.9 Ependymoma. A: Aspiration smear showing sheets of uniform round cells. **B**: Biopsy section showing sheets of uniform cells in a prominent perivascular arrangement.

FIGURE 22.10 Choroid plexus papilloma. A: Biopsy section showing papillary structures covered by round to cuboidal tumor cells. **B**: CSF showing clusters of round cells with hyperchromatic nuclei, consistent with choroid plexus carcinoma. **C**: Choroid plexus carcinoma showing compact papillary structures lined by anaplastic cells.

Medulloblastoma

Medulloblastomas occur in the cerebellum, most often in the first two decades of life, accounting for 25% of all primary brain tumors of this age group. Grossly, the tumors are well circumscribed, pale gray masses. They tend to disseminate through the subarachnoid space via CSF. In smears prepared from CSF or aspirates, the cells occur in aggregates with prominent nuclear molding. The cells are small but pleomorphic and have scanty cytoplasm. The nuclei are oval to spindle shaped and hyperchromatic with coarse chromatin (Fig. 22.11A). Rosette formation may be observed. Histologically, the tumors consist of sheets of small pleomorphic cells, showing rosette formation (Fig. 22.11B). The presence of glial and neuronal differentiation of these tumors is a unique feature distinguishing them from all other primary brain tumors. Clinically, patients present with hydrocephalus or signs of progressive cerebellar dysfunction. The high incidence of dissemination of the tumors in CSF necessitates radiotherapy of the entire neuraxis.

CNS Leukemia

The incidence of CNS involvement by acute lymphocytic leukemia ranges from 56% to 83%, and of acute non-lymphocyte leukemia 20%.[7,8] Close monitoring of CSF in leukemic patients is of importance in terms of preventing or treating leukemic involvement of the CNS. The cytologic features of all leukemic blast cells are identical regardless of the cell type, which should be identifiable in bone marrow smears. Blast cells are always isolated and are larger than small lymphocytes. They may show irregular nuclear contours with protrusions or notches and prominent nucleoli (Fig. 22.12).

Cerebral Lymphoma

Primary cerebral lymphoma is rare. The emergence of AIDS has resulted in a marked increase in incidence of primary CNS lymphomas, which are found in 5% of such cases.[9,10] Systemic lymphomas can involve the brain as lymphomatous meningitis, or less frequently, as parenchymal infiltration. Cerebral lymphomas may present as a solid mass or as a diffusely infiltrating lesion (Fig. 22.13A). The diagnosis can be established by CSF cytology or FNA (Fig. 22.13B).

Histologically, most cerebral lymphomas have a diffuse pattern of growth and are of large cell type. One of their most characteristic features is perivascular infiltration comprising concentric laminations (Fig. 22.13C).

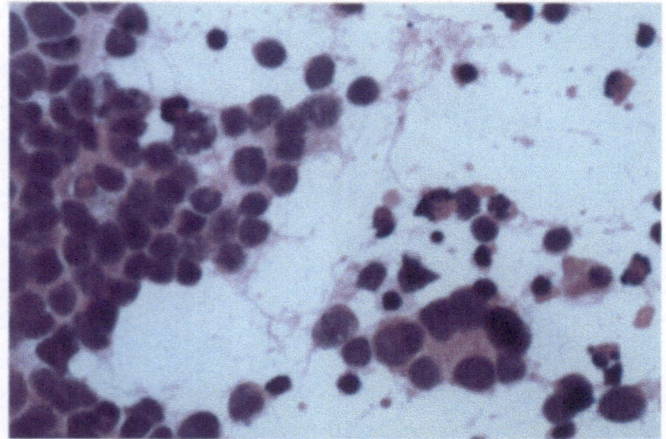

A

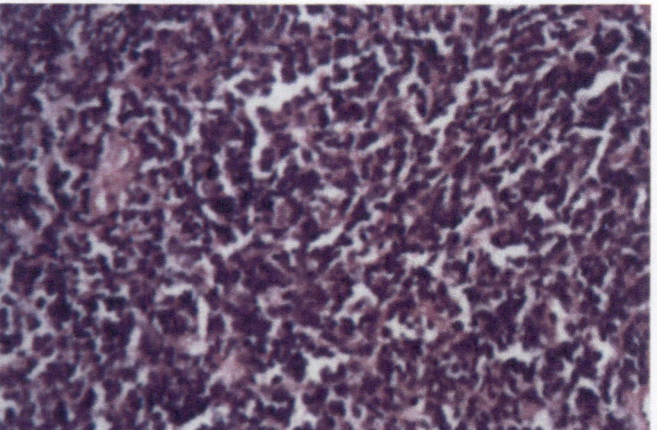

B

FIGURE 22.11 **Medulloblastoma. A**: Aspiration smear showing aggregates of small anaplastic cells with nuclear molding and rosette formation. **B**: Biopsy section showing sheets of small anaplastic cells.

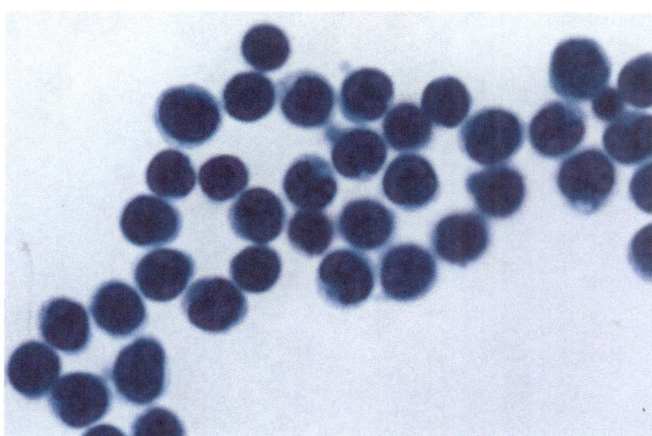

◄

FIGURE 22.12 **Acute lymphocytic leukemia in CSF.** Isolated monomorphic lymphoid cells with nuclear notches (cytocentrifuge preparation).

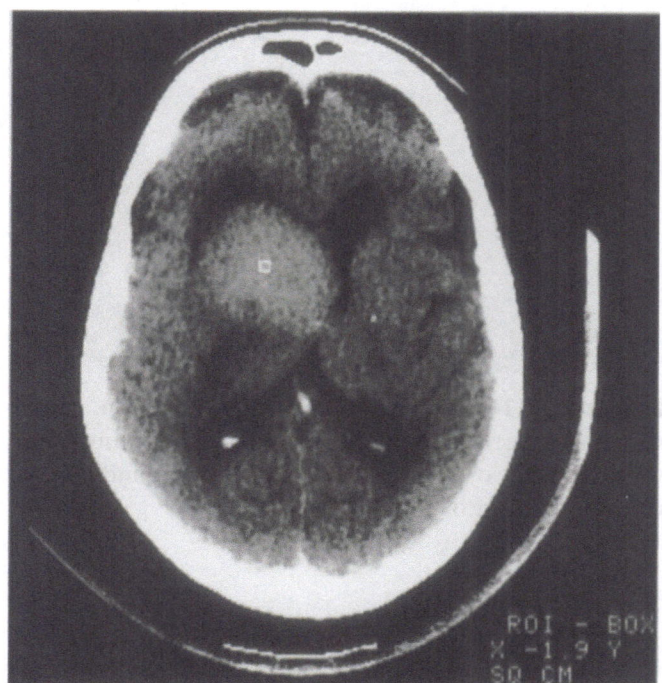

A

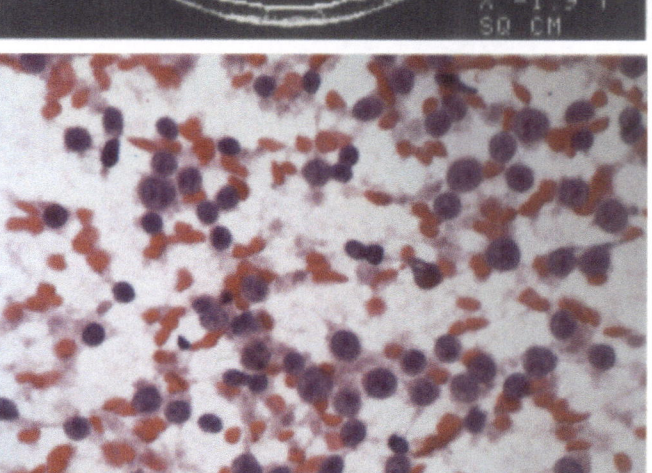

B

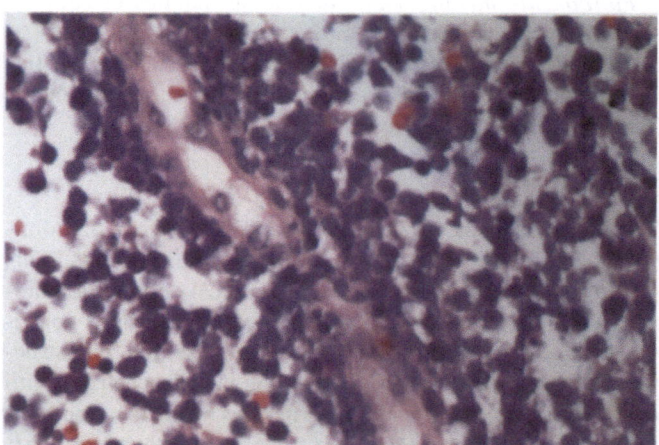

C

FIGURE 22.13 **Primary lymphoma of brain. A**: Well defined radiodense solid lesion in the right cerebral hemisphere (CT). **B**: Aspiration smear showing monomorphic large lymphoid cells occurring singly. **C**: Biopsy section showing sheets of large lymphoid cells around blood vessels.

Meningioma

Meningiomas arise from the specialized arachnoid cap cells, and most often occur in the anterior half of the cranium. They constitute about 20% of all primary intracranial tumors. Grossly, most meningiomas are solitary, irregularly shaped, bosselated solid masses adherent to the dura and indenting the brain. Most meningiomas can be treated successfully by surgical excision. Cytologically, the cells occur in rather loose sheets and aggregates. The cells have fibrillar cytoplasm with poorly defined borders. Intranuclear cytoplasmic inclusions may be observed. The nuclei are round to oval and have finely stippled chromatin (Fig. 22.14A). Histologically, there are three main histologic patterns.

Syncytial meningioma. Cellular whorls and nodules are characteristic features. Nuclei are round to oval, and may have intranuclear cytoplasmic inclusions.

Fibroblastic meningioma. Interlacing bundles of spindle-shaped bipolar cells.

Transitional meningioma. These tumors have characteristics intermediate between syncytial and fibroblastic meningiomas. Psammoma bodies are frequently found (Fig. 22.14B).

Midline Tumors

Tumors located in the midline of the brain occur predominantly in the area of the pineal and pituitary glands. This group includes pituitary adenoma, pineal tumors, craniopharyngiomas, ependymomas, and cysts of the third ventricle. Symptoms common to most of them are due to obstruction of the ventricular system, resulting in hydrocephalus with compression of vital midline structures. The location of a tumor is more critical than its cytologic or histologic grade.[11]

Pituitary Adenoma

Computed tomography can delineate a mass in the sella turcica (Fig. 22.15A). In aspirates or imprints the cells occur in cohesive sheets. They are round to polygonal and have well defined eosinophilic to basophilic cytoplasm. The nuclei are uniformly round with evenly dispersed stippled chromatin (Fig. 22.15B). In chromophobe adenoma, the cells tend to have scanty cytoplasm and round nuclei. Histologically, the tumor cells are arranged in sheets, cords, or nests having only a delicate vascular stroma (Fig. 22.15C). Immunocytochemistry, using antibodies to pitsuitancy hormones and electron microscopy, may help establish the diagnosis.

Craniopharyngioma (Rathke's Pouch Tumor)

Craniopharyngioma, a suprasellar tumor, may compress the pituitary (Fig. 22.16). The tumor is usually cystic. In direct aspiration of the cyst, the smears contain benign squamous epithelial cells and basaloid epithelial cells.

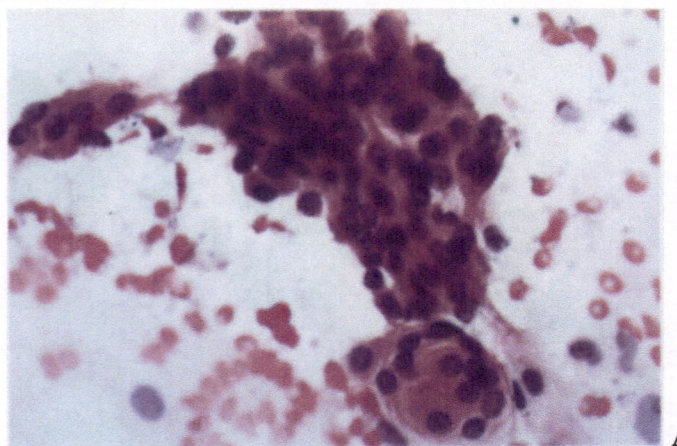
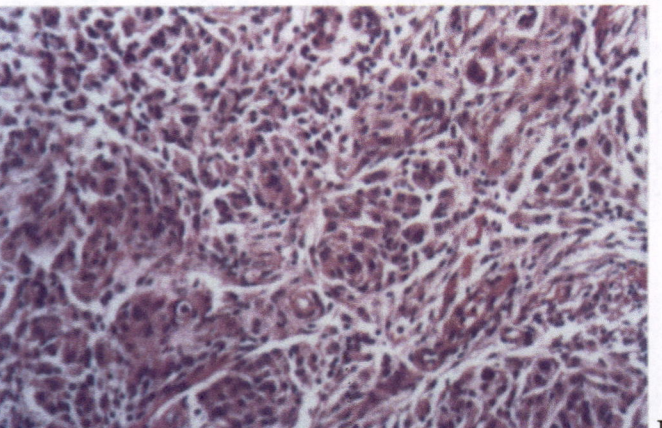

FIGURE 22.14 **Meningioma.** **A**: Aspiration smear showing whorls and loose aggregates of tumor cells with fibrillar cytoplasm. **B**: Interlacing bundles and whorled pattern of cells.

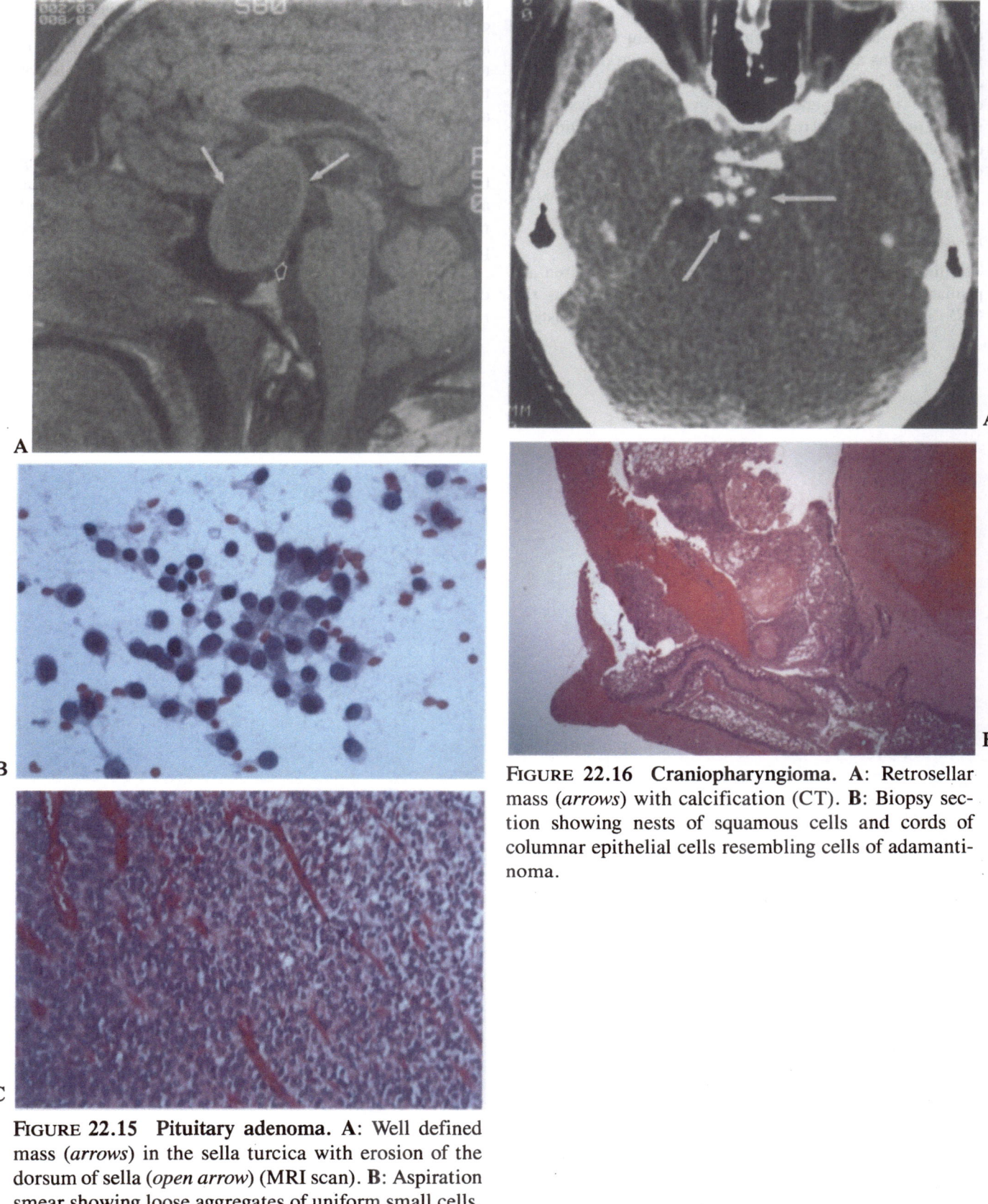

FIGURE 22.16   Craniopharyngioma. A: Retrosellar mass (*arrows*) with calcification (CT). B: Biopsy section showing nests of squamous cells and cords of columnar epithelial cells resembling cells of adamantinoma.

FIGURE 22.15   Pituitary adenoma. A: Well defined mass (*arrows*) in the sella turcica with erosion of the dorsum of sella (*open arrow*) (MRI scan). B: Aspiration smear showing loose aggregates of uniform small cells. C: Biopsy section showing sheets of uniform small cells and prominent vascular stroma.

Tumors of Pineal Gland

Germinoma is the most common neoplasm in the pineal gland. Glioma and pineoblastoma can occur in this site.[12] In aspirates or in CSF, the cells occur in loose aggregates and clusters. They are round to oval with scanty cytoplasm. The nuclei are large, round to oval, and hyperchromatic. Often the cells of germinomas resemble those of undifferentiated large cell carcinoma (Fig. 22.17).

Pineal germinomas may undergo extracranial metastasis.[13]

Metastatic Tumors

The most common neoplasms of the CNS in children are primary neoplasms, but up to 30% of the neoplasms of the CNS in adults are metastatic. The diagnosis of metastatic tumors of the CNS is one of the most rewarding applications of the FNA. Clinical data and CT or MRI may be of great assistance in interpreting the aspirates. Metastatic deposits tend to be multiple (Fig. 22.18). The cytologic features of metastatic carcinomas are usually similar to those observed at other anatomic sites, and are distinct from those of primary neoplasm of the CNS with rare exceptions.

Immunocytochemistry is of great help in distinguishing between anaplastic gliomas and carcinomas. Most gliomas are positive for glial fibrillary acidic protein (GFAP) and negative for cytokeratin. In contrast, most carcinomas are positive for cytokeratin and negative for GFAP.

The three most common primary sites of metastatic carcinomas in the CNS are lung, breast, and gastrointestinal tract.

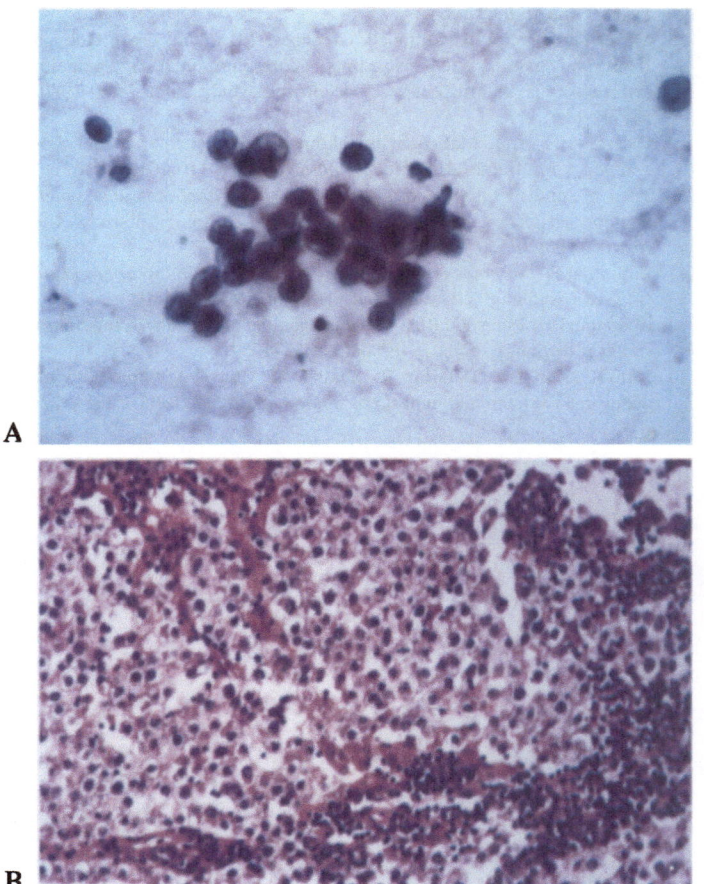

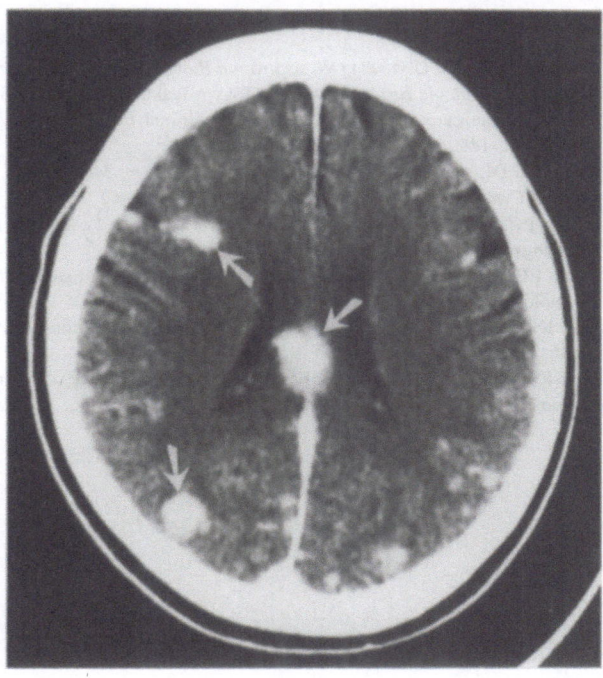

FIGURE 22.18   **Metastatic carcinoma in brain.** A contrast enhancement CT scan of the brain showing multiple nodular masses (*arrows*).

FIGURE 22.17   **Pineal germinoma. A**: Aspiration smear showing loose aggregate of tumor cells with large nuclei. **B**: Biopsy section showing sheets of large cells and intervening stroma with lymphocytic infiltration.

References

1. Koss LG, Woyke S, Olszewski W. *Aspiration Biopsy, Cytologic Interpretation and Histologic Bases*. New York/Tokyo: Igaku-Shoin; 1984;458.
2. Naylor B. The cytologic diagnosis of cerebrospinal fluid. *Acta Cytol*. 1964;8:141–149.
3. Rosenthal DL. *Cytology of the Central Nervous System. Monographs in Clinical Cytology 8*. GL Wied, (ed.). Karger, 1984;51–62.
4. Burger PC, Vogel FS. *Surgical Pathology of the Nervous System and its Coverings*. 2nd ed. New York: Wiley Medical; 1982.
5. Ilgren EB, et al. Ependymomas: A clinical and pathological study. Part 1 - Biologic features. *Clin Neuropathol*. 1984;3:113.
6. Kim K, Greenblatt S, Robinson M. Choroid plexus carcinoma. *Acta Cytol*. 1985;29:846–849.
7. Wolf RW, Masse SR, Conklin R, Freireich EJ. The incidence of central nervous system leukemia in adults with acute leukemia. *Cancer*. 1974; 33:863–869.
8. Meyer RJ, Ferreira PP, Cuttner J, Greenberg ML, Goldberg J, Holland JF. Central nervous system involvement at presentation in acute granulocytic leukemia. A prospective cytocentrifuge study. *Am J Med*. 1980; 68:691–694.
9. DiCarlo EF, et al. Malignant lymphomas and the acquired immunodeficiency syndrome. *Arch Pathol Lab Med*. 1986;110:1012–1016.
10. Yuen TS, et al. Primary central nervous system lymphoma in acquired immune deficiency syndrome: A clinical and pathological study. *Ann Neurol* 1986;20:566.
11. Rosenthal DL. *Cytology of the Central Nervous System. Monographs in Clinical Cytology 8*. GL Wied, (ed.). Karger, 1984;93–100.
12. Chapman PH, Linggood RM. The management of pineal area tumors: A recent re-appraisal. *Cancer*. 1980;46:1253–1257.
13. Kim K, Koo BC, Delaflor R, Shaikh BS. Pineal germinoma with widespread extracranial metastases. *Diag Cytopathol*. 1985;1:118–122.

23
Bone and Soft Tissue

Bone Tumors

This chapter focuses on bone lesions that clinically and radiologically are suspicious of being neoplasm and that require biopsy for diagnosis. The pathologic diagnosis of bone lesions, either by open biopsy or fine needle aspiration (FNA), requires a thorough knowledge of clinical and radiological data. Lesions in bone suitable for diagnosis by FNA are metastatic neoplasms, which are common. Primary tumors of bone are comparatively rare, although in some circumstances FNA may provide the diagnosis, an advantage in terms of cost effectiveness and optimal management.

Techniques

The traditional diagnostic approach to bone lesions is open biopsy or needle biopsy using an 18-gauge needle under fluoroscopic guidance. Fine needle aspiration of bone lesions is performed under local or general anesthesia, which enables the use of a thicker guide needle with stylet. When the guide needle is in the target the stylet is withdrawn and the fine needle is introduced into the target through the guide. Aspiration is then performed as in other organs.

Primary Bone Tumors

The discussion will be limited to the neoplasms in which cytology may be of diagnostic help.

Osteosarcoma

Osteosarcoma is the most common primary malignant neoplasm of bone, usually occurring in patients between 10 and 25 years of age. Most osteosarcomas involve the metaphysis of long bones (Fig. 23.1A, B). The neoplasm may be bony hard or soft and friable, depending on the proportions of bone, cartilage, and cellular stroma.

Histology. The typical osteosarcoma comprises a malignant spindle cell stroma accompanied by anastomosing bands of osteoid, with or without bone formation (Fig. 23.1C). Usually the tumors arise in the medullary cavity and may extend into the cortex, periosteum, and the neighboring soft tissue. The tumors usually abut on the epiphyseal plate, but rarely perforate it.

Cytology. The cells of osteosarcoma vary in shape and size. Aspirates contain spindle-shaped or polygonal cells that are isolated or arranged in loose aggregates. Their hyperchromatic nuclei show all the features of malignancy (Fig. 23.1D). Osteoid may not be identified in aspirates. The diagnosis is based on the presence of malignant stromal cells, supported by clinical and radiological data.

Chondrosarcoma

Most patients with chondrosarcoma are between 30 and 60 years of age. Chondrosarcoma differs from osteosarcoma by its lack of osteoid and bone formation by the tumor cells. Chondrosarcomas arise from the medullary cavity of the shafts of long bones and from pelvic bones, shoulder girdle bones, and temporal bone.

Radiologically, they present as osteolytic lesions with peripheral speckles of calcification (Fig. 23.2A). The 5-year survival rates for chondrosarcomas of low, moderate, and high grade, based on the degree of anaplasia, are 78%, 53%, and 22%, respectively.[1] Wide block excision is strongly recommended as treatment. Grossly, the tumors are lobular and glistening on section (Fig. 23.2B).

Histology. Chondrosarcomas comprise chondroblasts, with their multiple plump hyperchromatic nuclei, in a cartilaginous matrix. The essential diagnostic feature is the presence of atypical chondroblasts within lacunae. Bizarre tumor giant cells also may be present (Fig. 23.1C).

Cytology. The diagnostic cells are large multinucleated cells occurring singly and in small aggregates. They have abundant cyanophilic cytoplasm and plump round to oval nuclei with prominent nucleoli (Fig. 23.2D).

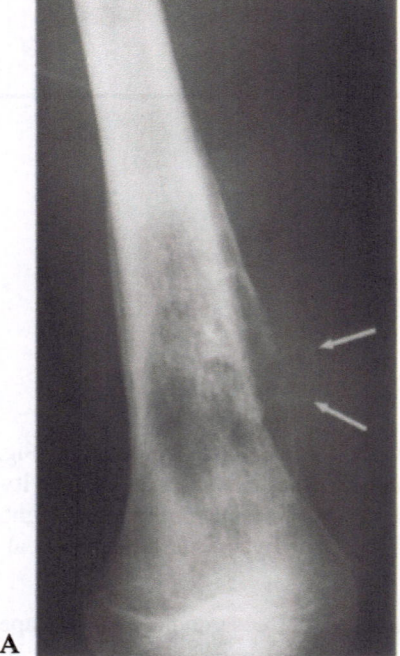

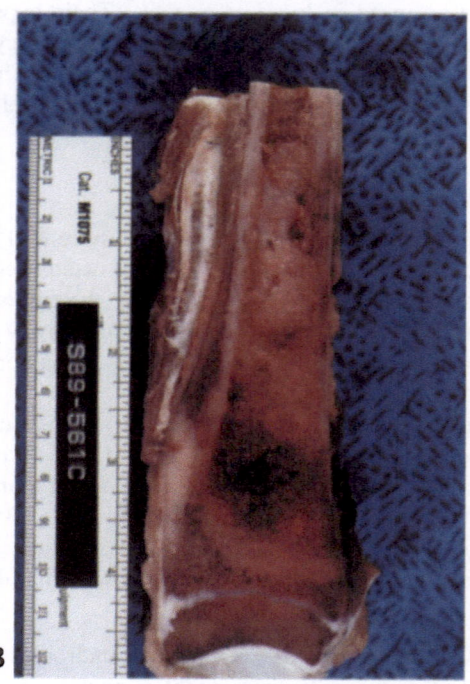

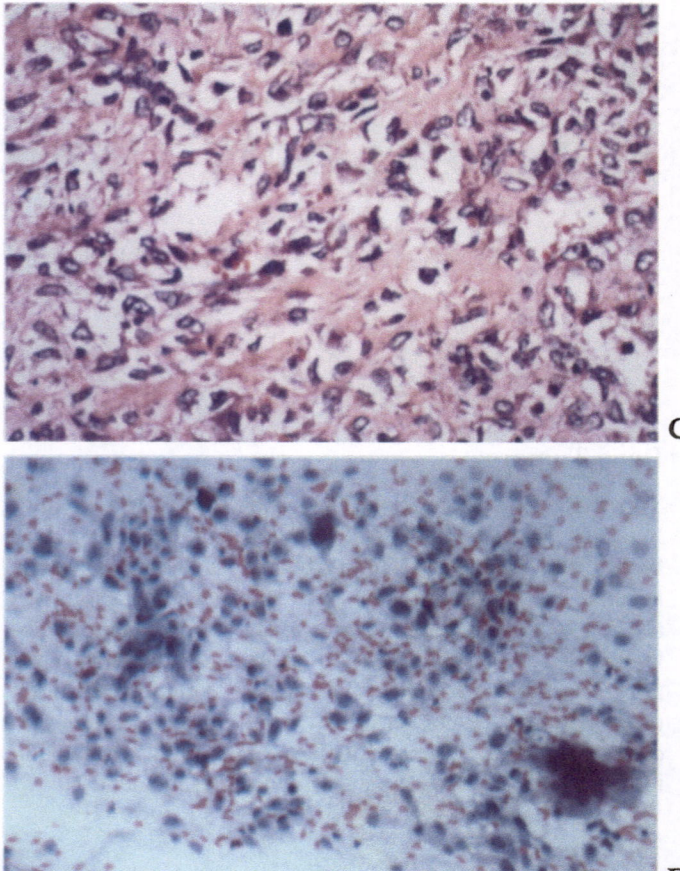

FIGURE 23.1   Osteosarcoma of distal tibia. A: Radiolucent lesion in the distal femur, with cortical destruction and spiculated periosteal reaction (plain radiograph). **B**: Amputated tibia showing the tumor extending to the proximal shaft, eroding the overlying cortex, and abutting on the epiphyseal plate. **C**: Histologic section showing spindle-shaped and pleomorphic mesenchymal cells and islands of osteoid. **D**: FNA smear showing pleomorphic cells in aggregates and singly and cyanophilic osteoid.

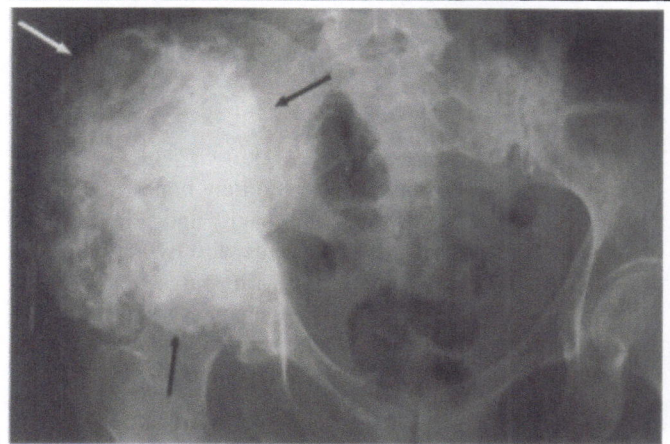

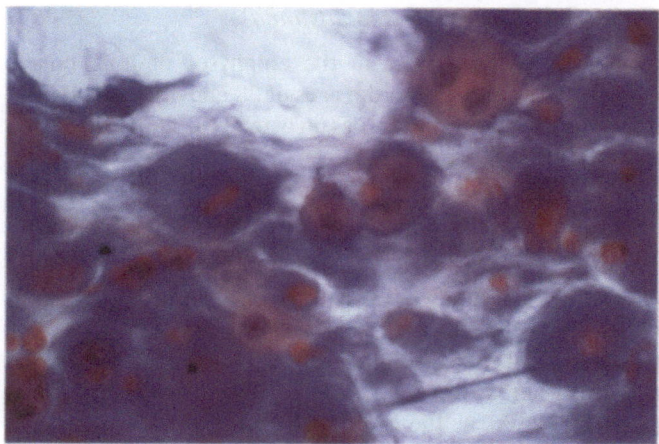

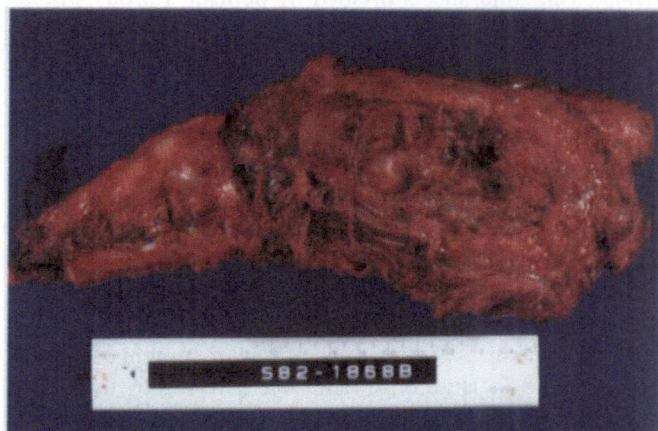

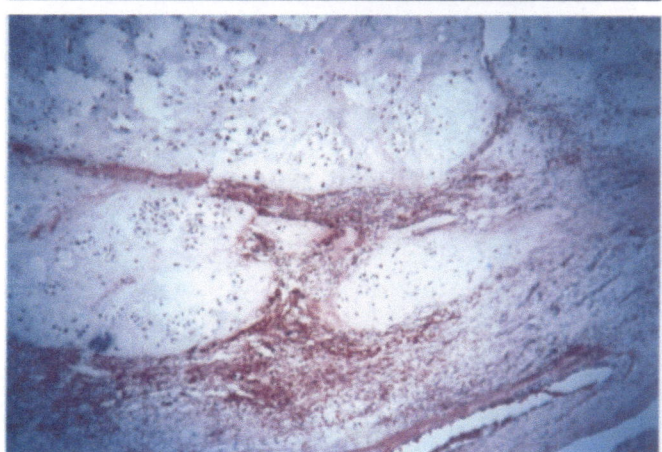

FIGURE 23.2   Chondrosarcoma. A: Radiograph of the pelvis showing a lobular destructive lesion with peripheral mottled calcification in the left ilium. B: Chondrosarcoma of rib showing a lobular mass with multifocal necrosis and glistening cartilaginous tissue. C: Histologic section showing chondroblasts with multinucleated lacunar cells. D: FNA smear showing multinucleated chondroblasts with cyanophilic cytoplasm.

Giant Cell Tumors (Osteoclastoma)

Giant cell tumors occur in the epiphyses of long bones. Almost all occur between the ages of 20 and 40 years. Radiologically, the tumor presents as an osteolytic, expansile lesion in an epiphysis (Fig. 23.3A).

Grossly, the tumors are solid, expansile, multilobular, and light brown on their cut surface. The overlying cortex is thin, without any periosteal new bone formation (Fig. 23.3B)

Histology. The tumors consist of regularly distributed multinucleated osteoclast-type giant cells and stromal cells. The tumor stromal cells are spindle shaped and have a single oval nucleus, whereas the giant cells may have 30 or more nuclei per cell. However, the basic tumor element is the stromal cells (Fig. 23.3C).

Cytology. Aspiration smears of giant cell tumors of bone consist of giant cells with multiple small round nuclei and small spindle-shaped tumor stromal cells occurring singly and in loose aggregates. Except for the occasional obviously sarcomatous lesion, microscopic evaluation as a predictor of biologic behavior is of little practical value. On the basis of 30% to 50% of giant cell tumors developing local recurrence and 5% to 10% distant metastasis after curettage, all giant cell tumors should be regarded as potentially malignant.[2-4]

Differential Diagnosis. Lesions simulating giant cell tumors are non-ossifying fibroma, chondromyxoid fibroma, chondroblastoma, solitary bone cyst, aneurysmal bone cyst, and osteoblastoma. Differential diagnosis should be based on radiological and clinical data and, in true giant cell tumors of bone, the salient microscopic feature of a regular distribution of giant cells and stromal cells.

Ewing's Sarcoma

Ewing's sarcoma occurs most often in long bones in children and adults. It arises in the medullary cavity and extends to the cortex and overlying soft tissue. Patients with Ewing's sarcoma present with bone pain and fever with leukocytosis, which simulate osteomyelitis. Radiographic changes are widening of the medullary cavity, cortical thickening, and a periosteal reaction imparting an onion skin appearance (Fig. 23.4A).

Histology. Ewing's sarcoma comprises uniform small cells arranged in solid sheets divided by delicate fibrous strands (Fig. 23.4B).

Cytology. The cells have scanty cytoplasm and round nuclei and occur singly (Fig. 23.4C). The periodic acid-Schiff (PAS) stain reveals cytoplasmic granules of glycogen, which distinguishes Ewing's sarcoma from lymphoma and metastatic neuroblastoma. Furthermore, cells of lymphomas and lymphoid tissue exhibit a positive reaction to leukocyte common antigen, and neuroblastoma cells exhibit a positive reaction to neuron-specific enolase and chromogranin. Ewing's sarcoma tends to spread widely and aggressively.

The 5-year survival after conventional treatment used to be only 5% to 8%. High dose radiation followed by multidrug chemotherapy has improved the 5-year disease-free survival to 25%.[5,6]

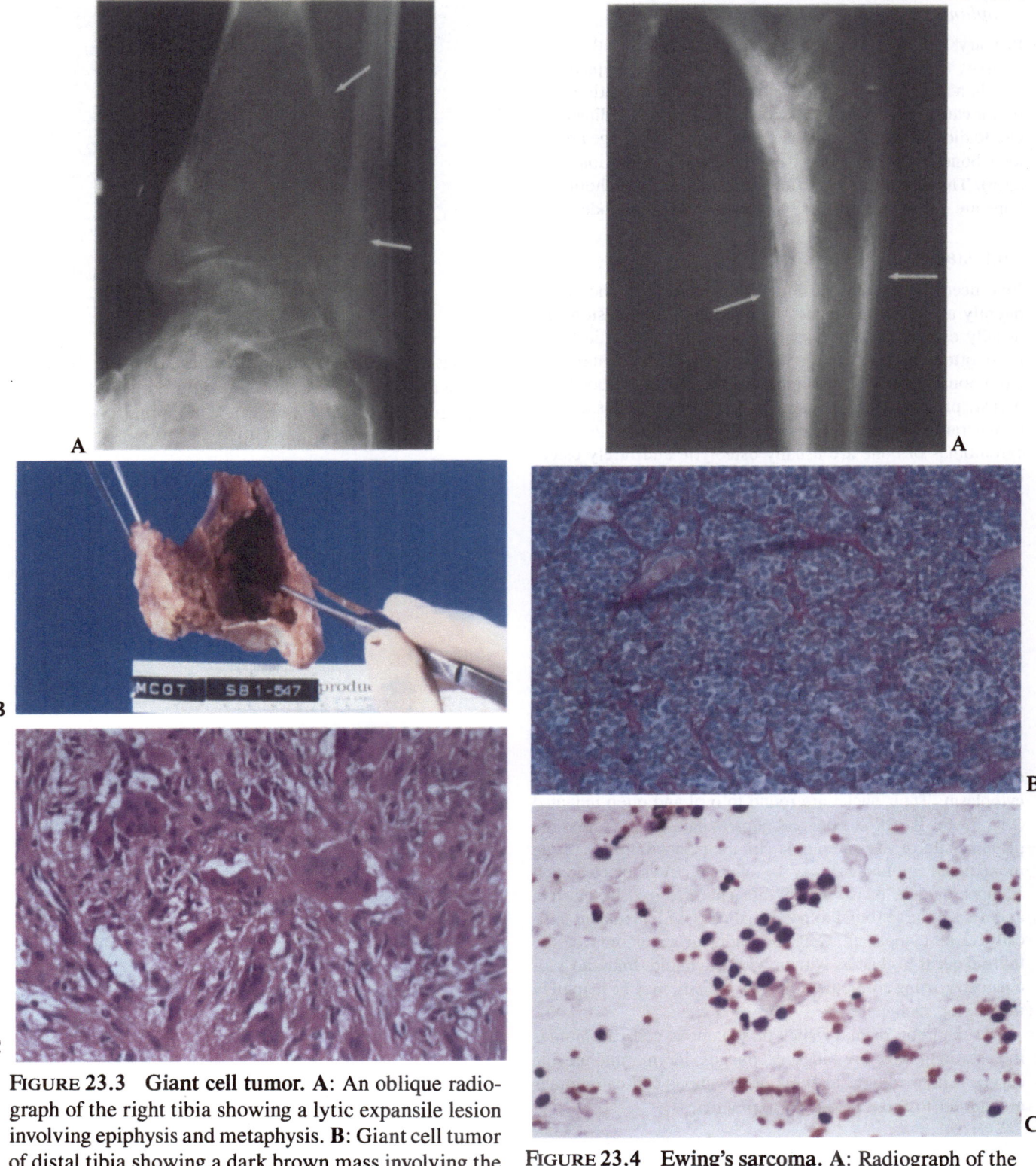

FIGURE 23.3   Giant cell tumor. A: An oblique radiograph of the right tibia showing a lytic expansile lesion involving epiphysis and metaphysis. B: Giant cell tumor of distal tibia showing a dark brown mass involving the epiphysis. C: Histologic section showing osteoclastlike giant cells intermixed with spindle-shaped stromal cells.

FIGURE 23.4   Ewing's sarcoma. A: Radiograph of the femur shaft showing an "onion-skin" periosteal reaction (*arrows*). B: Histologic section showing uniform small cells arranged in solid sheets separated by delicate fibrous stroma, with PAS-positive glycogen granules in the cytoplasm (PAS stain). C: Aspirate smear showing neoplastic cells with scanty cytoplasm and round nuclei occurring singly.

Lymphoma

Primary lymphoma of bone occurs in children and adults. Grossly, this tumor involves the metaphysis and diaphysis of long bones, producing medullary and cortical destruction. The tumor can extend into extraosseous soft tissues including muscle. Radiologically, lymphoma of bone involves a large area of long bone, with destruction and new bone formation (Fig. 23.5). The histologic and cytologic features of lymphomas of bone are similar to those of lymphomas of lymph nodes.

Metastatic Bone Tumors

Fine needle aspiration of tumors metastatic to bone is frequently a rewarding diagnostic procedure. Such lesions are usually carcinomas and usually widely distributed in bone, most often in vertebrae, pelvic bones, ribs, and humerus. Common sources of carcinomas metastatic to bone are breast, prostate, lung, kidney, and thyroid. Soft tissue sarcomas rarely metastasize to bone. Radiologically, metastatic carcinomas of bone are usually osteolytic and rarely osteoblastic except for prostate carcinoma. Aspirates of osteolytic lesions usually contain abundant neoplastic cells, whereas those of osteoblastic lesions usually contain far fewer.

Carcinoma is the most common type of cancer metastatic to bone and can usually be identified as such. However, it may be difficult to determine if a lesion is metastatic from a previously existing carcinoma or whether it originated from a second primary tumor. Immunocytochemistry may be of help in resolving this problem.

Adenocarcinoma is the most common neoplasm metastatic to bone, with the most common primary sites being the prostate and lung in men and the breast in women. The aspirated cells occur in clusters or in loose acinar form. They are round, columnar, or pleomorphic and have granular or vacuolated cytoplasm. Their nuclei are round to oval and often indented (Fig. 23.6). If radiological and clinical data do not reveal the primary site of the carcinoma, immunocytochemistry, using monoclonal antibodies, may be of help. Cells of clear cell adenocarcinoma of the kidney are characterized by clusters and nests of large round to polygonal cells with abundant optically clear cytoplasm. Cells of follicular carcinoma of the thyroid occur in clusters with or without colloid. Immunocytochemistry, using antibodies to thyroglobulin, may be helpful in identifying such cells.

The common primary sites of squamous cell carcinomas metastatic to bone are lungs, esophagus, larynx, and uterine cervix. The cytologic features of squamous cell carcinomas are similar to those of the primary sites.

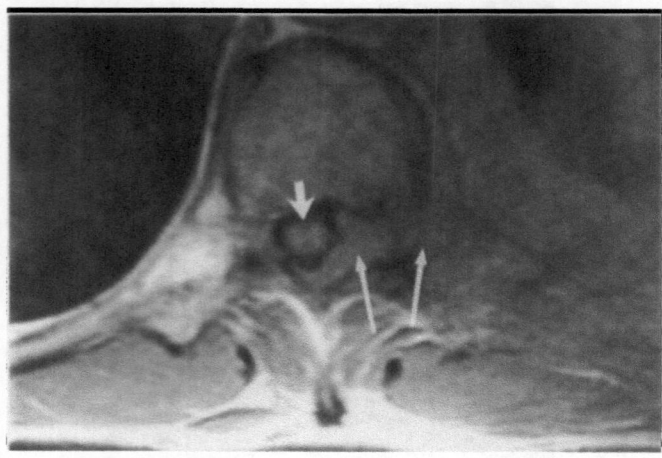

FIGURE 23.5 **Lymphoma of bone.** An axial thoracic MRI scan (SE500-20) showing lymphoma infiltrating the spinal canal (*long arrows*). The spinal cord (*short arrow*) is deviated to the right.

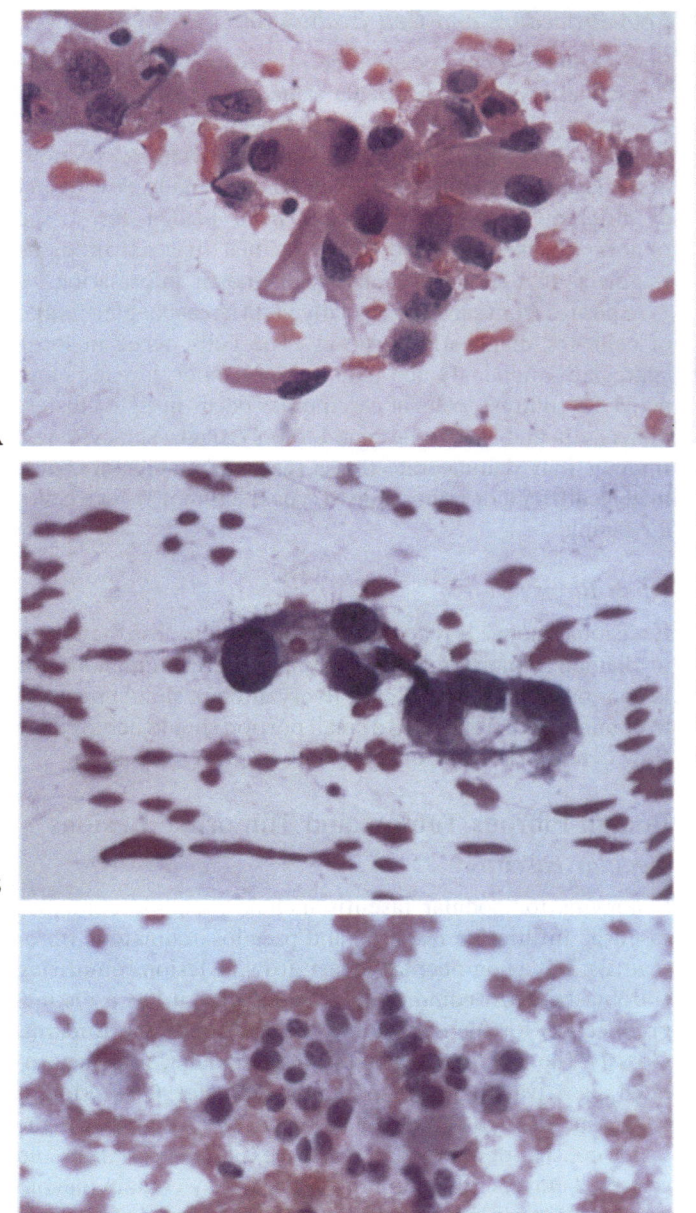

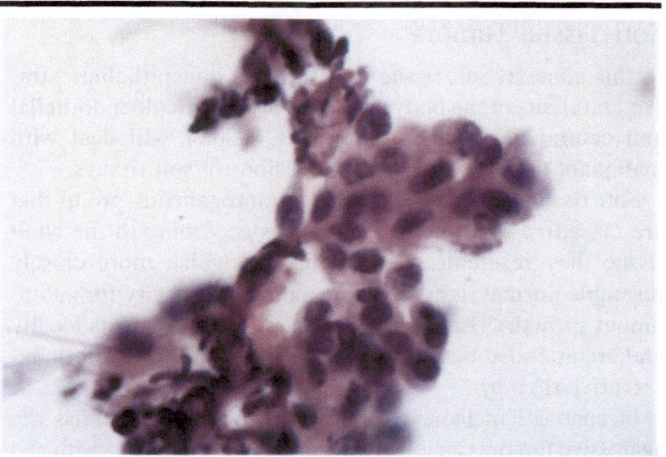

A

B

C

D

FIGURE 23.6   Metastatic carcinoma of bone. A: Cluster of adenocarcinoma cells with a columnar configuration (prostatic primary). **B**: Neoplastic cells occurring in loose aggregates and in tandem (breast primary). **C**: Metastatic clear cell adenocarcinoma in bone. Neoplastic cells, arranged in an acinar pattern, with optically clear cytoplasm (renal primary). **D**: Metastatic squamous cell carcinoma in bone. Syncytial aggregates of pleomorphic cells (lung primary).

Soft Tissue Tumors

In this context, soft tissue is defined as nonepithelial extraskeletal tissue of the body exclusive of the reticuloendothelial and central nervous systems. This chapter will deal with malignant tumors and tumorlike lesions of soft tissues.

Soft tissue tumors are a highly heterogeneous group that are classified on a histogenetic basis according to the adult tissue they resemble. Benign tumors, which more closely resemble normal tissue, possess a limited capacity for autonomous growth. They exhibit little tendency to invade locally and are attended by a low rate of local recurrence after conservative therapy.

In contrast, malignant soft tissue tumors or sarcomas are aggressive tumors capable of invasive or destructive growth and metastasis. To ensure total removal they require radical surgery.

Recent classifications of soft tissue tumors have been based principally on the line of differentiation of the tumor, that is, the type of tissue formed by the tumor rather than the type of tissue from which the tumor arose.

Grading of sarcomas is determined by a combined assessment of several histological features: 1) degree of cellularity, 2) cellular pleomorphism or anaplasia, 3) mitotic activity, 4) degree of necrosis, and 5) expansive, or infiltrative growth. Of these, the number of mitotic figures and the extent of necrosis are the two most important features.

Fine needle aspiration cytology can demonstrate the nature of soft tissue tumors in terms of whether they are benign or malignant and, in some cases, type of the tumor. Sometimes it is difficult to identify the true nature of these primary tumors by FNA cytology or even by ample open biopsy specimens. As with carcinomas, FNA cytology has a particularly useful role in identifying metastatic carcinomas or sarcomas.

Immunohistochemistry and electron microscopy are useful in classifying sarcomas; cytogenetics has little application, being impractical and expensive. For prognosis and therapeutic evaluation of sarcomas, the two most important features are grading and staging.

Clinical Features and Natural History

Soft tissue sarcomas can arise anywhere in the body and present as a soft tissue mass. Visceral sarcomas are discussed in each organ system. The four common anatomic sites of development of soft tissue sarcomas are the lower limbs (40%), trunk and retroperitoneum (30%), the upper limb (20%), and head and neck (10%). The relationship of a tumor to adjacent vital structures is all important in determining its resectability and can be assessed by various radiographic techniques, such as computed tomography (CT), magnetic resonance imaging (MRI), and arteriography. Size is also a significant prognostic factor in terms of resectability as well as the probability of developing distant metastasis. The overall survival rate of persons with soft tissue sarcomas is about 50%.[7]

FNA Procedure and Cell Evaluation

Fine needle aspiration can be performed readily on palpable superficial lesions. Fine needle aspiration of deeply situated lesions requires radiographic guidance. As much cellular material as possible should be obtained from multiple portions of the lesion by moving the needle forward and backward and in different directions. Aspirates from benign soft tissue tumors are likely to yield scanty cellular material or tissue fragments that do not provide any diagnostic information.

Aspirates from sarcomas usually yield a reasonable number of cells for diagnostic purposes. The cells occur in loose aggregates and singly and tend to be pleomorphic and elongated. In contrast, cells of carcinomas occur in tight clusters or syncytia and tend to be round to polygonal. The cytologic findings may demonstrate that a tumor is malignant, but it may be difficult or impossible to type the tumor from a cellular sample.

Open Biopsy

Excisional biopsy is recommended for lesions less than 3 cm in diameter. Incisional wedge biopsy is recommended for lesions over 3 cm in diameter. Every attempt should be made to obtain viable tissue, and a small portion should be saved for flow cytometric DNA analysis and electron microscopy.

Benign Fibrous Tumors and Tumorlike Lesions

Nodular Fasciitis

Synonyms for nodular fasciitis include pseudosarcomatous fasciitis, infiltrative fasciitis, and pseudosarcomatous fibromatosis. It is a non-neoplastic fast-growing lesion comprising fibroblasts. Most common in young adults, it has a distinct predilection for the trunk and volar surface of the forearm. Grossly, the lesion is a round to oval, nodular, nonencapsulated mass, usually less than 3 cm in diameter. On section, it is firm or may be soft and gelatinous. Microscopically, the lesion consists of interlacing bundles of plump fibroblasts and scattered chronic inflammatory cells. It may contain mucoid or myxoid material and mitotic figures.

Fibromatosis

Fibromatosis refers to a group of benign fibrous tissue proliferations and is divided into superficial and deep fibromatoses. Superficial fibromatoses, slowly growing and of small size, involve the palmar and plantar areas and the penis (Peyronie's disease). Deep fibromatoses are rapidly growing, of large size, and more aggressive. They occur in extraabdominal regions (extraabdominal desmoid), and in the pelvic and mesenteric abdominal spaces (intraabdominal desmoid), and in the abdominal wall (abdominal desmoid).

Grossly, superficial fibromatoses are small, firm nodules. Extraabdominal fibromatosis occurs in deeply seated muscles and aponeuroses, with a peak incidence between ages 25 and 35 years. They affect men and women with equal frequency. Abdominal fibromatosis (desmoid) arises from musculoaponeurotic structures of the abdominal wall and occurs in young women who are pregnant or within the first year postpartum.

Intraabdominal pelvic fibromatosis arises from the iliac fossa and may infiltrate the pelvic organs. It occurs in young women and is unrelated to pregnancy.

Microscopically, both superficial and deep fibromatoses are similar, consisting of interlacing bundles of fibroblasts with varying degree of collagenization. Chronic inflammatory cells or mitotic figures are usually not observed (Fig. 23.7).

Benign Fibrous Histiocytoma

Fibrous histiocytomas are benign tumors comprising a mixture of fibroblastic and histiocytic cells arranged in a storiform pattern. They occur most often in the dermis, where they may be referred to as dermatofibroma, sclerosing hemangioma, and cutaneous fibrous histiocytoma. Grossly, they are dome-shaped or elevated lesions, a few millimeters to a few centimeters in diameter.

Microscopically, cutaneous fibrous histiocytomas are well circumscribed, involving the dermis or subcutis, and consist of short, intersecting fascicles of fibroblastic cells with occasional "histiocytic" cells (refer to Chapter 2).

Deeply situated fibrous histiocytomas are less common and tend to be larger than cutaneous fibrous histiocytomas. They present as painless masses on a limb. Grossly, they are circumscribed, yellow or white masses.

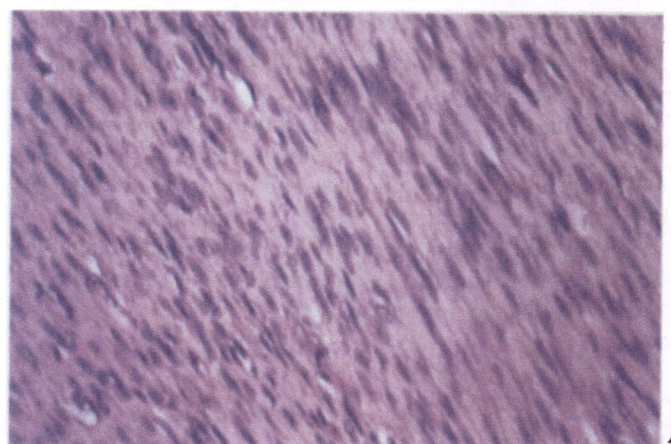

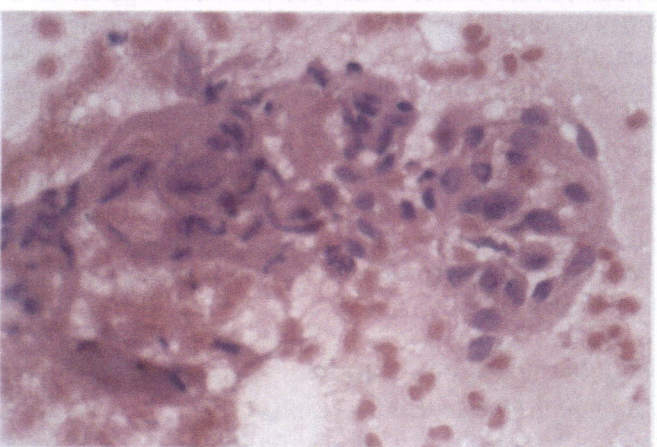

FIGURE 23.7 Fibromatosis. A: Elongated fibroblasts running in parallel. **B:** FNA smear showing elongated cells in loose aggregates.

Juvenile Xanthogranuloma (Nevoxanthoendothelioma)

Juvenile xanthogranuloma occurs exclusively in infants and young adults as a cutaneous lesion. The common anatomic sites are head, neck, and limbs, and they measure a few millimeters to a few centimeters in diameter. Grossly, they appear as red or brown nodules. The tumors tend to regress spontaneously. Microscopically, the neoplasm consists of sheets of histiocytes with scattered giant cells, including Touton-type giant cells. The neoplasm usually extends up to the epidermis and deep dermal layer (Fig. 23.8).

Dermatofibrosarcoma Protuberans

Dermatofibrosarcoma protuberans resembles a histologically benign fibrous histiocytoma, but it is more aggressive in terms of local infiltration and local recurrence after resection. Distant metastasis rarely occurs. This neoplasm usually presents during early or mid-adult life as a nodular cutaneous mass, usually about 5 cm in diameter. Most often it involves the trunk or upper limbs. Microscopically, the neoplasm infiltrates the dermis and subcutis and consists of plump fibroblasts arranged in storiform pattern. The cells are rarely pleomorphic. Mitotic figures are occasionally observed. Xanthoma cells, myxoid elements, or inflammatory elements may be present.

Malignant Fibrous Tumors

Malignant Fibrous Histiocytoma

Malignant fibrous histiocytoma (MFH), the most common soft tissue sarcoma of late adult life, is of uncertain histogenesis. It may arise from primitive mesenchymal cells that differentiate into three different cell lines: histiocytelike cells, fibroblastlike cells, and intermediate cells.[8] It occurs classically in the deep soft tissue and rarely in bone or other organs. The tumors usually present as a painless mass of several months' duration.

In aspirates, the cells occur in loose aggregates and singly. They are extremely variable in size and shape, with histiocytelike cells, fibroblastlike cells, and giant cells (Fig. 23.9A).

Grossly, the tumors are solitary, multilobulated, fleshy masses between 5 and 10 cm in diameter (Fig. 23.9B). Microscopically, the tumors are highly variable. In its classic form, the tumor consists of plump spindle cells arranged in short fascicles in a cartwheel or storiform pattern. Pleomorphic tumor giant cells, histiocytelike tumor cells, or an angiomatoid pattern may be present (Fig. 23.9C, D).

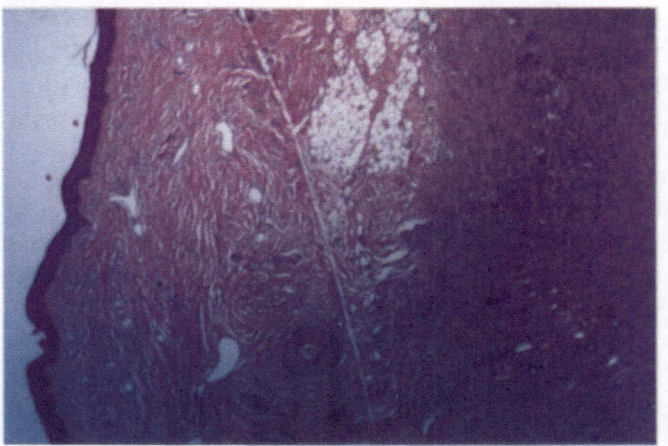

A

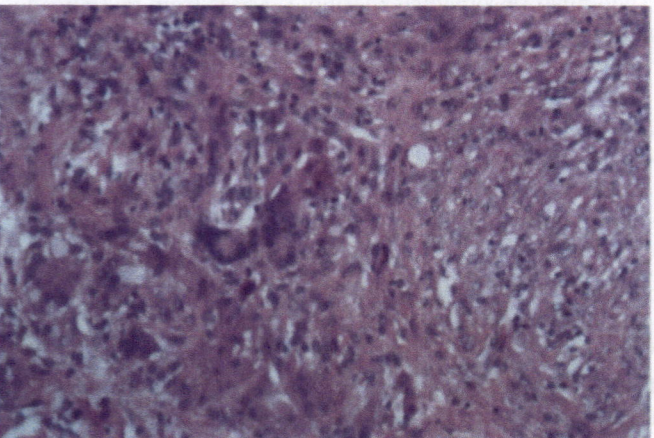

B

FIGURE 23.8   Juvenile xanthogranuloma. A: Sheets of histiocytes and giant cells in the subcutis. **B:** Higher magnification of the same lesion.

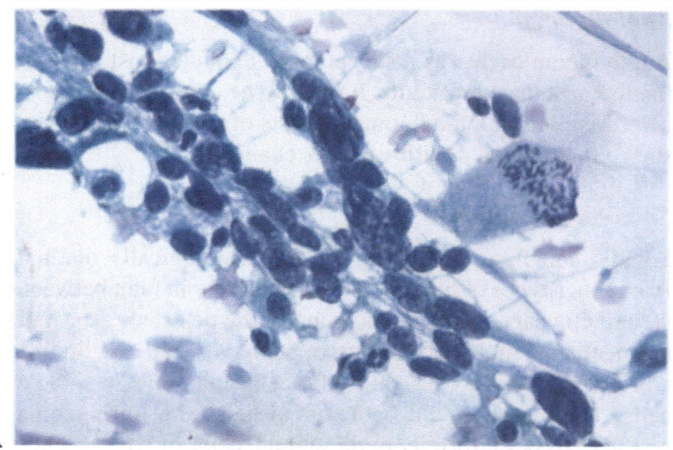

A

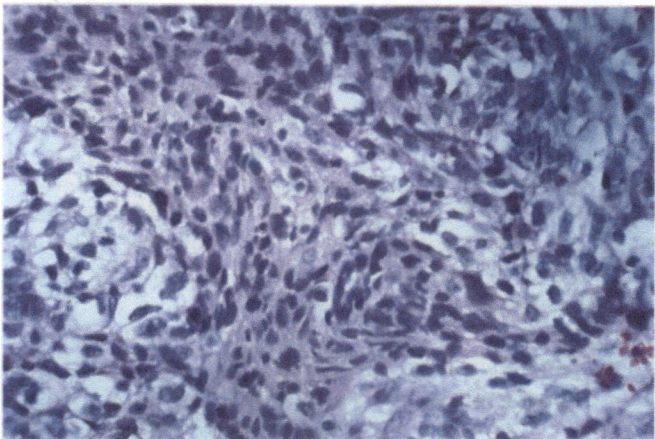

D

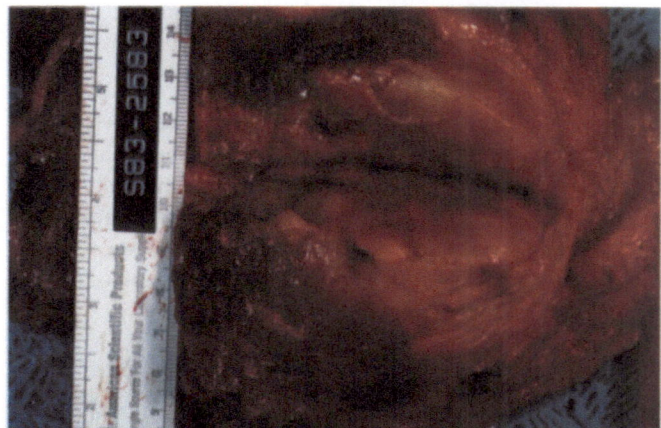

B

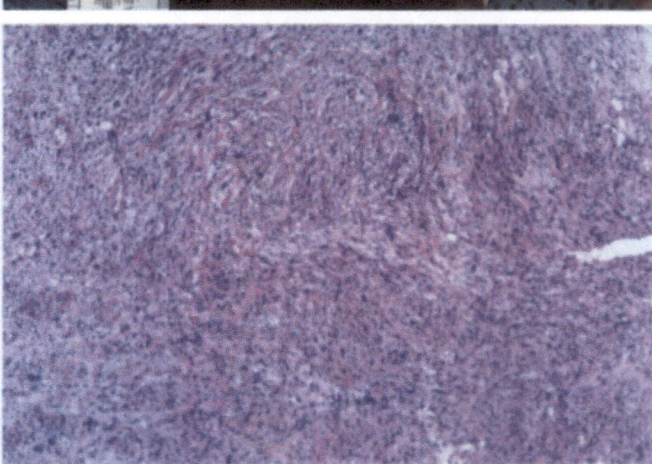

C

FIGURE 23.9 **Malignant fibrous histiocytoma. A**: Pleomorphic and elongated cells in loose aggregates (FNA). **B**: Malignant fibrous histiocytoma showing a large fleshy mass (gross). **C**: Histologic section of the tumor showing interlacing bundles of elongated and pleomorphic cells (storiform pattern). **D**: Fibroblastlike cells and histiocytelike cells in MFH.

Fibrosarcoma

Fibrosarcoma usually presents as a solitary palpable mass, 3 to 8 cm in diameter, and covered by intact skin. The most common anatomic site is a lower limb, followed by the upper limbs and trunk.

Grossly, it is a pale gray, fairly well circumscribed, firm mass. Aspirates contain elongated cells in loose aggregates and singly. The cells have scanty basophilic cytoplasm and elongated to spindle-shaped nuclei. Giant cells or bizarre cells are rarely observed (Fig. 23.10A).

Histologically, the fibrosarcoma shows a fasciculated growth pattern consisting of fusiform or spindle-shaped cells with varying amounts of collagen (Fig. 23.10B).

Benign Lipomatous Tumors

Lipoma

Lipoma is the most common tumor of mesenchymal origin. The common clinical manifestation is a slowly growing painless soft mass, most often in subcutaneous tissue of the trunk, neck, and upper thigh. Deep-seated lipomas are relatively rare, occurring in the retroperitoneum, anterior mediastinum, and paratesticular regions. Grossly, lipoma is a thinly encapsulated, lobular, doughy mass. Microscopically, lipomas consist of large, mature, adipose tissue cells arranged in a lobular pattern. They are thinly encapsulated. Malignant change in a lipoma is extremely rare.

Angiolipoma

Angiolipoma occurs as a subcutaneous nodule most often in the forearm in young adults. It tends to be tender and painful. Microscopically, angiolipoma consists of mature adipose tissue cells intermixed with vascular channels.

Spindle Cell Lipoma

Spindle cell lipoma is clinically and histologically distinct from other types of lipoma. It occurs mainly in men between 40 and 60 years of age and is found in the posterior aspect of the neck and shoulder. Microscopically, spindle cell lipoma consists of a mixture of mature fat cells and uniform spindle cells. The tumor should be distinguished from liposarcoma on the basis of uniformity of the spindle cells and the absence of lipoblasts.

Myelolipoma

Myelolipoma consists of mature fat and bone marrow elements. Myelolipomas are most common in the adrenal glands, occasionally occurring in the pelvis and mediastinum.[9-11] Most occur in persons older than 40 years. Grossly, the tumors are well circumscribed and soft, and grayish red on section. Microscopically, they comprise an irregular mixture of mature fat and bone marrow elements (Fig. 23.11).

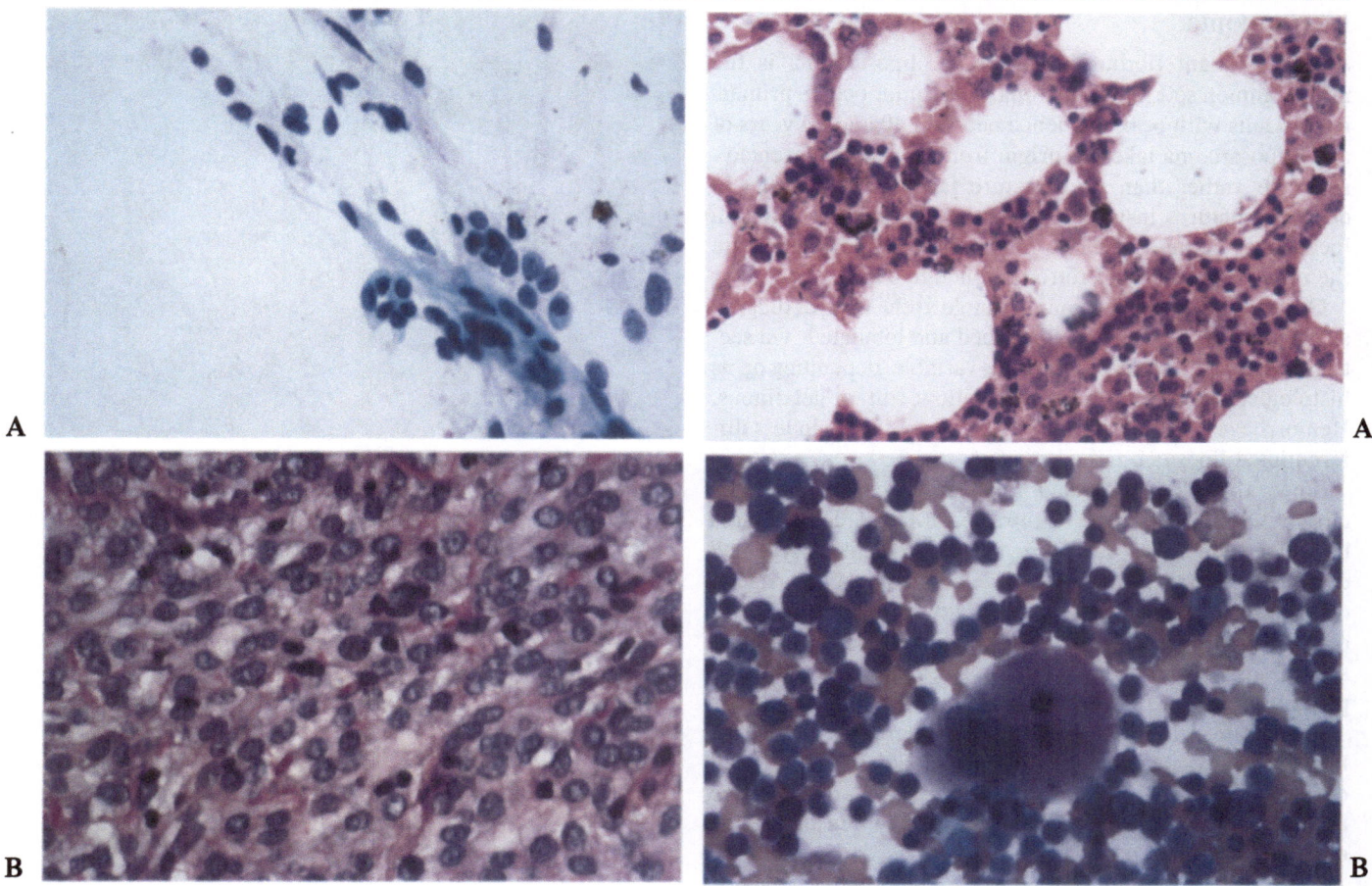

FIGURE 23.10 Fibrosarcoma. A: Cells in loose aggregates and singly (FNA). **B**: Histologic section of the same tumor showing elongated tumor cells running in parallel.

FIGURE 23.11 Myelolipoma. A: Fat cells and hematopoietic cells, reminiscent of marrow fat. **B**: FNA smear showing hematopoietic cells and megakaryocytes (Wright-Giemsa stain).

Liposarcoma

After malignant fibrous histiocytoma, liposarcoma is the most common soft tissue sarcoma. The tumor occurs primarily in adults with peak incidence between 40 and 60 years of age. Liposarcoma takes its origin from primitive mesenchymal cells rather than from mature fat cells and occurs in deeper structures instead of subcutaneous fat, the common location of lipoma. The two major sites of liposarcoma are the thigh–knee area and retroperitoneum.

Grossly, most liposarcomas are large at the time of diagnosis and tend to be well circumscribed and lobulated. On section, the appearance of the tumor is variable, depending on its histological composition. It is pale yellow, soft, or gelatinous. Hemorrhage and necrosis are frequently observed in less differentiated liposarcomas.

Since the clinical behavior of liposarcoma correlates closely with microscopic features, each liposarcoma should be widely sampled to determine the histological subtype and degree of differentiation. These are based on: 1) the stage of development of the lipoblasts, judged by the relative amounts of lipid in the cells and mucinous material in the extracellular spaces, and 2) the overall degree of cellularity and cellular pleomorphism (see Table 23.1).

In aspirates, the cells occur in loose aggregates. They are large and have abundant multivesicular cytoplasm and well defined cell borders. The nuclei are markedly variable in size and shape, depending on the types of liposarcoma and degree of differentiation.

Well Differentiated Liposarcoma

Well differentiated liposarcoma consists of mature fat cells, varying slightly in size and shape, and occasional lipoblasts with atypical hyperchromatic nuclei. Lipoblasts vary in size and shape and have cytoplasmic lipid droplets (Fig. 23.12). This subtype has the best prognosis of all types of liposarcomas.

Myxoid Liposarcoma

Myxoid liposarcoma is the most common type of liposarcoma and is less aggressive than round cell and pleomorphic liposarcomas. Grossly, the tumor is soft and gelatinous (Fig. 23.13A). Microscopically, the tumor consists of lipoblasts, delicate branching capillaries, and myxoid matrix (Fig. 23.13B).

Round Cell Liposarcoma

Round cell liposarcoma is a poorly differentiated form of myxoid liposarcoma, and is more aggressive than the usual myxoid liposarcoma. Microscopically, the tumor consists of relatively uniform round cells with vesicular nuclei and multivacuolated cytoplasm. Intercellular mucoid matrix and vascular components are less prominent (Fig. 23.14).

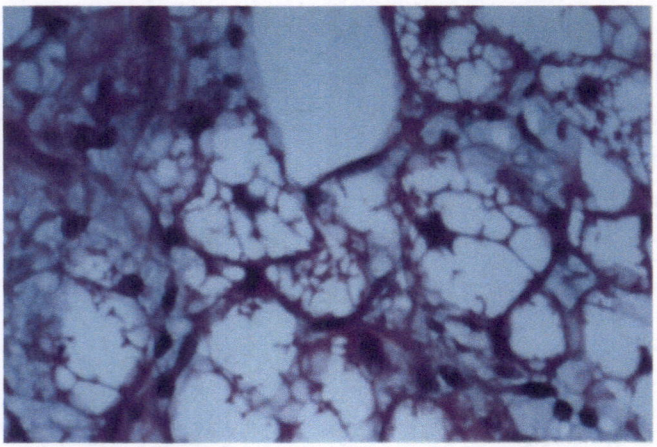

A

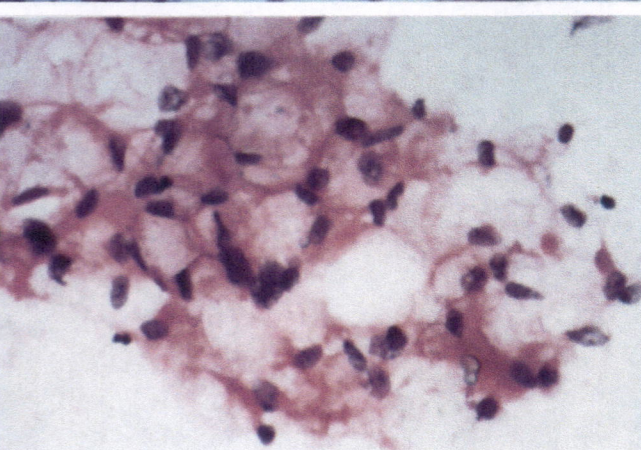

B

FIGURE 23.12 **Well differentiated liposarcoma. A:** Large fat cells with multivesicular cytoplasm and small hyperchromatic nuclei. **B:** FNA smear showing aggregates of fat cells with vesicular cytoplasm and hyperchromatic nuclei.

Table 23.1. The classification proposed by the Armed Forces Institute of Pathology.

1. Well differentiated liposarcoma
2. Myxoid liposarcoma
3. Round cell liposarcoma
4. Pleomorphic liposarcoma

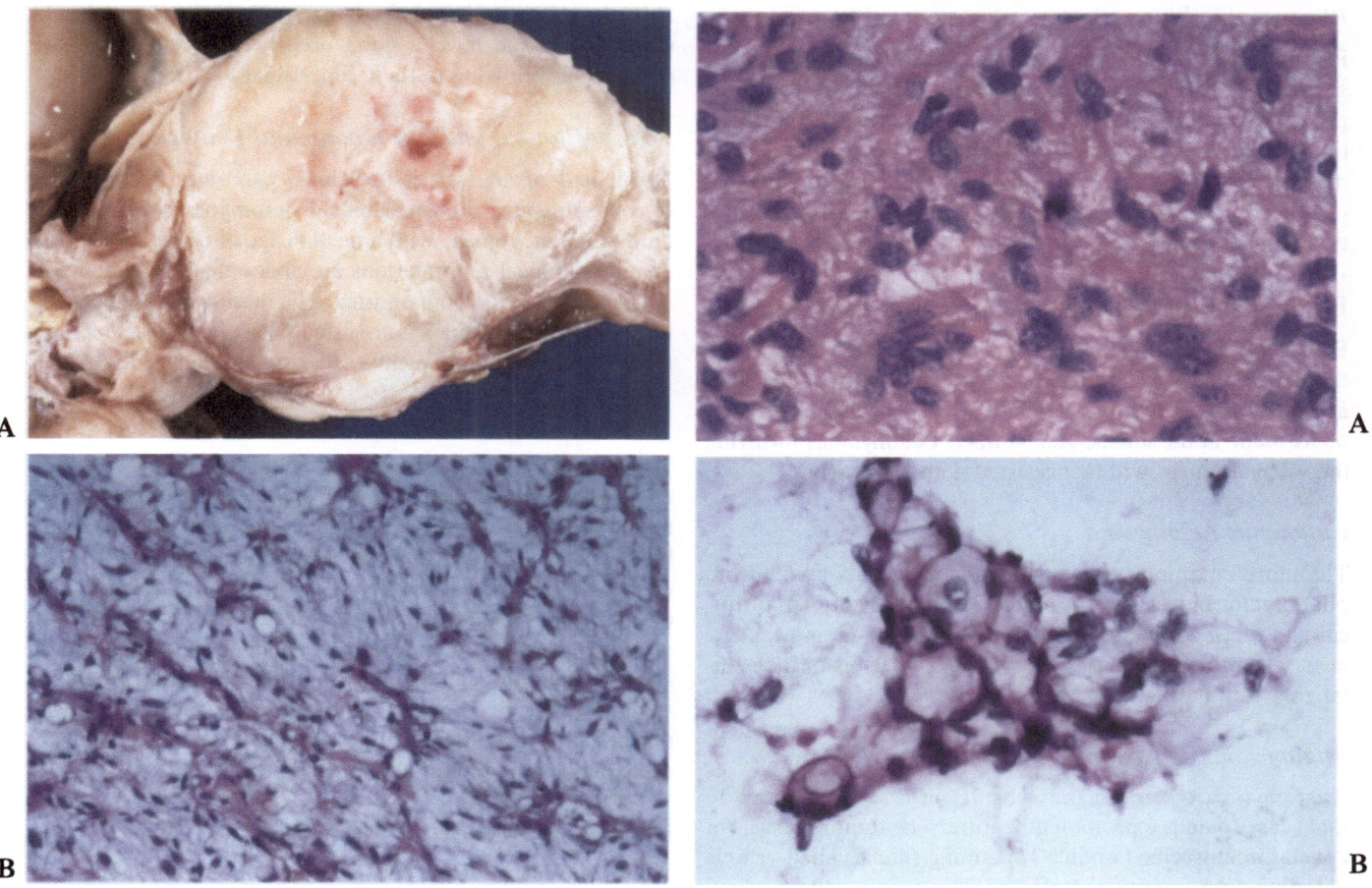

FIGURE 23.13   Myxoid liposarcoma. A: The tumor is soft and gelatinous (gross). B: Histologic section showing sheets of lipoblasts in a myxoid background with delicate branching capillaries.

FIGURE 23.14   Round cell liposarcoma. A: Sheets of round to polygonal lipoblasts. B: FNA smear showing aggregates of round lipoblasts.

Pleomorphic Liposarcoma

Pleomorphic liposarcoma is the most aggressive type of liposarcoma, with histologic characteristics of marked cellular pleomorphism and a disorderly growth pattern. Identification of lipoblasts or lipid droplets in cytoplasm by electron microscopy may be of help in distinguishing this tumor from pleomorphic rhabdomyosarcoma and malignant fibrous histiocytoma (Fig. 23.15).

Benign Tumors of Smooth Muscle

Benign tumors of smooth muscle occur most often in the genitourinary and gastrointestinal tracts, less frequently in the skin, and rarely in deep soft tissue. Ninety five percent of all leiomyomas occur in the female genital tract. Leiomyomas involving the visceral organs will be discussed with each organ.

Cutaneous Leiomyoma

The more common type, cutaneous leiomyoma arises from pilar erector muscles of the skin. The tumor is often multifocal and often associated with considerable pain and tenderness. The other type arises from the deep dermis of the genital zone and nipple.

Angiomyoma (Vascular Leiomyoma)

Angiomyoma occurs in the subcutis in a solitary form. In most cases pain is a prominent feature. The tumor consists of a well circumscribed nodule containing thick-walled vessels blending with smooth muscle.

Leiomyosarcoma

Leiomyosarcomas are less common than other types of sarcoma and occur most often in the uterus and gastrointestinal tract. Although all leiomyosarcomas of soft tissue are histologically similar, retroperitoneal and intraabdominal leiomyosarcomas are more aggressive and prognostically unpredictable. In contrast, leiomyosarcomas of cutaneous and subcutaneous tissue have a good prognosis because they are detected early owing to their superficial location.

Retroperitoneal and Intraabdominal Leiomyosarcoma

About half of all soft tissue leiomyosarcomas occur in the retroperitoneum. Retroperitoneal leiomyosarcomas occur more often in women, with a median age of 60 years.[12-14] The common clinical presentations are abdominal mass, abdominal pain, weight loss, or vomiting. The mass can be detected by CT. At surgery, the masses are usually large and often unresectable; commonly they involve other organs (Fig. 23.16A).

Histopathology and Cytology

The tumors comprise slender, elongated cells arranged in fascicles. The cells have distinct eosinophilic cytoplasm. The nuclei are hyperchromatic, elongated, centrally located, and blunt-ended ("cigar shaped"). Macronucleoli are not frequently observed. In most cases, mitotic figures average five or more per 10 high power fields (Fig. 23.16B). Glycogen can usually be demonstrated by the PAS stain in the cytoplasm. A stain for reticulin can demonstrate fine interstitial fibers. In aspirates, the cells occur in loose aggregates and singly. Cytoplasm is not prominent as in histologic sections. The nuclei are elongated and blunt-ended (Fig. 23.16C).

Differential Diagnosis

Less differentiated leiomyosarcomas may mimic malignant fibrous histiocytoma, fibrosarcoma, and malignant schwannoma. The electron microscopic features of leiomyosarcomas are pinocytotic vesicles and intercellular connections, basal lamina investing the entire cell membrane, and well oriented, thin myofilaments joined by dense bodies (Fig. 23.16D). Desmin, intermediate filaments characteristic of muscle tissue, can be demonstrated in tumors of muscle origin by immunohistochemistry.

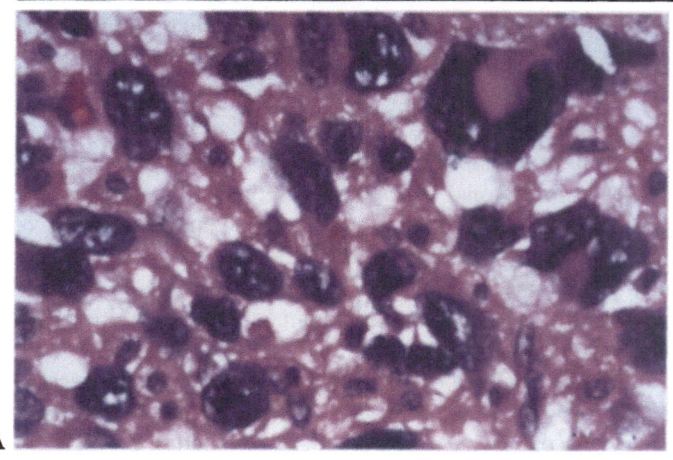

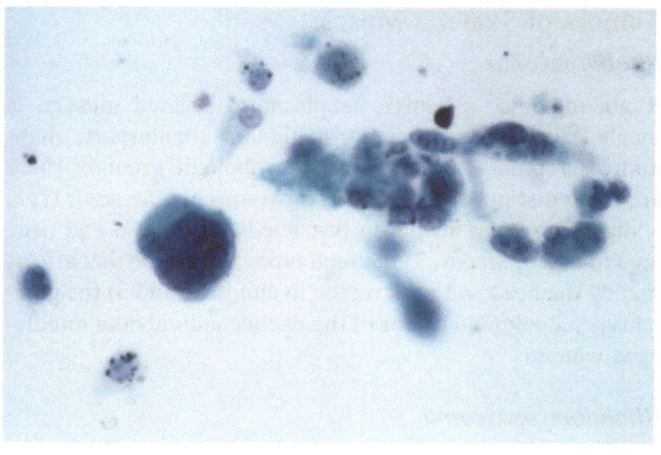

FIGURE 23.15 Pleomorphic liposarcoma. A: Giant cells and highly pleomorphic cells with no evidence of lipoblastic origin. **B**: FNA smear showing pleomorphic cells in loose aggregates.

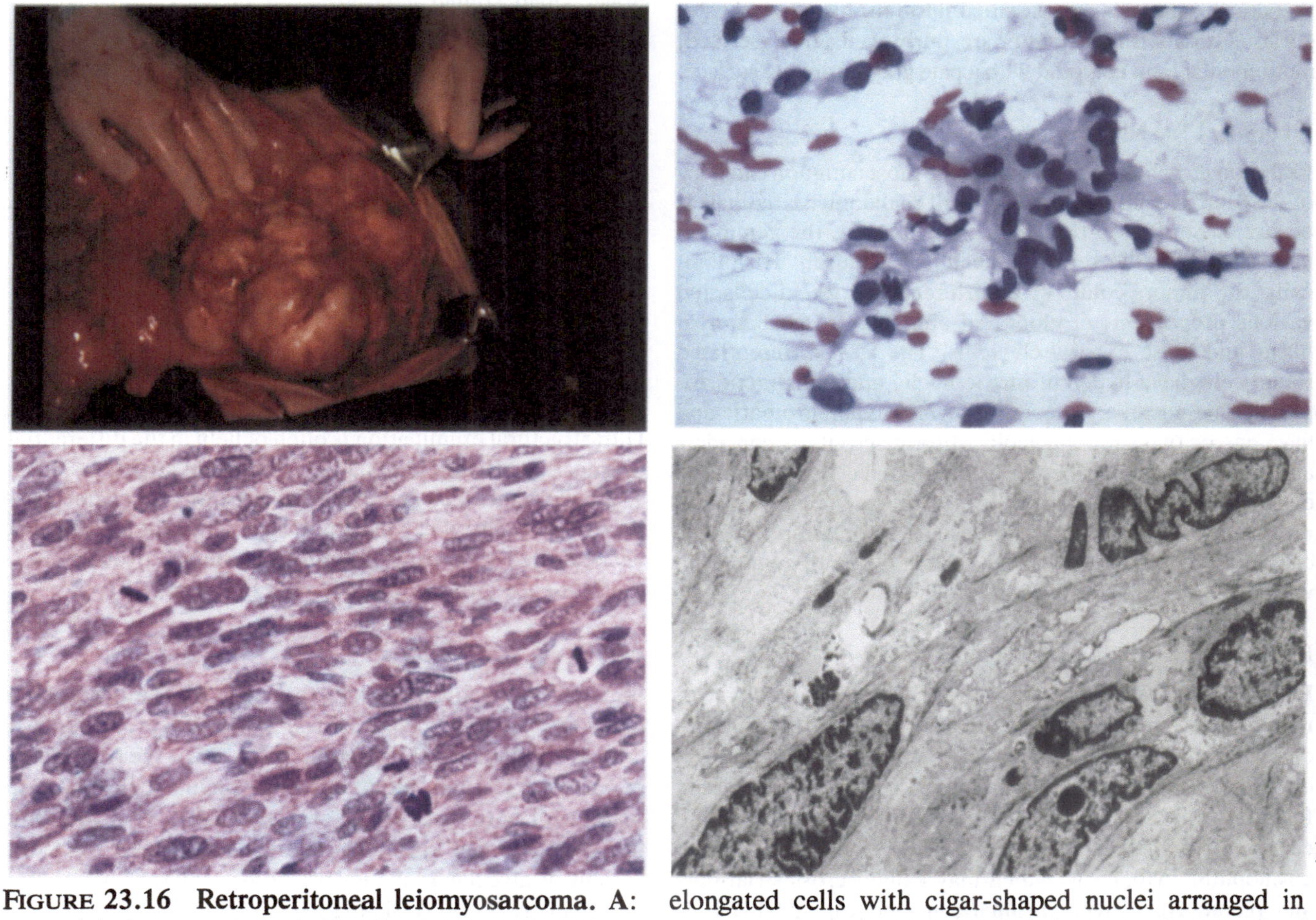

FIGURE 23.16 Retroperitoneal leiomyosarcoma. A: Large lobular mass (gross). **B**: Histologic section of the same tumor showing elongated cells arranged in fascicles. **C**: FNA smears from the same tumor showing elongated cells with cigar-shaped nuclei arranged in loose aggregates and singly. **D**: Electron micrograph of leiomyosarcoma showing nuclear grooves, thin myofilaments, and basal lamina.

Tumors of Skeletal Muscle

Rhabdomyoma

Rhabdomyoma, a benign neoplasm of striated muscle, is much less common than its malignant counterpart, rhabdomyosarcoma. On clinical and morphologic grounds, there are three distinct types of rhabdomyomas: 1) the adult type, a slowly growing neoplasm restricted to the head and neck area of older persons, 2) the fetal type, a rare type that affects mainly the head and neck region in children, and 3) the genital type, a polypoid tumor of the vagina and vulva of middle-aged women.

Rhabdomyosarcoma

Rhabdomyosarcoma is the most common soft tissue sarcoma of children and adolescents, composing 19% of all soft tissue sarcomas. The tumor occurs predominantly in infants, children, and adolescents. Based on their growth pattern, cellularity, degree of differentiation, and individual cell morphology, rhabdomyosarcomas are classified into four histological categories. Grossly, these tumors are fairly well circumscribed, multinodular, and polypoid with a pale gray glistening surface.

Embryonal Rhabdomyosarcoma

Embryonal rhabdomyosarcoma is the most common category of the four, accounting for 80% of all rhabdomyosarcomas. It occurs most often in the head and neck area, the genitourinary tract, and the retroperitoneum in children. Histologically, the tumors comprise undifferentiated round cells and various proportions of elongated and rounded rhabdomyoblasts and loose myxoid elements. The least differentiated round cells have hyperchromatic nuclei and indistinct cytoplasm. The nuclei are pleomorphic and hyperchromatic and have one or two small nucleoli. Mitotic activity is considerable (Fig. 23.17). The better differentiated cells are round to oval rhabdomyoblasts with eosinophilic cytoplasm, which rarely may contain cross striations and cytoplasmic vacuoles caused by deposits of glycogen. The nuclei are pleomorphic with prominent macronucleoli.

Pleomorphic Rhabdomyosarcoma

Pleomorphic rhabdomyosarcoma is the least common type of rhabdomyosarcoma, occurring most often in the limbs, especially the thigh, in adults. Grossly, it looks like skeletal muscle and often is confined within the compartment of a muscle fascicle. Microscopically, the tumor comprises pleomorphic cells with numerous giant cells. The cells have abundant eosinophilic cytoplasm, which may exhibit cross striations, and pleomorphic hyperchromatic nuclei (Fig. 23.19) It is almost impossible to distinguish pleomorphic rhabdomyosarcomas from malignant fibrous histiocytomas.

Botryoid-Type Embryonal Rhabdomyosarcoma

Botryoid-type embryonal rhabdomyosarcoma, a modified form of embryonal rhabdomyosarcoma, is characterized grossly by its polypoid shape reminiscent of a bunch of grapes. Microscopically, it is characterized by a relative sparsity of cells and an abundance of mucoid stroma in the submucosa. Commonly, there is a submucosal zone of increased cellularity, the "cambium layer" (refer to Chapter 17). With careful searching rhabdomyoblasts are frequently observed. Most botryoid rhabdomyosarcomas are found in the nasal cavity, nasopharynx, bile duct, urinary bladder, or vagina.

Alveolar Rhabdomyosarcoma

Alveolar rhabdomyosarcoma occurs predominantly in the limbs in an older age group. Microscopically, the tumor comprises small, round cells arranged in nests, separated by fibrous septa. The nests have a sparse and loosely cohesive central portion and a peripheral cell layer clinging to fibrous septa. The cells have eosinophilic cytoplasm and eccentric pleomorphic nuclei. Multinucleated giant cells are frequently observed. Cross striations are rarely found (Fig. 23.18). The prognosis of alveolar rhabdomyosarcoma is worse than that of the embryonal variety. Enzinger's studies showed 92% of the patients with alveolar rhabdomyosarcoma died from widespread metastasis within the first 4 years after diagnosis.[15] Lung and peripheral lymph nodes are the most common sites of metastasis.

Electron Microscopy

Ultrastructural examination is often of help in the differential diagnosis, revealing skeletal muscle-related structures, such as Z bands, and thick and thin myofilaments with characteristic A and I bands. Since these ultrastructural features may not be identified in poorly differentiated rhabdomyosarcomas, their absence does not exclude rhabdomyosarcoma.

Immunohistochemistry

Immunohistochemistry is of great value in the differential diagnosis of rhabdomyosarcomas. Myoglobin protein is specific for striated muscle differentiation, and is the first choice of markers. Desmin, an intermediate filament, is a specific marker for both smooth and striated muscle. It is probably the most reliable single marker for identifying the solid variant of alveolar rhabdomyosarcoma. Myosin, actin, and vimentin are less specific markers.

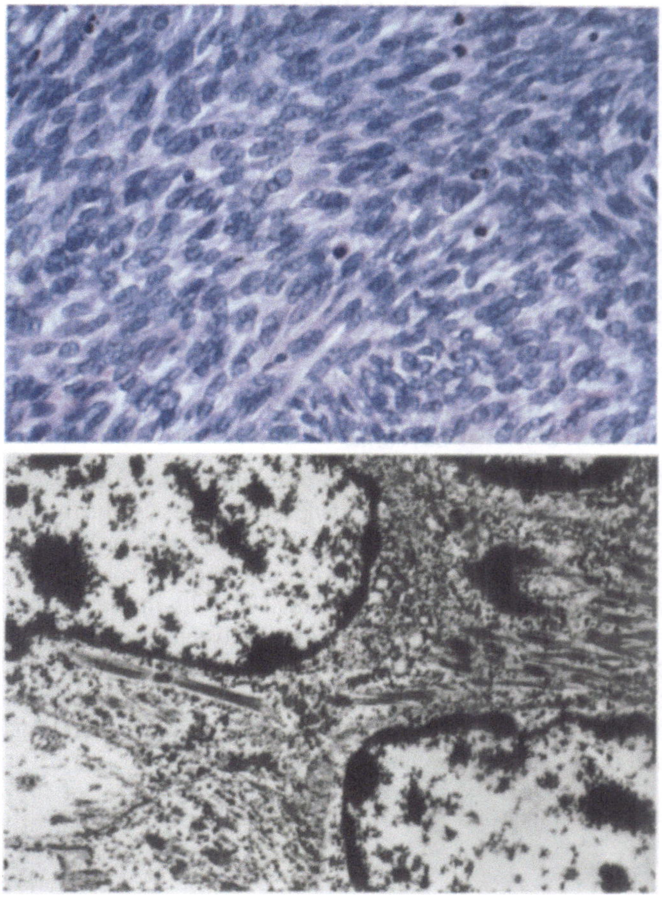

FIGURE 23.17 Embryonal rhabdomyosarcoma. A: Undifferentiated round to oval cells with frequent mitotic figures. **B:** Thick and thin myofilaments and Z band, characteristic of skeletal muscle cells.

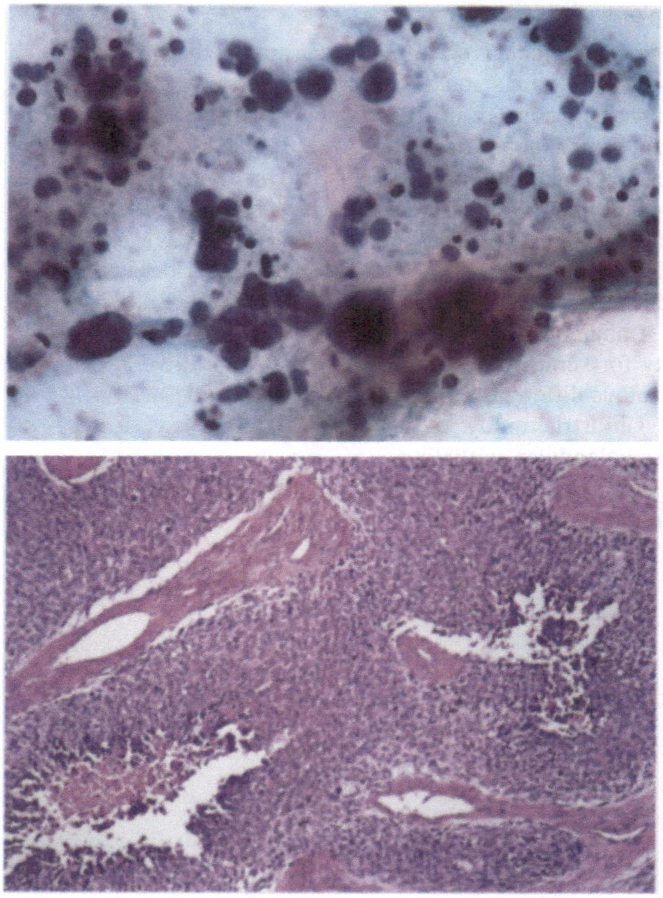

FIGURE 23.18 Alveolar rhabdomyosarcoma. A: Aspirate smear showing loosely cohesive pleomorphic cells. **B:** Histologic section showing round cells arranged in nests and sheets separated by fibrous septa.

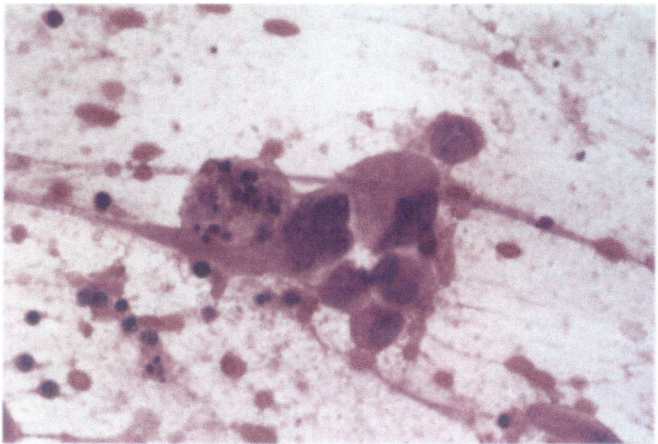

FIGURE 23.19 Pleomorphic rhabdomyosarcoma. FNA smear showing loose aggregate of pleomorphic cells with abundant eosinophilic cytoplasm.

Synovial Sarcoma

Synovial sarcomas occur most often around the knee and ankle joints of young adults. Microscopically, the tumor has a biphasic pattern resulting from the mixture of glandlike areas and sarcomatous stroma (Fig. 23.20). The tumors frequently exhibit calcification or osseous or cartilaginous metaplasia, which may be delineated radiographically. A reticulin stain demonstrates the biphasic nature of the tumor. Mucin stains demonstrate the presence of mucopolysaccharides in the spindle cells and PAS-positive glycoprotein in the epithelial foci.

Immunohistochemically, the tumor reveals strong reactivity for keratin in the epithelial areas, suggestive of carcinomatous differentiation from mesenchymal tissues.

Ultrastructurally, the epithelial elements have features of true glandular epithelium.

Synovial sarcoma can recur locally and metastasize to the lung and lymph nodes.

Tumors of Uncertain Cell Type

Granular Cell Tumor

Granular cell tumor, also known as granular cell myoblastoma, occurs most often in the tongue and skin. It has been seen, however, in the breast, larynx, bronchus, and gastrointestinal tract. The tumors are usually small, up to a few centimeters in diameter, and are poorly defined. Microscopically, the tumors consist of large cells with abundant eosinophilic PAS-positive granular cytoplasm, and small nuclei (Fig. 23.21). The strong immunoreactivity for S-100 and the ultrastructural features of reduplication of basal lamina and autophagic vacuoles suggest the tumor is of Schwann cell origin.

Alveolar Soft Part Sarcoma

Alveolar soft part sarcoma most often involves the deep soft tissues of the thigh and leg of young adults. Grossly, the tumor forms a large, well circumscribed, pale gray, firm mass. Microscopically, the tumor consists of nests of cells separated by delicate fibrous stroma. Detachment of cells in the central portion of the nests results in a typical alveolar pattern. The cells are large and have vesicular nuclei with prominent macronucleoli and granular cytoplasm. Mitotic figures are rarely observed (Fig. 23.22). These tumors are highly malignant and metastasize to the lung and other organs.

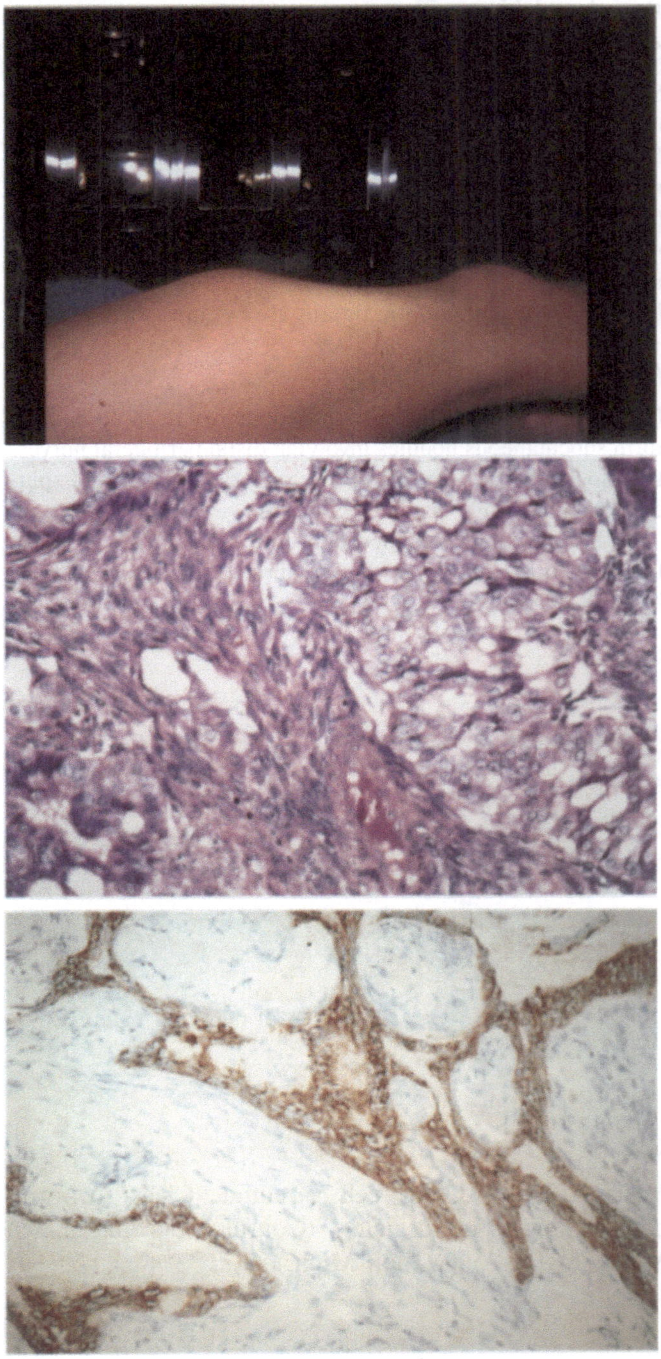

A

A

B

B

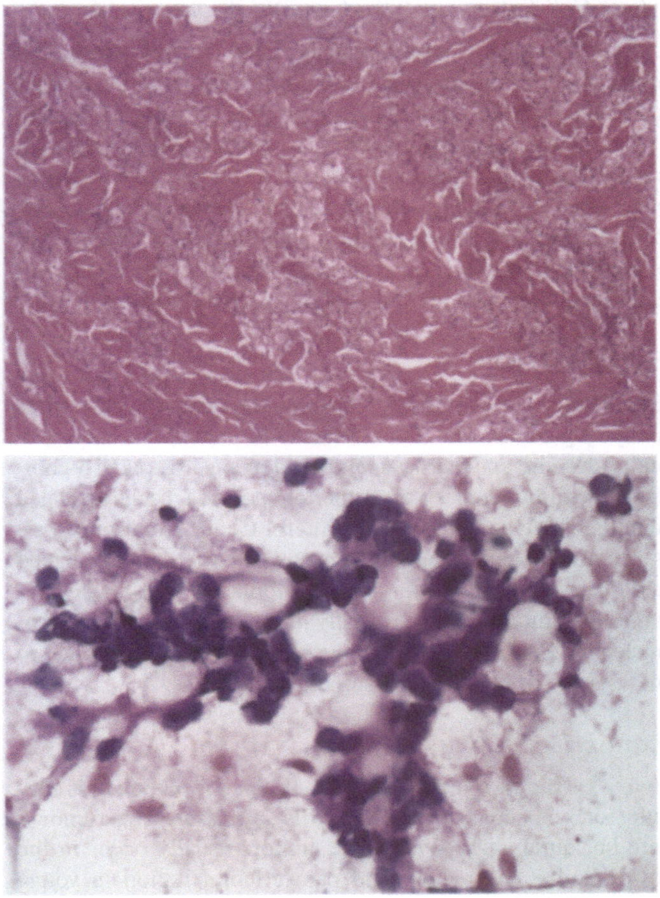

FIGURE 23.21   Granular cell tumor. A: Acidophilic cells arranged in nests. B: FNA smear showing tumor cells with acidophilic granular cytoplasm and round bland nuclei.

C

FIGURE 23.20   Synovial sarcoma. A: Tumor in the deep soft tissue of a lower limb. B: Histologic section of the same tumor showing its biphasic pattern, with epithelioid and spindle cell elements. (Courtesy of Sharon W. Weiss, M.D., Ann Arbor, Mich.) C: Immunostain of the section showing epithelioid cells selectively positive for cytokeratin. (Courtesy of Sharon W. Weiss, M.D., Ann Arbor, Mich.)

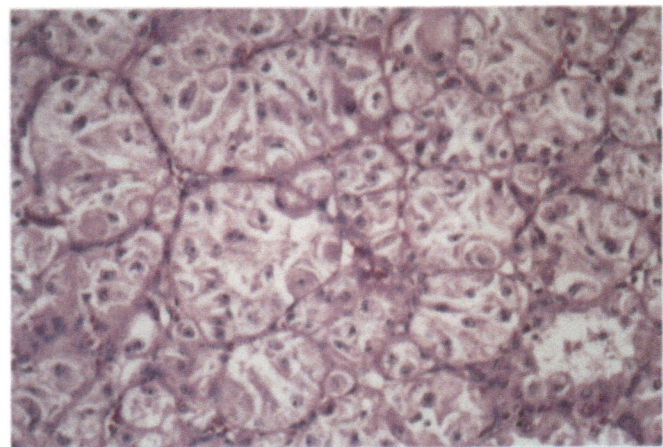

FIGURE 23.22   Alveolar soft part sarcoma. Tumor cell nests separated by delicate fibrous stroma. (Courtesy of Sharon W. Weiss, M.D., Ann Arbor, Mich.)

Clear Cell Sarcoma of Tendons and Aponeuroses

Clear cell sarcoma arises mainly from large tendons and aponeuroses of the limbs of young adults. Grossly, the tumors are well circumscribed and pale gray, and cut with a gritty sensation. Microscopically, the tumors consist of pale fusiform or cuboidal cells arranged in fascicles and solid nests. The nuclei are round to oval and have a single macronucleolus (Fig. 23.23). Multinucleated giant cells and intracellular and extracellular hemosiderin are frequently observed. The tumor cells usually exhibit immunoreactivity for S-100 protein.

Epithelioid Sarcoma

Epithelioid sarcoma usually occurs in the limbs of adolescents and young adults. The tumor tends to be superficial in the reticular dermis, aponeuroses, and tendon sheaths. Microscopically, the tumor consists of epithelioid polygonal cells arranged in nests with a nodular growth pattern. Central tumor necrosis is usually present. The cells are polygonal to spindle-shaped and have abundant eosinophilic cytoplasm. The nuclei are large, pleomorphic, and usually have a prominent macronucleolus (Fig. 23.24). The tumors tend to recur locally and to metastasize to regional lymph nodes and lungs.

Extraskeletal Ewing's Sarcoma

Ewing's sarcoma without evidence of bone involvement is considered as a primary neoplasm of the soft tissue. This tumor is rare but quite aggressive. These tumors usually occur in the lower limbs, chest wall, and paravertebral region in young adults. The tumor consists of small round cells arranged in sheets and nests. A perivascular arrangement of tumor cells frequently is observed. The cells have scanty cytoplasm that contains PAS-positive glycogen granules. Histologically, the tumor is similar to that of bone.

Peripheral Nerve Tumors

Schwannoma (Neurilemmoma)

Schwannomas are solitary and well circumscribed tumors, usually located close to peripheral nerves or spinal nerve roots. Histologically, the tumors consist of a highly cellular area with nuclear palisading (Antoni A area) and loose myxoid areas (Antoni B area), which are haphazardly intermixed. There may be Verocay bodies (eosinophilic bundles of cell processes) in between the areas of nuclear palisading (Fig. 23.25). Nuclear atypia and mitotic figures are not present.

Neurofibroma

Neurofibromas present as a solitary nodule or as multiple fusiform subcutaneous nodules involving distal peripheral nerves. Histologically, they consist of loose interlacing bands of spindle cells with wavy nuclei (Fig. 23.26).

Both schwannoma and neurofibroma can occur as a solitary localized form or as forms of neurofibromatosis (von Recklinghausen's disease).

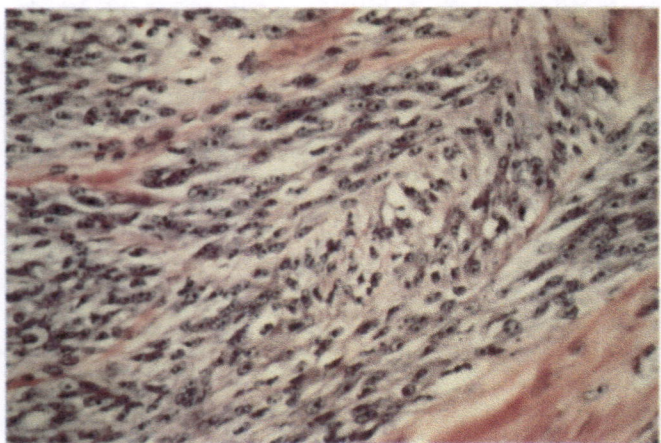

FIGURE 23.23 Clear cell sarcoma. Clear fusiform cells arranged in fascicles. (Courtesy of Sharon W. Weiss, M.D., Ann Arbor, Mich.)

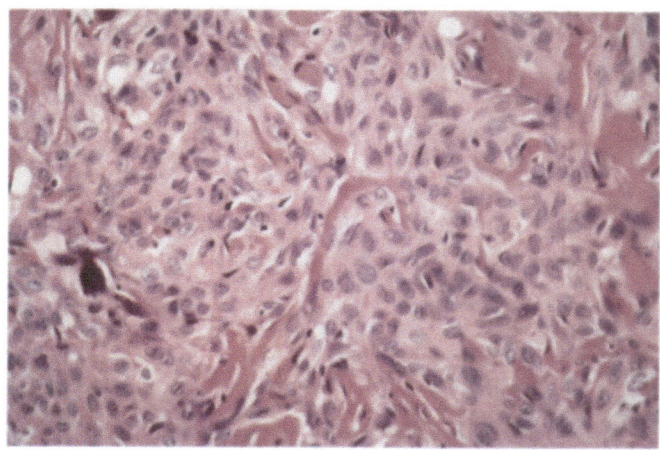

FIGURE 23.24 **Epithelioid sarcoma.** Epithelioid polygonal cells arranged in nests with a nodular growth pattern. (Courtesy of Sharon W. Weiss, M.D., Ann Arbor, Mich.)

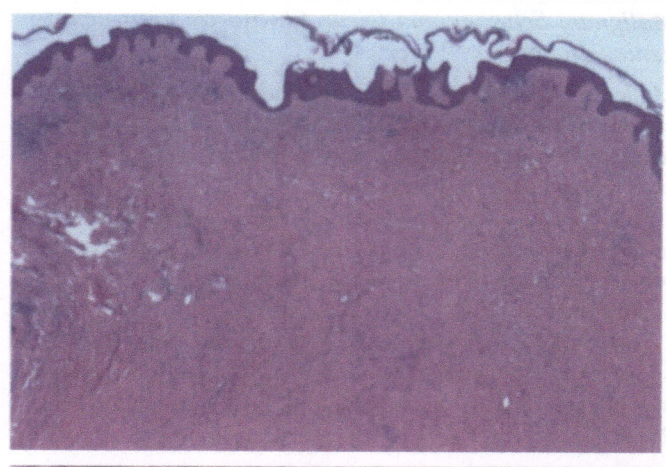

A

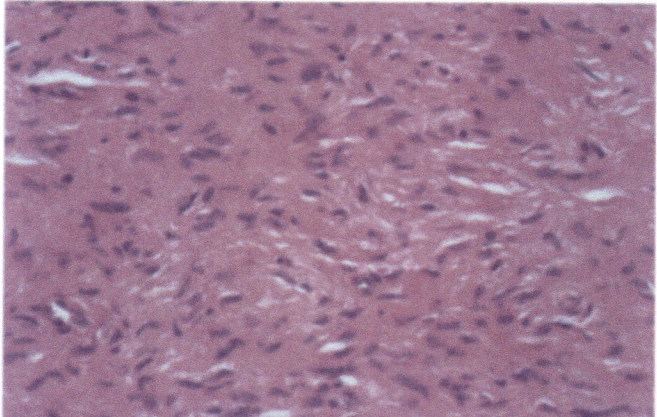

B

FIGURE 23.26 **Neurofibroma of skin. A, B**: Interlacing bands of wavy elongated cells.

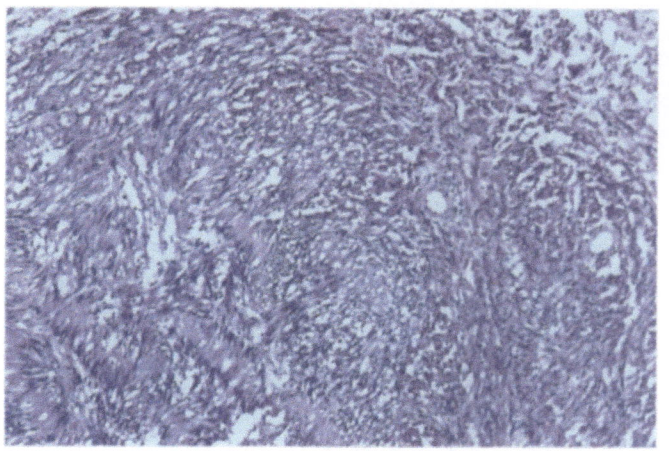

FIGURE 23.25 **Schwannoma (neurilemmoma).** Antoni A area, with pseudopalisading of tumor cell nuclei and Verocay bodies (*left*), and Antoni B area with a less cellular and more loose field (*upper right*).

Malignant Schwannoma (Neurofibrosarcoma or neurogenic sarcoma)

Malignant schwannoma arises as a large fusiform mass associated with a major nerve (Fig. 23.27A). In von Recklinghausen's disease, malignant schwannoma may develop within a preexisting neurofibroma.

Histologically, the tumor consists of elongated cells arranged in sweeping fascicles. The nuclei are irregularly shaped, with wavy or comma-shape forms in contrast to the symmetrical spindle-shaped nuclei of fibrosarcoma (Fig. 23.27B).

In aspirates, the cells occur in loose aggregates. They are spindle and elongated with a moderate amount of basophilic cytoplasm. The nuclei are spindle shaped and indented (Fig. 23.27C).

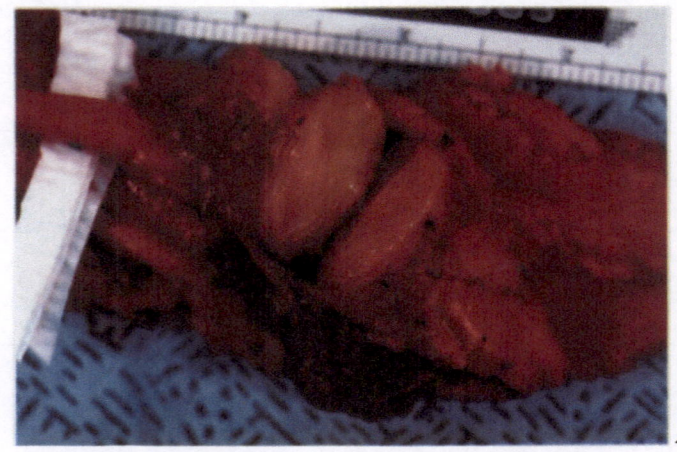

A

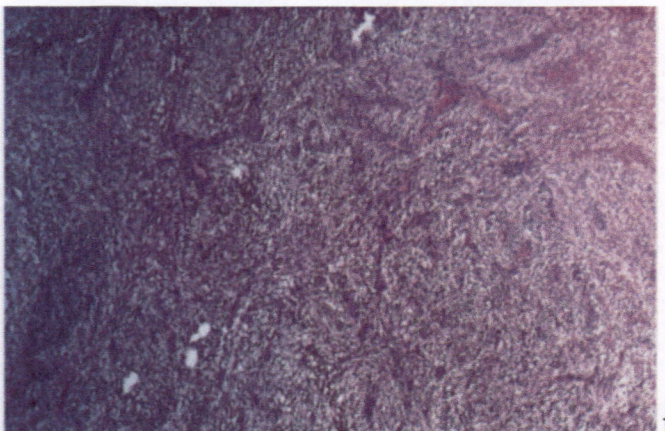

B

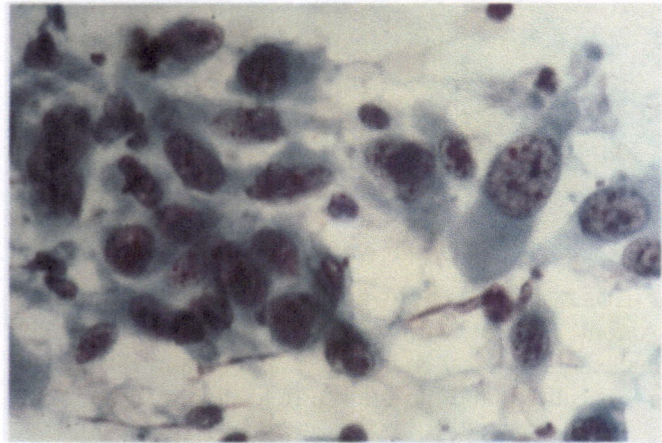

C

FIGURE 23.27 Malignant schwannoma involving a nerve. **A**: Fusiform mass associated with a peripheral nerve. **B**: Histologic section showing elongated cells arranged in sweeping foscicles. **C**: FNA showing spindle shaped neoplastic cells—loose aggregates.

References

1. Evans HL, Ayala AG, Romsdahl MM. Prognostic factors in chondrosarcoma of bone. A clinicopathologic analysis with emphasis on histologic grading. *Cancer.* 1977;40:818–831.

2. Bertoni F, Present D, Enneking WF. Giant-cell tumor of bone with pulmonary metastases. *J Bone Joint Surg [Am].* 1985;67:890–900.

3. Present D, Bertoni F, Hudson T, Enneking WF. The correlation between the radiologic staging studies and histopathologic findings in aggressive stage 3 giant cell tumor of bone. *Cancer.* 1986;57:237–244.

4. Rock MG, Pritchard DJ, Unni KK. Metastases from histologically benign giant-cell tumor of bone. *J Bone Joint Surg [Am].* 1984;66:269–274.

5. Bacci G, Picci P, Giteus S, Borghi A, Campanacci M. The treatment of localized Ewing's sarcoma. The experience at the Instituto Ortopedico Rizzoli in 163 cases treated with and without adjuvant chemotherapy. *Cancer.* 1982;49:1561–1570.

6. Pilepich MV, Vietti TJ, Nesbit ME, Tefft M, Kissane J, Burgert EO, Pritchard D. Radiotherapy and combination chemotherapy in advanced Ewing's sarcoma—intergroup study. *Cancer.* 1981;47:1930–1936.

7. Rosenberg SA, Suit HD, Baker LH. Sarcomas of soft tissues. In: *Cancer: Principles and Practice of Oncology.* Philadelphia: JB Lippincott Co; 1985;1243–1291.

8. Kim K, Goldblatt P. Malignant fibrous histiocytoma. Cytologic, light microscopic and ultrastructural studies. *Acta Cytol.* 1982;26:507–511.

9. McDonnell W. Myelolipoma of adrenal. *Arch Pathol (Chicago).* 1956;61:407.

10. Chen KTK, Felix EL, Flam MS. Extra-adrenal myelolipoma. *Am J Clin Pathol.* 1982;78:386.

11. Kim K, Koo B. Primary myelolipoma of mediastinum. *J Comp Tomogr.* 1984;8:119–123.

12. Russell WO, Cohen J, Enzinger FM. A clinical and pathological staging system for soft tissue sarcomas. *Cancer.* 1977;40:1562.

13. Ranchod M, Kempson RL. Smooth muscle tumors of the gastrointestinal tract and retroperitoneum. *Cancer.* 1977;39:255.

14. Yannopoulos K, Stout AP. Primary solid tumor of the mesentery. *Cancer.* 1963;16:914.

15. Enzinger FM. Alveolar rhabdomyosarcoma. An analysis of 110 cases. *Cancer.* 1969;24:18–31.

Index